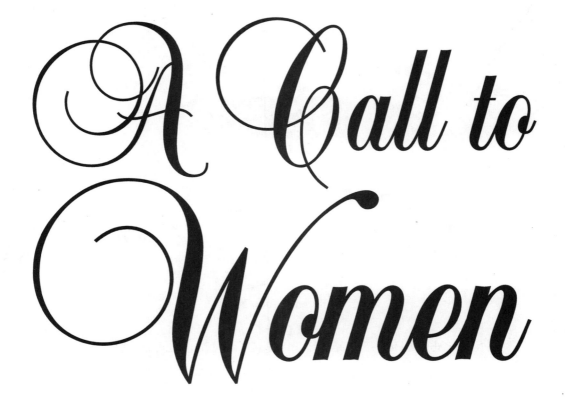

A Call to Women

THE HEALTHY BREAST
PROGRAM & WORKBOOK

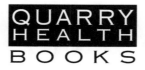

Fundamentals of Naturopathic Medicine
by Fraser Smith, ND

The Botanical Pharmacy: The Pharmacology of Common Herbs
by Heather Boon, BScPhm, PhD and Michael Smith, MRPharmsS, ND

Naturopathic First Aid
by Karen Barnes, ND

Vitamin C & Cancer
by Abram Hoffer, MD, PhD, FRCP (C) and Linus Pauling, PhD

Vitamin B-3 & Schizophrenia
by Abram Hoffer, MD, PhD, FRCP (C)

Hoffer's Laws of Natural Nutrition
by Abram Hoffer, MD, PhD, FRCP (C)

Dr Hoffer's ABC of Natural Nutrition for Children
by Abram Hoffer, MD, PhD, FRCP (C)

Masks of Madness: Science of Healing
by Abram Hoffer, MD, PhD, FRCP (C)
(Introduction by Margot Kidder)

A NATUROPATHIC GUIDE TO PREVENTING BREAST CANCER

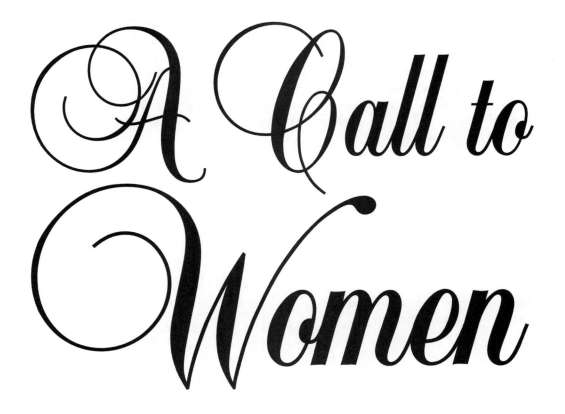

A Call to Women

THE HEALTHY BREAST PROGRAM & WORKBOOK

Sat Dharam Kaur, ND

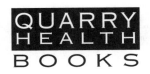

QUARRY HEALTH BOOKS

The author gratefully acknowledges permission to reprint and reproduce the following poems, exercises, and diagrams in this book: The United Nations Environment Program for three poems by the U.N. Environmental Sabbath Program; W.W. Norton & Company, Inc. for two poems by May Sarton, "Invocation to Kali, Part 2" and "Invocation to Kali, Part 5"; Gary Lawless for his poem beginning "when the animals come to us ..." from *First Sight of Land* (Blackberry Books); Susan Gibson for her poem "How Does One Write About Plutonium"; Broadway Books, a Division of Bantam Publishing Group, Inc., for the Rumi poems, translated by Coleman Barks from *The Illuminated Rumi*; architect Kal Kangas of Thunder Bay, Ontario, for the sauna diagram; the Reverend Harry Thor of the Congregation of Abraxas for the Unitarian prayer; Greenpeace for the chlorine pie chart and the alternatives to PVC chart; the Kundalini Research Institute and Yogi Bhajan for the Kundalini yoga exercises and breathing practices.

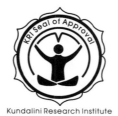

Kundalini Research Institute

The publisher gratefully acknowledges the support of the Book Publishing Industry Development Program of the Department of Canadian Heritage.

The nutritional, medical, and health information presented in this book is based on the research, training, and professional experience of the author, and is true and complete to the best of her knowledge. However, this book is intended only as an informative guide for those wishing to know more about health, nutrition, and medicine; it is not intended to replace or countermand the advice given by the reader's personal physician. Because each person and situation is unique, the author and the publisher urge the reader to check with a qualified health care professional before using any procedure where there is a question as to its appropriateness. A physician should be consulted before beginning any exercise program. The author and the publisher are not responsible for any adverse effects or consequences resulting from the use of the information in this book. It is the responsibility of the reader to consult a physician or other qualified health care professional regarding his or her personal care. It is a sign of wisdom, not cowardice, to seek a second or third opinion.

ISBN 1-55082-256-X

Design and type by The Right Type.

Printed and bound in Canada by AGMV Marquis, Cap-Saint-Ignace, Quebec.

Published by Quarry Press Inc., PO Box 1061,
Kingston, Ontario K7L 4Y5 Canada.
www.quarrypress.com

TABLE OF CONTENTS

LIST OF EXERCISES

CHAPTER 10 — *Spiritual Practices for Preventing Breast Cancer*

DEDICATION

To Lake Huron, who listened as I walked, and nursed me through my childhood,
may your waters become clean once again,

To the whales, who visited me often in my dreams and spoke to me through song,
may the oceans support your young,

To Yogi Bhajan, whose words and teachings have been the pillar of my life,
may there be many who continue your work,

To my husband and children, for your love, encouragement and tolerance,
may we support each other in our contributions to the world,

And to the women of the world, the guardians of life and growing things,
may we create a revolution to heal ourselves and the earth.

these breasts belong to you
they fill and empty
with the tides of your calling

ACKNOWLEDGMENTS

I WOULD LIKE TO ACKNOWLEDGE ALL THE PEOPLE who have contributed to the creation of this book from its conception to completion. Mireya Folch for the original incentive to write it; Chad Hollett and Melanie Gentles for volunteering time to help type; Pam McBurney, Sherry Leblanc, Marilyn Schaefer, Maren Drees, Rory Ford, Gurunater Kaur Khalsa, Moira Tobin, Raheem Habib, Laura McNeilly, Ann Ruebottom, Stewart Brown, Martha Ayim, Janet Miller, Hope Nemiroff, Mary Paterson, Hari Darshan S. Khalsa, and Nam Kaur Khalsa for helping to gather information and offering enthusiastic support. Bill Marshall for engaging conversations; Hari Nam Singh Khalsa for helping with the layout and the early printing; Sheila Cameron for taping the video for me; and Martha Ayim for helping to create the index.

Thanks to Dr Paul Saunders, Dr Deborah Gold, and the Canadian College of Naturopathic Medicine for allowing me to teach The Healthy Breast Program as part of a Continuing Education series and to lecture to third year students; and to the many third year students who enthusiastically helped establish The Healthy Breast Program as part of the clinic at the naturopathic college, despite their overwhelming schedules and commitments – especially Arvin Jenab, Kurt Stauffert, Jen Green, Jill Kelner, Dana Lerman, Vince Lurie, Kathleen Mercer, Cory Pustowka, Michelle Stapleton, and Stephen Tripodi. To all of the students who completed research projects on aspects of breast health, your work added to the completion of this manuscript, and I thank you.

Thanks also to Eli Neidert, Herman Adlercreutz, Greenpeace, Women's Network on Health and the Environment, the Canadian Cancer Society, the United Nations, and the World Wildlife Fund for kindly providing research materials. To Kal Kangas, for sharing his sauna design. To the women in my Healthy Breast Series, yoga classes, and my patients for sharing your lives with me. To the regulars who have come to the Guru Ram Das meditations and supported my prayers. To Susan Gibson for editing and offerings poems, and to Liz Zetlin for poetic offerings. To my husband Har Prakash for continual support, for child care, and for pushing me onward. To my sister, Lynda Orman for occupying my children, and to my children who have patiently left me alone as I typed, motivated me in my mission, and endured my absences. To my mother-in-law, Joan Ford, for hosting all five of us on our trips to Toronto. Thanks to my publisher, Bob Hilderley at Quarry Press for the sensitive and superlative re-organization of the book and Steve Knowles for the exquisite design and layout.

I would also like to acknowledge my mentors — people who have left their mark in my psyche because of their work and who have helped my becoming. These are Yogi Bhajan, Guru Ram Das, Marion Woodman, Carl Jung, Rilke, Rumi, Coleman Barks, Robert Bly, Rachel Carson, Sandra Steingraber, Theo Colborne, David Suzuki, Bella Abzug, Susun Weed, Joanna Macy. Thank you all for preparing the ground.

To all of you who will take The Healthy Breast Program and share it — I thank you.

Finally I would like to acknowledge the Great Spirit who fed and nurtured me continuously throughout this remarkable project. It has been a privilege to listen and obey.

A GRAND STATEMENT made by Marshall McLuhan in his *Interior Landscape* keeps coming back to me when I think about women and cancer. "Must we continue to mow down the Kennedy's," McLuhan asked in 1969, recognizing that we are living in a collective society where everything you do affects me and everything I do affects you. We are all responsible, all culpable. The same can be said about the cancer dilemma. We are the cause of the present state of affairs but we are also the cure.

Cancer is a very expensive illness, an 'industry' whose treatment costs have almost reached the five billion dollar mark annually in North America. Cancer is big, big business and access to the 'market' — in other words, our bodies — is fiercely fought over. Yet over the past 40 years, treatments have barely improved and survival rate is no better. And the greatest and most recent increase is in hormone-dependent cancers of the breast, prostate, and testicles. Every 12 seconds a woman dies of breast cancer.

This realization was brought home to me during two conferences on breast cancer held during 1999, the Second World Conference on Breast Cancer in Ottawa and another in Hamilton. The common theme of both conferences was that our current social and economic system is the ultimate cause of cancer. Thirty years ago the World Health Organization declared that up to 90% of all cancers are caused by pesticides, radiation, and other toxic chemicals in our environment. Dr Samuel Epstein, whose research was key to banning DDT, pointed out that all of us now carry more than 500 different compounds in our cells, none of which existed before 1920, and that "there is no safe dose for any of them." For Sandra Steingraber, special advisor on cancer prevention to the President of the United States and author of the best selling *Living Downstream*, cancer has "become a human rights issue" which can only be tackled with "old fashioned political organization." That is why "scientists are now going directly to the public" in order to expose "the deception at the heart of the chemical industry, namely that these pesticides are necessary." Although the earth has been made "chemically addicted" and all life is being poisoned, Steingraber states there are signs of change. For example, drycleaning fluid, which can cause many cancers including bladder cancer, may be completely phased out in the foreseeable future. And organic farming has become a multi-billion dollar business.

Another sign of change is the growth in the popularity of alternative and complementary medicine offering a different approach to the cancer dilemma through prevention. *The New England Journal of Medicine* reported in 1993 that one-third of American citizens were using alternative medicine and annually spending over 10 billion dollars out of pocket on visits to alternative medicine practitioners. A follow up survey in 1998 in the *Journal of the American Medical Association* reported that between 1990 and 1997 Americans increased their visits to alternative medicine practitioner by 43%. The total visits were 427 million in 1990, 629 million in 1997.

Among alternative and complementary health care practices, naturopathy has gained wide-spread respect. When I practiced as a Naturopathic Doctor in Ontario for 13 years, I taught my patients how to take responsibility for their own health — to ask their doctors questions about their health and to work with practitioners who followed the seven principles of naturopathic medicine, whether they were medical or naturopathic doctors.

1) Identify and Treat the Causes

2) First Do No Harm

3) Doctor as Teacher

4) Treat the Whole Person

5) Emphasize Prevention

6) Support the Healing Power of the Body

7) Physician Heal Thyself

There are now several naturopathic colleges training in these principles. One such doctor educated at the Canadian College of Naturopathic Medicine is Sat Dharam Kaur who has applied her skills in an exceptional way by writing this definitive text on breast cancer prevention using the naturopathic model.

The Healthy Breast Program and Workbook is not a book you can skim in one session; you might have to sit with it a dozen times to grasp all the information and the scope of the book. But starting with the first chapter you can begin to put your health in order and prevent breast cancer. And the medical information and advice for prevention found throughout the book make this an indispensable resource and companion for all women, in poor or good health. I also love the fact that Dr Kaur is spearheading Rachel Carson Day on May 27th each year, honoring the woman that alerted us to the poisoning of our environment. She never lets us lose site of our need to clean both our bodies and our environment. Focusing on only one or the other will never be enough.

Fully aware that her book is asking a great deal from you in terms of taking on personal responsibility for your own breast health, Dr Kaur uses an extremely gentle and loving approach. You can see her smiling through the lines on the page and embracing you when you read a particularly difficult passage. These things are palpable through the whole text and make me weep just thinking about her care and concern for her readers and for the planet. And weep we must if we are to get in touch with our feelings for ourselves and for others. For the pain we have caused ourselves and our children and grandchildren. Weeping is not a sign of weakness but a sign of caring. A call to action. A call to women.

I am often drawn to the *Greek play Lysistrata*, written by Aristophanes in the fifth century BC, about the role women played in ending the Peloponnesian War by withholding sex from their men folk. Women of our new millennium may establish a similar victory in the war against cancer by withholding our considerable buying power. Stop rewarding industry that pollutes our air, soil, and water and begin to reward clean and pure products, organic goods, and companies that care for the environment. Involve yourself with simple acts of activism and kindness that will ripple across the planet. That is how I see our larger mission as modern-day warriors. I know Sat Dharam Kaur has the same vision. And I trust you will be amply rewarded by participating in her Healthy Breast Program.

— *Carolyn Dean* MD, ND

INTRODUCTION

A Call to Women

IN THE FALL OF 1996 I BEGAN TEACHING the Healthy Breast Program because I felt it was necessary for women to become proactive in the prevention of breast cancer. From my studies of naturopathic medicine, I had some knowledge to share, and while I was a student, I had watched one friend in her early thirties die of breast cancer. My inability to help her at the time stimulated the writing of this book ten years later.

As I read more articles over the years about breast cancer, I was not only astounded by the connection between the deteriorating environment and cancer development in our age but also angered by the cover-up of this knowledge. My passion to communicate this knowledge grew. I started to visualize women all over the world getting together in small groups — supporting each other, educating each other, claiming their identities, preventing the disease in themselves, and taking an active role in preserving the environment. I felt inter-species grief resonating in my heart. The grief of mothers unable to nurse their young and unable to nurture themselves because the soil, the air, and the water have become inhospitable to life. The grief of bald eagles who see the shells of their offspring shatter unnaturally beneath their weight; the grief of St. Lawrence beluga whales dying of cancer, their carcasses hazardous waste because of the chemicals they contain. I heard the painful cries of future generations robbed of children because their hormones have been tampered with. It is the feminine principle, the right to raise offspring, that is being violated. The waters of life have been poisoned along with the earth and breath of Gaia. Breast cancer is the call to arms. Arms of action, arms of prayer, arms of holding and joining, arms held up in resistance to complacency, convenience, and denial, arms united. We each have two arms. Together we are one body.

This call to arms has many facets. Breast cancer reminds us that we must be honest with ourselves and in our relationships — that we speak our truth and follow our inner guidance. Breast cancer draws the anger out of us — anger at God, anger at ourselves for having surrendered pieces of our wholeness we must now retrieve, anger at the political, corporate, and industrial forces that have got us in to such an insane environmental mess, anger at the unconscious ease of convenience. The breast cancer epidemic offers us a path of purification that we sorely need. Each of us must choose when to plant our feet upon that path — before or after a diagnosis. I believe that the only way out of the global breast cancer epidemic is through a path of purification. To me this includes honoring the soul and our unique abilities, being mindful of what and how we eat, releasing toxic emotions, cleansing the body, adopting a spiritual practice which is suited to our individual make-up, and realizing that it is our duty to make the environment safe and sacred once again.

It became clear to me as I was writing this book that we must shift from our present attitude of domination to cooperation and facilitation. We have been trying to dominate nature with our agricultural practices and it is making us, wildlife, and the planet sick. We have been trying to dominate the body with the overuse of antibiotics, the birth control pill, hormone replacement therapy, chemotherapy, and invasive treatments. The body has its own intelligence. It is much more fruitful to work with, rather than against, the body's processes: assist the liver in detoxification; enhance elimination with fiber and probiotics; balance the glands with herbs and meditation rather than cut them out, shut them down, or replace them with drugs; fortify the immune system with nutrition, herbs, visualization, and yoga before we immobilize it with chemotherapy and radiation. This is a naturopathic medical approach which recognizes the inherent ability of the body to heal itself when given the means to do so.

We have been trying to dominate each other with marketing hype and consumerism. The driving force behind domination is greed. Greed is destroying the Earth, our home, and destroying us. We must move from greed to living simply, realizing the consequences of our actions. What we do to the Earth, we do to ourselves. Breast cancer is evidence of that. Governments are not acting in the best interests of planetary ecology. We cannot rely on "them" to take care of us or the earth. Industry continues to spew out billions more tons of chemicals each year into the environment while insisting that it does no harm. Countries explode nuclear weapons and nuclear power plants malfunction. There is no other Earth but the one we live on. Is there anywhere safe?

Where can my children go?

Before we buy a product, we can consider how the air, earth, water, and wildlife were affected in the production of it, if it can be recycled or not, and whether it is safe to burn or bury. Most of the things we use are not. As our population expands, so does our toxic landfill. Before we eat our food, drink our water, and flush our toilets, we can ask these same questions. Then we do what we can to create positive change. We can accomplish a lot together. We are the guardians of the fertility of the Earth. All of us.

I feel a responsibility to do what I can in my own lifetime and to help others do the same. And so this book has been born. My prayer is that you will take it, use it yourself, share it with your daughters, sons, husbands, partners, friends, and lovers, teach someone else and perhaps start your own Healthy Breast Program. And that all over the world women will say no to food that is not organic, to plastic, to nuclear power, to chlorine, to anything that nature cannot take back into herself to nurture something else. We have broken the cycle of creation with our toxic waste. We must mend it.

I believe that women can turn things around. We stand united. We say no. We shall remain conscious rather than bowing to convenience. We hear the voices of the beluga whales, the polar bears, the Lake Apopka alligators, the Baltic seals, the bald eagles, Great Lakes salmon, and the voices of each other pressing us on, asking us to please help and act now. We act with the welfare of future generations of all species in our minds and hearts. We can and must make a difference.

The Healthy Breast Program & Workbook

The following 11 suggestions summarize the components of The Healthy Breast Program that will be discussed in greater detail chapter-by-chapter. For a comprehensive list of the "Actions for Prevention" recommended in each chapter, see the list at the end of chapter 11.

1) Determine your hereditary, reproductive, lifestyle, hormonal, environmental, dietary, psychological, and spiritual risks for developing cancer. Complete The Breast Health Balance Sheet provided.

2) Get to know your breasts through self-examination and mapping. If you have high risk factors for breast cancer or suspect a problem during self exams, use thermography, the AMAS test, and other diagnostic procedures annually to ensure that no cancer is present. These may indicate the presence of very small cancers that are easier to treat. Use mammography biannually after the age of 50, and before age 50 when there is suspicion of cancer.

3) Gain an understanding of your endocrine or hormone system, especially the link between estrogen and breast health. Monitor your hormone levels yearly, checking estradiol, estrone, estriol, the ratio of C2 to C16 estrogen, serum IGF-1 and 2, progesterone, TSH, T4, T3, reverse T3, and melatonin using saliva testing.

4) Decrease your exposure to known carcinogens and toxins. Become active in your home and community in protecting yourself from environmental toxins and in restoring the health of our environment. Use nontoxic body and home care products.

5) Detoxify. Do a liver cleanse for at least six weeks, once or twice a year, or on an ongoing basis if you have breast cancer or live in a particularly polluted area. Do a parasite cleanse for three months, once or twice a year, while simultaneously cleansing the intestines with a fiber formula or enemas and using probiotics (good bacteria). Make saunas a part of your life, having at least one each week (two 20-minute periods with a cool shower in between). Do a sauna detoxification program with supervision every 1–5 years.

6) Activate your lymphatic and immune systems. Exercise at least four hours a week and rebound daily for from 5–30 minutes. Practice the exercises for lymphatic cleansing at least three times weekly. Use one of the herbal formulas for lymphatic cleansing for at least three months twice yearly, or continuously if you have breast cancer. Practice skin brushing and have alternating hot and cold showers daily. Activate your immune system with one of the immune herbal formulas each winter, as needed, or continuously if you have breast cancer.

7) Follow a preventative dietary regime, including increasing your consumption of foods with high phytoestrogen content. Try the Healthy Breast Diet and the recipes for breast health included in this book. Supplement your diet with vitamins, minerals, and other nutrients in consultation with your health care professional. Develop a daily supplement schedule.

8) Develop assertiveness and release anger rather than storing it. Practice techniques using imagery and visualization.

9) Live your life in harmony with your true nature, making the most from your gifts and doing what makes you feel happy and fulfilled. Make time for play and being. Practice a relaxation, meditation, or breathing exercise for at least 11 minutes 1–5 times daily, including before bed. Develop a spiritual practice that suits you and helps you stay in touch with your soul. Include prayer in your life.

10) Monitor your program daily and yearly. Make adjustments as necessary. Maintain with your physician a Breast Health Data Sheet.

11) Develop a positive relationship with your body and breasts and put your well-being ahead of family and job responsibilities. Make your health a priority today, so that you can enjoy your family, work, and leisure time tomorrow. Simplify your life, consume less, enjoy more. Throughout this book, various mental, emotional, physical, and spiritual exercises encourage this process. Of special value are the Kundalini Yoga exercises which integrate mind, body, and soul in the pursuit of good health, not only for our breasts but for our whole being.

Using This Program

This book was written to be used in one of two ways. You can take the information and use it for yourself, making the changes in your life that are possible at this time. It may take several years to absorb and act on some of the suggestions presented in these pages. My hope is that you will come back to it year after year, taking in a little more each time. It may seem overwhelming at first. Skim through the book to begin. Glance at the glossary of terms in chapter 13. Stop and take breaks as you read through the environmental section. Drink some water. Take rescue remedy. Call a friend and cry. Breathe deeply. Find support. Focus on hopeful, positive change and transformation and the role you can play. Do the best you can and only what you can. Please don't stress yourself about following the program. Your life, how you feel about yourself and your personal direction, are more valuable than any program. This is only a guide — it is up to you to feel comfortable with it and adapt it to your particular set of circumstances.

You may also use this program in a group. It will be more powerful this way and the group support will make the information easier to digest. Consider gathering some women together and going through the chapters one at a time. I have taught five versions of this over the last three years, meeting once a month with women for three hours at a time over nine months. I like the gestation time of nine months — it is a womanly rhythm and works well if you start in September and continue until May. You don't have to cover all the details in each chapter. Focus on enough to get an overview, on the experiential exercises and on group sharing. Keep the momentum going. If you are in a group, please take action on the environmental links to breast cancer in your area. Figure out what you can do together. Make waves. Let us bring about a tidal wave of personal and global transformation.

This program is continually evolving. As I work with patients and groups and integrate breast cancer research, I add and subtract. You can keep abreast (!) of changes and link up with women worldwide who are following The Healthy Breast Program by contacting my website at www.healthybreastprogram.on.ca.

How to Begin a Kundalini Yoga Kriya or Meditation

Kundalini Yoga is a sacred science that has existed for thousands of years in India and was brought to North America in the last 30 years by Yogi Bhajan. Traditionally a mantra (or sacred sound) is used before practising Kundalini Yoga. The purpose of this is threefold:

1) the mantra helps to shift us from our former activities and mindset and prepare us to practise yoga;

2) it connects practitioners together in a group through sound;

3) it acts energetically to protect and guide us while practising Kundalini Yoga and links us to teachers of the past.

The mantra that is used worldwide among practitioners of Kundalini Yoga is ONG NAMO GURU DEV NAMO. ONG refers to the infinite creativity of the universe as it manifests through time and space. NAMO means "I bow" or humble myself. GURU literally means darkness/light and refers to the dispelling of darkness and bringing of light, which may occur through a teacher. DEV means "invisible" or "transparent," so in this case the teacher is invisible. NAMO again means "I bow."

The whole translation of the mantra could be read as "I bow to the creativity of the universe as it manifests through time and space; I bow to the invisible teacher inside and out." The mantra is not specific to any religion. It can be used by anyone in preparation to practise Kundalini Yoga and to elevate one's mental state or consciousness.

Sit cross-legged with the eyes closed and the palms pressed flat together against each other in front of the center of the chest with the thumbs touching the sternum. The position resembles hands in prayer. Close your eyes and focus them up as though looking at a point between your eyebrows. The spine should be straight with the chin pulled back slightly.

Take a deep breath in through your nose. Repeat the following mantra in the musical pattern below as you breathe out:

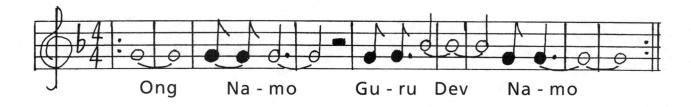

Ong   Na - mo   Gu - ru Dev   Na - mo

Do it with a clear, strong voice, from your heart, as though you are linking with your inner teacher.

Repeat the mantra 3–5 times in this way.

Then begin the yoga exercises.

What Are Your Risk Factors for Developing Breast Cancer?

Exercises

Contents

*B*reast cancer is a multifaceted disease with many contributing causes and a complex array of interactions between these causes. It would be convenient if we could say with certainty that an individual woman's breast cancer was caused by exposure to a particular chemical or to radiation, by an excess of dietary fat or increased estrogen levels, by an emotional turmoil or grief. Most of the time we do not know the cause. We do know, however, many contributing factors that predispose a woman to breast cancer. Although some are not, many of these factors are within our control. And while there is no specific 'cure' for breast cancer, just as there is no one cause, we can do much to prevent the disease by changing our lifestyle, cleaning up our environment, and participating in various regimes for healing.

There are many factors that help to protect us from breast cancer. With educated determination, women can decrease their risk factors. Women can also unite to create global reform in phasing out toxic chemicals, especially organochlorines. Women can press governments to discontinue the use of nuclear power and find viable alternatives. We can take our breast health into our own hands and help to heal our sisters and our planet at the same time. The growing incidence of cancer among women, especially in North America, makes this a pressing task.

Incidence Rates

Present statistics suggest that approximately one woman in nine in Canada and one in eight in the United States will develop breast cancer at some point in her life. In the 1920s a woman's risk was one in 20.[2] Women with no identifiable risk factors have a lifetime risk of breast cancer of about one in 16 through to the age of 80.[1] Breast cancer is a leading cause of death for women ages 35 to 50 living in Canada and the United States. The estimated number of new cases of breast cancer in Canada and the USA in 1998 was 19,300 and 180,300, respectively. The

estimated number of deaths from breast cancer in Canada and the United States in 1998 was 5,300 and 43,900, respectively.[3,4] Breast cancer is much less common in other parts of the world, implying that dietary, environmental, and lifestyle factors play a large role in its occurrence. The following chart compares breast cancer age-standardized incidence rates per 100,000 women in several countries between the years 1988–1992.[5]

Country	Incidence per 100,000 Women
USA (whites)	90.7
USA (blacks)	79.3
Canada	76.8
Denmark	73.3
England / Wales	68.8
Czech Republic	45.1
Ecuador	26.8
China	26.5
Japan	24.3
Africa	20.4

In Canada the incidence has steadily climbed from 76.8 per 100,000 women in 1988–1992 to 108.2 per 100,000 women in 1998.[6] A similar increase in incidence rates has been seen in studies of American women.

Causes of Breast Cancer

Any 'cure' for breast cancer must treat the causes of this disease, not simply eliminate the cancerous tissue through surgical intervention or chemotherapy, though these procedures may be necessary once the cancer has advanced to a critical stage. From an understanding of the causes, we can begin to devise strategies to reduce the risk of developing cancer. These risks can be placed in several categories, ranging from hereditary through environmental to spiritual factors. A brief overview of these factors is presented here, followed by a more comprehensive discussion of hereditary, reproductive, lifestyle and health care risks in this chapter. Subsequent chapters will focus on understanding and addressing hormonal, environmental, dietary, psychological, and spiritual risks.

Hereditary

We cannot change our genes but we can influence gene expression through lifestyle and environment. Inheriting the genes linked to breast cancer accounts for less than 5% of cases of the disease. By following the breast health program in this book, you can significantly decrease the likelihood of breast cancer even if you have the genes associated with the disease.

Reproductive

Reproductive factors refer to questions of whether we have children and how many children we have and whether we nurse them or not. Many women find that they do not have a lot of control over if and when they have a child, nor should we have children simply for the sake of breast health. We must consider our emotional health, relationship stability, financial security, and life circumstances. Having a child is not a guarantee against developing breast cancer, although it helps. Earlier child-bearing will have positive biological effects for mother and child.

Lifestyle and Health Care Factors

Lifestyle and health care factors linked to breast cancer are also under our control. Usually we have a little room in our lives to develop a relaxation program of some kind, to create an exercise routine, and to do annual cleansing. The challenge for many women is to put themselves first, making these goals a priority in the face of family, social, or work demands.

Hormonal Factors

There are many hormonal links to breast cancer and profound interactions between the environment and our glands. Generally hormonal and environmental links to breast cancer have been downplayed and underestimated. This is partly because large financial interests are at stake if these connections are revealed (chemical manufacturers and pharmaceutical companies). We have a degree of control over hormonal links through the choices we make about using birth control pills, fertility drugs, and hormone replacement therapy. We also need to do more subtle, routine testing of glandular function, specifically monitoring the estrogen quotient, C2 and C16 estrogen ratio, IGF-1, progesterone, melatonin, and thyroid function, including reverse T3. We need to acknowledge the profoundly debilitating effects our chemically toxic environment is having on our glandular health and work to eliminate these toxins form our bodies and from our environment.

Environmental Factors

The links between our environment and breast cancer are overwhelmingly evident, though for many years I could not bear to know this intellectually and emotionally. I believe our culture is in a collective state of denial about what we have done and continue to do to the environment. Denial breeds evil. The only way we will heal ourselves and the earth is by shaking off that denial and taking personal responsibility. We must each look at how we contribute to the environmental crisis, clean up our little corner of the earth, and take a stand together against the chemical, plastic, pulp and paper, and nuclear industries — and the political machinery that support them.

Dietary Factors

Here is where we can make a great deal of difference to our breast health. We now know which foods promote breast cancer and which ones prevent or even reverse it. Foods can be medicine. There is a growing trend supporting organic farming methods, and as this continues, breast cancer may decline somewhat. For our physical and spiritual health, it is important that we make a connection to the soil that grows our food — plant a garden, use window boxes, link up with an organic farm and work in the fields. Part of our sickness is due to our alienation from nature and our broken link to the creative cycle. We have become uprooted from the soil that nourishes us. We can utilize and develop farming methods that replenish the soil rather than trying to dominate and control nature with chemicals.

Psychological Factors

Psychological factors linked to breast cancer are mostly about denying who we really are, ignoring or bottling up our true feelings, and assuming the role of the 'pleaser' in our attempts to feel loved. Healing comes from connecting to our deepest desires and callings, courageously creating our own path and honoring our intuition. Healing also comes from developing assertiveness, releasing anger, and resolving conflict.

Spiritual Factors

I think of serious illness as a path of purification so that eventually we'll relate to our soul. Illness is sometimes the messenger sent to wake us up. Our spiritual selves need to be nourished just as our mind, emotions, and body do. No longer can we separate these parts of ourselves, feed one or two occasionally, and hope to stay healthy. They all need to be taken care of. We take care of our spiritual self when we connect to what is meaningful for us, live with a sense of purpose, express our creativity, laugh and have fun, and develop some sort of regular checking-in process. We can call this a spiritual practice. It may consist of prayer, meditation, yoga, dreamwork, martial arts, writing, creative activity, or all of these. Mostly it's a listening process — paying attention to the inner voice that guides our life and actions day to day, connecting to the great mystery.

The Breast Health Balance Sheet Exercise

The following table or 'balance sheet' on pages 23–26 summarizes the risk factors for breast cancer explained throughout the rest of the book. It also outlines those factors that protect us from breast cancer. Make checkmarks beside the risk factors and protective factors that are true for you. The bracketed numbers to the right of some entries refer to how much that risk factor increases your likelihood of having breast cancer; that is, (+2) means your risk doubles, (+3.6) means it increases your risk over three and a half times. If the number is beside a protective factor, it means that it decreases your risk by that amount. We are always in a state of flux and we do have a lot of control as to what happens to our bodies.

Come back to the balance sheet at least once a year to see what progress you have made in adopting a breast health/cancer prevention program. If you feel overwhelmed on your first read through, put it aside and come back to it another day. Things you may not understand initially will be explained in later chapters of this book in their appropriate section. Fill in what you can and return later.

(To calculate your 'body mass index', take your weight in kilograms and divide by the square of the your height in meters. To determine your waist-to-hip ratio, divide your waist measurement by your hip measurement.[7])

Hereditary Factors

Mother or Sister with Breast Cancer

Having a mother or sister with breast cancer increases risk 1.5 to 3 times above the one in eight susceptibility.[8] This is probably the risk factor most overestimated by women.[9] Increased age of the mother when diagnosed reduces the risk for the daughter. Women whose mothers were diagnosed before the age of 40 have about double the usual risk.[10,11] This doubling of risk may be due to a daughter's exposure to similar breast carcinogens as her mother, common dietary habits, and/or a genetic predisposition. Genetic mutations account for about 2–5% of total breast cancer incidence, and the influence of heredity decreases as a woman grows older.[12] Generally women with inherited genetic mutations have a 59% chance of developing the disease by age 50 and an 80% chance by age 65. The predominant genes connected with the expression of breast cancer are BRCA-1 and BRCA-2. Only 0.5% of all women have these genetic weaknesses.[13] Genetic susceptibility combined with environmental factors increases risk dramatically. Nevertheless, being proactive about preventing breast cancer will decrease genetic susceptibility.

▶ **Action for Prevention:** Avoiding the other risk factors wherever possible, actively participating in environmental reform, strengthening immunity, and adopting a health-promoting lifestyle can prevent breast cancer, even when the genetic predisposition exists. ◀

Female Relatives with Ovarian or Endometrial Cancer

If you have a first, second, or third degree relative with ovarian or endometrial cancer, then you are at greater risk for breast cancer.[14]

▶ **Action for Prevention:** Follow The Healthy Breast Program when you are at higher risk because of relatives with ovarian, endometrial, or prostate cancer. ◀

Brother or Father with Prostate Cancer

One study indicates that having a brother with prostate cancer increases breast cancer risk fourfold.[15] Others demonstrate increased risk with either a brother or father diagnosed with prostate cancer. Plausible theories for this include inherited genetic mutations,[16] similar dietary

• The Breast Health Balance Sheet •

Risk Factors		Protective Factors	
Hereditary			
Mother or sister with breast cancer	(+2)	No family history of breast cancer	
Relative with ovarian or endometrial cancer		No family history of ovarian or endometrial cancer	
Brother or father with prostate cancer	(+4)	No family history of prostate cancer	
Light-skinned		Dark-skinned	
Body mass index > 23		Body mass index < 22.8	
Over 5' 6" tall		Under 5' 6" tall	
Weight > 154 lbs.	(+3.6)	Appropriate weight; weight < 153 lbs.	
Waist to hip ratio >.81	(+7)	Waist to hip ratio < .73	
Reproductive			
No children or children after 30		Gave birth before age 20 or 30	
No breast-feeding		Breast-fed kids for at least 6 months	(-.25)
No children		More than one child	(-.5 with 5 kids)
Lifestyle and Health Care			
Aging		Use antioxidants and anti-aging supplements	
Exercise less than 4 hours weekly		Regular exercise (4 hours weekly)	(-.60)
< 2 bowel movement per week	(+4.5)	2 or more bowel movements daily	
Use beta-blockers, Prozac, Elavil, Haldol, steroids, Reserpine, hydralazine, Tagamet spironolactone, metronidazole, vincristine, Nitrofurazone, Valium, Xanax, nitrogen mustard, procarbazine, cholesterol-lowering drugs, Claritin, Atarax.		Use herbal, nutritional, homeopathic, and naturopathic recommendations when possible instead of prescription drugs. Educate yourself on the side effects of medications before taking them.	
Dental problems: mercury fillings, infection		Replace fillings with ceramic, clear infection	
Immune deficiency, allergies		Follow immune-strengthening program	
Annual mammograms (from radiation exposure)	(+.5)	Monthly breast self exam reduces risk of dying of breast cancer; use AMAS test	(-.2)
Cigarette smoking increases risk		No smoking; avoid secondhand smoke	
Alcohol increases risk (> 3 drinks/week)		Avoid alcohol or have minimally	
Exposure to light at night decreases melatonin production, increases risk		Meditate shortly before bed, sleep in the dark	
Use commercial hair dyes		Use henna or natural hair dyes	
Have breast implants		No breast implants; have them removed	
Wear a tight-fitting bra		Go braless or use looser cotton bra	
Mineral and enzyme deficiency		Eat organic, replace minerals and enzymes	

• The Breast Health Balance Sheet •

Risk Factors		Protective Factors	
Parasitic infection		Do parasite cleanse once or twice yearly	
Liver toxicity		Do liver cleanse once or twice yearly	
Bowel toxicity		Do bowel cleanse once yearly; replace flora	
Use of antibiotics		Avoid antibiotics, deal with candidiasis	
Chemical toxins accumulate in fat tissue		Use saunas regularly or sauna detox yearly	
Poor lymphatic circulation		Use skin-brushing, rebounding, exercise	
Hormonal Factors			
Estrogen quotient is .5–.8		Estrogen quotient is 1.2–1.3	
Low ratio of C-2 to C-16 estrogen	(+5)	High ratio of C-2 to C-16 estrogen	
Early onset of menstruation (<11)	(+2)	Early onset of menstruation (>14)	
Late menopause	(+2)	Early menopause (<45)	
Menstrual cycle <25 days	(+2)	Menstrual cycle 26–28 days	
Menstrual cycle >30 days	(+2)		
Low progesterone (see symptoms)	(+5.4)	Normal progesterone	
Fibrocystic breasts	(+1.8)	Healthy breasts	
Increased testosterone		Normal testosterone	
Increased prolactin		Normal prolactin	
Increased growth hormone		Avoid dairy with bovine growth hormone	
Increased insulin levels	(+3)	Normal insulin levels	
Women whose mothers had high estrogen levels during pregnancy		Protect yourself and fetus from environmental estrogens while pregnant	
Unbalanced thyroid; iodine deficiency		Correct thyroid function; use seaweeds	
High blood levels of IGF-1	(+7)	Normal blood levels of IGF-1	
Decreased melatonin levels		High melatonin; meditation practice	
Sleep with light on at night		Sleep in a dark room	
Birth control pills used before age 20 or for more than 5 years before age 35	(+3)	Natural fertility methods such as sympto-thermo or Justisse method, condoms.	
Use of fertility drugs in past		Avoidance of fertility drugs	
Post-menopausal and >50 lb. overweight		Post-menopausal and not overweight	
Estrogen replacement therapy, especially when used for more than 5 years		No estrogen replacement therapy, or have stopped for > 5 yrs.	
Former use of the drug DES or your mother took it while pregnant	(+.4)	No DES; avoid drugs in pregnancy	
Environmental Factors			

• The Breast Health Balance Sheet •

Risk Factors		Protective Factors	
Exposure to radiation		Miso and seaweeds 3× weekly	
Fly frequently		Fly seldom	
Live within 50 mi. of nuclear reactor		Live > 50 mi. from nuclear reactor	
Continuous exposure to electricity and electromagnetic fields		Live in the country with few electrical devices	
Work in electrical trade	(+.7)	Work away from excess electricity	
Install, repair telephones	(+200)		
Sleep within 2½' of electrical devices		Sleep > 3' away from electrical devices	
Sit < 2' from front, < 4' from sides of computer video display terminals		Sit further from computer video display terminals and use them < 20 hours weekly	
Use an electric blanket		Use cotton, wool, down blankets	
Exposure to pesticides: food, lawn, farm, golf courses, public areas		Eat organic, avoid pesticides	
Live in industrialized area		Live away from industry & pesticide sprays	
Exposure to petrochemicals, gas stations		Use car less	
Exposure to formaldehyde		Choose products without formaldehyde	
Exposure to benzene		Avoid benzene	
Exposure to organochlorines	(+10)	Recognize and avoid organochlorines	
Use of chemical or industrial cleansers		Use of non-toxic cleansers	
Exposure to carcinogens		Recognize and avoid known carcinogens	
Live near a hospital incinerator		Live away from a hospital incinerator	
Live near a PVC recycling plant		Live away from a PVC recycling plant	
Use plastics		Avoid plastics, use glass, wax paper, cardboard, butcher paper	
Live near a chemical plant		Live away from a chemical plant	
Live near a toxic waste site or dump		Decrease waste; live away from a toxic waste site or dump	
Live near a sewage treatment plant		Use a composting toilet, live away from a sewage treatment plant	
Use chlorine bleach		Use non-chlorine bleach	
Drink chlorinated water		Drink ozonated or filtered water	
Dry-clean clothing		Avoid dry-cleaning; use natural detergents	
Dietary			
High fat consumption; > 30% total calories		Low fat consumption; < 15% total calories	
Low fiber; < 10 grams daily		High fiber; >30 grams daily	(-.30)
Eat meat weekly		Vegetarian	(-.30)
Use dairy products		Use organic soy milk, no added oil or sugar	

• The Breast Health Balance Sheet •

Risk Factors	Protective Factors
Eat sweets, sugar products	Have 2 or more fruits daily
Use processed food	Use whole, unrefined foods
Use bread products regularly	Use beans, whole grains
Drink coffee	Drink herbal teas, e.g., red clover, dandelion, taheebo, mint
No soy products	Soy products daily (avoid if allergic)
No orange fruits and vegetables	Use 2 foods high in vitamin A daily
Use vegetable oils, animal fat, margarine and cooked oils; have low essential fatty acids	Use unheated flaxseed and olive oil
Minimal fruits and vegetables	Use 6–9 servings of fruits and vegetables/day
Eat mostly cooked food	50–85% raw food
No brassicas (cauliflower, cabbage, broccoli)	Raw brassicas daily
High salt intake	Low sodium / high potassium
Overly acidic body	Keep pH of urine and saliva at 6.2–7.2
Use of plastic food containers and wraps	Use glass, ceramic containers
Psychological	
Unresolved Conflict	Resolve conflict; find solutions
Deny, bury, repress or hold on to anger	Express anger constructively and let it go
Ignore one's own needs; please others	Define your needs; become assertive
Feel alienation	Find or create your community
Death of a loved one or loss of a relationship within the previous one to five years	Express your grief; find reasons for living, find something or someone to love
Stress and the inability to relax	Regular relaxation breaks
Living a life following someone else's script rather than one's own	Follow your deep desires and callings; create your path
Spiritual	
Hopelessness, despair	Spiritual counseling, therapy, prayer, yoga
Lack of a sense of purpose	Develop a meaningful life, find your passion
Lack of joy	Laugh, play, have fun
Loss of faith	Create a relationship with your soul
Foiled creative fire	Express your creativity
Ignore intuition	Awaken and follow your intuition
Lack of support	Find at least one supportive person, support group or spiritual group
Other Factors	

histories, or siblings who have common exposures to environmental estrogen-mimickers, which can initiate both prostate and breast cancer. A fourth link may be the blood levels of insulin-like growth factors 1 and 2 (or IGF-1 and IGF-2), which when elevated dramatically increases risk of both breast and prostate cancer.[17] Yet another explanation may be that brothers and sisters are exposed to similar environments in utero, when hormone-related cancers may originate, only to develop decades later.[18]

Light-Skinned Women

Light-skinned women are slightly more likely to develop breast cancer than women with dark skin, although black women are more likely to die from it.[19,20] The reasons for the higher mortality rate in black women are at least partially due to lower socioeconomic status.

Tallness or Obesity

Larger women who are over 5 feet 6 inches tall and weigh more than 154 pounds are 3.6 times more likely to get the disease.[21] The more body fat we have, the more estrogen we will produce. Our fat cells convert adrenal hormones into estrogen and this process becomes more efficient as we grow older, particularly after menopause.[22] Researchers have found that the avoidance of weight gain and accumulation of central body fat during adulthood decreases the risk of both endometrial and post-menopausal breast cancer. The risk of breast cancer is lowest in lean women (body-mass index <22.8) who exercise at least four hours per week in their leisure time and are active in their work.

▶ **Action for Prevention:** Weight management is a necessary component of a breast cancer prevention program. ◀

Waist-to-Hip Ratio

Body shape and fat distribution influence risk. If your waist-to-hip ratio is greater than .81 as opposed to under .73, you have a sevenfold increase in likelihood of getting breast cancer. Dietary changes include decreasing or eliminating unhealthy fats (animal fat, margarine, cooked oils, chemically processed and refined oils) and stabilizing blood sugar and insulin levels by choosing carbohydrate foods with a low glycemic index. Chronic high levels of insulin in the blood cause fat to be deposited around the waist and is directly related to increased risk of breast cancer. Post-menopausal women who are more than 50 pounds overweight are 1.5 times more likely to develop breast cancer.

▶ **Action for Prevention:** Follow the dietary guidelines of The Healthy Breast Program. ◀

Reproductive Factors

Having Children Early

Having children before the age of 20 or even 30 is generally protective against breast cancer. The shorter the time between the onset of menstruation and a woman's first full term pregnancy, the less the risk of breast cancer. This is because breast cells complete their maturation process only with a full-term pregnancy. Partially matured breast cells have unstable DNA that is more susceptible to the process of cancer. When breast cells become matured by pregnancy, they stabilize and are less affected by menstrual cycle hormones, developing resistance to breast cancer. Menopause ends this protective phase.[23,24,25]

During pregnancy, the hormone estriol (a weak, short-acting, protective estrogen) is secreted by the placenta at about 1000 times the level that exists in the body before pregnancy. After a first pregnancy, there continues to be an elevated ratio of estriol to estradiol. Serum estriol concentration may be increased 14 to 25% for many years following a first pregnancy. Estriol is able to bind to estrogen receptors in breast cells and competitively prevent the stronger estrogens, estradiol and estrone, from binding where they would promote cell division and consequent tumor growth.[26] The plant estrogens work in a similar way to protect our breasts.

▶ **Action for Prevention:** Have children before age 30 and closer to age 20 if possible. It will decrease your breast cancer risk and be healthier for your children. The younger you are when you conceive, the less vulnerable your breasts will be and the lighter will be the toxic load you pass on to your children through breast milk. ◀

Breast-Feeding

The longer the period of breast-feeding, the lower the risk of breast cancer for the mother but the higher the risk for the child. Women who nurse for at least six months after the age of 20 reduce their risk by 25%.[27,28] Nursing for just two months offers some protection. Considering the high toxicity of organochlorines towards breast tissue and their presence in human breast milk, breast-feeding is one way of diminishing the concentration of these chemicals in our bodies.[29] Protection is given to the mother but the chemicals are passed on to the child. Breast milk contains about 3% fat, and as it is made, the blood carries pollutants to the breasts from fat reserves throughout the body. Breast milk has been found to contain at least 17 pesticides, 13 furans, 65 PCBs, 10 dioxins, and 30 other organochlorines. All of these chemicals contain chlorine and are hormone disruptors. Contaminants in breast milk can affect the development of our children's kidneys, liver, central nervous system, and immune system.[30,31] Exposure to DDT and DDE is linked to behavioral changes in children. In 1976, 25% of samples of breast milk in the U.S.A. were found to contain PCB concentrations exceeding the legal limit, above 2.5 parts per million. Had it been bottled and sold as food it would have been banned as being too contaminated. In only six months of breast-feeding, an infant in Canada, the United States, and Europe receives the maximum recommended lifetime dose of dioxin and five times the allowable limit of PCBs set by international standards for a 150-lb adult.[32] In the Arctic, infants take in seven times more PCBs (spread by wind and water currents and ending up in animal fat) than southern Canadian or American babies and are suffering from chronic ear infections and weakened immune systems.[33]

Generally, the concentration of organochlorine chemicals in breast milk increases with the age of the mother and the amount of sport fish consumed, and decreases dramatically the longer a woman breast-feeds and the more children she nurses.[34] A 1998 study by David Josephy, Professor of Biochemistry at the University of Guelph, found that all samples of breast milk from 31 nursing mothers living near Guelph, Ontario contained aromatic amines capable of causing breast cancer in rats. These toxic substances are present in plastics, dyes, pesticides, pharmaceutical drugs, industrial waste, air, water, tobacco smoke, and some foods.[35] Guelph lies in the 'golden triangle' in southwestern Ontario, less than a hundred miles from Lake Ontario. The dioxin level in the Great Lakes was zero in the 1920s, while today it is upwards of 3200 parts per trillion.[36,37] Our breast milk contains dioxin, one of the most toxic substances known, and a potent endocrine disruptor.

I have thought much about this very sobering issue. On the one hand, breast-feeding is good for the mother and good for the baby as it introduces beneficial bacteria to the intestinal tract, decreases allergies, provides superior nutrition, immune strength, emotional bonding, and security. On the other hand, we release our toxic inventory of environmental chemicals into our children's small bodies when we nurse, particularly the first child.

One way of releasing these chemicals before we conceive is through the regular, intensive use of saunas. The Finnish people have used these for many generations and have significantly lower breast cancer rates than surrounding Scandinavian countries.[38] We could eliminate most of the body's burden of toxic chemicals before having a child. Subsequent generations would not accumulate the toxins from the previous generation, which have been found to persist for five generations in animal studies. Surely this is prevention. Other ways to release toxins stored in fat tissue may be through using homeopathic preparations. A German homeopathic company called Phonix has made three specific homeopathic combinations for detoxification that have been used for the last 15 years. Testing on three individuals found that these formulas used in sequence for two months caused a 78% reduction in blood levels of certain environmental chemicals.[39] The formulas used were C-23, which helps to eliminate fat soluble toxins through the liver and gallbladder; C-26, which assists in removing water-soluble toxins through the kidneys; and C-3, which improves the elimination of toxins through the lymphatic system. These are available in Canada from Bona Dea Ltd. in Waterloo, Ontario (tel. 519-886-4200.)

While we breast-feed, we can express as much milk as possible between nursings in the first few months and discard it. Most of the fat in milk is supplied at the end of a feeding, with a higher sugar content present in the milk at the beginning of a feeding. We could express a little milk after we nurse our infants, then throw it away. We can protect ourselves and our children by eating organically grown food, limiting animal products, filtering our water, using unbleached paper, using non-freon refrigerators, and using glass containers for food and water storage rather than plastic ones.

▶ **Action for Prevention:** Adopt a chemical free lifestyle (including avoiding animal fat) as early as possible in life and cleanse the body before conceiving. Detoxify weekly and annually with saunas, homeopathic preparations, and liver and bowel cleansers. Breast-feed your children for at least six months. ◀

Greater Number of Children

Having a greater number of children may reduce breast cancer risk.[40,41] Women who have five or more children have a 50% less risk of breast cancer than women with no children.[42]

Lifestyle and Health Care Factors

Age

The risk of breast cancer increases with age. In Canada in 1992 the incidence per year of breast cancer in women was .35/1000 for those aged 30 to 39 years, 2.2/1000 for those aged 50 to 59 years, and 4.0/1000 for those aged 70 to 79 years.[43]

▶ **Action for Prevention:** Take antioxidants regularly or get them from your food to slow down the aging process and to protect your DNA from damage. ◀

Exercise

Women who exercise at least four hours per week in their leisure time (to the point of sweating) and are active in their work are less likely to develop breast cancer. There is a 37–60% reduction in risk with this amount of exercise. This effect is more pronounced among pre- rather than post-menopausal women.[44,45]

Increased physical activity through adolescence protects against adult breast cancer, even at moderate levels. One study found that if girls engaged in any one of four specific activities, they were less likely to be diagnosed with breast cancer later in life. These activities included walking to school, biking to school, competitive training, or vigorous household chores.[46]

Long term exercise decreases estradiol and progesterone secretion, delays the onset of menstruation in girls, and can prevent ovulation. Exercise also enhances the metabolism of estrogen, promoting more of the 'good' estrogen.

▶ **Action for Prevention:** Regular exercise (four hours weekly) is part of a prevention program. We can encourage our daughters to develop a regular exercise program before puberty (age 10 onward) that they can maintain for life. ◀

Prescription Drugs

Regular use of some prescription drugs has been found to increase breast cancer risk in animal studies. Beta-blockers (such as Atenolol), the antidepressants Prozac and Elavil,[47] the antipsychotic drug Haldol,[48] and steroids all may increase risk. Reserpine, a drug commonly used to lower blood pressure, increases the blood concentration of prolactin, which can stimulate breast cancers to develop. Another drug that lowers blood pressure is Hydralazine, also known as Apresoline. Women who take this drug for more than five years can double their risk of breast cancer.[49] Spironolactone (Aldactone) is a diuretic used to lower blood pressure which may increase breast cancer risk. Two different antibiotics may increase breast cancer risk — Metronidazole (Flagyl),[50] which is used as an anti-fungal agent, and Nitrofurazone,[51] used to treat skin wounds and stomach ulcers. The tranquilizers Valium and Xanax increase prolactin levels, which stimulates the growth and development of invasive breast cancer. When tumors are already present, these drugs will accelerate their growth.[52] Unfortunately, these two medications are commonly given to cancer patients to decrease anxiety. Actual anti-cancer drugs may elevate breast cancer incidence 15 or more years after their use. Nitrogen mustard, vincristine, and procarbazine have been linked to increased future risk of breast cancer.[53] Cholesterol-lowering drugs consisting of fibrates and statins such as Pravachol (pravastatin) have been found to cause breast cancers in rodents; one study found that women taking pravastatin had 12 times the rate of breast cancer than women who were not taking the drug.[54] Tagamet, a drug commonly used to treat indigestion and ulcers, increases the level of 'bad' estrogen that promotes breast cancer and decreases the 'good' estrogen. It can cause breast enlargement in men who use it and is linked to increased breast cancer risk.[55] Antihistamines such as Claritin and Atarax may promote the growth of already existing cancers.[56]

This list of prescription drugs that may increase breast cancer risk is alarming, to say the least. As a society we have learned not to question the medications given to us for various disorders. Fortunately, safe alternatives exist for most, if not all, of the above drugs.

▶ **Action for Prevention:** Find a practitioner who uses natural substances such as herbal, nutritional, and homeopathic formulas and alter your diet and lifestyle to deal with health ailments. Use pharmaceutical drugs only if your symptoms cannot be controlled through natural means. Educate yourself on the side effects of prescription drugs and herbal remedies before you take them. ◀

Dental Problems

Many medical doctors and alternative health practitioners, particularly in Germany, are aware of chronic degenerative diseases being linked in part to problems with the teeth. Each tooth is associated with an acupuncture meridian and organ. If there is a low grade infection, mercury toxicity, or root canal associated with a particular tooth, it may manifest as a problem in another area of the body. The teeth are commonly sites of bacterial or parasitic infections. Dr Thomas Rau, Medical Director of the

Paracelsus Clinic in Lustmuhle, Switzerland, believes that in about 90% of breast cancer patients there is a dental component to their illness. Root canals in particular may harbor bacteria and toxins that enter the bloodstream from the tooth root. These circulate through the body, causing depressed immunity and potentially infecting or producing inflammation in another body part. Practitioners who use electrodermal screening, thermography, or applied kinesiology can sometimes determine whether this is a problem. Treatment may include the use of homeopathic remedies, extraction of the infected tooth, or removal and replacement of mercury amalgam fillings with ceramic or porcelain fillings, followed by mercury detoxification. The plastic replacement fillings can act as weak estrogens, as they usually include phthalates and bisphenol-A. I believe they should not be used.

▶ **Action for Prevention:** Take care of your teeth, brushing and flossing regularly. Visit a dentist who does not use mercury amalgam fillings and who can test for low grade infections that may not show up on an x-ray. Try to avoid root canals. ◀

Immune Deficiency and Allergies

Persons with illnesses suggestive of immune deficiency such as allergies or chronic viral infections have a greater susceptibility to breast cancer. Specific conditions can be treated effectively with naturopathy, homeopathy, and Chinese medicine to improve immune function.

▶ **Action for Prevention:** If your immune system is weakened, follow an immune-strengthening program using herbs, diet, and nutrients. ◀

Constipation

Women who do not have at least two bowel movements per week increase their risk of breast cancer. One study has shown that women with two or less bowel movements per week had 4.5 times the risk of pre-cancerous breast changes than other women who had bowel movements more than once daily.[57] Part of a breast cancer prevention program, therefore, includes encouraging at least two bowel movements daily.

▶ **Action for Prevention:** Drink 8–10 glasses of water daily, use wheat bran, flaxseeds, and 6–9 servings of fruits and vegetables daily to up your fiber content and encourage more regular bowel movements. Exercise four hours weekly and practice rebounding daily.

Monthly Breast Self-Exams

Approximately 90% of all breast cancers are found by women who notice changes in their own breasts.[58] Women who practice breast self-exams detect their cancers earlier with less likelihood of finding positive lymph nodes and have smaller tumors than women who do not perform breast self-exams.[59] Monthly breast self-exams are able to reduce breast cancer deaths by 20–30%, by providing early detection before the cancer has become invasive.[60]

▶ **Action for Prevention:** Perform monthly breast self-exams, map your breast topography and keep a written record of your findings to stay in touch with your breasts. Teach your daughters to do the same. ◀

Cigarette Smoking

Cigarette smoking increases the risk of breast cancer and is dose dependent. Women are more likely to die of the disease if they are smokers.

▶ **Action for Prevention:** Stop smoking and avoid secondhand smoke. Consult an acupuncturist, naturopathic doctor, or self-help group to help you stop smoking. ◀

Hair Dyes

Roughly 40% of American women between the ages of 18 and 60 dye their hair every month or two, and may continue this practice for decades. Chemicals from permanent and semi-permanent dyes are easily absorbed through the scalp. Some of the carcinogenic substances found in hair dyes, detergents, and preservatives include diaminotoluene, diaminoanisole, 4-ethoxy-m-phenylene sulfate [4-EMPD], para-phenylenediamine, artificial colors (C1 disperses Blue 1, D&C Red 33, HC Blue No. 1), dioxane, diethanoloamine, triethanolamine, ceteareth, laureth, polyethylene glycol, DMDM-hydantoin, imidazolidinyl urea, quarternium 15, nitrosamines, and formaldehyde. Women who start to use hair dyes in their twenties are more at risk than women who begin to dye their hair in their thirties or forties — in short, hair dyes represent a cumulative toxicity. It is the darker shades of dyes that contribute most to increased breast cancer risk. Hairdressers who apply these dyes have higher than normal rates of bladder cancer as well.

In the last several years there has been a movement towards safer hair dyes. Some lines that are safe include Igora Botanic, VitaWave from California, and Paul Penders hair coloring products.[61]

▶ **Action for Prevention:** Avoid hair dyes containing carcinogenic substances. Use henna or natural dyes instead. ◀

Breast Implants

There are two main types of breast implants that have been in use since the late 1960s — one uses silicone gel wrapped in either a seamless silicone outer envelope or casing made of polyurethane foam; the other uses a saline solution injected into a silicone pouch that has been surgically inserted into the breast. Silicone gel implants were banned in the United States in 1992, while saline filled implants are still readily available. Some of the problems associated with silicone gel implants include rupture and leakage of the silicone into the body, an increase in autoimmune and rheumatoid diseases, and a higher breast cancer incidence in women with the implants. Polyurethane foam, of which the casings of many of the implants were made, degrades in breast tissue as it releases a potent carcinogen, 2,4-toluene diisocyanate (TDI) which then is converted into another carcinogen, 2,4-diaminotoluene (TDA). Both TDI and TDA are able to induce breast cancer in rodents. TDA is found in the urine, blood, and breast milk of women with implants containing polyurethane foam.[62]

▶ **Action for Prevention:** Avoid breast implants and consider surgical removal if you already have them. ◀

Wearing a Bra

Women who wear their bras more than 12 hours a day increase their risk of breast cancer by a factor of 6. Underwire bras make this worse. The lymphatic system is one of the body's mechanisms that protects our breasts through removing cellular debris. For it to function properly, there needs to be movement of the breasts. Tight bras restrict movement, while going braless offers protection.

▶ **Action for Prevention:** Don't wear a bra unless you have to; take it off as soon as you are able to; use a cotton stretchy bra without underwires if you can. ◀

Summary

Many practical actions for avoiding or ameliorating the risk of developing breast cancer from hereditary, reproductive, and lifestyle or health care risks are within our control. Strategies for preventing cancer arising from hormonal, environmental, dietary, psychological, and spiritual factors will be presented in the following chapters. As we develop our understanding, we can return to The Breast Health Balance Sheet and choose to eliminate risk factors while gradually incorporating protective strategies.

Further Reading

Colborn, Theo, D. Dumanoski, J. Peterson Myers. *Our Stolen Future*. New York, NY: Penguin, 1996.

Epstein, S. and D. Steinman. *The Breast Cancer Prevention Program*. New York, NY: Macmillan, 1997.

Lee, John R. *What Your Doctor May Not Tell You About Menopause*. New York, NY: Warner Books Inc., 1996.

Steingraber, Sandra. *Living Downstream: An Ecologist Looks at Cancer and the Environment*. Reading, MA: Addison-Wesley Publishing Co. Ltd., 1997.

References

1. Harris, J.M. Lippman, et al. Breast Cancer. *New England Journal of Medicine*, 1992;327:319-28.
2. Thornton, J. *Human Health and the Environment: The Breast Cancer Warning*. Washington, DC: Greenpeace, 1993.
3. Cancer Facts and Figures - 1998. American Cancer Society.
4. Canadian Cancer Statistics 1998. Toronto, ON: National Cancer Institute of Canada, 1998:13.
5. Canadian Cancer Statistics 1998:55.
6. Canadian Cancer Statistics 1998:34.
7. MacDonald, P. Effect of obesity on conversion of plasma androstenedione to estrone in post-menopausal women with and without endometrial cancer. *Am J Obstet Gyneco*,1978;130:448.
8. Willett, W. The search for the causes of breast and colon cancer. *Nature*, 1989;338:389-93.
9. Breast Cancer Risk Factors: Are They Taken Too Seriously? *Health Facts*, September 1993.
10. Anderson, D. A genetic study of human breast cancer. *J Natl Cancer Inst*, 1972;48:1029.

11. Ottman, R. Practical guide for estimating risk for familial breast cancer. *Lancet*, 1983;2:556.

12. Breast cancer: A reassuring look at your odds, *Health*, January 1993.

13. Fackelmann, K. Breast cancer Risk and DDT: No Verdict Yet. *Science News*, April 23, 1994.

14. Tulinius, H., Egilsson, V., Olafsdottir, Gudrider, Sidvaldason. Risk of prostate, ovarian, and endometrial cancer among relatives with breast cancer. *BMJ*, Oct.10,1995.855-857.

15. *Lifetime Health Letter*, University of Texas. October, 1992.

16. Payson, R.A. Regulation of a promoter of the fibroblast growth factor 1 gene in prostate and breast cancer cells. *J Steroid Biochem Mol Biol.* 1998 Aug;66(3):93-103.

17. Li, S.L. et al. Expression of insulin-like growth factor (IGF)-II in human prostate, breast, bladder, and paraganglioma tumors. *Cell Tissue Res*, Mar;291(3):469-79.

18. Ekbom, A. Growing evidence that several human cancers may originate in utero. *Semin Cancer Biol*, 1998. Aug;8(4):237-44.

19. Saltzstein, S.L. The association of ethnicity and the incidence of mammary carcinoma in situ in women: 11,436 cases from the California Cancer Registry. *Cancer Detect Prev.* 1997;21(4):361-9.

20. Paskett, E.D., et al. Cancer screening behaviors of low-income women: the impact of race. *Women's Health*, 1997. Fall-Winter;(3-4):203-26.

21. Breast cancer and body shape, *Annals of Internal Medicine*, 1990;112:182-86.

22. MacDonald, P. Effect of obesity on conversion of plasma androstenedione to estrone in post-menopausal women with and without endometrial cancer. *Am J Obstet Gyneco*,1978;130:448.

23. Hoy, C. *The Truth about Breast Cancer*. Don Mills, ON: Stoddart, 1995.

24. Love, S. *Dr. Susan Love's Breast Book*. Don Mills, ON: Addison-Wesley Publishing Co.,1995:128.

25. Kelly, P. *Understanding Breast Cancer Risk*. Philadelphia, PA: Temple University, 1991.

26. Ungar, S. What about Estriol? *Menopause News*, March/April 1998 Vol.8 Issue 2, Madison Pharmacy Associates Inc.

27. *New England Journal of Medicine*, 1993;328:176.

28. Chris, J. Women who breastfeed. *American Health*, April, 1994.

29. Galetin-Smith, Pavkov, S. and Roncevic, N. DDT and PCBs in human milk: implication for breast-feeding infants. *Bulletin of Environmental Contaminant Toxicology.* 1989;43:641-646.

30. Allsopp, M., R. Stringer, P. Johnston. Unseen poisons: Levels of organochlorine pollutants in human tissues. Exter, UK: *Greenpeace Research Laboratories*, Dept. of Biological Sciences, University of Exeter, 1998:33.

31. Yurko, J., J. Millington. Increased breast milk toxicity in women of the Arctic: causes and methods for reduction. Toronto, ON: *Canadian College of Naturopathic Medicine*, April, 1999.

32. Colborn, Theo, D. Dumanoski, J. Peterson Myers. *Our Stolen Future*. New York, NY: Penguin, 1996: 107.

33. Colborn, Theo, D. Dumanoski, J. Peterson Myers. *Our Stolen Future*. New York, NY: Penguin, 1996:107.

34. Steingraber, Sandra. *Living Downstream: An Ecologist Looks at Cancer and the Environment*. Reading, MA: Addison-Wesley Publishing Co. Ltd., 1997:238.

35. Toxins found in breast milk, Owen Sound Sun Times, Dec. 26, 1998. From research published in the Dec. 20 edition of *Chemical Research in Toxicology.*

36. Greenpeace. *Death in Small Doses. The Effects of Organochlorines on Aquatic Ecosystems*. 1992.

37. Coleman, C., D. Lerman. Environmental toxins in breast milk. Toronto, ON: *Canadian College of Naturopathic Medicine*, April 1999.

38. Moller Jensen, O, B. et al. *Atlas of Cancer Incidence in the Nordic Countries*. Helsinki, Finland: Nordic Cancer Union, 1988.

39. Translation of a German study presented to me by Bernd Rohlf from Bona Dea Ltd., Dec. 8, 1999. The original study was done by Dr. Maiwald of Wurzburg, Germany.

40. Kelsey, J. and M. Gammon. The epidemiology of breast cancer. *A Cancer Journal for Clinicians*, 1991;41:146-65.

41. Willet, W. The search for the causes of breast and colon cancer. *Nature*, 1989;338:389-93.

42. LaCecchia, C.L. et al. Reproductive factors and breast cancer: An overview. *Soz Praventivmed*, 1989;34:101-107.

43. Health Canada. Clinical practise guidelines for the care and treatment of breast cancer: a Canadian consensus document. *Can Med Assoc J*, Feb. 10, 1998;1158 (3 Suppl)S3.

44. Thune, Inger, T. Brenn, E. Lund, M. Gaard. Physical activity and the risk of breast cancer, *New England Journal of Medicine*, May 1, 1997;336(18):1269-1275, 1311.

45. Jancin, B. Exercise study may point to hormones as the breast cancer culprit. *Family Practise News*. 1994;Nov.1;5.

46. Marcus, P.M., et al. Physical activity at age 12 and adult breast cancer risk (United States). *Cancer Causes Control*, 1999;Aug;10(4):293-302.

47. Brandes, L.J. Stimulation of malignant growth in rodents by antidepressant drugs at clinically relevant doses. *Cancer Research*, 1992;52:3796-3800.

48. *Physician's Desk Reference*, Montvale, N.J.: Medical Economics Data Production Company, 1996:1577-1579.

49. Williams, R.R., et al. Case-control study of anti-hypertensive and diuretic use by women with malignant and benign breast lesions detected in a mammography screening program. *Journal of the National Cancer Institute*, 1978;61:327-335.

50. Danielson, D.A., et al. Metronidazole and cancer. *Journal of the American Medical Association*, 1982;247(18):2498-2499.

51. Erturk, E., et al. Transplantable rat mammary tumors induced by 5-nitro-2-furaldehyde semicarbazone and by formic acid 2[4-(5-nitro-furyl)-2-thiazolyl]hydrazyde. *Cancer Research*, 1970;30:1409-1412.

52. Stoll, B.A. (ed.) Psychosomatic factors and their growth from *Risk Factors in Breast Cancer*. Chicago: Yearbook Medical Publishers, 1976:193.

53. *Breast Cancer: Research and Programs*, National Cancer Institute, June, 1993.

54. Newman, T.B. and S.B. Hully. Carcinogenicity of lipid -lowering drugs. *Journal of the American Medical Association*, 1996;275(1):55-60.

55. Smedley, H.M. Malignant breast change in man given two drugs associated with breast hyperplasia. *Lancet*,1981;2:638-639.

56. Fackelmann, K.A. Do antihistamines spur cancer growth? *Science News*, 1994, May 21:324.

57. Petrakis, N.L. & E.B. King. 1981. Cytological abnormalities in nipple aspirates of breast fluid from women with severe constipation. *Lancet*, 1981;ii:1203-1205.

58. Ross, W.S. *Crusade: The Official History of the American Cancer Society.* New York: Arbor House, 1987:96

59. Smigel, K. Perception of risk heightens stress of breast cancer screening. *Journal of the National Cancer Institute*, 1993;85(7):525-526.

60. Gastrin, G., et al. Preliminary results of primary screening for breast cancer with incidence and mortality from breast cancer in the Mama program. *Sozial- und Praventivmedizin*, 1993:38(5)280-287.

61. Epstein, S. and D. Steinman. *The Breast Cancer Prevention Program.* New York, NY: Macmillan, 1997:226-231

62. Epstein, S. and D. Steinman. *The Breast Cancer Prevention Program.* New York, NY:Macmillan, 1997:133-141.

Getting to Know Your Breasts

Exercises

Contents

Intimately linked with nurturing, sexuality, and motherhood, your breasts are perhaps the part of your body that you have the most feelings about, positive and negative. Many of us ignore those feelings and lack understanding as to how our breasts work and what affects them. We are often ignorant of the various breast conditions that show up as lumps or pain at different times in our lives and are hesitant to perform breast self-exams because of what we may find. This chapter will help you to become familiar with your breasts by understanding their anatomy and physiology through breast exploration and self-examination, and through a description of various breast ailments and diseases, including cancer. Diagnostic tests for breast cancer are described so you can become fully aware of these procedures, and various supplements, homeopathic remedies, and breathing exercises are recommended for prevention and treatment of breast ailments and diseases.

Breast Anatomy and Physiology

The normal function of our breasts is to secrete milk, providing food for our infants after they are born. They are also a source of sexual attraction and stimulation. Found between the second and sixth ribs, and extending from the sternum to the axilla, or armpit, the breasts rest upon the pectoralis major muscles. Each breast has a nipple located at its tip and a surrounding circular area of pigmented skin called the areola.

The mammary glands found in each breast are specialized tissue, being modified sweat glands surrounded by adipose (fatty) tissue. It is the amount of fatty tissue that determines breast size and shape. During puberty the ovaries produce estrogen which initiates the growth of the mammary glands and adipose tissue.

Resembling the branches of a tree, each mammary gland is composed of 15–20 lobes. The lobes are subdivided into smaller lobules which contain the glandular alveoli. After pregnancy and delivery, the hormones of prolactin (luteotropin) and oxytocin, secreted by the pituitary gland, stimulate the mammary glands in the breasts to secrete milk.

I think of this 'tree' in our breasts as being a hidden tree of life. Breast milk is its fruit. Normally breast milk sustains life. Today chemical pollutants and radiation

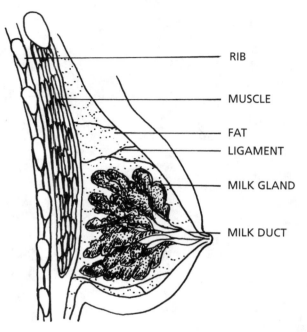

- RIB
- MUSCLE
- FAT
- LIGAMENT
- MILK GLAND
- MILK DUCT

poison the fruit, just as our air, water, soil and many planetary life forms are poisoned. The breast cancer epidemic is but a symptom and symbol of our planet in crisis and of its poisoned and dying tree of life.

Ways of Knowing Your Breasts

Many of us feel vulnerable around our breasts. We may have celebrated their gentle expansion during puberty or felt shame and discomfort. We may perceive them as being too large or too small, too noticed or not noticed enough. We often judge our bodies based on the images that television, film, and advertising gives us, causing many women to reshape their breasts through implants or surgery. We may feel that they are touched too much or want them to be touched more. We may be uncomfortable with the way they move when we exercise or their tenderness before menstruation. We may lament the fact that we could not or did not breast-feed our children long enough or we may have disliked the breast-feeding experience. Our breasts are intimately connected to our capacity to nurture others and ourselves and to the nurturing we received from our mothers.

Most of us experience an element of fear connected to our breasts because of the risk of breast cancer. Many women consider their breasts a liability. Often this fear causes us to cut ourselves off from our breasts psychically. Our fear prevents us from touching our breasts and from befriending them. In its wisdom, our mind sometimes expresses symptoms in parts of our bodies we deny in order to gather our attention. This can be the catalyst that moves us towards wholeness and integration.

Positive and Negative Associations with Your Breasts Exercise

Using an unlined sheet of paper, about 18 x 24 inches, or using the space below, draw a picture of your breasts as you experience them. Use colored markers, pastels, or crayons to express feelings you have about your breasts, including emotions or past traumas you associate with your breasts. Include cysts, scars, or tumors, and sensations you feel within them. Beneath the drawing divide the page in two. On the left hand side, write all the positive associations you have with your breasts. On the right hand side, write the negative associations you have. If you are in a group, share your drawings and experiences with one another. Sit in a circle and let each group member speak about some of the ways she has related to her breasts in the past or present. If there are more than 15 women, break into small groups of five to do this.

Breast Drawing

Positive Associations

Negative Associations

Befriending Your Breasts Exercise

Lie down in a comfortable place. Imagine you are relating to your breasts as though they were a close friend. Bring compassion and acceptance to your fingers. With one hand, begin to touch your breasts in a loving, exploring way, leaving your analytical mind out of it. Allow the quality of touching to welcome your breasts to the rest of your body. Invite them in. Reclaim them. Explore their topography, being sensitive to the different textures beneath your fingers. Notice how it feels when you dance lightly over the surface of your breasts, and when you press in deeply. As you press deeply, trace the boundaries of your ribs beneath. Move your breasts around, squeezing or massaging them as you do so. Touch your nipples and notice their sensitivity. As you touch one breast and then the other, notice any emotional differences you experience between them. Be aware of your breathing as you continue to explore your breasts, allowing it to slow down and deepen. Release the tension you might be holding in your abdomen. Let go of any fear you experience and bring your awareness to the present moment and to the sensitive exploration of your breasts. Spend an equal amount of time on either side. Go slowly. Continue for 10 minutes.

Breast Self-Examination (BSE) Exercise

Once we have developed a healing tactile relationship with our breasts, we can begin to perform regular breast self-exams. Many women experience fear at the thought of a breast self-exam and are reluctant to perform them on a regular basis. Other women have a hard time distinguishing between various kinds of lumps and feel confused and frustrated with breast self-exams. The key to success is familiarity through repetition. Each of you will have your own unique 'breast topography'; once a familiarity with what is normal for you is gained, variations from the norm are more easily noticed. Be patient and persist.

A monthly breast self-exam is helpful, usually best performed a few days after your period begins or at the same time each month if your periods have stopped.

Breast self-examination consists of two stages: the visual exam and palpation.

The Visual Exam

Stand before a mirror. With each of the following positions, observe your breasts in the mirror. Each position highlights a different part of your breast. Be watchful for any dimpling, puckering, bulging irregularities, or changes in size. Look for any changes in your nipples such as nipple inversion or displacement to one side. Notice any changes in skin texture or color. Take the time to be thorough and bring tenderness to it. The positions are as follows:

1) Place your hands on your hips and apply pressure. Examine the contour of your breasts, noticing any irregularities.

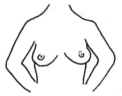

2) Slowly raise both arms over your head, stretching them up high. Examine your breasts and the underarm area, or axilla.

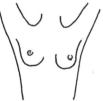

3) With your arms above your head, clasp your hands together and bring them down behind your head. Pull your elbows back and squeeze your hands together. Look for any changes in the appearance of your breasts and the axilla.

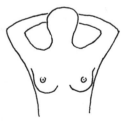

4) Bring your palms flat together in front of your forehead with your elbows out to the sides. Press your hands together. Examine your breasts.

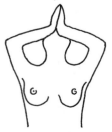

5) Bend forward from your hips until your nipples point down, resting your hands on your knees. In the mirror, observe the contour of your breasts for any irregularity.

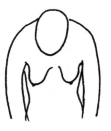

Palpation

The second stage of BSE is palpation — gently but firmly feeling the breasts to detect any unusual thickening or lumps. There are a number of accepted palpation methods. The three most commonly used are illustrated as follows.

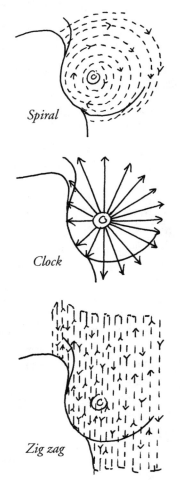

Spiral

Clock

Zig zag

Hold the first two or three fingers of one hand close together. Use the pads of those fingers to palpate the opposite breast. Make small circles with your fingers as you press towards the ribcage, moving the skin with your fingers. Use three levels of pressure on your breast so that you may detect lumps at various depths. For each position, start with gentle pressure, followed by moderate pressure and then press deeply enough so that you can feel the ribs beneath your breasts. Follow one of the patterns diagrammed above and use it consistently. Keep your breathing slow and relaxed.

Some women prefer to do their breast examination while in the shower, placing the hand of the examined side behind the head. If you have larger breasts, you may find it more efficient to lie down for a BSE. Place a towel or pillow under your shoulder to support and stabilize the breast that you are examining; the hand of the examined side rests behind your head. The opposite hand is then used to palpate your breast. Following either of the patterns above, slowly and thoroughly palpate each breast, being aware of any lumps or changes in lump size from your previous breast self-exam.

Breast tissue extends from the collarbone to just below the fold of skin under your breast, and from the middle of your chest to your side and armpit, so be sure to palpate this whole area, as in the drawing below. Also palpate the area above the collarbone, known as the supraclavicular area. Occasionally, breast cancer may be detected through persistent swollen lymph nodes in this area or in the nodes in the armpit. As you complete your exploration of each breast, squeeze your nipple to notice any discharge. Any unusual or bloody discharge warrants further examination with your medical doctor. A persistent nipple discharge on only one side may be due to cancer 4–21% of the time, particularly if it is bloody.[1]

Several studies have shown that women who do not palpate their breasts are twice as likely to have lymph node involvement at the time of a breast cancer diagnosis. Women who include a thorough visual exam of their breasts are twice as likely to find tumors smaller than 2 cm at the time of diagnosis. Although breast self-exams do not reduce the risk of breast cancer, they can reduce the risk of dying from breast cancer as tumors are detected sooner and treatment can begin earlier in the course of the disease.[2] We can encourage each other to be vigilant by performing monthly breast self-exams.

▶ **Action for Prevention:** Become an expert at performing monthly breast self-exams. Take time to explore and befriend your breasts at least once weekly. ◀

Mapping Your Breast Topography Exercise

It is difficult to detect from month to month what changes have occurred in our breasts, particularly if we have fibrous and lumpy breasts to begin with. If we map our breast topography with notations about size of lumps, location, texture, shape, moveability, and tenderness, we provide ourselves with a comparative study. It then becomes easier to notice when there has been a shift. We can take our maps to our health practitioners and more accurately describe our concerns or ask questions.

Using the following key with abbreviated notations, draw the topography of your breasts on the diagram on page 41 as you perceive it from your breast self-exam. As your breasts change in time, or as you become more proficient at breast self-exams, change your map accordingly. Use a ruler in centimeters to estimate the size of any lumps. Superimpose an imaginary clock over your breasts to describe the location and specify in which quadrant you find the lump — upper right (URQ), upper left (ULQ), lower right (LRQ) or lower left (LLQ).

Draw any lumps and document beside them the following characteristics:

SIZE:	size of lumps in cm, both length and width.
LOCATION:	where it is located on the imaginary clock (i.e. 2:00); how far outward from the nipple (i.e. 6 cm); and in which quadrant of which breast (i.e. upper left quadrant ULQ of the left breast LB).
TENDERNESS:	tender (T), non-tender (NT), and describe the quality and severity of the pain (achy, bruised, needle-like, cramping, pulling, tearing, burning, throbbing).
SHAPE:	regular shape with smooth edges (R), irregular (I).
TEXTURE:	hard (H), soft (S). Circle which of the following best describes the overall texture of your breasts: smooth granular lumpy cystic fibrous.
MOVEABILITY:	freely moveable (FM), fixed (F). For example, if you find a small, tender, regular shaped, soft, freely moveable lump, you would draw its location and write: *1 cm, 3:00, T, R, S, FM* beside it.
LYMPH NODES:	underarm L R supraclavicular swelling hardness # of nodes palpable. Circle which area of nodes has swelling or hardness and indicate the number of nodes you are able to feel.
NIPPLE DISCHARGE:	no yes L R nonbloody bloody

Eighty percent of all breast lumps are benign. The lumps which are non-tender (NT), irregular (I), hard (H), and fixed (F) are the ones most likely to be breast cancer. However, there are exceptions. Bring any lump to your doctor's attention for further investigation. Be particularly attentive to lumps that persist for more than two menstrual cycles and do not disappear after your period. Follow up testing might include fine needle aspiration, thermography, the AMAS blood test, an ultrasound, a mammogram, or a biopsy.

Now map your breast topography monthly, as you do your breast self-exams, using copies of this breast map as your guide.

Breast Ailments

From your self-examination, you may discover various ailments other than cancer. I think of breast ailments as occurring on a continuum. Many of them are linked to high estrogen and low progesterone levels, thyroid and other hormonal imbalances, environmental toxins, lymphatic congestion, stress, weakened immunity, a diet too high in fat, disturbances in liver function, and/or deficiencies of key nutrients such as magnesium, iodine, vitamin B6, vitamin E, coenzyme Q10, and essential fatty acids. There is an association between some benign breast diseases and breast cancer, so it makes sense to improve our breast health through natural methods should any of the following breast ailments be present. Protective and therapeutic nutrient supplement regimes are recommended here, though the homeopathic remedies which follow in this chapter, as well as Traditional Chinese Medicine formulas described in subsequent chapters, may also help to prevent breast cancer.

BREAST MAP

Photocopy this page, map your breast topography on it monthly and record any changes.

Date:_____

Palpate the area contained within the dotted lines on your own breasts and draw what you find using the notations on the previous page. Check your map each month, making changes as needed.

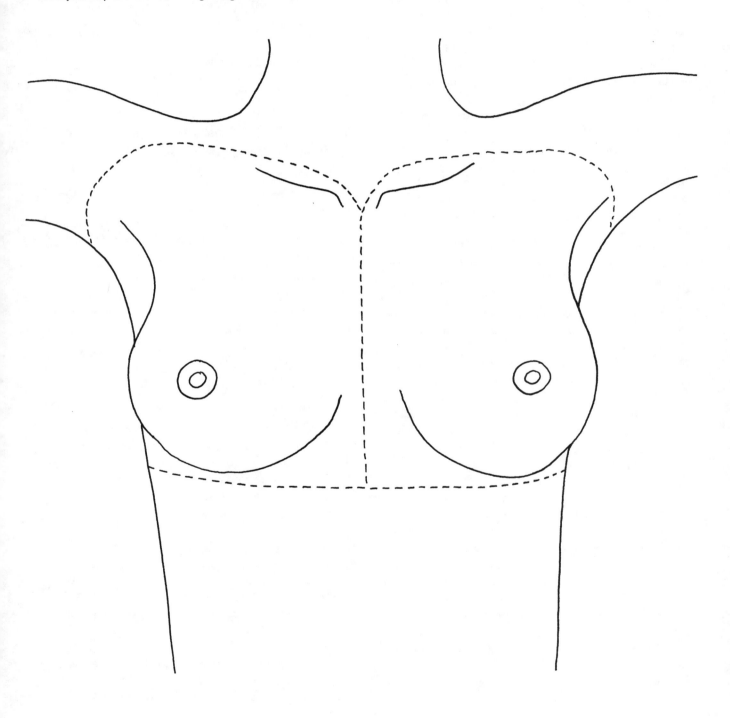

Premenstrual Breast Pain and Swelling

During a breast self-exam your breasts may feel swollen and tender. Roughly 35% of all pre-menopausal women experience swollen, tender breasts one to two weeks before their periods. If you are one of these women, you may also experience weight gain, abdominal bloating, and swelling of the face, hands and ankles. The symptoms are caused by an increase in the hormonal secretion of aldosterone from the adrenal glands. The triggers for aldosterone production include stress, excess estrogen, and a deficiency of dopamine, a brain neurotransmitter.

Dopamine levels in the brain are depleted when there is a deficiency of magnesium and B6. Vitamin B6 promotes the production of dopamine in the hypothalamus, which then inhibits the release of the hormone prolactin. Increased prolactin causes breast swelling.

Premenstrual breast pain and swelling is improved with extra magnesium and vitamin B6. Low magnesium in the body causes the adrenal glands to enlarge and release more aldosterone, resulting in increased fluid retention and weight gain. Pumpkin seeds are one of the highest dietary sources of magnesium. We can eat them daily with cereal, snacks, or added to salads. Low vitamin B6 levels in the body also decrease the kidney's ability to get rid of sodium and thus water is retained. Sufficient B6 helps to increase progesterone levels, which reduces breast swelling. Too much sugar can cause water retention due to the increased secretion of insulin from the pancreas. Thyroid imbalance, iodine deficiency, and an overgrowth of intestinal yeast (candidiasis) can also cause premenstrual breast pain and swelling.

In Traditional Chinese Medicine, breast swelling is believed to occur due to 'stagnation of liver energy and blood'. The energetic function of the liver is to allow for the free flow of energy outward in all directions. The liver is the organ most vulnerable to stress. Repressed anger, depression, frustration, excess stress, alcohol, and unhealthy fats are some of the things that disturb the liver's ability to circulate energy and blood. Aerobic exercise, expressing emotions, regular deep breathing, and relaxation are ways to relieve liver stagnation.

It may be difficult to determine the exact cause of your premenstrual breast pain and swelling, but you can experiment with B6 and magnesium for a few months to see if there is improvement. Include more sea vegetables containing iodine in your diet. Decrease your consumption of fats to less than 15% of your total caloric intake, with the exception of flaxseed oil and extra virgin olive oil. Increase aerobic exercise to four hours weekly and develop a regular relaxation or meditation practice. Other therapies that I have seen work are the Chinese patent formula Xiao Yao Wan, which circulates the liver energy; the Hoxsey Formula, a lymphatic cleanser; a balanced ratio of Omega 3 and Omega 6 essential fatty acids; and vitamin E. In many women, the homeopathic remedy Folliculinum 9CH, taken on days seven and 21, relieves breast swelling by stimulating progesterone production.[3] Increasing progesterone through the use of herbs like chaste tree berry or by using a natural progesterone cream is also effective.

Supplements and Dosages

Vitamin B6: 50 mg 3x daily with meals as well as a B complex.

Magnesium: 150 mg 2x daily with calcium, with meals.

Xiao Yao Wan: 8 small pills 3x daily between meals to assist liver function.

Hoxsey Formula: 15–30 drops 3x daily between meals starting 7 days after your period begins and stopping at the onset of your period. It can be toxic in high dosages and should not be used in pregnancy. It works on improving lymphatic circulation.

Evening Primrose Oil: 2 g daily, combined with twice as much flaxseed oil; or balanced oil with 2:1 Omega 3: Omega 6 fatty acids.

Vitamin E: 600 IU daily.

Folliculinum: 9 CH – one dose on the seventh day and another on day 21 of the menstrual cycle; an extra one on day 14 if necessary.

Fibrocystic Breast Disease

If you notice soft, tender, moveable cysts in your breasts that are predominant one to two weeks before your period and diminish after your period, you may have a condition called fibrocystic breast disease. It commonly affects 20–40% of pre-menopausal women between the ages of 20 and 50 years.

Fibrocystic breast disease, like breast cancer, is increasing in frequency. In 1928 an autopsy series reported a 3% incidence,[4] while in 1973 an autopsy report quoted an 89% incidence.[5]

The cysts are cyclic, vary in size, and are often painful, freely moveable and multiple, occurring in both breasts. Twenty percent of women with this condition are able to feel swollen lymph nodes in the underarm area as well. The condition is more severe before the menstrual period and is thought to be due to an increased estrogen to progesterone ratio. Some researchers have also suggested it is linked to an upset in the ratio between estrone and estriol,[6] or an underactive thyroid. Yet others suggest that it may be due to high estradiol and low testosterone. Clearly it is related to hormonal imbalance. It may also relate to nutritional deficiencies in vitamins E and B6, iodine, coenzyme Q10, or essential fatty acids. Sluggish bowels, an overburdened liver, and a diet too high in fat are also implicated.

Supplementation with vitamins E and B6 helps to increase progesterone and decrease estrogen,[7] and these are used in the treatment of fibrocystic breast disease. When estrogen levels rise from both internal and external sources, prolactin levels are also increased. Prolactin is a hormone released from the anterior pituitary gland that stimulates the enlargement of breast tissue. A low fat diet will help to lower estrogen and prolactin levels and decrease premenstrual breast pain.[8]

Another nutrient of importance in maintaining breast health is coenzyme Q10. A 1998 study found that women with benign breast tumors (fibrocystic breasts and fibroadenomas) as well as women with breast cancer had lower plasma levels of coenzyme Q10 than did women with normal breasts. The more severe the breast disease, the greater the deficiency.[9] Vitamin B6 and the amino acid tyrosine (also needed for proper thyroid function) are utilized in the formation of coenzyme Q10 in our bodies.

Low thyroid function may cause an increase in prolactin levels. When the thyroid gland needs a boost, TRH, a hormone from the hypothalamus, causes both a release in thyroid-stimulating hormone and prolactin from the anterior pituitary gland. Prolactin can be measured using a saliva test. Thyroid function can easily be tested by taking the underarm temperature before rising in the morning on days 2 to 7 of the menstrual cycle. Temperatures at or below 36.5°C or 97.8°F may indicate low thyroid function, even though blood tests for the thyroid gland appear normal. Increased progesterone may enhance thyroid function, and a deficiency of progesterone can suppress thyroid function. Interestingly, the thyroid gland may be underactive due to a deficiency of iodine, and supplementation with one of several forms of iodine has been shown to improve fibrocystic breast disease as well. The amino acid tyrosine is also needed to make thyroid hormones.

Kelp tablets, Lugol's Solution (sodium iodide), or aqueous molecular iodine are often helpful in alleviating fibrocystic breasts. Dr William Ghent of Kingston, Ontario and his colleagues found that Lugol's Solution improved fibrocystic breasts in 70% of patients after several months, with less than 5% of the women experiencing side effects (changes in thyroid function and acne). Aqueous molecular iodine caused a faster improvement in a greater number of women with fewer side effects and complete disappearance of pain and cysts within five months. Aqueous iodine is more easily absorbed into breast tissue than sodium iodide.[10] The action of aqueous iodine does not affect the thyroid gland while other forms of iodide stimulate the thyroid. Dr Jonathan Wright has used iodine to increase estriol levels in women, creating a more favorable estrone to estriol ratio which would decrease estrogen-related breast disease. Bernard Eskin, MD, found that iodine deficient rats were more prone to breast cysts and breast cancer and that aqueous molecular iodine could reverse the cysts better than sodium iodide.[11] In breast tissue, iodine is only found in the terminal and intralobular duct cells, which are the areas most prone to fibrocystic changes and breast cancer. Ghent and his colleagues believed that iodine deficiency made the cells of the terminal and intralobular ducts more sensitive to estrogen stimulation and thus more vulnerable to cancer.[12] Perhaps the iodine sensitizes the estrogen receptor to estriol (the protective estrogen) rather than to estradiol or estrone.

There is a strong association between methylxanthine consumption and fibrocystic breast disease. Methylxanthine is found in coffee, black tea, green tea, cola, chocolate, and caffeinated medications and has been shown to promote the growth of cancer cells in the mammary gland of rats. Fibrocystic breast disease often improves when women stop using foods or drugs containing methylxanthines.[13,14]

Since the liver is the main site for estrogen breakdown, any factor that interferes with proper liver function may lead to estrogen excess, and disturb the ratio of estrone to estriol, which in turn may promote breast disease. Specifically, when the liver is inefficient at converting the harmful estrogens (estradiol, estrone, C16-hydroxyestrone) to the harmless estrogens (estriol, C2-hydroxyestrone), the risk for fibrocystic breast disease and breast cancer increases. Environmental estrogens also contribute to estrogen excess and fibrocystic breast disease. Many factors can get in the way of proper liver function: chemicals in food, bowel toxicity, allergies, decreased immunity, polluted air and water, environmental chemicals and toxins, nutritional deficiencies, use of drugs or alcohol, stress, lack of exercise, and a high fat diet. Improving liver function with herbs (milk thistle, dandelion, schizandra, globe artichoke, barberry, chelidonium, rosemary, turmeric) and nutritional supplements (NAC, B complex, choline, methionine, vitamins E and A, magnesium, calcium, zinc, and flaxseed oil) can help fibrocystic breasts.

In Traditional Chinese Medicine, fibrocystic breast disease is linked to stagnation of liver energy and blood which has occurred long enough to cause local accumulations, particularly if the diet is high in phlegm producing foods, such as fat, dairy, sugar, and wheat products. Treatment is geared toward activating the liver energy and blood and removing the accumulation. Typical herbs used to accomplish this are bupleurum, paeonia lactiflorae, angelica sinensis, atractylodes, and ginger.

Fibrocystic breast disease and breast cancer have been linked to the Western diet and bowel function. Women having less than three bowel movements per week have a risk of fibrocystic breast disease four to five times greater than women having at least one a day, for two reasons. First intestinal bacteria linked to high fat and meat based diets can break apart an estrogen complex (called a glucuronide conjugate) formed in the liver that would ordinarily be excreted in the stools. The estrogen is then reabsorbed through the wall of the large intestine and becomes active in the body. High fiber, plant-based diets which increase the frequency of bowel movements prevent this from occurring. Second, fecal bacteria can make three types of estrogen from dietary cholesterol, the precursor of estrogen hormones. These three estrogens (estrone, estradiol, and 17-methoxyestradiol) can be absorbed back into the body.[15] Fatty foods (particularly in meat) promote the growth of harmful bacteria in the large intestine that accomplish these two tasks and will also slow down bowel transit time. This partially explains the link between fatty foods, fibrocystic breast disease, and breast cancer.

Women wishing to protect themselves from fibrocystic breast disease and breast cancer should drastically reduce fats found in meat, dairy, and fried food, and restrict their fat intake to olive oil, flaxseed oil, and a few nuts and seeds. Diets high in fiber from unrefined starch sources promote bowel movements. Fiber also acts as an intestinal barrier to the re-absorption of estrogens. Freshly ground organic flaxseeds, psyllium, wheat bran, and legumes are especially beneficial high fiber foods.

Women whose breast cyst biopsies reveal ductal or lobular proliferation, or atypical hyperplasia (33% of biopsied patients) have a risk of developing breast cancer four times higher than age-matched controls.[16] Otherwise, women with cystic breasts have a subsequent breast cancer risk of 1.8.[17] Fibrocystic breast disease can be a precursor for later breast cancer.[18]

You can reverse fibrocystic breast disease with naturopathic methods. Consider the following supplements and actions for prevention.[19]

Supplements and Dosages

Vitamin E, mixed tocopherols: 600 IU daily.

Beta Carotene: 25,000–40,000 IU daily.

Kelp tablets and/or Iodine in one of the following forms:

a) aqueous molecular iodine – 0.07 to 0.09 mg per kg of body weight daily for 6 months (preferred type of iodine but only available by prescription from a medical doctor);

b) Lugol's Solution (sodium iodide) — 5 to 10 drops daily, depending on body weight.

Evening Primrose Oil: 2–3 g daily, combined with twice as much flaxseed oil.

Vitamin B6: 50 mg 3x daily with meals and a B complex.

Coenzyme Q10: 60–200 mg daily.

Progesterone Cream, if indicated by low amounts in saliva: 2 oz per month or 15–20 mg per day.

Xiao Yao Wan: 8 pills 3x daily; and / or

Milk Thistle or Dandelion Tincture: 25 drops 3x daily for liver support.

Dietary use of **Turmeric, Soy and Rosemary.**

Hoxsey Formula: 15–30 drops 3x daily starting 7 days after your period begins and continuing until the next period. (The Healthy Breast Formula may be used as a substitute).

Folliculinum 9 CH: one dose on the seventh day and another on day 21 of the menstrual cycle; an extra one on day 14 if necessary.

Correct homeopathic treatment may also help fibrocystic breast disease, as will the Chinese herbal formulas found in subsequent chapters.

I usually start a patient on two or three of these therapies and add or subtract as symptoms call for it.

▶ Actions for Prevention:

1) Decrease your exposure to environmental estrogens.

2) Reduce unhealthy dietary fats to less than 15% of total calories, but do use flaxseed oil and olive oil.

3) Increase consumption of fresh fruits and vegetables, fiber, and phytoestrogens; decrease or eliminate meat.

4) Eliminate methylxanthines found in coffee, black tea, and chocolate.

5) Drink 8 or more glasses of water daily to promote bowel movements and elimination.

6) Assist liver function with herbs and nutritional supplements.

7) Correct thyroid function and iodine deficiency.

8) Normalize estrogen to progesterone ratios; and estrone to estriol levels.

9) Achieve appropriate weight and reduce body fat to 20–22%; maintain a regular exercise program.

10) Correct essential fatty acid deficiency with a 2:1 Omega 3: Omega 6 ratio.

11) Correct deficiencies of vitamin E, B6 and coenzyme Q10. ◄

These strategies are discussed in later chapters and are the same strategies that will prevent breast cancer. Continue for at least 5 months before evaluating their effectiveness.

Fibroadenomas

This is a tumor commonly seen in younger women and is the third most frequent of all breast diseases after fibrocystic breast disease and breast cancer. Unlike fibrocystic breast disease, the tumor is not cystic, but is constantly present. It is not malignant, although its presence indicates the possibility of a higher risk for breast cancer later in life. The lump is firm, smooth, round, and moveable, like a marble under the skin. If a fibroadenoma breaks down on its own, it can develop into calcifications or microcalcifications. These may be associated with the development of breast cancer. Sometimes a mammogram or biopsy is recommended to confirm that the lump is a fibroadenoma and not breast cancer.

Conventional medical treatment indicates fibroadenoma removal under local anaesthetic. Naturopathic treatment is similar to that for fibrocystic breast disease with an increase in coenzyme Q10 (200–300 mg per day) and the inclusion of more Chinese or Western herbs that assist tumor breakdown. Some of the Chinese herbs used to break down hard tumors are *Bombyx batryticatus, Pericarpum Citri reticulatae viride, Sparganium, Taraxicum mongolicum, and Curcuma zedoaria.* Western herbs used to accomplish the same thing are burdock root, marigold flowers, goldenseal, echinacea, European mistletoe, phytolacca, red clover, cleavers, and wild indigo. Individually prescribed homeopathic remedies are also helpful. Survey the list at the end of the breast ailments.

Mastitis

Mastitis is an inflammation of the breast and milk duct systems, usually due to infection caused by bacteria entering a fissured or cracked nipple. It most often occurs in a first-time mother after childbirth and during breast-feeding. A duct becomes blocked with thick milk that feeds bacterial growth. Symptoms include breast pain with heat and redness, a hard swelling, fever, and possibly swollen cervical and/or axillary lymph nodes. It may occur due to poor nipple preparation in the final two to three months of pregnancy, breast engorgement due to incomplete emptying, excessive suckling by the newborn, not drinking enough water, or stress. Western medicine treats this condition with antibiotics and surgical drainage if necessary. I have healed my own mastitis in 24–48 hours several times with increased fluid intake, warm compresses, and frequent nursings, along with the following supplements.

Supplements and Dosages

Vitamin C: 500 mg every 2 hours.

Homeopathic Phytolacca 30K: 3 pellets hourly, away from food and dissolved under the tongue.

Hoxsey Formula: 15 drops every 2 hours.

Goldenseal/Echinacea Herbal Tincture: 15 drops every 2 hours.

Intraductal Papillomas

Intraductal papillomas are relatively uncommon, small, benign tumors occurring on the lining of the nipple ducts of the breast. Frequently they are too small to feel. The main symptom is a watery, pinkish, or bloody discharge from the nipple. Surgical removal of the affected ducts is the standard treatment. The tissue must be biopsied since a bloody discharge from the nipple, especially if it occurs in only one breast, can be due to malignancy.

Breast Calcifications

Calcifications in the breast are felt as small, hard, regular shaped tumors. They may have originated from old fibroadenomas that you had as a teenager which have calcified. They may also be calcifications in a blood vessel that occurs with aging. As we age, calcium leaves our bones and may collect in other tissues such as the joints and arteries, particularly if our bodies are overly acidic. Calcium in the bloodstream acts as a buffer for an overly acidic body. Check the pH of your urine and saliva in the morning for several days to see if your body is too acidic. You can purchase pH paper at a drug store and some health food stores. A normal range for both of these is 6.4 –7.2. If you consistently fall below that range, then increase your alkalinity by consuming more fruits and vegetables and less meat, protein, and grain. You can also create more alkalinity by taking a calcium-magnesium supplement before bed, increasing your water intake, relaxing, and practicing deep breathing.

Eighty percent of calcifications are not linked to breast cancer. A few are. If they are clustered close together, are very small, and don't seem to be in other parts of the breast, they are more likely to be pre-cancerous. A biopsy will tell. If there are a lot of them spread throughout both breasts, they are less likely to lead to cancer. Calcifications should be monitored closely every few months to be sure there is no change in size or shape, which might indicate cancer.[20]

The homeopathic tissue salt Calc fluor 6X may be helpful in alleviating calcifications. Generally women with calcifications should be diligent in adopting a cancer prevention diet and lifestyle, following many of the guidelines in this book.

Breast Cancer

Most often breast cancer is felt as a hard, irregular-shaped, non-tender lump that feels as though it is attached to the underlying tissue. There may be puckering of the skin near the lump site, bloody nipple discharge, and/or changes in nipple size and shape.

Evidence shows that cancer cells are often present 10 years before the mass is finally detectable, having grown to a size one centimeter in diameter and consisting of one billion cells. The time required for one cell to divide into two cells is called doubling time, and the rate varies between 21–100 days depending on the type of breast cancer. More aggressive cancers have a faster doubling time.

Breast cancer begins with changes in the DNA of the breast cell initiated by a variety of causative agents, including chemicals, radiation, free radicals, toxic minerals, electromagnetic fields, genetic defects, drugs, viruses, and stress. Ordinarily the cell has the capacity to repair its DNA, bolstered by a healthy diet and lifestyle. Cells from our immune systems also constantly survey the body, on guard for disfigured, pre-cancerous cells. When DNA repair is unable to keep up with breast cell genetic damage, the cell repeats or accentuates the damaged DNA

as it divides and reproduces itself. Excess estrogen contributes to the faster multiplication of breast cells and accelerates the rate at which the damaged cells form a tumor, though it may not be the original cause of the genetic defect. The hormone IGF-1 also promotes breast cell multiplication and tumor growth.

When the clump of aberrant cells spreads out from the tissue of origin to the surrounding area, it is classified as invasive cancer. This is the growth phase of the tumor, promoted by estrogen and IGF-1 and kept in check by melatonin and possibly progesterone. The tumor starts to recruit blood vessels to gain its nourishment. Environmental estrogens may help it to do this. Soy, green tea, and turmeric help to prevent the formation of this blood supply, known as angiogenesis. Single cancer cells can separate from the original tumor and travel through the blood to the rest of the body. They can migrate to the liver, lungs, bone marrow, or brain and multiply to form another tumor, or metastasis, of the original deranged breast cell.

The body tries to put a halt to this process by attacking breast cancer cells in the lymph nodes, and sending out white blood cells to patrol the blood to seek and destroy any wandering cancer cells. Melatonin levels increase in an attempt to halt the cancerous process. Unlike normal cells, cancer cells lose the signal to die after they reproduce. They are on a narcissistic mission of self-perpetuation at the expense of their host. Over time, they can interfere with processes essential to life.

There are approximately 30 types of breast cancer and a series of grades or levels, indicating severity. Generally they are divided into two categories: lobular vs. ductal. Over three quarters of all breast cancers are ductal; this category includes mucinous, papillary, and combination cancers. Lobular cancers are more difficult to treat. Breast cancers that are neither lobular nor ductal include Paget's disease and inflammatory carcinoma.

The stages of breast cancer are ranked to reflect the severity of the disease or threat to life, and are labeled Stage 0, I, II, III, or IV.

Stage 0:   Stage 0 is carcinoma in situ, which most often does not progress to invasive cancer. Five-year survival with a ductal cancer is 95%.

Stage I: Stage I is when the tumor is less than 2 cm and there is no lymph node involvement. Five-year survival with a ductal cancer is 85%.

Stage II: Stage II occurs when the tumor is less than 2 cm with lymph node involvement, or when the tumor is between 2–5 cm with no affected lymph nodes. Five-year survival with a ductal cancer is 65%.

Stage IIB: Stage IIB is when the tumor is 2–5 cm with positive nodes, or when the tumor is bigger than 5 cm. Five-year survival with a ductal cancer is 55%.

Stage III: Stage III is when the tumor is larger than 5 cm with positive lymph nodes. Five-year survival with a ductal or lobular cancer is 40%.

Stage IV: Stage IV occurs when the cancer has metastasized to a distant site or the diagnosis is inflammatory carcinoma. Five-year survival is 10%.

When breast cancer occurs in a younger woman, it usually follows a more aggressive course than cancer occurring in a post-menopausal woman.

Diagnostic and Predictive Tests for Breast Cancer

If you suspect from your self examination that you may have a serious breast ailment or cancer, there are a variety of medical tests recommended by different medical bodies such as the American Medical Association or the Canadian Medical Association to assist in diagnosis. When a breast lump or change in breast texture is found, the Canadian Medical Association, for example, recommends the following procedure for physicians to follow.

1) Begin the investigation with a history, physical exam, and usually mammography.

2) Find out how long the lump has been noticed, whether any change has occurred and whether there is a history of biopsy or breast cancer. Establish the individual's risk factors for breast cancer.

3) From the physical exam, identify the features that might differentiate malignant from benign lumps.

4) Use mammography to clarify the type of lump and detect lesions in either breast.

5) Use fine needle aspiration to detect whether the lump is solid or cystic. When it is solid, obtain cells to examine them further.

6) Ultrasound can be used instead of fine needle aspiration to distinguish a cyst from a solid tumor.

7) If any doubt remains as to whether the lump is benign or malignant, do a biopsy.

8) During a surgical biopsy, attempt to remove the whole lump in one piece with a margin of surrounding normal tissue.

9) Alternatively, a core biopsy can usually establish or exclude cancer, reducing the need for a surgical biopsy.

10) Thermography and light scanning are not recommended as diagnostic techniques, and MRI is not routinely recommended at this time.

11) Choices of procedure depend upon the experience of the diagnostician and the technology that is available.

12) These diagnostic procedures should be completed quickly, informing the patient throughout.

13) Even when cancer is not found, follow up surveillance may be recommended.[21]

Women over 50 are advised to have a yearly mammogram, while women under 50 years of age are not. Mammograms are controversial, however, because they expose a woman to more radiation, which has a cumulative effect, and over time can cause breast cancer. Until we have safer diagnostic tools, such as laser mammography, these recommendations are very useful and should be considered. But how do we detect early, nonpalpable breast cancer in women under 50 and in women over 50 when annual mammograms fail to show any abnormality? Three additional testing procedures — the AMAS test, Immunicon test, and thermography — may help to fill those gaps and can be used to complement (not replace) the above guidelines. Both of these tests as well as the conventional tests listed above are described below.

The AMAS Blood Test (Antimalignin Antibody in Serum)

This is a non-specific cancer-screening test that measures antimalignin, an antibody found elevated in the serum of people with cancer. Malignin is found in the cell membranes of all cancer cells, and some of our white blood cells make antimalignin antibody in response to its presence. The antimalignin antibody is found increased in 93–100% of cases when a person has an active, nonterminal malignancy. In other words, the test is very effective in detecting small (1mm), previously undiagnosed tumors, but will not tell you where the cancer is. It is not useful for late stage cancer. It is elevated no matter where the site of the cancer and for all cell types. The test results in very few false positives — only 5% in serum kept frozen for more than 24 hours and less than 1% in serum tested within 24 hours of blood being drawn. False negatives are found in 7 percent of cases.

The antimalignin antibody is normal in 96% of cancer patients who no longer have evidence of disease and in persons with no previous history of cancer, but will also be normal in people with terminal cancer. The AMAS test can be positive one to 19 months before a cancer is detected clinically.

In a study of 1,175 breast cancer patients, it was found that one month to 30 years after treatment, clinical remission of breast cancer is correlated with the return of elevated AMAS values to normal values approximately 95% of the time. This is particularly useful for women who have had a lumpectomy and are considering chemotherapy and/or radiation.[22] If their AMAS levels are normal after the lumpectomy, no further allopathic treatment is required. It is also useful for naturopathic doctors using herbal, homeopathic, and dietary methods with cancer patients to monitor progress and know when remission has been achieved.

It makes sense for this test to be used more frequently in breast cancer monitoring. Rather than expose ourselves to hazardous radiation from mammograms, women under 50 can use it as an annual screening test,[23] along with thermography. If the test results are positive, a mammogram can be used to follow it up. All women, especially those who have worked in the electrical, chemical, nuclear, or plastics industries, can consider having the test done annually. The AMAS test can also be used to monitor a cancer patient's progress and response to treatment.[24]

Keep in mind that it is not foolproof. There are a few false negatives and false positives and this test should be used as a guide rather than as a test for confirming the presence of cancer. I have heard from several people for whom this test was inaccurate.

The test can be ordered from Oncolab Inc. (36 The Fenway, Boston, MA 02215, tel. 617-536-0805 or 1-800-9-CATest, fax. 617-536-0657). The cost of the test is approximately $135.00 (USA currency).

▶ **Action for Prevention:** Consider having the AMAS or the Immunicon test done annually if you are under 50. If you are over 50, also consider the AMAS test annually, as it can pick up the presence of any cancer when it is only 1 mm large, which is more sensitive than a mammogram. If a positive result comes back, then have a mammogram to determine where the cancer might be. ◀

The Immunicon Test

A new blood test has been developed by Immunicon Corporation that can detect one tumor cell among 20 million white blood cells. In studies on more than 60 breast cancer patients from two major American medical centers, the test was able to detect small numbers of tumor cells in the blood of women with very early stage breast tumors and greater numbers in those with advancing disease. Over a 12-month study of a group of patients, it was found that when the disease process worsened or when patients did not respond to treatment the numbers of tumor cells increased. When treatment was effective, the number of tumor cells dropped. In a few women thought to be in complete remission, tumor cells were found and further examination showed that they were indeed relapsing. The blood test will be positive when there are as few as 1,000 tumor cells in the entire circulation.[25] The test is presently available only to clinical researchers. For more information, contact the web site, www.immunicon.com or Immunicon Corporation (tel. 215-938-0100 or fax. 215-938-0437).

Thermography

Thermography was inaccurate 20 years ago and its use lost favor. Today, efficiency has improved with the use of new ultra-sensitive high-resolution digital infrared devices. Thermography measures subtle changes in the temperature at the surface of the body. Because cancerous tumors have an increased blood supply, they are slightly hotter than the surrounding areas in which they are found. This difference in temperature is measurable, particularly when both breasts can be compared. Any area of increased heat can then be investigated further with a mammogram or with the more general AMAS blood test.

Thermography measures physiology, unlike a mammogram, which detects changes in anatomy. Often the physiological changes precede the anatomical changes. As a physiological test, thermography demonstrates heat patterns that are strongly indicative of abnormality, although not authoritative. It has been estimated that thermal imaging is three to five years ahead of mammography as a risk indicator. Canadian studies done at the Ville Marie Breast Center in Montreal have found that thermograms were positive for 83% of breast cancers compared to 61% for clinical breast exam alone and 84% for mammography. The 84 % sensitivity of mammography was increased to 95% when infrared thermographic imaging was added.[26]

It is women under 50 who can most benefit from the

use of thermography. Breast cancers tend to grow significantly faster in women under 50. The average tumor doubling time for women under 50 is 80 days; for women between 50–70, it is 157 days; and for women over age 70, it is 188 days. The faster a tumor grows, the more infrared radiation it generates, and therefore the more likely it will be picked up with thermography.[27] Breast cancer patients with abnormal thermograms tend to have faster-growing tumors which are more likely to metastasize.[28] Abnormal thermograms are associated with large tumor size, high grade and positive lymph nodes.[29] This information, grim as it is, can be used to encourage a patient to do everything possible to prevent a recurrence.

Thermography is noninvasive, safe, with no risk of cumulative radiation, and takes about 10 minutes to perform. Its success depends on strict protocols being followed, as there are many variables that can influence body temperature, such as the ambient room temperature, type of floor covering, type of equipment utilized, and the presence or absence of windows. We need more doctors and technicians trained in the use and interpretation of thermography available in breast cancer screening centers, as they are, for instance, at the Ville Marie Breast Center in Montreal. I would advocate annual thermography in women under 50 in conjunction with the AMAS or Immunicon test as a screening procedure. Mammography can be used if cancer is suspected. Women over 50 can use mammography with the other two tests for higher diagnostic efficacy.

In Canada, thermography is available at the Ville Marie Medical Center in Montreal, QC (tel. 514-933-2778) or at Northside General Hospital in North Sydney, NS (tel. 902-794-8521). For a directory of where thermography is available in the United States, see the September 1999 issue of *Alternative Medicine*.

▶ **Action for Prevention:** If you are under 50, have annual thermography screening with the AMAS test. If you are over 50, consider a yearly mammogram along with the above two tests. ◀

Mammography

A mammogram is an x-ray of the breast that can pick up lesions as small as 0.5 cm, which you are usually not able to feel. (The AMAS test can detect that cancer is present when a tumor is only 1 mm in size and thermography can discern an abnormality when it is smaller than 0.5 cm.) Mammography can detect approximately 85% of all breast cancers.[30] In contrast, an experienced physician can detect 61–92% of breast cancers through a breast exam,

depending upon the physician.[31] However, mammograms are not ideal diagnostic tools for several reasons: if a woman has dense breasts, a lump may not be visible through the tissue; mammograms will miss up to 25% of tumors in women 40–49 years old.[32] Mammograms are less accurate in picking up lesions in smaller breasts; and they expose us to doses of radiation which are cumulative and over time can increase our risk of breast cancer. It can take 40 years for cancer to show up after exposure to radiation, so for women under 50, annual mammograms increase risk. I remember Rosalie Bertell, an expert on the effects of radiation, say that for some women (who are particularly susceptible to radiation), even one mammogram was too many. This is particularly applicable to women with a family history of breast cancer who are already at risk. To use diagnostic tools that increase risk doesn't make sense. Often mammograms provide women and their doctors with a false sense of security if nothing is found – overall, mammograms will miss cancers 9–20% of the time, especially in younger women with dense breasts.[33]

Approximately 5% of all mammograms are read as positive for cancer. Of these, 97.5% will be false positives – there will really be no cancer present. In other words, out of every 100 mammograms read as positive or suspicious of cancer, only two or three will actually turn out to be cancer. This is why it is so critical to have a biopsy after a 'positive' mammogram – otherwise surgery may be performed when it is entirely unnecessary. The AMAS and Immunicon tests are also useful to separate the false positives from actual positive cases. Women will experience extreme anxiety in the waiting period while other testing is done to confirm or disprove the diagnosis.

On the other hand, mammograms do prolong lives with earlier detection of breast cancer, resulting in less invasive treatments. Statistically, mammography reduces the death rate by 30% in women over 50 who have annual mammograms because tumors are detected earlier.[34] It increases the death rate from cancer 30–50% when performed annually in women under 50 since women accumulate radiation toxicity.[35]

A mammogram is recommended if you find a lump and need an accurate diagnosis. Mammograms are not conclusive; if the lump is there and persists but the mammogram looks fine, it is imperative to have another test to find out what kind of mass it is. This test might be an ultrasound, fine needle aspiration, biopsy, or the AMAS or Immunicon test. Trust your body's signals and insist on thorough testing until you come to a conclusive diagnosis.

▶ **Action for Prevention:** If you are under 50, have a mammogram only as needed for diagnosis of a suspected lump. Use the AMAS or Immunicon test annually. If you are over 50, have an annual mammogram, or as another option, use the AMAS or Immunicon test and thermography on alternate years instead of a mammogram. ◀

Computed Tomography Laser Mammography

X-ray mammograms may soon be a thing of the past. Computed tomography laser mammography uses state-of-the-art laser technology operating in the near infrared aspect of the electromagnetic spectrum to image the breasts. In combination with sophisticated computer systems, 4mm thick slice planes of the breast are reconstructed giving an almost 3D representation of the breast and its internal structures. The results are then stored on a CD-Rom, accessible to patients and their doctors.

Laser mammography is painless, unlike the big squeeze used in x-ray mammography. It also poses no risk because ionizing radiation is not used. It is just as accurate when used on younger women with dense breasts as with older women, unlike x-ray mammography. It can easily be used when a woman has breast implants. It can distinguish between a cyst and a solid lesion, potentially eliminating the need for fine needle aspiration or biopsy. It is expected to pick up tumors as small as 2 mm, making it more sensitive than traditional mammography.

A woman lies on a scanning bed and places a breast in a chamber. The laser rotates 360° around the breast collecting data from the way ultra-short light pulses travel through breast tissue. Benign and malignant breast tissues have different optical properties that can be translated into images through computerized technology. Cancer cells are highlighted on the screen, usually eliminating the need for biopsies. At present, clinical trials are being conducted at the Nassau County Medical Center in Long Island, New York and at the University of Virginia. FDA approval for commercial use of the machine is expected in 2000. Clinical trials are planned for two locations in Toronto in the near future — at Princess Margaret Hospital and King Medical Center. If laser mammography proves to be at least as accurate as traditional mammography through comparative studies, then commercial testing should be available by September 2000.[36,37]

Ultrasound

Ultrasounds are used to distinguish cysts from solid tumors. They are harmless and do not expose us to radiation. Cancers and fibroadenomas are solid, while cysts are hollow and filled with fluid. If the ultrasound demonstrates that the lump is filled with fluid, a biopsy is not necessary. If it shows that the mass is solid, then a biopsy must be carried out to determine whether it is a fibroadenoma or cancer.

The ultrasound can be carried out before a mammogram when a cyst is suspected. If it is a cyst, there is no need for a mammogram, and a woman is spared radiation exposure.

▶ **Action for Prevention:** Use an ultrasound to confirm the presence of a cyst, and if a cyst is not present, choose one or more of the other tests to rule out breast cancer. ◀

Fine Needle Aspiration

Fine needle aspiration is easy to perform, painless, and can be carried out in a doctor's office. A needle is inserted into the tumor and some fluid is removed. If clear fluid is removed and the tumor dissolves, it was a simple cyst. If the fluid is bloody, cancer with a cystic component may exist, and the fluid is sent for analysis. If no fluid is obtained, a biopsy must be performed. Fine needle aspiration is the least invasive, fastest, and most inexpensive way to diagnose breast cancer when a physician is skilled in the technique. Dr William Hindle of the Breast Diagnostic Center in the Women's and Children's Hospital in Los Angeles believes that fine needle aspiration should be performed on all palpable breast masses. Ninety percent of the time a diagnosis is established with this technique. The combination of physical exam, fine needle aspiration, and mammography establishes an accurate diagnosis 99% of the time.[38]

▶ **Action for Prevention:** Use fine needle aspiration when appropriate as a diagnostic tool for breast cysts that may have a cancerous component. ◀

Biopsy

A biopsy will confirm or negate the presence of cancer if the above tests have not been definitive. A sample of tissue is taken in one of two ways and then analyzed. The first method is called open surgical biopsy and is ideally performed as a lumpectomy, as though the diagnosis of cancer had already been made. This reduces the need for a second surgery should the first demonstrate breast cancer, and reduces scarring. The whole mass should be removed with a margin of normal tissue so that a pathologist can be sure that all the edges of the cancer have been taken out, and nothing remains.

The second method is called a core biopsy. For a large palpable mass, one to six slender cores of tissue are taken from different sites within it. It is most accurate for lesions over 2.5 cm in diameter and is much less invasive than an open surgical biopsy.

▶ **Action for Prevention:** Use a core or open surgical biopsy to confirm or rule out breast cancer if other tests are inconclusive. ◀

Breast Cancer Tumor Markers

Medical practitioners sometimes use blood tests to look for tumor markers indicative of breast cancer recurrence, although their use is controversial. Specialized labs are needed to do this testing. Tumor markers that are used in the follow-up care of invasive breast cancer include the CEA, CA 15-3, and the C-erbB-2. In a study of 250 breast cancer patients who all underwent mastectomies, one of these three tumor markers was the first sign of recurrence in approximately 70% of the women, detectable about four months before clinical symptoms. These particular tumor markers are more sensitive in picking up metastases to the liver or bone than they are in detecting a local recurrence.[39] Another study of 550 breast cancer patients found that the CEA and CA 15-3 were effective independent prognostic factors for relapse or survival.[40]

A fourth tumor marker is CD24 which is expressed on breast cancer cells in a particular pattern different from its expression on benign breast lesions. CD24 expression increases with the histological grade of the tumor. It may be a useful marker for tracking breast cancer and its metastasis.[41]

Possible Use of Hair to Diagnose Breast Cancer

Studies done at the University of New South Wales, in Sydney, Australia and published recently in the journal *Nature* found that hair from women with breast cancer had a different molecular structure than hair from healthy women. An x-ray technique called synchrotron x-ray scattering found that all samples from 23 breast cancer patients showed identical changes in scattering patterns. Samples taken from 28 healthy subjects, on the other hand, were normal in 24 of the women. A single pubic hair was taken from five women who had a family history of breast cancer or who had earlier been found to have a mutation of the BRCA1 gene that is associated with a higher risk of breast cancer. Three of these women had the same pattern as breast cancer patients while two showed a partial change.

Although the sample size in these studies is small, the preliminary research suggests that in the future we may be able to assess breast cancer risk and assist in diagnosing breast cancer through the use of pubic hair samples.

Other Predictive Tests

The following tests may also be useful in assessing breast cancer risk (though not in diagnosing breast cancer) and can guide us in using intervention strategies to improve health. See the Resource Directory at the back of the book for information about these laboratories.

1. Urinary or salivary estradiol, estrone, estriol and the estrogen quotient (order from Aeron Labs, DiagnosTech International Inc., ZRT).
2. Ratio of C-2 to C-16 estrogen in urine (DiagnosTech).
3. Salivary progesterone (Aeron Labs, DiagnosTech, ZRT).
4. Salivary melatonin (Aeron Labs, DiagnosTech).
5. Blood TSH, free T4, free T3, reverse T3, antimicrosomal and antithyroglobulin antibodies (Meridian Valley Laboratory or DiagnosTech).
6. Saliva IGF-1 and IGF-2 (DiagnosTech).
7. Urinary equol, daidzen, enterolactone and enterodiol (may become available from DiagnosTech).
8. Stool and blood glucuronidation rate.

▶ **Action for Prevention:** Consider carrying out some of the above tests annually to detect your susceptibility to breast cancer. Make appropriate changes in your diet, lifestyle or supplement schedule to move towards more favorable values, thus protecting you from a breast cancer diagnosis. ◀

Homeopathic Symptom Pictures and Remedies

Homeopathy is an art and a science that relies on the principle of 'like cures like'. A given substance, which in the crude form may cause a particular set of symptoms, can stimulate the body to heal when it is used in the diluted or 'potentized' form. Individual remedies are prescribed based on the totality of a person's symptoms, known as the 'symptom picture,' which includes details about a particular illness, food preferences, emotional well-being, body temperature, and times of aggravation, among others.

What follows is a brief introduction to homeopathic symptom pictures and remedies that have an affinity with the breasts. These can be prescribed for breast ailments and as an adjunct to standard breast cancer treatment.

A full homeopathic case-taking should occur before choosing one of these or a different remedy. Since it takes years of training and experience to be a good homeopath and to prescribe correctly, search for a qualified homeopathic or naturopathic medical professional to advise you.

Apis (Honeybee): A hard, stony, or open cancer of the breast with stinging, burning pains, often where there has been a history of mastitis. The nipples may be drawn in. May accompany ovarian cysts, particularly on the right side. There can be swelling of the face or breast, with a rosy hue. The patient feels better from cold air or applications and worse from heat. She is generally not thirsty. Sadness and weeping, seemingly without cause, with much worry and fidgeting. Can be very irritable, suspicious, jealous, and without joy.

Arsenicum album (Arsenic Trioxide): Rapid weight loss, with parchment-like dryness of the skin and a waxy paleness. Feels chilled. Anxiety felt in the stomach with no desire to see or smell food. May have sensation of burning anywhere, or burning discharges, as though on fire. Rotten body odor. Very fearful of death, with extreme anxiety, restlessness, insomnia and despair of recovery followed by weakness and exhaustion. Thinks it useless to take medicine. Fear of being alone. Great sadness and weariness of life, with suicidal tendencies. Feels worse between 1:00 and 2:00 p.m. and just after midnight, between 1:00 and 2:00 a.m.

Asterias rubens (Red Starfish): Useful for flabby women with a red face. Cancer around the nipple, which is retracted. There may be a darkened red spot which ulcerates, oozing a smelly, watery liquid. The skin over the sternum is swollen and painful. The lymph nodes under the arms are swollen, hard and knotted, and may ache. There may be acute tearing, piercing or sharp pains in the breast, particularly at night. The pains may travel down the left arm to the little finger, and are worse with motion. There may be numbness of the hands and fingers of the left side. There can be increased sexual excitement. Feels as though the left breast is drawn inward. Breast swelling and pain, as though before the period, more often in the left breast.

Baryta iodata (Iodide of Baryta): Breast cancer after a traumatic injury. Hard swelling of the axillary glands.

Belladonna (Deadly Nightshade): Red streaks in the breast that radiate outwards and may feel hot and throbbing, particularly with mastitis. Breasts feel heavy, hard, and red. Pains that both come and go suddenly and are made worse by motion and worse when lying down.

Glands may be swollen, tender, and red. No anxiety or fear. May experience delusions or hallucinations. Pupils may be dilated.

Bromium (Bromine): Hard cancer of the breast, with stitching sensation from the breast to the axilla, particularly in the left side. Feels worse with any pressure over the breast and at night. Stony, hard enlarged lymph nodes. Often a hard, irregular tumor in the left breast, firmly attached to the surrounding tissue. There may be piercing pains around the tumor, made worse from pressure and worse at night. The face may appear grayish, old, and emaciated. Depressed, with low spirits, particularly before menstruation. Menstrual periods may cease. Palpitations with nausea or headaches. Weakness in the legs. Enlarged veins and hemorrhoids. Feels worse from being overheated, in the evening until midnight and feels better from any kind of motion. She is also sensitive to a draft of cool air.

Bufo (Toad Poison): She is anxious about her health and desires solitude. Bothered by noise and music. Mental confusion and memory loss. Child-like regressed mental state. Easily laughs or cries inappropriately. Feels worse in a warm room and on awakening. Breast cancer, with redness and swelling along the course of the lymphatic vessels. Burning pains in the breasts with yellow blisters that form around the tumor. The blisters may contain a yellow, watery discharge. There may be sharp pains, made worse by walking or sitting too long. Sensation of burning in the ovaries, vagina, and uterus.

Calcarea carbonica (Carbonate of Lime): Cancer occurring in obese women with a tendency to swollen glands and increased perspiration, particularly around the head at night. For women who fear misfortune or loss of reason. Forgetfulness and confusion with an aversion to work or exertion. Pale, chalky skin, with a tendency to take cold easily. The breasts may be tender and swollen pre-menstrually. A breast tumor can be very sensitive and painful to the touch. Swollen glands. Menstrual periods may be too early, heavy, and long.

Calcarea oxalata (Oxalate of Lime): Cancer of the left breast, with intense, agonizing pain.

Carbo animalis (Animal Charcoal): Late stage of cancer with emaciation. There is darkened bluish loose skin around the tumor or red spots on the skin. Sensation of burning or stinging and drawing towards the axilla with hard axillary lymph nodes that may appear purplish. A hard, purplish lump the size of a hen's egg may form in the breast. The tumor is more often left-sided and can be in the nipple. Burning, ulcerating cancer surrounded by hardened, dark tissue. There may be an offensive discharge. This remedy helps to palliate the pains that occur in cancer, particularly stinging, burning pains. Spirits are low and despondent. Feeling of weakness with every menstrual period. There may be night sweats and a faint, empty sensation in the pit of the stomach.

Chimaphila umbellata (Pipsissewa): Useful for women with very large breasts. A hard, painful breast cancer. The nipple is retracted and the woman may feel sharp pains in the tumor and the axilla. The cancer may be open with ragged edges that are turned outward, discharging offensive pus. This remedy is also used when there is a painful tumor in young, unmarried women. The glands may be enlarged.

Cistus canadensis (Rock Rose): The patient who needs this remedy is extremely sensitive to cold and may feel cold in various parts, particularly the abdomen. She may feel exhausted with both physical and mental exertion. She may have a hard tumor in the breast as well as many small, hard tumors in the glands in the neck. The glands may be hard and inflamed. All the mucous membranes throw out a yellowish, thick, offensive discharge. May have dryness, cracking and bleeding on the hands and the ends of the fingers, worse in the winter and from washing in cold water. Itching of the skin and mucous membranes. Feels better from heat.

Clematis (Virgin's Bower): Fears being alone, and yet hates company. A hard cancer in the left breast, which is very painful as the moon becomes full and with touch. The glands may be hot, painful and swollen. She feels worse at night and cannot stand to be uncovered. Stitch-like pain in the shoulder and axillary nodes. There may be inability to urinate completely, with dribbling after urination.

Condurango (Condor Plant): A hard cancer of the whole breast, skin, and axillary nodes. The tumor is immovable, with severe, tearing, or piercing pain. The nipple is retracted and the skin is purple and wrinkled in spots. There may be a smelly discharge of pus and blood and much falling away of dead tissue. Emaciation. May have painful cracks in the corners of the mouth.

Conium (Poison Hemlock): Weakness of body and mind, with trembling. Sadness and depression. Difficulty walking, with a sudden loss of strength. Dizziness when lying down and when turning over in bed. Eyes are sensitive to light and water easily. Terrible nausea and heartburn, which is worse when going to bed. Weakness after

stools. The breasts may be hard, shrunken and painful to the touch. They may also be enlarged and painful premenstrually. Hard, stony, irregular breast tumors, with sharp, pricking, stinging, or shooting pains and occasional twinges. The tumor may be as large as a teacup. Sensation of great heaviness in the breast. Feels worse before and during every menstrual period. Swollen, hard, painful axillary lymph nodes, with a sensation of numbness down the arm. Cancer may occur after a blow, bruise, or injury to the breast. May have bone metastases. Ailments may occur from repressed or excessive sexual activity. Feels worse in cold weather. May wake from sleep with pain. Sweats easily upon falling asleep or closing one's eyes.

Graphites (Black Lead): Useful in obese, chilly women with fair skin. Cancer arising from old scars which have remained after repeated abscesses. The nipple is cracked and painful. Swollen, hard glands in the neck. There may be skin eruptions, or blisters around the nipple, with discharge. Tendency to be constipated. May have cracking in the ends of the fingers and dry skin generally.

Hepar sulphuris calcareum (Calcium Sulphide): Mastitis, breast abscess, or breast cancer with stinging or burning pain around the edges of the mass. There may be small pimples or ulcers surrounding the cancerous tissue. Ulcerating cancer that bleeds at the slightest touch. Cancer may discharge pus, which smells like old cheese. Itching of the nipples during menstruation. The glands are easily enlarged and hard. Yellow skin and complexion. Hypersensitivity to cold and pain, and intolerant to touch. Easily irritated personality; quarrelsome, hard to get along with and nothing pleases her. Cracking of the skin on the hands and feet.

Hydrastis canadensis (Goldenseal): Hard, immovable cancer, firmly attached to the surrounding tissue. Mottled and puckered skin around the tumor. The mass can be as large as a small egg, and may be ulcerating. More often occurs in the left breast, with hard axillary nodes. Nipple retraction. Sensation of a cutting pain, like knives. Can have a thick, yellow, ropey discharge from any mucous membrane. There may be an empty feeling in the stomach with no desire for food and a stubborn constipation.

Lachesis (Bushmaster Snake Poison): Used for women who are very talkative and may be jealous or suspicious. Cannot bear tight clothing around the waist or throat. May have hot flashes, fainting spells, and headaches during menopause. May feel worse after falling asleep, waking with a start. Breast cancer with tearing, piercing pains and a constant feeling of pain and weakness in the left shoulder and arm. The cancer may be open with a dark, bluish-red appearance, containing black streaks of decomposed blood.

Lapis albus (Silico-fluoride of Calcium): Breast cancer with intense burning, shooting, stinging pains and swollen glands. Persistent pain in the breasts. No ulceration. May have a thyroid goiter. Glands are not hardened but feel more elastic. Profuse bleeding from any part.

Lycopodium (Club Moss): Hard breast tumor, more often on the right, with stitching and cramping pain, causing her to walk around and bringing tears. Feels better in the open air. Defined areas of redness on the face. Abdominal bloating with much gas, especially after bread, cabbage and beans. Feels full after eating just a little. Craves sweets and warm food and drink. Emaciation and weakness. She looks thin, withered, and dry. Feels worse between 4:00 to 8:00 p.m. Sadness and lack of confidence with a fear of being alone. Spells or writes the wrong words or syllables.

Mercurius (Quicksilver): Breast cancer with a feeling of rawness or soreness. The glands are easily swollen, particularly after becoming cold. Increased sweating and drooling at night. The skin is almost always moist. Very sensitive to changes in temperature. Feels worse at night and worse with perspiration. Trembles easily. Foul smell to the breath and bodily secretions. Very thirsty for cold drinks.

Natrum muriaticum (Table Salt): For breast ailments that occur after the separation, loss, or death of a loved one, which she has never recovered from emotionally. She may have difficulty expressing grief and be unable to cry. She prefers to be alone and does not like to be consoled. May have underlying feelings of guilt. May crave salt.

Nitric Acid: Hard breast cancer, with soreness of the nipple. Feeling of hard knots in the breasts. Swollen glands in the neck and axilla. Pessimistic personality; one who holds grudges, is spiteful, hateful, and unmoved by apology. Likes to eat fatty and salty foods, and is generally not thirsty. She is sensitive to cold and always chilly.

Phosphorus: Used for fibrocystic breast disease and fibroadenomas. Inflammation around the tumor, with much pain, made worse by exposure to air. Stitching pain in the breast. Ulcerating breast cancer that bleeds very easily. Hot nipples. Often indicated in tall, slim women who find it difficult to gain weight. For women who are quick to startle and become easily excited. Thirst for very

cold water. May have a history of lung and throat complaints, such as pneumonia and laryngitis.

Phytolacca (Poke Root): Used for fibrocystic breast disease and for breast tenderness, which is worse before and during the menstrual period, along with irritability. The breast can be hard, painful with a purple discoloration, as with a breast abscess or mastitis. The nipple may be cracked, very sensitive and inverted. There may be a bloody, watery or milky discharge from the breast. Tumors are more often right-sided, and can be the size of a hen's egg. There may be ulceration. Swollen axillary lymph nodes, with heat and inflammation. Pain extending down the arms. There may be a shooting pain in the right shoulder, with stiffness and inability to raise the arm.

Pulsatilla (Windflower): For women who love fresh air, despite feeling chilly. They cry easily and are emotionally dependent on others. Indicated for all lumps occurring in the breasts of young girls. The lumps may be very painful, and can affect the arm of the corresponding side. Useful when the periods have stopped or are late. Generally there is a lack of thirst, despite a dry mouth. They dislike fatty foods.

Scirrhinum: Enlarged axillary glands. Hard breast cancer. Feels chilly but desires cold drinks.

Sepia (Cuttlefish Ink): For women who are irritable and indifferent to loved ones. They may be very sad, crying easily. A hard breast tumor with the sensation that the breast is enlarged. May have stitching or burning pain. The liver may be sore and painful. Yellow, earthy complexion on the face, perhaps with brown mottling. The urine may smell rotten and contain clay-like deposits. The uterus may be prolapsed, with a feeling of a weight pushing down in the pelvis. She generally feels much better with exercise.

Silicea (Silica): For women who are generally chilly and sensitive to cold air. Lack of stamina. Very cold, sweaty feet. Very sore nipples that ulcerate easily, and may be retracted. Hard tumors in the breasts.

Tarentula cubana (Cuban Spider): Breast cancer when the surface is dark and bluish, with severe burning, stinging pain. Particularly useful to ease pain in the last stages of illness, before death.

Left-Sided and Right-Sided Remedies

Many of these remedies are associated with the left or the right side:

Left-Sided Remedies	Right-Sided Remedies
Asterias rubens, Bromium, Calcarea oxalata	Apis, Arsenicum album, Lycopodium, Phytolacca
Carbo animalis, Clematis, Lachesis, Hydrastis canadensis	

Other remedies can be left- or right-sided, including Baryta iodata, Belladonna, Bufo, Calcarea carbonica, Chimaphila umbellata, Cistus canadensis, Conium, Graphites, Hepar sulph., Lapis albus, Mercurius, Natrum muriaticum, Nitric acid, Phosphorus, Phytolacca, Pulsatilla, Sepia, Silicea.

▶ **Action for Prevention:** Use appropriate homeopathic remedies for breast ailments, while keeping the whole person in mind. ◀

Summary

With this basic understanding of the anatomy and physiology of our breasts, including some of the symptoms and remedies for breast ailments, we are ready to explore the mysteries of our endocrine system and the many hormones that affect breast health.

References

1. Canadian Medical Association. Clinical practise guidelines for the care and treatment of breast cancer. *Can Med Assoc J.* Feb. 10, 1998;158(3 Suppl)S5.
2. Harvey, B.J., A. Miller, C. Baines, P. Corey. Effects of breast self-examination on the risk of death from breast cancer. *Canadian Medical Association Journal.* Nov.1, 1997:157 (9), 1205-1212, 1225-1226.
3. Tetau, Max. Folliculinum and the premenstrual syndrome. *Dolisos Newsletter.* #10.
4. Sem, B.C. Pathologico-anatomical and clinical investigations of fibroadenomatosis cystica mammae, and its relation to other pathological conditions in mammae especially cancer. *Acta Chir Scand.* 1928;64(suppl 10):1-484.
5. Kramer, W.M., B.F. Rush, Jr. Mammary duct proliferation in the elderly; a histopathologic study. *Cancer* 1973;31:130-137.
6. Vishnyakova, V.V., N. Murav'yeva. On the treatment of dyshormonal hyperplasia of mammary glands. *Vestn USSR Akad Med Sci.* 19666;21:26-31.
7. London, R.S., G.S. Sundaram, M. Schultx et al. Endocrine parameters and alpha-tocopherol therapy of patients with mammary dysplasia. *Cancer Res.* 1981;41:3811-3813.
8. Rose, D. Low fat diet in fibrocystic disease of the breast with cyclic mastalgia: a feasibility study. *Am J Clin Nutr,* 1985;41:856.
9. Jolliet, P., et al. Plasma coenzyme Q10 concentrations in breast cancer: prognosis and therapeutic consequences. *Int J Clin Pharm and Therapeutics.* 1998;36(9):506-509.
10. Ghent, W.R., B.A. Eskin, D. Low, L.P. Hill. Iodine replacement in fibrocystic disease of the breast *CJS.* 1993;36(5):453-460.
11. Eskin, B.A. Iodine metabolism and breast cancer. *Trans NY Acad Sci.* 1970;11:911-947.
12. Ghent, W.R., B.A. Eskin, D. Low, L.P. Hill. Iodine replacement in fibrocystic disease of the breast *CJS.* 1993;36(5):453-460.
13. Minton, J. Caffeine, cyclic nucleotides and breast disease. *Surgery* 86,1979:105.
14. Brooks, P. Measuring the effect of caffeine restriction on fibrocystic breast disease. *J Reprod Med,* 1981; 26:279.
15. Goldin, B., H. Adlerkreutz, J. Dwyer, et al. Effect of diet on excretion of estrogens in pre and post-menopausal women. *Cancer Res,* 1981;41:3771-3773.
16. Peters, F., W. Schuth, B. Schevrich, M. Breckwoldt. Serum prolactin levels in patients with fibrocystic breast disease. *Obstet. Gynecol,* 1984;64:381-5.
17. Ciatto, S., et al. Risk of breast cancer subsequent to proven gross cystic disease. *Eur Jour Cancer,* 1990;26(5):555-557.
18. Modan, B., et al. Breast cancer following benign breast disease - a nationwide study. *Breast Cancer Research and Treatment,* 1997;46(1):45.
19. Guiltinan, J. Naturopathic management of fibrocystic breast disease. *The Journal of Naturopathic Medicine,* 1997;7(1):95-98.
20. Love, S. *Dr. Susan Love's Breast Book.* New York, NY: Addison-Wesley Publishing Co. 1995:130-131.
21. Health Canada. Clinical practise guidelines for the care and treatment of breast cancer: a Canadian consensus document. *Can Med Assoc J.,* Feb. 10, 1998;1158 (3 Suppl)S3.
22. Abstract #3318. Scientific Proceedings. *87th Annual Meeting of the American Association for Cancer Research.* Washington, DC., 1996, April 20-24.
23. Botti, C., A. Martivetti, S. Nerini-Molteni, L. Ferrari. Anti-malignin antibody evaluation: a possible challenge for cancer management. *Int J Biol Markers,* 1997, Oct.-Dec;12(4):141-7.
24. Requisition for AMAS Determination and information sheet from Oncolab, Boston; 1-800-9-CATest.
25. Ultra-sensitive breast cancer blood test developed. PRNewswire. Huntington Valley, PA., Feb. 20, 1999.
26. Infrared imaging as a useful adjunct to mammography. *Oncology News International,* Sept., 1997:6(9).

27. Leandro, P. Position paper on digital infrared imaging of the breast. http://www.meditherm.com/breasthealth/research.htm. 1999:1-7.

28. Head, J.F., F. Wang, R.L. Elliott. Breast thermography is a noninvasive prognostic procedure that predicts tumor growth rate in breast cancer patients. *Ann N Y Acad Sc*, 1993:Nov.30;698:153-8.

29. Sterns, E.E., B. Zee, S. SenGupta, F.W. Saunders. Thermography. Its relation to pathologic characteristics, vascularity, proliferation rate, and survival of patients with invasive ductal carcinoma of the breast. *Cancer*. 1996:Apr 1;77(7):1324-8.

30. Love, S. What we really know about breast cancer and HRT. *Alternative Therapies*, Sept, 1997:3(5)82-90.

31. Health Canada. Clinical practise guidelines for the care and treatment of breast cancer: a Canadian consensus document. *Can Med Assoc J.*, Feb. 10, 1998;1158 (3 Suppl)S5.

32. Whitaker, Julian. Preventing breast cancer: Let's clear up the confusion on mammograms. *Alive*, April, 1999:16-17.

33. Love, S. *Dr. Susan Love's Breast Book*. Don Mills, ON: Addison-Wesley Publishing Co.,1995:128.

34. Love, S. What we really know about breast cancer and HRT. *Alternative Therapies*, Sept, 1997:3(5)82-90.

35. Clorfene-Casten, Liane. Breast Cancer: *Poisons, Profits and Prevention*. Monroe, ME, Common Courage Press, 1996:107.

36. Turnbull, Barbara. Laser detects breast cancer. *Toronto Star*. Jan. 27, 2000:A2.

37. Grable, R. Medical optical imaging: A status review. http://www.imds.com/moi.htm. July 1997:3.

38. Hindle, William. Fine needle aspiration of a palpable breast mass: current technology and techniques. Ottawa, ON: World Conference on Breast Cancer, oral presentation, July, 1999.

39. Molina, R., et al. C-erbB-2, CEA and CA 15.3 serum levels in the early diagnosis of recurrence of breast cancer patients. *Anticancer Res*, 1999:Jul-Aug;19(4A):2551-5.

40. Ebeling, F.C., et al. Tumor markers CEA and CA 15-3 as prognostic factors in breast cancer - univariate and multivariate analysis. *Anticancer Res*, 1999:Jul-Aug;19(4A0:2545-50.

41. Fogel, M. et al. CD24 is a marker for human breast carcinoma. *Cancer Letters*, 1999:Aug 23;143(1):87-94.

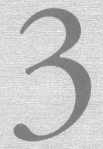
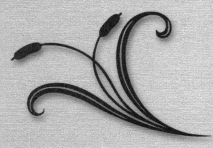

Understanding the Hormone Puzzle

Exercises

Contents

In order to understand the cause of breast cancer and the means of preventing this disease, we need to familiarize ourselves with the hormone so linked to breast cancer — estrogen — and its interaction with other hormones of the endocrine system.

What Is a Hormone?

A hormone is a chemical messenger which moves through the bloodstream, potentially affecting every cell of the body. Different hormones are produced by different glands. They can be fast or slow acting and help to maintain a constant environment inside the body, despite outside changes. Hormonal secretions can be rhythmic, tied to the solar and lunar cycles, instantaneous, or active over very long periods of time, such as the action of growth hormone throughout childhood. Hormones are able to act by binding to particular receptors in or on the cells of their target tissues. The receptor has an affinity for that particular hormone. The hormone then affects the cell nucleus to create a specific protein, which acts as an enzyme with a characteristic action. The action causes a shift in the body's metabolism (see diagram on p.64).

The collective actions of glands and hormones is termed the endocrine system. The function of the endocrine system is profoundly affected by what we feel and think, as well as by the environment around us and by what we put into our bodies as food and drink. Today more than ever before, environmental chemicals, radiation, electromagnetic fields, and contaminants in food are disrupting our hormones.

Hormones work in concert. Like musicians in an orchestra, they are dependent upon one another to produce the music that sings through the body. Any imbalance in one hormone is likely to make the whole symphony sound out of tune.

What Are the Parts of the Endocrine System?

There are nine main endocrine glands in our bodies. Other organs such as the liver, stomach, intestines, kidneys, and heart also manufacture hormones. The chart on the next page briefly summarizes the name, location, and function of each of the main endocrine glands. In direct and indirect ways, they can be involved in the development of cancer.

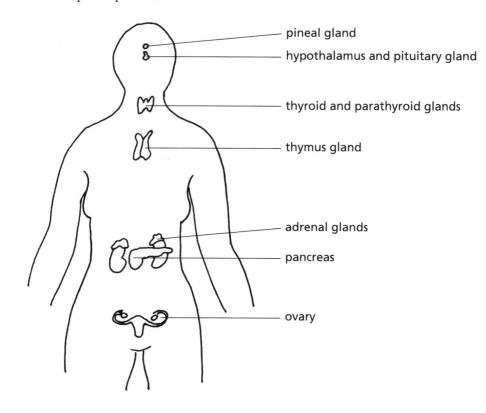

- pineal gland
- hypothalamus and pituitary gland
- thyroid and parathyroid glands
- thymus gland
- adrenal glands
- pancreas
- ovary

Estrogen Balance

Estrogen refers to a class of hormones or hormone-like substances that have particular physiological effects, as outlined below. Estrogen comes into our bodies from five possible sources.

1) Our bodies make it. Three types of estrogen are made primarily by the ovaries, each with slightly different activities. They are known as estradiol (E2), estrone (E1), and estriol (E3). Estrogen is also made by the placenta during pregnancy (estriol) and the adrenal glands and fat cells after menopause (estrone). Estradiol and estrone promote breast cancer, while estriol is generally protective. The liver can convert estradiol and estrone to estriol.

2) We get it from a class of foods and herbs called *phytoestrogens*. Certain plants such as soy, flaxseeds, legumes, mung bean and clover sprouts, pumpkin seeds, wild indigo, licorice root, mandrake, bloodroot, thyme, yucca, hops, verbena, turmeric, yellow dock, and sheep sorrel contain components that act like weak estrogens. Phytoestrogens protect us from breast cancer by displacing the body's estrogens from their receptor sites. These are discussed in chapter seven.

3) We take it in from the environment. Some environmental chemicals, known as *xenoestrogens*, are able to mimic estrogen in our bodies and lead to an estrogen excess. Because we have inefficient mechanisms for breaking them down, they tend to persist in our bodies for life. Their cumulative and synergistic effect promotes breast cancer. These chemicals are present in some pesticides, plastics, petrochemicals, detergents, solvents, chlorinated water, lice shampoos and other sources discussed in chapter four.

4) Synthetic estrogens. We are exposed to these when we take the birth control pill, fertility drugs, and/or hormone replacement therapy during menopause. Their effects also promote breast cancer.

5) We consume estrogen when we eat animal products such as meat, poultry, dairy and fish. These animals may naturally contain estrogen, may have been injected or fed estrogen to increase fat or milk production, or have accumulated xenoestrogens in their fat from environmental sources or pesticide residues over their lifespan. A meat and dairy based diet promotes breast cancer. Although fish oils protect us from breast cancer, contaminants present in many sources of fish promote it.

Gland	Location	What Its Hormones Do
Hypothalamus	in the brain behind the eyes	Controls the secretions of the pituitary gland, body temperature, hunger, thirst and sexual drive.
Pineal Gland	in the center of the brain	Responds to light, dark and electromagnetic energy. Affects cell division, sleep. Inhibits cancer, slows down the aging process, protects the thymus gland, may help depression.
Pituitary Gland	in the brain behind the eyes	Controls bone growth and regulates the other glands. Often called the "master" gland.
Thyroid Gland	at the front of the throat	Controls the rate of fuel use in the body, sensitivity to heat and cold, supports immune function.
Parathyroid Glands	behind the thyroid	Control the level of calcium in the blood.
Thymus Gland	in the upper part of the sternum	Co-ordinates white blood cells and the immune system. Shrinks with age.
Adrenal Glands	on top of the kidneys	Controls salt and water balance in the body and our reactions to stress.
Pancreas	near the stomach	Controls the level of sugar in the blood.
Ovaries (women)	on either side of the groin	Control sexual development and egg production.
Testes (men)	behind the penis	Control sexual development and sperm production.

Estrogen and the Cancer Process

Cancer requires several sequential cellular events to occur before it can manifest in a body, events estrogen can influence.

1) The first step in the cancer process is for a mistake to be made in the duplication process of the cell's genetic material. Inside a human cell nucleus are approximately 80,000 genes situated on 23 pairs of ribbon-like strands called chromosomes. Each gene is composed of smaller bits of DNA, the same way words are composed of letters. (Think of the chromosome as being the sentence). A dividing cell must faithfully reproduce approximately one billion bits of genetic information. Mistakes can be made when pieces of DNA are inserted in the wrong spot, are duplicated incorrectly, or are missed altogether. The likelihood of a mistake being made is higher if the cell has been exposed to a carcinogen capable of damaging the DNA. Carcinogens include intense sunlight, toxic chemicals, radiation exposure, cooked or rancid fats and oils, and toxic minerals such as arsenic, cadmium, and lead. Mistakes in DNA replication also occur by chance.

2) When genetic mistakes occur, the cell may fix them with repair mechanisms, or it may die shortly after being reproduced. Both of these processes are overseen by tumor suppressor genes, which are responsible for either activating repair mechanisms, calling a halt to cell replication when mistakes have been made, or ordering cell death. Occasionally the tumor suppressor gene itself has a mutation that makes it incompetent at its task and the aberrant cell survives, reproducing itself. We have many tumor suppressor genes but our primary one is called p53 and is the most commonly mutated gene in human cancer, playing a role in about 60% of tumors. Typically, cancer cells divide too frequently and lack mechanisms for controlled, programmed cell death.

3) In a good scenario, if the mutated cell survives, components of our immune system would recognize it as 'non-self' and destroy it before it became a larger tumor. When the immune system is weakened because of stressors, pollutants, glandular imbalances, poor nutrition, or emotional and spiritual factors, the renegade cell will continue to divide and reproduce, forming a cancerous tumor. Some cancer cells are particularly aggressive, reproducing quickly and requiring a very strong immune system to counteract them. Immune enhancers include many vitamins, minerals, and herbs.

4) The doubling time for breast cancer cells can range between 21–100 days. This means that during this span of time the cells will double in number. A mass of 100 billion cells is about the size of a golf ball and can take three to more than ten years to form. If cancer cells have a short doubling time and are particularly aggressive, pharmacological doses of melatonin administered before bed can slow down the doubling time and help to stabilize the cancer.[1]

5) When a cancerous tumor attains the size of a pinhead, it sends out chemical signals that cause small blood vessels to encircle it, providing it with nutrients and carrying away waste. This increased blood supply encourages the tumor to grow to a large size. Soy products, green tea, and turmeric help to prevent the formation of new blood vessels that feed the cancer.

6) As the tumor grows it can release clumps of cancer cells into the blood stream or into the lymphatic system from where they can colonize other bodily organs or tissues. This process is called metastasis. The most common sites for breast cancer metastases include the liver, bones, brain, and lungs.

Estrogen promotes cell division, especially in tissues that have a high number of estrogen receptors, such as the breasts and uterus. When estrogen activates the cellular DNA, it causes the cell to divide and multiply more quickly. As more division occurs, more mistakes can be made, and the cell can become a wild variant of the original parent cell. The action of a carcinogen or a chance mistake in DNA replication, combined with the increased cell division that estrogen and its mimickers promote, creates breast cancer. If our immune systems are unable to control the cancerous growth, it acquires a life of its own, on a different track from the rest of the breast tissue.

The Production of Estrogen

The ovaries begin to produce estrogen during puberty — when a girl is anywhere between 10–14 years of age. During a single menstrual cycle, the ovaries produce increasing amounts of estrogen from the first day of the period leading up to the day of ovulation in an effort to prepare the uterus for a possible pregnancy. Estrogen levels peak just before ovulation. After ovulation, estrogen levels drop for a few days and then increase less dramatically between days 18–23, followed by a gentle decline until the end of the menstrual cycle. The monthly rise in estrogen levels is the link that puts some women at higher risk for breast cancer. The more menstrual periods a woman has in her lifetime (early onset of menstruation and late menopause), the greater amount of estrogen she will be exposed to in her lifetime, and the more likely her chances are of developing breast cancer. Women with ovarian failure who produce little or no estrogen or whose ovaries have been removed have a very low incidence of breast cancer. Men also have very little breast cancer because their estrogen levels are low.

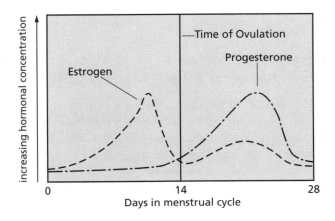

The Kinds of Estrogen

The body produces not one but three main types of estrogen: estradiol (E2), estrone (E1), and estriol (E3). Estradiol, produced by the ovaries, is the strongest of the three, being 1,000 times more potent in its effects on breast tissue than estriol. Hence high amounts of estradiol are linked to a greater risk of breast cancer. Estrone is also linked to increased breast cancer risk and is the form of estrogen synthesized in our fat cells after menopause. Estradiol can be converted in the body to estrone, and vice versa. Estriol is the weakest of the three and generally exerts a protective effect, except when supplemented in very high amounts. Estriol is produced in the ovaries and is also a breakdown product of estradiol and estrone, synthesized in the liver. The normal ratios present of circulating estrogens are: 10–20% estradiol (E2), 10–20% estrone (E1), and 60–80% estriol (E3).[2] In a woman who is not pregnant, the ovaries produce 100–200 mcg per day of estradiol and estrone.

Of the three forms of estrogen, then, estradiol and estrone are linked with increased breast cancer risk,[3] particularly in post-menopausal women. Estriol, a short-acting weak estrogen, is associated with decreased risk except when given at

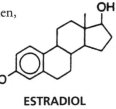

ESTRADIOL

very high concentrations.[4] Estriol is synthesized in the liver as a breakdown product of estradiol and estrone. Women who excrete more estriol in their urine have a lower risk of breast cancer.[5] Cancer remission in patients receiving endocrine therapy occurs only when estriol levels increase.[6] Estriol protects the breasts from the tumor-producing effects of estradiol and estrone.[7] During pregnancy, estriol is produced in large quantities by the placenta and becomes the dominant estrogen as ovarian production of estradiol and estrone decreases. All estrogens compete for the same receptor sites, so estriol exerts its protective effect when it binds to breast cell receptors, preventing the attachment and action of estradiol and estrone.

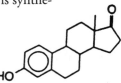

ESTRONE

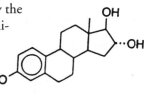

ESTRIOL

The types of food we eat can facilitate or block the conversion of estradiol and estrone to estriol. Improving liver function with specific nutrients also assists this conversion. The use of iodine compounds or sea vegetables may increase estriol levels in pre- and post-menopausal women. More research is needed in these areas, since generally the more estriol our body makes, the more we are protected from breast cancer. There is, however, a risk in too much estriol. If we were to take high amounts (5–15 mg daily) from external sources, it can act like estradiol, causing increased division of breast cells, possibly promoting cancer.[8,9]

In a pregnant woman, there is a dramatic shift in the three estrogen ratios. The placenta takes over estrogen production from the ovaries and produces estriol in milligram quantities, while estrone and estradiol are made only in microgram amounts, with there being the least estradiol.

After menopause estrone continues to be made when a hormone from the adrenal glands called androstenediol is converted in body fat and muscle cells to estrone. Thus the more fat cells we have after menopause, the more estrogen we are exposed to 'in house'. Some obese women produce more estrogen after menopause than thin women make before menopause. Women who are overweight are more at risk for breast cancer, although the increased estrogen protects them from osteoporosis. Paradoxically, the better a woman's bone density, the greater her risk of breast cancer.

Too Much Estrogen

Breast cancer is caused in part by the action of a carcinogen in the presence of too much estrogen without the opposing balance of its partner hormone, progesterone. In the last 50 years, industrial societies have been bathed in a sea of carcinogens and estrogens from the increased use of environmental chemicals and synthetic hormones. Environmental chemicals accumulate in the fat tissue of animals. When we consume animal products, we increase our estrogen exposure even more.

Target Sites and Effects of Estrogen

Estrogen acts only when it is able to bind to specific receptor sites in the cells of target organs or tissues. The target sites for estrogen include the breasts, uterus, ovaries, vagina, skin, bone, brain, fat cells, liver, and blood vessels, with most of it going to the breasts and uterus. It also has an effect on the body as a whole. The chart on page 63 illustrates estrogen's effect on its target sites.

Estrogen's Partner — Progesterone

Progesterone is secreted by the ovaries and acts in tandem with estrogen. It is also secreted in large amounts by the placenta during pregnancy. Like all hormones, it attaches to a receptor molecule before affecting cells of its target tissues. Estrogen and progesterone sensitize each other's receptors so that when the amounts of one are high, the other also increases. Mostly their actions are antagonistic to one another. Progesterone protects us from estrogen excess. A woman with low progesterone is more likely to be diagnosed with breast cancer than a woman with normal levels. Low progesterone may lead to menstrual irregularities or spontaneous abortions during pregnancy. We must also be cautious about having too much progesterone, for progesterone can be converted into estrogen, and a few types of breast cancer are stimulated by progesterone. Generally, estrogen is responsible for the growth of tissues, while progesterone is linked to the maturation of tissues. During pregnancy the high levels of progesterone are what causes the breast cells to mature and become more stable and less susceptible to cancer. The target tissues and functions of progesterone are outlined in the table on page 63.

When Estrogen Is Unbalanced

We need adequate but not excessive amounts of estrogen for good health. When we have either too little or too much, we may experience the following ailments:

Too Little Estrogen	Too Much Estrogen
Amenorrhea (lack of menses)	Dense or cystic breasts
Infertility	Irregular or excessive periods
Early menopause	Breast cancer
Hot flashes, vaginal dryness, low libido	Uterine cancer
Osteoporosis (loss of bone density)	Endometriosis

Circulation of Estrogen and Its Binding to Receptors

As estrogen circulates through the body in the bloodstream, it hooks onto a carrier molecule called sex-hormone binding globulin, also known as SHBG. This carrier molecule shuttles estrogen through the bloodstream to the target organs where it can bind to an estrogen receptor located in a cell and exert an effect particular to its target site. Estrogen is not active until it binds to a receptor. At any given time, most estradiol is bound to SHBG, so that only a portion of it can bind to an estrogen receptor in a breast cell. Estriol, on the other hand, has a lower affinity for binding to SHBG and a greater percentage is available for biological activity.[10] The more estrogen receptors we have in our breast cells, the more vulnerable our breasts are to cancer.

Exposure to environmental chemicals that mimic estrogen increases the levels of estrogen receptors in breast cells and has caused an increased incidence of breast cancer in post-menopausal women with estrogen-dependent tumors.[11]

Estrogen fits into the receptor site much as a key might fit into a lock. Once it attaches to the estrogen receptor, it becomes active in the cell and binds to the DNA in the cell nucleus. It activates proteins that direct cell division, which speeds the rate of DNA replication and increases the likelihood that a genetic mutation will occur. If the mutation is not repaired, cancer can begin as the mutant cells continue to divide. Here comes the catch. Estrogen receptors have been called 'promiscuous' — they will attract not only the real estrogen but also its impostors. Even when the impostors have only a slight resemblance to estrogen. Some of its impostors are strong enough to activate the DNA in the same way that estrogen is able to, while other impostors just occupy the receptor sites so that estradiol can't attach — all the seats are taken. Estrogen's impostors can act in a harmful or protective way.

Target Sites	Effects of Estrogen
Breasts	Stimulates duct development in puberty and pregnancy, causes breast cells to multiply. Increases risk of breast cancer. Ensures adequate milk production.
Uterus	Causes uterine growth at puberty. Causes increased cell production and thickening of the uterine lining so that it can support a pregnancy. Increases risk of endometrial cancer.
Ovaries	Causes release of an egg each month during ovulation.
Vagina	Causes vaginal growth at puberty. Retains vaginal thickness and lubrication.
Skin	Encourages formation of collagen, which gives structural support to the skin. Causes growth of underarm and pubic hair. Causes pigmentation of the nipples and areolae.
Bone	Increases bone density by inhibiting breakdown of bone.
Brain	Affects sexual desire.
Fat	Causes fat to be deposited on thighs, hips, and breasts; increases body fat generally.
Liver	Site of estrogen breakdown.
Blood Vessels	Encourages formation of HDL ('good' cholesterol) and keeps arteries free of plaquing. Increases blood clotting
Rest of Body	Causes salt and fluid retention; depression and headaches; impairs blood sugar control. Causes loss of zinc and retention of copper; can interfere with thyroid hormone. Reduces oxygen levels in all cells; increases risk of gallbladder disease; increases risk of auto-immune diseases.

Target Site	Effects of Progesterone
Uterus	Prepares uterus for implantation. Maintains the development of the placenta. Protects against endometrial cancer.
Breasts	Responsible for breast enlargement or 'ripening' during pregnancy. Develops milk-secreting cells during pregnancy. Protects against fibrocystic breast disease. Helps protect against breast cancer, in most cases.
Kidneys	Acts as a natural diuretic.
Brain	Restores libido. Acts as a natural antidepressant.
Adrenal Glands	Helps to normalize blood sugar levels. Acts as a precursor to adrenal hormones.
Bone	Builds bone and protects us from osteoporosis by stimulating osteoblasts.
Thyroid	Facilitates action of thyroid hormone, raises body temperature.
Fat cells	Helps to use fat for energy.
Rest of Body	Normalizes zinc and copper levels; normalizes oxygen levels in the cell.

Sufficient melatonin, a hormone produced by the pineal gland, acts to decrease the production of estrogen receptors, thus allowing lower levels of estrogen to get into the breast cell to initiate cell division and potential cancer. Melatonin acts as a kind of breaker switch for estrogen and has been used in breast cancer treatment for this reason. The effects of melatonin and means of activating this hormone against cancer are described later in this chapter.

Estrogen's Impostors

We now know that the plant estrogens, or phytoestrogens as they have been called, are able to occupy the receptor sites in the target cells and exert a variety of effects. One of the ways that soy, for instance, decreases a woman's risk of breast cancer is by filling the breast cell receptor sites so that the body's estradiol cannot bind. The soy estrogen is too weak to exert a harmful estrogenic effect on the breast cell. However, it has been found to act as a weak estrogen on bone tissue in a positive way and protect us from osteoporosis by preventing bone loss. It also protects the heart and blood vessels by causing more HDL or 'good' cholesterol to be made. It is as though it exerts selective activity depending on the target organ and the body's need. The plant estrogens are rapidly broken down in the body, and do not accumulate in our tissues over time. So far, the action of soy and other plant estrogens seems to be towards good health.

The other not-so-good impostors are the environmental estrogens, or xenoestrogens. They are sometimes also called estrogen-mimickers or hormone disruptors because they affect other hormones as well as estrogen, particularly thyroid hormone. The environmental estrogens include many pesticides, plastics, commercial detergents, drugs, fuels, and chlorine-based chemicals called organochlorines. Some environmental estrogens bind to the 'promiscuous' estrogen receptor sites in the target cells and affect the DNA in the same way that estrogen does. They may either cause mutations in the genes that regulate cell division or cause abnormal cell growth — in either case the breast cell multiplies out of control and its DNA is altered in the process.

Xenoestrogens can stimulate breast cells to produce new blood vessels needed for tumor growth and spread.[12] Unlike the plant estrogens, environmental estrogens tend to accumulate to high levels in our bodies because they resist breakdown by our detoxification pathways. We store them in our fat cells. Most of the environmental estrogens are foreign chemicals unknown to biological systems before the 1940s. Because we have inefficient mechanisms for breaking down and eliminating them, they can persist in our bodies for decades. The action of environmental chemicals is synergistic – several together have a much stronger estrogenic effect than a single chemical. Thus we are chronically exposed to higher 'estrogen' levels than our bodies are used to. This is the basis for the environmental

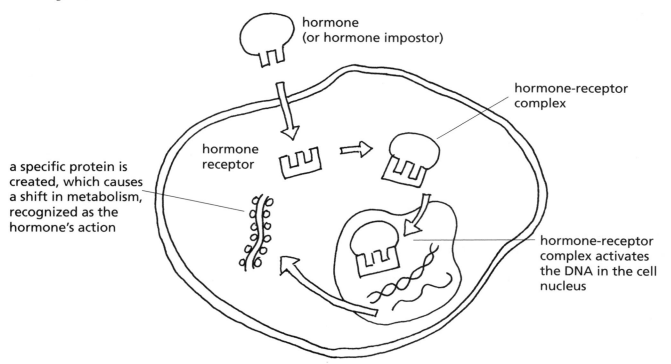

hormone
(or hormone impostor)

hormone-receptor
complex

hormone
receptor

a specific protein is
created, which causes
a shift in metabolism,
recognized as the
hormone's action

hormone-receptor
complex activates
the DNA in the cell
nucleus

link to breast cancer. Animal and human studies support this theory, although there are conflicting studies and many unanswered questions. Hence part of the dramatic rise in breast cancer rates over the last five decades is not so much due to female hormones but to the environmental chemicals that mimic female hormones and our body's inability to eliminate them.

▶ **Action for Prevention:** We can look at this piece of the hormone puzzle and help protect ourselves from breast cancer by:

1) Decreasing our exposure to the xenoestrogens and carcinogens in general. We must become active in fighting the production and use of these chemicals, and remove them from our homes and environments.

2) Increasing the phytoestrogens and other protective foods in our diets.

3) Strengthening immunity using vitamins, minerals, herbs, and nutritional substances as well as through psychological and spiritual growth.

4) Increasing our own melatonin levels through a meditation or visualization practice.

5) Enhancing the body's detoxification ability through improving liver function.

6) Improving elimination through the colon and skin (saunas) to decrease our load of "in house" estrogens, environmental estrogens, and toxins. ◀

Each of these measures will be discussed in further detail in subsequent chapters.

Breakdown of Estrogen

Estrogen is metabolized, or broken down, in the liver where it is bound to another substance called glucuronic acid. This process is called glucuronidation. The glucuronide complex passes from the liver into the bile, then into the intestines and out through the stool.

During the breakdown of estradiol and estrone in the liver, two mutually exclusive products, or metabolites, are formed through the actions of particular enzymes. These metabolites are known as the C-2 metabolite (2-hydroxyestrone) or 'good estrogen' and the C-16 metabolite (16-hydroxyestrone) or 'bad estrogen'. The ratio between these represents, to a large degree, the activity of estrogen in our bodies. It has been found that breast cancer patients have significantly lower ratios of the C-2 estrogen metabolite compared with the C-16 metabolite, in

contrast to women without breast cancer, who have higher ratios. This ratio is a significant factor predictive of breast cancer and might be used by women in annual testing to determine risk.[13]

The only structural difference between the C-2 and C-16 metabolites is the location of an -OH molecule. Their actions, however, are completely different. The C-2 metabolite is inactive and exerts no further estrogenic effect. The C-16 metabolite remains active as a hormone and if it is not eliminated it is able to enter the breast cell, activating the genes that enhance breast-cell proliferation and perhaps triggering gene mutations. Women with breast cancer and women with a family history of breast cancer tend to have nearly five times as much of the C-16 metabolite as other women.[14,15,16]

We know that a class of plant chemicals called indoles are able to promote the conversion of estrogen to the C-2 metabolite and inactivate the C-16 metabolite, thus protecting us from breast cancer. The active phytochemical, or plant chemical in the indoles is indole-3-carbinol. The indoles are found in the brassica family, which includes cabbage, broccoli, Brussels sprouts, kale, cauliflower, bok choy, kohlrabi, mustard and turnips. The indoles are destroyed through cooking so these foods should be consumed raw as much as possible or lightly steamed. We can eat them twice daily for added protection or take a supplement containing at least 300 mg of indole-3-carbinol daily. A mixture of cabbage, carrot, and beet juice would also suffice. Approximately one third of a head of cabbage daily will convert most of the estrone to the C-2 metabolite. Raw Brussels sprouts and savoy cabbage are the highest sources of indole-3-carbinol. Raw brassicas have the potential to inhibit the production of thyroid hormones by interfering with iodine uptake. This is ameliorated if we include sea vegetables in our daily diet.

We know that certain environmental xenoestrogens promote the formation of the C-16 metabolite,[17,18] while substances such as reduced glutathione, N-acetyl-cysteine, soy, turmeric, schizandra, and milk thistle assist the liver in its detoxification of environmental chemicals and will help to prevent the formation of the C-16 metabolite.

▶ **Action for Prevention:** When we examine this piece of the estrogen puzzle, we see that we can increase our protection from breast cancer by consuming raw foods from the brassica family, along with sea vegetables, avoiding xenoestrogens, and assisting the liver with the above substances. ◀

Elimination of Estrogen

Estrogen by-products are excreted through our urine and stools. Urinary estrogen is eliminated completely, but the estrogen journeying down the intestines can be recycled to be used again, thereby adding to our cumulative estrogen exposure. Sometimes there is a high level of an enzyme present in the intestines called beta-glucuronidase (made by certain intestinal bacteria) that separates the estrogen from the glucuronide complex made by the liver. The more of this enzyme that is present, the more free estrogen will be reabsorbed back into the bloodstream through the intestinal wall.[19,20] Once in the blood, it circulates and can re-attach to estrogen receptors in breast cells and promote breast cancer. It serves double or even triple time. This process is more likely to occur when we have a diet high in saturated fat and meat, which encourages the presence of specific bacteria and the increased production of the enzyme beta-glucuronidase. A diet high in fiber (in wheat bran, psyllium, and legumes) and in the plant lignans, found in high amounts in flaxseeds, discourages the recycling of estrogen. Hence a low-fat, high fiber vegetarian diet which includes wheat bran and psyllium is part of a breast cancer prevention program. Women who eat this way have a bacterial balance in their large intestines that converts very little excreted estrogen into the absorbable form. Consequently, more estrogen is eliminated from the body. Vegetarians excrete two to three times more estrogen in their stools than non-vegetarians.[21] Circulating estradiol and estrone levels are 50% higher in meat-eaters than in vegetarians.[22] One study with rats found that equal amounts of wheat bran and psyllium provided maximum protection against breast cancer tumors, rather than either fiber alone. Beta-glucuronidase activity was especially lowered by the psyllium.[23]

In studies on rats a natural, non-toxic substance called calcium D-glucarate was able to prevent the separation of estrogen from the glucuronide conjugate so that the estrogen was eliminated and not reabsorbed into the bloodstream. When rats were fed calcium D-glucarate after treatment with a carcinogen that would stimulate breast cancer, tumor development was inhibited by over 70 percent.[24] Unfortunately, this has not been replicated in studies on women – one study found no change in estrogen levels after supplementation with calcium D-glucarate.[25] It is possible to measure the amount of harmful beta-glucuronidase activity in women through a stool test to see whether dietary changes or supplementing with wheat bran and psyllium are warranted.

▶ **Action for Prevention:** So, looking at this last piece of the estrogen puzzle we are able to decrease our risk of breast cancer by avoiding meat and saturated fat, consuming a high fiber vegetarian diet with the addition of wheat bran, psyllium, legumes, and flaxseeds, and ensuring that we have two or more bowel movements daily. From an understanding of estrogen metabolism we can recognize that there is much we can do to prevent breast cancer. We can become proactive in protecting our breasts. ◀

Estrogen Quotient

Some research has demonstrated that a mathematical formula, called the estrogen quotient, is also a valuable index for predicting breast and endometrial cancer. Six epidemiological studies of estrogen quotients found higher estrogen quotients (more estriol in relation to estradiol and estrone) in populations with a lower risk of breast cancer.[26,27] A few studies do not support this link.[28] The estrogen quotient is determined by:

$$\text{Estrogen quotient} = \frac{\text{Estriol}}{\text{Estrone} + \text{Estradiol}}$$

It is the functional ability of the liver that influences these estrogen ratios, and improving liver function will increase both the amount of C-2 estrogen and estriol, decreasing risk.

In one study, 34 pre- and post-menopausal women without breast cancer showed an estrogen quotient of 1.2 to 1.3, respectively, while 26 pre- and post-menopausal women with breast cancer had an estrogen quotient of 0.5 to 0.8, respectively. The estrogen quotient of the women with breast cancer was about half of that of the women free of cancer.[29] An estrogen quotient below 0.8 is associated with an increased risk of breast cancer, while an EQ value above 1.0 is linked with a decreased incidence of breast cancer.

Estriol can be manipulated in the body through diet, supplements, and normalization of the thyroid gland. Improving liver function will increase estriol levels and shift the hormone balance to a higher, more favorable estrogen quotient. Jonathan V. Wright, MD, at the Tahoma Clinic in Kent, Washington, has successfully used iodine compounds to improve the estrogen quotient in pre- and post-menopausal women. One of his methods has been to use 5 to 7 drops of Lugol's solution (sodium iodide) daily with regular monitoring of the thyroid gland. We may increase our levels of estriol by using sea vegetables in our diets and phytoestrogens like soy and flaxseeds. Improving liver function as outlined in chapter five may also increase estriol levels, since it is synthesized in the liver during the breakdown of estradiol and estrone. Research is needed to assess the foods, nutrients, and herbs that increase estriol.

Dr Wright has developed a hormone replacement therapy for women that mimics urinary proportions seen in populations with a lower incidence of breast cancer. His formula contains all three estrogens in a 1:1:8 ratio, that is 10% estradiol, 10% estrone, and 80% estriol. For women that must use hormone replacement therapy this balance of estrogens offers at least some protection against breast cancer due to its high estriol content.[30]

The measurement of estriol, estrone, and estradiol can be obtained from urine or saliva. A simple urine test called the sex hormone profile can be ordered through Meridian Valley Clinical Laboratory in Kent, WA by a naturopathic or medical doctor (tel. 253-859-8700). A saliva test can be ordered from the following labs: Aeron Life Cycle Clinical Laboratory in San Leandro, CA (tel. 510-729-0375 or 1-800-631-7900); DiagnosTech International Inc., in Osceola, WI (tel. 715-294-2144 or 1-888-342-7272); ZRT Laboratory, in Portland, OR (tel. 503-469-0741. See the resource directory at the back of this book for complete addresses.

▶ **Action for Prevention:** Check your ratio of C2 estrogen to C16 estrogen and your sex hormone profile yearly through a saliva or urine test to evaluate your balance of estrogens and risk of breast cancer. This can be used as a routine annual test to assess women at risk for breast cancer, followed by work at prevention with diet changes and nutrient supplementation. ◀

Early Onset of Menstruation, Late Menopause

Higher breast cancer risk is associated with early onset of menstruation (before age 11) in women and late menopause. The more menstrual cycles a woman has, the more estradiol her ovaries produce over her lifetime and consequently the greater is her risk of breast cancer. Therefore either late onset of menstruation, pregnancy, breastfeeding or early menopause will reduce the number of menstrual cycles and decrease overall estradiol.[31] Studies on women in the West have shown that if a girl begins to menstruate before the age of 11, she increases her lifetime risk of breast cancer.[32]

One of the factors associated with early onset of menstruation and late menopause is dietary fat. Young girls raised on a high-fat diet begin menstruating about four years earlier than girls eating low-fat starch-based meals — at twelve rather than sixteen years.[33] The hypothalamus, a center in the brain that governs glandular function, signals the onset of puberty depending on three factors in a young girl — her weight, percentage of body fat and activity level. The ovaries are stimulated to produce estrogen particularly when she reaches a certain weight. Menopause begins about four years later for women consuming a high-fat diet compared to those on a low-fat diet — at 50 rather than 46 years.[34] The increased years of menstruation are caused by the extra estrogens produced as a result of high dietary fat intake.[35] Early onset of menstruation and late menopause are each linked with roughly twice as high a risk of developing breast cancer relative to women with a shorter menstrual life.[36,37]

The age of onset of menstruation has become younger in the last century. In the 1800s the average age was 16–17, compared to 11–12 today. This seems to be a product of industrialization, due in part to electric light at night, increased dietary fat, the consumption of hormones in animal products, and exposure to environmental estrogen-mimickers. Some organochlorines have been linked to early onset of menstruation.[38] Today, many girls are entering puberty one year earlier from the dates recognized in current medical texts, which state that only 1% of girls show signs of breast development and pubic hair before age eight.[39]

A *Pediatrics* study found that a large proportion of American girls have one or both of these characteristics at age seven and 1% of all girls now have one or both of them at age three. African-American girls show the first signs of sexual development about a year earlier than white girls. The study found that the average age of onset for puberty was just under nine for African-Americans and was just over 10 for whites, whereas medical texts note that puberty begins between 11 and 12, on average.[40] It has been found that early puberty is linked with higher estradiol levels that persist into early adult life.[41,42,43]

A *New Scientist* study demonstrated that the girls with the highest prenatal exposure to environmental estrogens such as PCBs and DDE entered puberty 11 months earlier than girls with lower exposures. The mothers of these girls were exposed to the chemicals through normal diet and environmental sources, not from environmental accidents or other abnormally high exposures.[44]

When a girl's periods begin, her ovaries produce more estrogen and progesterone and there is also an increase in the production of growth hormone and other hormone-like substances called insulin-like growth factors, or IGF-1 and IGF-2.[45] Higher levels of insulin-like growth factors are linked to higher breast cancer incidence.

If we are speeding up sexual development with our use of environmental chemicals that mimic estrogen, then it would stand to reason that we are also increasing these girls' risk of breast cancer later in life by increasing their lifelong exposure to estrogen — from their own bodies and from the environment.[46,47] This is compounded by the increased exposure to radiation from nuclear power plants and weapons. At the present time, one woman in eight will develop breast cancer in her lifetime in North America. Women my age (42) have almost three times the rate of breast cancer as our great-grandmothers did when they were the same age. What will it be for my daughter, whose breasts are just beginning to bud at age 10? And her daughters, granddaughters, and great-granddaughters? If we aren't able to stop the environmental causes, and if women are still able to conceive, it will be one woman in three. This is a frightening thought. We must act now to protect future generations. It is our duty.

► **Action for Prevention:** Do not consume animal products while pregnant or breast-feeding. Do what you can to stall puberty in your daughters by keeping lights out at night, eating organic food, eliminating or drastically reducing animal products in their diets, giving them flaxseed oil regularly while limiting other fats, and protecting them from environmental exposure to estrogen-mimicking chemicals. Become aware of and fight the use of these chemicals. This is the call to arms, the call to women. We must protect the fertility of ourselves, other species, and the earth. ◄

Shorter Menstrual Cycles

Women who have menstrual cycles shorter than 25 days have double the risk of breast cancer. This is due to more doses of estradiol, which is produced in greatest concentrations at mid-cycle. Women whose cycles are longer than 30 days are also at twice the risk.[48] These women are exposed to more doses of estradiol because the estrogen-secreting phase of their menstrual cycle is prolonged.[49] Menstrual cycles can usually be normalized with the use of appropriate Chinese or Western herbs and homeopathy.

► **Action for Prevention:** Consult a practitioner of Traditional Chinese Medicine, a naturopath, herbalist, or homeopath to help you regulate your periods. Decrease your breasts' ability to absorb estradiol by eating plants rich in phytoestrogens, which bind to breast cell receptors and prevent estradiol, estrogen replacement therapy and organochlorine estrogen-mimickers from entering the breast cell where they could promote cancer. These plants include tofu and soy products, flaxseeds, lentils, dried beans and their sprouts, pumpkin seeds, and herbs such as red clover, licorice root, turmeric, and fenugreek. ◄

Birth Control Pills

Birth control pills have variable effects on breast cancer. When used before the age of 20 or if used for more than five years before the age of 35, they can triple the likelihood of developing breast cancer.[50,51] Although birth control is a dilemma for many, natural methods that focus on an awareness of the body are safer. The Justisse method is one such program and a woman can seek out a Justisse educator for guidance.

The birth control pill is also an environmental hazard. When women on the Pill urinate, the urine contains estrogenic substances that end up in the wastewater of sewage treatment plants. Fish exposed to this water show hormonal abnormalities.

► **Action for Prevention:** Do not use the birth control pill for longer than five years or before the age of 20; preferably, avoid it altogether. Investigate other methods of birth control such as the Justisse method, and the use of condoms and the diaphragm. ◄

Hormone Replacement Therapy

Estrogens prescribed for menopausal and post-menopausal women have been linked to 8% of breast cancers, especially when used for more than five years.[52] Even when estrogen is combined with progestin (synthetic progesterone), women have increased risk of the disease. However, when natural progesterone derivatives are used alone there seems to be increased protection from breast cancer.[53] The risk of having breast cancer diagnosed in a woman increases for every year that she has been on hormone replacement therapy. There will be an extra 12 cases of breast cancer by the age of 70 for every 1000 women who start taking hormones at age 50 and continue until age 70. When a woman stops hormone replacement therapy, the risk is reduced and is greatly diminished after five years.[54]

► **Action for Prevention:** Maintain your calcium status from age 35 onward, ensuring 800–2000 mg daily depending on age, pregnancy and breast-feeding. Consult Dr Gaby's book, *Preventing and Reversing Osteoporosis*, and Dr John Lee's book, *What Your Doctor May Not Tell You About Menopause*, for alternatives to estrogen replacement therapy in reversing osteoporosis. If you are at high risk for heart disease, adopt the dietary guidelines in this book and supplement with vitamin E, magnesium, coenzyme Q10, and grapeseed. Consult a naturopathic doctor for a full program in reducing risk for heart disease and in dealing with menopausal symptoms. Consider the use of Chinese or Western herbal formulas and natural progesterone cream for menopausal symptoms. Avoid hormone replacement therapy except as a last resort and continue it for less than five years. Make sure your hormone replacement therapy contains estriol to offset the tumor enhancing effects of estradiol and estrone, as outlined in Dr Gaby's book, as well as natural progesterone cream, as described by Dr Lee. Increase your estriol levels naturally with the inclusion of sea vegetables (for iodine), flaxseeds, soy products, and other phytoestrogens. ◄

Fertility Drugs

Women who have taken fertility drugs to induce pregnancy may have a higher risk of breast cancer, as may fertile women who took the drugs to become egg donors. Fertility drugs are used to increase a woman's estrogen levels in order to enhance ovulation and release more eggs. The number of prescriptions written for Clomiphene citrate, the most frequently used fertility drug, has nearly doubled in the United States since the beginning of its use in 1967. Infertility is on the rise in men and women, as it is in animal populations exposed to estrogen-mimicking chemicals. The long-term answer is not more fertility drugs that add to the breast cancer epidemic, but to rid the planet of the chemicals that are causing the problem to begin with. There have been relatively few studies on the long-term effects of fertility drugs, although a National Institute of Health study was begun in the U.S.A. in 1994 and results are expected in the year 2000.[55] It is probable that women who have difficulty becoming pregnant already have an increased risk of breast cancer, either because of exposure to environmental estrogens or DES that rendered them infertile, or because they are older and have not yet had a child. When doctors prescribe fertility drugs to these already-at-risk women, they may be compounding that risk.

► **Action for Prevention:** Before you intend to conceive, detoxify your liver, colon, and whole body using the methods outlined in the Healthy Breast Program or other detoxification regimes. Avoid all stimulants, including coffee, and follow an organic vegetarian diet for three months. Before you resort to fertility drugs to become pregnant, consult with a practitioner of Traditional Chinese Medicine or a naturopathic doctor. There are many natural ways to increase fertility without putting yourself at risk. ◄

DES

Women who took the drug DES (diethyl stilbestrol) have a 44% increased risk of breast cancer and their daughters are also more vulnerable.[56] DES was given to pregnant women beginning in the 1940s through to the 1970s to prevent miscarriage. A synthetic chemical that mimicked estrogen, it was considered a wonder drug in its time and was prescribed liberally by doctors. In the daughters of the women to whom it was given, there is increased incidence of clear-cell vaginal cancer, malformations of the reproductive tract, infertility, and a reduction in T-helper cells and T-killer cells, which are essential components of our immune systems in their surveillance against cancer. DES exposed women are more likely to develop autoimmune diseases as they age. All this 20 or more years after initial exposure. Apparently, the timing of the exposure in utero is more important than the amount that the mother received. The fetus is most sensitive to estrogen-mimicking chemicals early on in pregnancy, between the sixth and the sixteenth week when the reproductive organs are developing. Women whose mothers took DES before the tenth week of pregnancy have a greater chance of developing vaginal or cervical cancer while those exposed after the twentieth week of pregnancy are spared reproductive tract deformities. DES seems to sensitize the developing fetus to estrogens, making the individual more likely to develop certain cancers later in life, such as those of the breast, ovaries, uterus, and prostate. DES also has effects on the brain and the pituitary gland. In animal studies, exposure to DES or higher than normal levels of estrogen at a sensitive time in utero caused permanent and dramatic changes in brain structure and behavior. Female rodents exposed to excess estrogen before or just after birth (think breast-feeding) showed a more masculine pattern of reproductive behavior, causing them to act more like males with a decrease in feminine mating patterns.

In studies of women exposed to DES in utero, there was a higher than average rate of bisexuality and homosexuality. There are also higher rates of depression, anorexia, anxiety, and phobias in women and men exposed to DES.[57]

► **Action for Prevention:** If you are pregnant, take stock of your environment. Learn whether there are industries, farms, toxic waste sites, plastic recycling plants, or sewage treatment plants around you that are releasing organochlorines, dioxin, furans, pesticides, formaldehyde etc., or if these are in your water supply. If possible, for the first four months of your pregnancy, move to a less polluted area. Filter your water using a reverse osmosis or charcoal filter. Avoid animal products and fish. Don't overdo it on the phytoestrogens during pregnancy, which the diet in this book recommends to prevent breast cancer; instead, eat more beans and nuts and less tofu. Use more almond milk and less soy milk during pregnancy and breast-feeding. ◄

High Estrogen Levels During Pregnancy

Women born to mothers with high estrogen levels during pregnancy are at increased risk of breast cancer when they reach adulthood.[58,59] It is probable that high levels of estrogen include the body's natural hormones.

Plant estrogens protect females from breast cancer when ingested from before puberty onward. Their effectiveness lies in the fact that they act as weak estrogens and can bind to estrogen receptor sites on breast cells. This leaves fewer sites for the body's tumor-enhancing estrogens (estradiol and estrone) or environmental estrogens to attach to.

We do not know how high amounts of plant estrogens during pregnancy or breast-feeding affect infants over their lifespan. The fetus is much more sensitive to hormonal stimulation and excess estrogen, particularly before four months of pregnancy. The blueprint for the child's sexual development and possibly orientation are laid down in utero. The effects of excess estrogen may not visibly manifest until years later. Therefore, we should be cautious about quantities of phytoestrogens consumed during pregnancy and lactation, both for mother and child, until we know that high amounts are safe.

In Australia in the 1940s, widespread infertility and stillbirths affected sheep that fed on pastures of clover. The epidemic became known as 'clover disease'. Clover contains an estrogen-mimicker that was making the sheep sterile. Women who consume large amounts of soy products tend to have longer menstrual cycles. This is good breast cancer prevention but may make a woman slightly less fertile. Some scientists believe that plant estrogens are a form of self-defense for the species involved — eventually the predator becomes infertile and the plant is able to rebound back from overgrazing. It confers a survival advantage to the plant.[60]

In summary, if you are trying to conceive or are pregnant, don't over-consume soy products, flaxseeds, and other phytoestrogens. They are fine in moderation but should not be the dietary mainstay. Use instead a variety of beans, grains, vegetables, fruits, nuts, and seeds.

Some scientists are concerned about the use of soy formulas in infants. Although they have been used for thirty years without noticeable effects, the daily exposure to infants of the plant estrogens in soy (called isoflavones) is 6–11 times higher on a body-weight basis than the dose that exhibits hormonal effects in adults. The amount of these phytoestrogens that circulate in the infant's blood are 13,000–22,000 times higher than plasma estradiol concentrations in early life. Though they are weak estrogens, soy formulas may have hormonal effects on young children that we have been unaware of so far, although one study demonstrated that four-month-old infants did not yet have the intestinal bacteria needed to convert genistein into its active phytoestrogen, equol. Long-term follow-up studies are needed to assess the benefits or harmful effects of soy formulas in infants.[61] In the meantime, it makes sense to vary the substitutes for breast milk, so that it is not exclusively soy-based. Alternatives are almond milk and organic goat milk. Recipes using these products are included in this book.

► **Action for Prevention:** Avoid using, ingesting, or inhaling all chemicals while pregnant. Eat organic food and avoid animal protein while pregnant, including milk. If you are not breast-feeding your child, or are supplementing breast milk, be cautious about only using soy-based formulas because of their possible hormonal action. Use almond milk and organic goat milk as alternatives. Drink filtered water and attach a filter to your shower. ◄

Reducing Estrogen Production to Protect Our Breasts

From an understanding of estrogen metabolism, we can recognize that there is much we can do to prevent breast cancer. We can become proactive in protecting our breasts. There are several points during the production of estrogen where we can exert a protective influence.

► **Action for Prevention:**

1) Rid our bodies of environmental chemicals before we conceive through the intensive use of saunas, homeopathic formulas, and a liver and bowel detoxification program so that we do not pass on our accumulated load of environmental estrogens to our children.

2) Stall puberty in girls by encouraging athletic activity, utilizing diets high in phytoestrogens such as soy and flaxseeds (in Japan, girls reach puberty at age 14–17), limiting their consumption of meat and fat to minimize estrogen intake and re-absorption from the intestines, decreasing exposure to environmental estrogens or "xenoestrogens", increasing elimination of xenoestrogens through improving liver function and the regular use of saunas.

Decrease exposure to light and electromagnetic fields at night to increase melatonin production. Prevent obesity in our daughters, since puberty is partially triggered when a certain level of fat is present in a young girl's body.

3) Encourage higher circulating amounts of estriol and lower amounts of estradiol through vegetarian diets high in phytoestrogens, fiber, the brassica family (cabbage, broccoli, Brussels sprouts, cauliflower, kale), sea vegetables, and through normalizing or improving thyroid and liver function.

4) Decrease dietary fats with the exception of flaxseed oil, extra virgin olive oil and uncontaminated cold water fish oils and encourage women to watch their weight, particularly after menopause. ◄

These preventative procedures will be discussed in greater detail in subsequent chapters.

Low Progesterone

Women with low progesterone have a tenfold increase in all cancers and experience 5.4 times more breast cancer than women with normal progesterone.[62] Estrogen and progesterone are both produced by the ovaries. Many women have high estrogen levels and low progesterone, which Dr John Lee believes may be linked to hormone-disrupting chemicals affecting ovary development during the embryo stage.[63] Studies have shown that environmental chemicals can suppress progesterone synthesis in other mammals.[64] Estrogen dominance causes uterine cells to multiply faster and stimulates breast tissue, resulting in breast swelling and tenderness. Progesterone decreases the rate at which breast cells multiply, eliminates breast tenderness, and stops uterine cells from multiplying. High estrogen without the opposing balance of progesterone is linked to elevated rates of breast cancer. Synthetic progestin does not protect from breast cancer,[65] while natural progesterone (made from wild yam or soy) may offer protection. One clinical trial has shown that breast cancer patients who were given progesterone had an improved disease-free and overall survival rate.[66]

A 1999 study found that progesterone caused a 90% inhibition of cell growth in breast cancer cells in a laboratory setting when the cells were progesterone receptor positive. These cancer cells were exposed to 10 microM of progesterone for 72 hours, a dosage comparable to that seen in a pregnant woman's blood during the third trimester of pregnancy. After 72 hours, 48% of the cells had undergone apoptosis (self-destruction) and another 40% showed signs of disintegration. Progesterone had no

effect on breast cancer cells that lacked the receptors for it.[67] This study would seem to indicate that progesterone might be a powerful hormonal treatment for progesterone receptor positive breast cancer.

Maybe not. In a study published in the journal *Cancer Research* in February 2000, Dr John Wiebe from the University of Western Ontario found that breakdown products of progesterone could act either to stimulate or to inhibit breast cancer. A particular enzyme called 5alpha-reductase is 30 times more prevalent in breast cancer cells than in healthy breast cells. When surgically removed cancerous tissue from the breasts of six women was incubated with progesterone over eight hours, the metabolites of progesterone were recovered and identified. The enzyme 5alpha-reductase transformed progesterone into a metabolite called 5alpha-pregnane-3,20-dione (5alphaP) that stimulated breast cancer. A second enzyme known as 3alpha-HSO pushed progesterone to a metabolite called 3alphaHP that directly inhibited breast cancer cell growth.[68] The deciding factor in this process is the quantity of 5alpha-reductase in the breast cell — if there is a lot of it (which there is in cancer cells), progesterone may be contraindicated. If there isn't, as in healthy breast cells, progesterone may be protective. The long and short of it is that we have contradictory studies on the use of progesterone with breast cancer patients. For the time being, we should err on the side of caution. However, progesterone supplementation exerts a protective effect in the absence of breast cancer, particularly in premenopausal women.

The most accurate test for progesterone levels is a salivary hormone test, available from Aeron Lab in San Leandro, CA (tel. 800-631-7900 or fax. 510-729-0383) or from DiagnosTech International Inc. in Osceola, WI (tel. 715-294-2149). This test is best done between days 20–23 of your menstrual cycle when progesterone should be highest, counting from the first day of your previous period. When supplementing with progesterone cream, it is important to monitor how the body responds to a particular dosage, as this will vary between individuals. Saliva progesterone levels should not exceed 0.5 ng/ml.[69]

Progesterone levels higher than this may cause a decrease in the number of estrogen receptors. While this may be beneficial for breast cancer prevention, it may increase the risk of osteoporosis and cause emotional problems. In its metabolic pathway, progesterone can become converted to estradiol, although this seems to happen only in a small subset of women. It is possible (I have seen it occur once so far) that estradiol levels will rise with an excess of progesterone, which would then increase breast cancer risk. If you are using progesterone cream or oral progesterone, you should consider follow-up testing of saliva levels of both progesterone and estradiol to ensure that both hormones stay in a favorable range. Testing could occur two months after beginning use and then every six months thereafter.

Many products are available now that claim to contain natural progesterone but which in fact only contain diosgenin, a component in wild yam, which must be converted through a lab process to natural progesterone in order to have an effect. The body does not convert it to progesterone.[70] Other products actually do contain progesterone. Dr John Lee suggests that the ideal amount is 400–500 mg of progesterone per ounce, which delivers the physiological amount that the ovaries normally produce when dosages of ¼–½ teaspoon are taken daily or for a portion of one's menstrual cycle. Three products, which contain the recommended amount, are OstaDerm by Bezwecken in Beaverton, OR; Pro-Gest by Prof. Tech Serv., Inc. in Portland, OR; and Wild Yam Cream by Enrich International in Orem, UT. For more information on the benefits and usage of natural progesterone, consult Dr Lee's excellent book, *What Your Doctor May Not Tell You about Menopause.*

Herbs which have been traditionally used to stimulate the production or availability of progesterone include chaste tree berry, yarrow, lady's mantle, mugwort, white deadnettle, elecampagne root, helonias root, wild yam root, birth root, black haw root bark, saw palmetto berry, Jamaican sarsaparilla root, Dong quai root, and marigold flowers.[71] However, David Zava and his co-workers tested over 150 various herbs, foods, and spices for progesterone bioactivity and found that none of the substances increased salivary progesterone in women, although many of them were able to bind to progesterone receptors in vitro. By far the strongest of these was bloodroot (Sanguinaria canadensis). Bloodroot, mistletoe, mandrake, and juniper were also all found to inhibit the proliferation of both estrogen receptor positive and estrogen receptor negative cell lines. Bloodroot[72] and mistletoe have a long history of use in treating breast cancer. Zava's testing included chaste tree berry, mugwort, sarsaparilla, helonias root, saw palmetto and yarrow. In his test, they did not raise progesterone levels.[73] This does not mean that they are ineffective — they may have a mechanism of action not apparent in his type of testing, perhaps requiring a period of several months to work.

Other researchers have found that consistent use of chaste tree berry will raise progesterone levels. It acts by stimulating the pituitary gland to secrete luteinizing hormone, which in turn signals the ovaries to make progesterone.[74] It is a slow-acting tonic requiring at least three months of daily use with permanent improvement occurring after about a year.[75] Another herb called stoneseed has also been found to stimulate progesterone secretion.[76]

Zava did not test lady's mantle (*Alchemilla vulgaris*), white deadnettle (*Lamium album*), elecampagne (*Inula helenium*), birth root (*Trillium pendulum*), and black haw (*Viburnum prunifolium*). Further testing (particularly of lady's mantle and birth root) remains to be done to see whether any of these herbs will increase progesterone levels. Testing should allow for several months of usage before assessing increases in hormone levels.

Vitamins which help increase progesterone include vitamin B6 and vitamin E. Vitamin B6 has been shown to reduce serum estrogen and raise progesterone levels.[77] Vitamin E enhances the absorption of progesterone. Minerals that assist in progesterone production are boron, zinc, and selenium. Increasing levels of boron in the diet will raise blood levels of both estrogen and progesterone, which is why it is an important nutrient in helping to maintain bone density. Zinc supplementation has resulted in lowered blood levels of estrogen and higher progesterone as well.[78] Animal studies have shown that selenium supplementation can increase plasma progesterone levels.[79] I suspect that iodine levels may also have a bearing on progesterone, as the ovaries contain high amounts of iodine. Hair analysis is an accurate method to test our levels of these particular trace minerals.

Melatonin has been found to stimulate the production of progesterone, and some, though not all studies, have found that melatonin levels are higher during the luteal phase (latter half) of the menstrual cycle when progesterone levels are highest.[80]

Another innovative tool that may increase progesterone is the homeopathic remedy Folliculinum 9CH. Dolisos Laboratory found that it reduced premenstrual symptoms and breast swelling in women when given on days seven and 21 of the menstrual cycle.[81] As far as I know, their research did not measure progesterone levels in these women, but instead rated symptoms. This would be important research to continue – we could monitor salivary progesterone in menstrual cycles with and without the use of Folliculinum to evaluate its effect. It is a simple and inexpensive therapy.

Eating soy foods will raise progesterone levels. One study found that the number of progesterone receptors in breast cells increased significantly in women who consumed soy regularly.[82]

Progesterone levels are highest during pregnancy, when the hormone is produced by the placenta and causes growth and permanent maturation of breast cells. Mature breast cells are more resistant to cancer. If an abortion or miscarriage halts the pregnancy, this ripening process of breast cells also stops as progesterone levels drop. The breast cells stay in a transitional state, still susceptible to cancerous changes. Therefore, carrying one's first pregnancy to term and allowing the breast cells to mature fully confers protection. Some scientists believe that having an abortion actually increases risk. The younger a woman is when she has a child, the more protection she gains.

▶ **Action for Prevention:** When you are pregnant for the first time, realize that you will decrease your breast cancer risk by having the child rather than terminating the pregnancy. If you have premenstrual breast tenderness, fibrocystic breast disease, or breast cancer, have your progesterone levels checked through a salivary hormone test. If it is low, take vitamins B6 and E and increase your foods or supplements containing zinc, boron, and selenium. Evaluate mineral status yearly using hair analysis. Increase soy foods. Consider using one or more of the progesterone-enhancing herbs and work with a practitioner familiar with their use. Use the natural progesterone cream only if the other therapies are unsuccessful at raising progesterone, as the cream is not curative – it only supplies you with progesterone for its duration of use. ◀

High Prolactin

Prolactin is a hormone secreted by the anterior pituitary gland. Its job is to stimulate breast cells to produce milk. There is a link between high prolactin levels and breast cancer,[83] and increased prolactin contributes to denser breast tissue, which may result in fibrocystic breasts.[84] In pregnancy, prolactin levels are lower during the first trimester, which may help to protect women from breast cancer during this period.[85] High prolactin may be linked to an underactive thyroid; indeed, serum prolactin levels are increased in about 40 percent of patients with primary hypothyroidism. Melatonin decreases the stimulating effects of prolactin on breast cancer cells. Prolactin can be measured in saliva and this test is available from DiagnosTech International Inc. in Osceola, WI (tel. 715-294-2144 or 888-342-7272).

▶ **Action for Prevention:** Screening for prolactin levels may show susceptibility to breast cancer. Normalize thyroid function to lower prolactin. Avoid dairy. ◀

Increased Growth Hormone

Growth hormone is secreted by the pituitary gland and regulates normal growth and development. Some forms of growth hormone stimulate milk production, which is why they are given to cattle in the United States. In some animal experiments, growth hormone is stronger than prolactin in stimulating breast development.[86] Girls who had a growth hormone deficiency and were given the hormone experienced accelerated development of breast tissue.[87] Growth hormone stimulates the ovaries to produce estradiol, causing puberty to occur earlier.[88] Growth hormone is the main regulator of circulating IGF-1, and higher levels of IGF-1 increase breast cancer risk. Therefore, increased growth hormone might increase breast cancer risk through at least three mechanisms: indirectly by increasing circulating IGF-1; indirectly by stimulating estradiol production by the ovary, leading to earlier puberty and increased estradiol long-term; and directly by enhancing growth of breast tissue.

Many American children are drinking milk from cows who have been given growth hormone. They will receive the hormone in their milk and this is likely to cause earlier onset of puberty, accelerated breast development, and increased risk of breast cancer.

▶ **Action for Prevention:** Ban the use of growth hormone in agricultural practice and keep your children away from dairy products. ◀

Increased Testosterone

Several studies have demonstrated a link with elevated testosterone levels and risk of breast cancer. In women, small amounts of testosterone are normally secreted by the adrenal glands and function to enhance libido. Like estrogen, testosterone binds to a carrier molecule in the blood known as sex hormone binding globulin, or SHBG. As long as either hormone is bound to this protein, it cannot attach to a receptor site and is inactive. Increased levels of testosterone displace estrogen from the carrier molecule so that more is available to bind to receptor sites, where it can promote breast cancer.

Unbalanced Thyroid

Women who have an underactive or unbalanced thyroid gland may have a higher risk of breast cancer. The thyroid gland makes two hormones, thyroxine (T4) and triiodothyronine (T3), from iodine and the amino acids tyrosine and phenylalanine. Their job is to regulate cell metabolism. T3 is the more active thyroid hormone, and as the T4 circulates through the blood it is converted to T3 in many tissues, especially the liver. Some of the T4 is converted to a variant of T3 called reverse T3, or RT3. Reverse T3 is inactive in the cell but is able to bind to T3 receptor sites and block T3 activity. This is more likely to occur after a significant stressor such as childbirth or during a chronic illness.

A condition called Wilson's syndrome can occur when there is an excess of RT3, due to the liver's inability to make the conversion of T4 to T3. The enzyme required to make this conversion is dependent upon the mineral selenium and the amino acid, cysteine. Wilson's syndrome can be suspected when the underarm temperature before rising is consistently below 97.8°F. It can be confirmed with a blood test from Meridian Valley Clinical Laboratory or from DiagnosTech International Inc. which measures T3 and reverse T3. When the ratio of T3 to reverse T3 is less than 10:1, the patient has Wilson's Syndrome and may manifest symptoms of hypothyroidism such as feeling cold, low energy, hair loss, dry skin, weight gain, anxiety, insomnia, depression, memory loss, headaches, and PMS, although other thyroid blood tests remain normal.[89,90] Iodine, zinc, selenium, copper, and flaxseed oil improve the conversion of T4 to T3 and elevate the ratio of T3 to reverse T3. Selenium specifically is needed for a particular enzyme that converts T4 to T3. Desiccated thyroid also improves this ratio, as does using T3 alone.

According to Dr John Lee, excess estrogen inhibits thyroid function, while progesterone facilitates the action of thyroid hormone.[91] I have found this to be true in working with patients. One study has shown that plasma T3 concentrations were reduced significantly in both early and advanced breast cancer, and that TSH levels were elevated in women with advanced breast cancer — both signs of hypothyroidism.[92] Another study demonstrated that women with breast cancer were more likely to have autoimmune thyroid disorders than women who were healthy.[93] Yet a third study revealed a correlation between hyperthyroidism and breast cancer.[94] Other studies have not supported these findings. Since environmental chemicals skew thyroid function, it is not surprising that women with breast cancer may have thyroid abnormalities. Yearly monitoring of thyroid function would reveal any imbalance.

Two minerals that the thyroid needs to produce its hormones are iodine and selenium; and the incidence of breast cancer is higher in areas where the soil is deficient in these minerals. It has been theorized that breast cells are more sensitive to stimulation from estrogen when iodine is deficient. Hair analysis is one way of assessing iodine and selenium deficiencies. Liberal use of sea vegetables such as kelp, dulse, nori, hiziki, and wakame delivers iodine to the body. The thyroid gland absorbs 80 times more iodine than any other tissue but contains only 20% of the body's iodine content, the rest being found in the skeletal muscles, liver, central nervous system, pituitary gland, breasts, and ovaries. The thyroid has the highest selenium concentration per gram of tissue than any other organ.[95] Selenium is most abundant in Brazil nuts, sunflower seeds, sesame seeds, barley, brown rice, red Swiss chard, tuna, wheat germ and bran, and brewer's yeast.

Dr Max Gerson used a form of iodine called Lugol's Solution, half strength, in a dosage of three drops six times daily as well as desiccated thyroid in his cancer patients, believing that it restored the electrical potential of the cell and enhanced cellular activity. It is crucial that the thyroid gland be operating efficiently in cancer patients because it maintains the body's normal temperature. Enzymes within the whole body work best at a particular temperature and pH. If temperature and pH are not maintained at optimal levels, there will be multiple enzyme deficiencies, and a decrease in the body's ability to fight cancer cells. Thyroid hormones affect the basal metabolic rate, which is the rate of oxygen consumption in the body at rest. This can be measured as either the number of kilocalories of heat energy produced or the volume of oxygen consumed per square meter per hour. Cancer cells do not thrive when there is an abundance of oxygen. So, it is plausible that women with hypothyroidism are more prone to breast cancer in part because of decreased tissue oxygenation.

Gerson believed that the temperature and basal metabolic rate of cancer patients is often disturbed, being either very high or low with a corresponding high or low iodine content of the blood. He was able to normalize either of these extremes with supplemental iodine.[96] Dr Jonathan Wright, as noted previously, uses iodine to normalize the estrogen quotient in pre- and post-menopausal women.

Iodine therapy and thyroid metabolism must be monitored closely. With too much iodine, the thyroid can become overactive. Natural substances to normalize an underactive thyroid include bee pollen, spirulina or chlorella algae, wheatgrass, oats, watercress, kelp, and the herbs bladderwrack, saw palmetto berries, damiana leaf, guggul, and globe artichoke.[97] Coconut oil massaged into the soles of the feet nightly may also improve thyroid function.

Other nutrients that support the thyroid are the amino acids tyrosine and L-carnitine, and the trace minerals chromium, zinc, copper, selenium, manganese, gold, and fluorite. Some individuals may need bovine desiccated thyroid to normalize thyroid function. One reliable source of this is from the firm Atrium (800-522-6461 or 815-648-4200).

Environmental Chemicals and Thyroid Function

The thyroid gland is vulnerable to environmental chemicals. Synthetic chemicals may disrupt the thyroid and the adrenal glands just as much as they interfere with the reproductive organs. According to Linda Birnbaum, head of the U.S. Environmental Protection Agencies Health Effects Research Laboratory, the thyroid gland is the most frequent target for synthetic chemicals.[98] Even very low levels of PCBs and dioxins can disrupt thyroid function in the mother and fetus, causing permanent neurological damage in the developing baby that may manifest as learning disabilities, attention problems, and hyperactivity throughout childhood and adult life. It has been estimated that at least 5% of babies in the United States are exposed to quantities of environmental chemicals that would cause neurological damage.[99] We cannot continue to destroy our air, water, soil, and offspring with environmental pollutants: the consequences of environmental chemicals to humans are devastating — they cause widespread loss of human potential, decreased quality of life, impair the health of future generations, cause increased costs to health, education, and social services, inflict stress and despair on individuals and the family unit, and lead to increased crime as affected individuals cannot cope in schools and work environments.

Thyroid Function in Wildlife

The thyroid glands in wildlife are also affected. For example, Florida panthers that prey on fish-eating raccoons are having trouble reproducing. They have high levels of sperm abnormalities, low sperm count, impaired immunity, undescended testes, and disturbed thyroid function. It is believed that hormone disruption by PCBs and DDE and other chemicals are the cause of their decline. Great Lakes salmon eggs have lower levels of thyroid hormones than eggs from Pacific salmon living in less polluted waters. Adult salmon and herring gulls in the Great Lakes have thyroid gland enlargement, evidently caused by chemicals in their environment that block the action of thyroid hormones, and not caused by a deficiency of iodine.[100] When a mixture of DDT, PCBs, mirex, and photomirex, all abundant contaminants in the Great Lakes in the 1970s, was fed to ringed doves, they experienced disruption in their normal courtship and breeding cycle. The adult birds became hyperactive. They spent less time feeding their young, were erratic in their incubating habits, and their nesting success dropped by up to 50%. Their inattentive behavior was associated with thyroid abnormalities.[101] In my own naturopathic practice in Toronto, I frequently see women with under-functioning thyroid glands who do not easily respond to appropriate therapies. I now suspect that part of the cause is hormone disruption from chemical toxicity.

Chemicals can exert direct effects on the thyroid gland in one of several ways: they can inhibit the ability of the thyroid gland to trap iodine (thiocyanate and perchlorate do this); they can block the binding of iodine and the coupling of iodothyronines to form the thyroid hormones, thyroxine (T4) and triiodothyronine (T3) (sulfonamides, thiourea, methimazole, and aminotriazole do this); they can inhibit thyroid hormone secretion (lithium and an excess of iodine do this); they can increase the metabolism of thyroid hormones so that they are used up faster where they are needed in the body (many drugs do this – phenobarbitol, benzodiazepines, calcium channel blockers, and steroids; PCBs and organochlorine pesticides such as chlordane, DDT, and TCDD do this as well).[102]

Another cause of thyroid imbalance is physiological or psychological stress. Techniques in stress management and practice of the alternate nostril series of breathing exercises described in The Healthy Breast Program are ways to normalize the thyroid when its imbalance is due to stress.

There are several ways to test thyroid function. The simplest way is to take your underarm temperature in the morning before getting out of bed. A normal temperature is between 97.8° and 98.2°F with fluctuations that occur with your menstrual cycle. If your temperature is consistently lower than this, chances are you have an underactive thyroid. If your temperature is often higher than 98.2°, your thyroid may be overactive. Regular blood tests for thyroid function may or may not show a deficiency, even when your temperature is low. A specialized blood test that measures T3 and reverse T3 may reveal a thyroid disorder when a regular test does not. This test is available when ordered by a naturopathic or medical doctor from Meridian Valley Clinical Laboratory in Kent, WA (tel. 253-859-8700) or DiagnosTech International Inc. (715-294-2144).

▶ **Action for Prevention:** Check your thyroid function annually with a temperature test, If it is low, follow-up with a blood test that measures TSH, T4, T3, reverse T3, and thyroid autoantibodies. If it is underactive, consume sea vegetables, use kelp and dulse powder as seasonings on your food, and regularly use bladderwrack, bee pollen, spirulina or chlorella algae, wheatgrass, oats, watercress, saw palmetto berries, damiana, guggul, and/or globe artichoke. Ensure adequate intake of iodine, selenium, zinc, and flaxseed oil. Make sure your progesterone and adrenal hormone levels are normal. Massage coconut oil into the soles of your feet nightly. Detoxify annually following the guidelines in this book or using other methods to remove hormone-disrupting chemicals. Work with a naturopathic doctor and a medical doctor to normalize any thyroid dysfunction. Establish routine sauna use. Actively participate in reducing environmental damage due to chemicals through the choices you make as a consumer and through activism. This is a critical time. We are all needed to work together in restoring the earth. ◄

High Insulin Levels

Women with high insulin levels have a breast cancer risk almost three times higher than women with normal levels.[103] Too much insulin can stimulate the growth of an already existing breast cancer. Insulin levels are often high in women who are overweight, particularly if they carry their weight above their waists. Contributing factors to high insulin levels include overconsumption of sugar, alcohol, and carbohydrates with a high glycemic index (see The Healthy Breast Diet chapter for this index), lack of exercise, and an excess of saturated fat and Omega 6 essential fatty acids.[104]

Insulin is released from the pancreas in response to high levels of glucose in the blood. Its job is to bring down these levels and to help the glucose get into your cells where it can be used for energy. Chronic high insulin levels lead to obesity, and obese children have higher insulin levels than lighter children. Children whose insulin levels are high will usually maintain those levels throughout life, unless dietary measures are used to intervene. High insulin levels in the blood occur when insulin cannot get into the cells, a process called insulin resistance, which can ultimately lead to diabetes. Several mechanisms contribute to insulin resistance, one of them being the types of fat that we eat. Insulin resistance increases with consumption of Omega 6 fatty acids (vegetable oils) and saturated fat from animal products and improves with exercise and consumption of the mineral chromium, alpha lipoic acid, and Omega 3 fatty acids, which include flaxseed oil and fish oils. The trace mineral chromium helps to regulate insulin levels, is used in the

prevention and management of both hypoglycemia and diabetes, and decreases sugar cravings. It is a common deficiency and can accurately be measured in a hair analysis. The usual dose is 200–600 mcg per day.

► **Action for Prevention:** Keep your insulin levels low by avoiding sweets, alcohol, refined carbohydrates, and saturated fats. Exercise regularly. Decrease insulin resistance with the use of chromium, alpha lipoic acid, and flaxseed oil. Eat foods with a low glycemic index. ◄

High Insulin-like Growth Factors-1 and 2 (IGF-1 and IGF-2) Levels

Insulin-like Growth Factors-1 and 2 (IGF-1 and IGF-2) are natural hormones responsible for growth and development. They are stimulated by growth hormone from the pituitary gland and are produced by the liver. Our levels of IGF-1 are low at birth, rise during childhood, peak at puberty, and decline as we age. Both insulin and IGFs cause cells to hypertrophy, or enlarge. The structures of IGFs are similar to that of insulin, and when insulin levels fluctuate, so do the levels of IGFs. Circulating total and free IGF-1 levels are low when insulin levels are low.[105] The Harvard Nurse's Study found that women whose blood contained slightly higher levels of IGF-1 had a sevenfold increase in breast cancer risk, making it one of the highest predisposing factors to the disease. Women with breast cancer have increased blood levels of IGF-1. Higher levels of IGF-1 also increase risk of prostate and lung cancers.[106]

IGF-1 binds to its receptor sites on breast cell membranes and acts synergistically with estradiol to increase cell division and promote breast development during puberty as well as breast cancer later in life.[107] It is a highly potent stimulator of breast cells and causes massive multiplication of growth when added to breast cell tissue cultures. It promotes the growth and invasiveness of malignant cells. Insulin-like Growth Factor-1 protects breast cancer cells from cell death, or apoptosis, and in so doing, interferes with the effects of chemotherapy. Receptors for IGF-1 have been found in 90% of breast cancer cell lines and in most biopsies of breast cancer tumors.[108,109] Higher estrogen levels may make the breasts more sensitive to the growth-promoting effects of IGF-1 by increasing the number of IGF-1 receptor sites in the breasts.[110] Whatever the mechanism, it is clear that estrogen enhances the response of breast cells to the IGFs.

IGF-1 levels are higher in pre-menopausal breast cancer patients (compared to post-menopausal patients) and are higher in women with breast cancer recurrence. One of the effects of Tamoxifen is to reduce IGF-1 levels. The probability of survival is greater in breast cancer patients with plasma IGF-1 levels less than 120 ng/ml.[111]

The insulin-like growth factors are carried in the blood on one of seven binding proteins.[112] When the concentration of these binding proteins increases, the availability and activity of the IGFs decreases. Binding proteins affect the biological activity of IGFs, and can either increase or decrease their cancer-promoting activity or act independently from them. The binding protein IGFBP-3 in particular is able to inhibit breast cancer cell growth. Future therapies for breast cancer may include natural or synthetic substances that increase these binding proteins, so that there is less free IGF available to stimulate cell growth.

Moderate consumption of alcohol increases the liver's production of insulin-like growth factors, although IGF production declines in heavy drinkers as alcohol-related liver damage prevents their formation.[113]

Interestingly, animal studies have shown that the thyroid hormone, T3, exerts a direct effect on IGF-2. Hypothyroidism was associated with higher levels of circulating IGF-2.[114] We see over and over how our hormones act in concert and an imbalance in one is likely to affect many others. We are sitting on the edge of a hormonal disaster as we continue to use hormone-disrupting chemicals. Since growth hormone stimulates IGF-1, any substance we ingest that contains growth hormone will increase our baseline levels of IGF-1. This currently poses several concerns. In the United States, cows are given bovine growth hormone to increase milk production by approximately 10%. The milk of these cows contains a tenfold increase in IGF-1 beyond the milk of cows not given growth hormone. Because the IGF-1 is not protein bound, it is easily absorbed across the intestinal wall, and its digestion is blocked by casein present in the milk. This leads to higher levels of IGF-1 in the person ingesting the milk, which in turn leads to increased growth and stimulation of breast cells. IGF-1 has been found to selectively accumulate and concentrate in breast cells. We would expect that this will lead to earlier breast development in girls who consume milk containing bovine growth hormone and an increased risk of breast cancer. Higher circulating levels of IGF-1 are linked with a sevenfold increase in breast cancer and a fourfold increase in prostate cancer.

A current health fad is to take bovine colostrum, containing growth hormone, to encourage fat loss, build muscle mass, or stimulate immunity. Any person who does this will simultaneously increase their cancer risk by increasing circulating IGF levels. Colostrum is meant for newborns who need rapid growth, not for adults.

Higher serum levels of IGF-1 are associated with increased breast cancer risk in pre-menopausal women.[115] We can have our blood or saliva levels of IGF-1 and 2 checked annually, beginning at puberty, and change our diets, avoiding foods that dramatically raise blood sugar and insulin levels. If we lower plasma IGF-1 levels, we may reduce the risk of developing breast cancer in high risk groups; slow the progression of early stage breast cancer; lower the risk of recurrence; and increase the probability of survival. Serum or saliva levels of IGF-1 and 2 may be one of several predictive tests indicative of breast cancer risk. IGF-1 can be measured in saliva using a test from DiagnosTech International Inc. in Osceola, Wisconsin (715-294-2144 or 888-342-7272).

▶ **Action for Prevention:** Have your saliva or serum levels of IGF-1 and 2 checked annually and adopt a diet using carbohydrates with a lower glycemic index. These include most beans, barley, the Brassica family, green beans, tomatoes, sea vegetables, powdered greens, cherries, plums, grapefruit, peaches, apples, and pears. Include flaxseed oil and chromium in your diet or supplement schedule. Avoid sweets. Eliminate or drastically reduce saturated fat. Aim for a 2:1 ratio of Omega 3 to Omega 6 fatty acids. ◀

Decreased Melatonin

Degeneration of the pineal gland and decreased melatonin production cause women to be more vulnerable to breast cancer. Melatonin is a hormone secreted by the pineal gland. It acts to modify the function of the nervous system, glandular system, and immune system. The pineal gland translates changes in external light into chemical signals that impose a circadian rhythm upon the body, which helps orchestrate many, if not all of the other body rhythms. In a 24-hour cycle, the highest level of melatonin production occurs during the night at about 3:00 a.m., while we are asleep in the dark. Exposure to light or electromagnetic radiation at night reduces these levels. Electromagnetic fields from clocks, radios, electric blankets, and anything else within two and one half feet of us while we sleep will inhibit melatonin production. We can protect ourselves by ensuring that we and our children sleep in a darkened room with closed curtains, away from electrical devices and outlets.

We have our peak levels at age 15 and have half of our highest levels at age 45 with a gradual decline after that. As melatonin levels decrease with aging, we are more vulnerable to disorders associated with disturbances in the body's rhythms, such as sleep disorders, hormonal imbalances, and cancer. Youthfulness and longevity are linked to high levels of melatonin secretion. Some of the health benefits ascribed to producing or taking melatonin on a regular basis are improved sleep, increased libido, resistance to viral infections, improved energy, and prevention of jet lag.

Melatonin is found in lower amounts in the blood of people with cancer, with circulating hormone levels in the blood being 30–40% lower in cancer patients than in people who are cancer free at similar ages.[116] Autopsies of cancer victims reveal shrinkage and decreased weight of the pineal gland.[117] Melatonin is one of the body's first lines of defense in response to malignant breast cell growth. Increased melatonin keeps abnormal breast cancer cells under control, while a deficiency of melatonin allows breast tumors to form. Patients with aggressive breast tumors have lower levels of melatonin than women with a low rate of malignant cell growth.[118]

Melatonin inhibits the growth of breast cancer cells through several mechanisms:

1) Melatonin can directly kill breast cancer cells.

2) Melatonin inhibits the production of tumor growth factor, thereby thwarting tumor growth.

3) Melatonin stimulates the differentiation of cancer cells, shifting them towards normal cells.

4) Melatonin improves the individual's immune system to fight against the tumor.[119]

5) Melatonin decreases the ability of cancer cells to attach to basement membranes, preventing invasive cancer.[120]

6) Melatonin helps to regulate cell division and multiplication.

7) Melatonin decreases the number of estrogen receptors in breast cells, thereby decreasing estrogen's effect on breast cells. It also competes with estrogen for the existing receptor sites.

When a small breast tumor begins to form, the pineal secretes more melatonin in an attempt to control it. If it fails to control the process and breast cancer is initiated, pineal exhaustion sets in and blood levels of melatonin decrease as the tumor grows in size. The critical nighttime level is particularly low.[121]

If the breast tumor metastasizes and spreads through the body, the pineal makes a last, valiant attempt to stop the cancer from spreading by sending large amounts of melatonin into the bloodstream. Usually the prognosis is poor, but occasionally the pineal's efforts are successful

and the cancer retreats. Older people may have less success because the pineal has deteriorated due to aging. Supplementation with melatonin often results in stabilizing cancer so that it ceases to grow, or can actually cause tumors to regress.[122] Women with late stage breast cancer achieved partial remission lasting an average of eight months when they were given high doses of melatonin in the evening (20 mg per day). Patient improvement and tumor regression has been directly correlated with a rise in blood melatonin levels. It has an added benefit of decreasing anxiety.[123] If melatonin is prescribed, all doses should be taken at bedtime, since morning administration has been found to stimulate cancer growth in animal studies, while evening dosing inhibits cancer.[124]

Melatonin has been shown to prevent chemically caused breast tumors in studies on rats. This may be due to its powerful antioxidant effect. It is a stronger antioxidant than vitamin C, vitamin E, or beta-carotene and is unique in that it can permeate any cell in any part of the body, so its antioxidant action is widespread.[125] This is good news for us in our chemically polluted world – if we can stimulate our own bodies to increase melatonin levels, we will improve our protection against chemical toxicity.

Melatonin decreases the stimulating effect of the hormone prolactin (secreted by the pituitary gland) on breast cancer cells. Prolactin can promote the growth of breast tumors and increase the activity of estrogen. Women with breast cancer and low melatonin levels tend to have higher secretions of prolactin around noon. It seems that melatonin is involved in the complex timed release of other hormones, including prolactin.[126] Hypothyroidism is also often linked to higher prolactin levels.

Melatonin levels vary during a woman's menstrual cycle, and melatonin itself may stimulate progesterone secretion, though research is conflicting.[127] Progesterone protects us from breast cancer. Some studies, though not all, show that melatonin levels are low at ovulation and increase premenstrually three to sixfold, reaching their peak at menstruation.[128]

Melatonin affects the number of estrogen receptors in breast cells – higher amounts of melatonin will cause a decrease in the numbers of estrogen receptors. It inhibits the replication of breast cancer cells in the laboratory by regulating cell division and multiplication.[129] It's as though this pineal hormone flips a breaker switch to turn off estradiol's activity on the breast cell. It may actually even lower estrogen levels.[130]

Melatonin also competes with estrogen for the estrogen receptor sites, thus inhibiting estrogen's activity on breast cells in several important ways. It has been found to be highly effective at blocking estrogen-receptor positive breast cancer cells but only minimally effective in inhibiting cancer cells that were not estrogen-sensitive. Melatonin increases the effectiveness of Tamoxifen when used along with it and improves patient response to chemotherapy. It can reduce the toxicity of chemotherapeutic drugs but does not prevent hair loss or nausea. It can, however, help prevent weight loss during chemotherapy treatments.

Cancer cells have rapid, uncontrolled cell division and multiplication. The pineal gland and melatonin help to reset timed cell division to its normal levels. There is a close relationship between the function of the pineal, pituitary, and thymus glands, each of them playing a role in cancer prevention and immune fitness. Melatonin stimulates the thymus gland and the activity of natural killer cells, which directly target and destroy cancer cells. A hormone from the thymus gland called thymosin, which improves immune function, is regulated in part by melatonin. A 240% increase in natural killer cells has been observed after melatonin supplementation.[131] This means that the immune system has more than double the ability to directly annihilate cancer cells when melatonin levels are high. Stress can interfere with the ability of enzymes to repair DNA damage within the cell, while correct melatonin levels can enhance DNA repair. Melatonin can reverse shrinkage of the thymus gland caused by psychological and physiological stress.[132]

Interestingly, melatonin is a molecule that is present in many life forms, including plants. It is synthesized in humans from the amino acid tryptophan, which is first converted to serotonin in the pineal gland and then to melatonin. Melatonin production is dependent on vitamins B3 and B6, calcium, magnesium, and zinc. Vitamin B6 in particular is needed for the conversion of tryptophan to serotonin. Melatonin's effectiveness in the body is at least partially dependent on glutathione, an amino acid complex important for the liver's detoxifying ability and immune health. We can supplement with N-acetylcysteine or reduced glutathione to ensure adequate glutathione levels, or eat plenty of the cystine containing foods listed in chapter seven.

One of the ways we can promote melatonin production is by ensuring an adequate dietary supply of tryptophan. Tryptophan is the least abundant amino acid in foods. Animal studies have shown that increased amounts of dietary L-tryptophan can cause a fourfold elevation in blood melatonin levels. Some of the food sources of tryptophan are as follows:[133]

Food	Serving	Tryptophan (mg)
Spirulina, dried	3.5 oz	929[134]
Soy Flour	1 cup	683
Soy Nuts	1/2 cup	495
Cottage Cheese	1 cup	312
Soy Protein Powder	1 oz	312
Tofu, raw, firm	1/2 cup	310
Tuna	3 oz	291
Tempeh	1/2 cup	234
Salmon	3 oz	231
Cashews	20 whole	215
Oatmeal flakes	1 cup	200
Miso	1/2 cup	197
Navy Beans, boiled	1 cup	187
Kidney Beans, boiled	1 cup	182
Great Northern Beans, boiled	1 cup	175
Lentils, boiled	1 cup	160
Mung Beans, boiled	1 cup	154
Chick Peas, boiled	1 cup	139
Pumpkin seeds	122 seeds	122
Hummus	1 cup	116
Wheat Germ	1/4 cup	110
Soy Milk	1 cup	103
Collards, boiled	1 cup	100
Egg	1 medium	100
Sunflower Seeds	1 oz	99
Brazil Nuts	8 nuts	74
Organic Raisins	7 tbsp	60
Spinach	2 cups raw	50
Sweet Potato	1 small	50
Yogurt	1 cup	50

Tryptophan can be purchased in capsule form as 5-HTP. Usually the dosage is 100–200 mg, 2–3 times daily. If you follow The Healthy Breast Diet, you will consume more than enough tryptophan to optimize your melatonin levels. Be sure to take vitamin B6 as well.

We can ingest melatonin itself in a variety of foods. One study found that an average of 100 grams of fruit or vegetable contained the following amounts of melatonin: banana, 47 ng; tomato, 25 ng; cucumber, 9 ng; beetroot, 0.1 ng. The "Sweet 100" variety of tomatoes contains about five times more melatonin than wild tomatoes.[135] Rice, corn, barley, ginger, daikon radish, oats, pineapple, watercress, citrus, halibut, turkey, carrots, celery, broccoli, and cottage cheese are also purported to contain melatonin, although I could find no studies giving amounts.[136]

Certain herbs contain melatonin. Praveen Saxena, a horticulture professor at the University of Guelph, with a team of graduate students found that the amount of melatonin in some herb samples tested higher than commercial preparations of melatonin sold presently in the United States. The Chinese herb Hunaqqin (Scutellaria baicalensis) tested highest with 7.11 ug/g of melatonin, followed by the flowers of St. John's wort with 4.39 ug/g (the leaves contained only 1.75 ug/g), and the fresh green leaves of feverfew which contained 2.45 ug/g of melatonin.[137]

Finally, we can stimulate our own bodies to produce melatonin through the regular practice of meditation or breathing exercises, particularly before bed. In his book, *Self-Healing: Powerful Techniques*, Ranjie Singh, PhD, demonstrates particular breathing and meditation techniques that are able to raise melatonin levels within minutes when practiced correctly. Regular practice of breathing exercises reverses the degeneration of the pineal gland, providing us with a constant source of melatonin within our own bodies for life. Stimulating our own bodies to produce melatonin is much more reliable and empowering than taking supplemental melatonin. Singh found that practitioners were able to raise their melatonin levels from 50% to 10 times higher with an average of three times higher than baseline levels. Cancer patients experienced an average increase in melatonin levels of 230% or over double their baseline levels.[138]

► **Action for Prevention:** There are ways to take care of the pineal gland and melatonin production through lifestyle practices, diet, and herbal and nutritional supplementation. The way many of us live is geared to upset pineal function and we should attempt to balance our lifestyle before resorting to any "quick fix". Here are guidelines for taking care of your pineal gland:

1) Avoid shift work. It confuses your body's rhythms and will interfere with melatonin production.

2) Spend at least 20 minutes outside in natural light (without sunglasses) in the early part of the day. This may help melatonin levels to be higher at night.[139]

3) Sleep in a dark room, with no light shining in from the street. Melatonin production is lower when we are exposed to light at night. Low intensity light (50 lux) is acceptable but levels of 500 lux or higher suppress melatonin release. If need be, wear a mask over your eyes as you sleep.

4) Keep regular hours, preferably going to bed early and getting up early.

5) Avoid excessive exposure to electromagnetic radiation, which interferes with melatonin production. Do not sleep within three feet of an electrical outlet or device.

6) Exercise regularly. One hour daily on a stationary bicycle can double or triple melatonin levels.[140]

7) Ensure adequate consumption of foods high in tryptophan or melatonin, along with vitamins B3, B6, calcium, magnesium, zinc, and NAC or foods containing cystine (see chapter seven). Consider supplementation with 5-HTP or St. John's wort.

8) Avoid the other factors which interfere with pineal function — alcohol, caffeine, recreational drugs, nicotine, intense electromagnetic fields, bright lights and medications such as beta-blockers, diazepam, haloperidol, chlorpromazine, and ibuprofen.

9) Practice a meditative or breathing exercise one or more times daily, particularly before bed.

10) If you have breast cancer, especially if it is estrogen receptor positive, consider supplementing with 5–20 mg of melatonin one half hour before bedtime (8:00–10:00 p.m.) with medical supervision. If you are at high risk for breast cancer, use 3–9 mg of melatonin nightly as prevention.

11) Monitor melatonin levels annually through saliva testing. (DiagnosTech International Inc. or Aeron Labs). ◄

Melatonin and Ultradian Breath Rhythms

Breathing exercises can help to prevent cancer by reducing stress, regenerating the pineal gland, balancing the glands in general, and raising melatonin levels.

Ordinarily we breathe predominantly through one nostril at a time for about a 90 to 120 minute period, and then breathe through both nostrils for approximately 20 minutes. This is followed by predominance of the other nostril for another 90 to 120 minutes. This cycle occurs throughout the day and night, and is known as an ultradian rhythm (one that occurs more than once in a 24 hour cycle). Other physiological and psychological processes governed by ultradian rhythms include the desire to eat and drink, sleep, dreaming and wakefulness, aspects of the immune system, breast-feeding, hormonal secretions, stress reactions, attention and concentration, cell replication, and mood changes. These are governed by the same 90 to 120 minute periods as the breath cycle.[141] As the breath cycle comes into balance through practicing breathing exercises, the other ultradian rhythms normalize as well.

When the left nostril is dominant, the right hemisphere of the brain exhibits more activity.[142] The right hemisphere is linked to creative thought, intuition, non-linear thinking, a sense of timelessness, and appreciation of art, music, and poetry. With left nostril dominance the parasympathetic nervous system is activated, causing us to feel more relaxed. Blood pressure will often decrease with left nostril breathing. When the right nostril is dominant, the left hemisphere of the brain shows more activity. The left hemisphere is related to linear thinking, assertiveness and aggressiveness, concentrated study, athletic activity, mathematical problem solving, and logic. With right nostril dominance the sympathetic nervous system is activated, causing us to feel more alert and charged, ready for action.[143] Right nostril breathing will often elevate blood pressure slightly and prepare us for intense physical activity, study, or assertive exchanges.

The twenty-minute period when both nostrils are dominant is a time of integration between the hemispheres. This is often the time when we want to daydream, fantasize, reflect, have a break from what we were doing, move around, or process emotional material. It is the time of reconciliation between mind and body, when we are more open to receive and pay attention to the messages from the body. It is the time when we are primed to receive intuitive impulses, inner guidance, and connect to our spiritual selves. During this twenty-minute break, we are more apt to recognize emotions we have suppressed.

The Twenty-Minute Break

Western society chronically neglects the body's need for a twenty minute break every two hours or so. We replace these times of potential integration with addictions such as coffee, cigarettes, alcohol, work, television, sugar or excess food, and recreational drugs, which compound the problem. These addictions further alienate us from the messages our bodies send us, from our emotional truths, and from our spiritual identities. Evidence suggests that ignoring the psychological and physiological need to relax fosters hormonal imbalances and increased cell replication leading to cancer.

Melatonin and Breathing Exercises

When we develop and practice a slow, meditative breath, melatonin levels increase throughout the body as the pineal gland responds with renewed vigor.[144] One of the functions of melatonin is to regulate cell division and multiplication. When the pineal gland is not functioning properly, there will be increased cell division and multiplication and a greater likelihood of cancer. We know that cell division is linked with the breath cycle through ultradian rhythms, so that normalizing the breath cycle can help to normalize cell division. The complete process of cell division typically takes between 1½ to 2 hours, with a 20-minute critical period of time when molecules called "cyclins" accumulate in the cell to determine if and when it will divide. The mechanism for this is likely linked to the release of melatonin from the pineal gland. We can help to prevent breast cancer by keeping our melatonin levels high through an evening meditation practice.

The Need for Regular Relaxation

When we are chronically stressed, the breath cycle becomes derailed. Most often it speeds up, so that the nostril shift will occur within a shorter period. We may also become dominant in one nostril, rarely breathing through the other. This can lead to over dominance in one hemisphere of the brain, problems occurring particularly on one side of the body and dominance of either the parasympathetic or sympathetic nervous system. We lose our pre-programmed equilibrium. It is no wonder that breast cancer often occurs after a period of chronic stress.

Many of us live very busy lives with little time for genuine relaxation, self-reflection, meditation, prayer, or solitude. Relaxation is a necessary component of any healing process. When we relax, we activate the parasympathetic branch of the autonomic nervous system, which promotes healing. Stress is a component of almost all illness, and relaxation and meditation help to decrease the physiological effects of stress.

One of the best ways to maintain the body's equilibrium despite stress is through breathing exercises, or pranayams, as they are termed in yoga. Many of the body's timed cyclical processes revolve around the breath cycle. We often forget that every process in the body has its own rhythm. Our bodies are subjects of time, bound to the solar, lunar and planetary cycles. Our minds more easily approach the timeless. Breathing exercises can synchronize our bodily processes with the great universal rhythms and lead our minds into a state of timelessness.

This need for regenerating rest and relaxation has been declared by the United Nations Environmental Sabbath Program in the poem at the bottom of this page.

Discovering Your Ultradian Rhythms Exercise

As you sit wherever you are, take your right thumb and place it against your right nostril, closing the nostril. Take a breath in and out of the left nostril only and notice how easily the air goes in and out. Does it feel freely open or a little clogged? Now take the left thumb and block the left nostril, breathing in and out through the right nostril only and noticing how open it feels. Which one seems more open? This is your dominant nostril at this time. If both nostrils seem equally open, your body may be orchestrating its 20-minute break.

1) Choose one day this week when you will be able to check your nostril dominance quickly like this every half-hour. Record nostril dominance on the sheet on page 83, using L for left, R for right and B for both. Observe the pattern. There will be fluctuations depending on your activities. It's a very flexible system but look for the pattern. The pattern should average out to be 90–120 minutes one nostril, 20 minutes both nostrils, and 90–120 minutes the other nostril. Record also what type of activity you were engaged in during the nostril dominance and what body-mind signals you receive that signify it is time for you to take a break. If you are consistently dominant in one nostril or your nostril shifts occur in less than 90 minutes most of the time, you especially need to practice the breathing exercise below to regain equilibrium. Try it once daily for 40 days and then recheck your nostril dominance throughout the day to see if you've normalized your cycle.

2) Begin checking nostril dominance at whatever time you get up in the morning and record left (L), right (R), or both (B) in the column with the heading *Nostril*. Jot down what you were doing when you checked your nostril dominance, as specific activities have an influence on right or left nostril dominance. For example, under the *Activity* column you might write 'having breakfast', 'watching a movie', or 'working on the computer'. The next column is designed to help you pay attention to what body-mind signals you receive when it's time for you to take a break. These will be recorded every two hours or so and might include 'yawning, poor concentration, need to stretch, thirst, daydreaming, deep sighing.' The final column will list ways in which you can practically honor those signals, given your schedule and work. It might include 'going for a walk, practicing the alternate nostril series, consciously breathing deeply while in the midst of activity, bathroom break, visualization, meditation, personal prayer, creative activity, journaling, inner listening …'

3) Then your task following this exercise is to integrate more of the rejuvenating activities into your life during the 20-minute periods when your body-mind signals you to do so. For expansion on this idea, read *The Twenty-Minute Break* by Ernest Rossi. Keep in mind that this 20-minute period of rejuvenation is a psychological and physiological necessity. You deserve it.

We who have lost our sense and our senses — our touch, our smell, our vision of who we are, we who frantically force and press all things, without rest for body or spirit, hurting our earth and injuring ourselves: we call a halt.

We want to rest. We need to rest and allow the earth to rest.

We need to reflect and to rediscover the mystery that lives in us that is the ground of every unique expression of life, the source of the fascination that calls all things to communion.

We declare a Sabbath, a space of quiet: for simply being and letting be; for recovering the great, forgotten truths; for learning how to live again.[145]

• Ultradian Rhythm Cycle •

Time	Nostril	Activities	Body-Mind Signal to Rejuvenate	Ways to Rejuvenate
6:00 am				
6:30				
7:00				
7:30				
8:00				
8:30				
9:00				
9:30				
10:00				
10:30				
11:00				
11:30				
12:00 pm				
12:30				
1:00				
1:30				
2:00				
2:30				
3:00				
3:30				
4:00				
4:30				
5:00				
5:30				
6:00				
6:30				
7:00				
7:30				
8:00				
8:30				
9:00				
9:30				
10:00				
10:30				
11:00				

Diaphragmatic Breathing and the Alternate Nostril Series Exercise[146]

To restore your breath cycle, normalize the body's ultradian rhythms and keep your melatonin levels elevated, practice the following breath series once or twice daily for 12 minutes at a time. One of the practice periods should be an hour before bedtime. If you have cancer, consider practicing this, a similar breath series, or other relaxation technique four or five times daily to restore your ultradian rhythms and normalize cell division. It is no coincidence that several religious traditions utilize prayer five times daily as part of their practice, such as the Muslims and Sikhs. These prescribed breaks would help to normalize ultradian rhythms at the appropriate times and contribute to physical and spiritual renewal. You can design your own spiritual practice consisting of a combination of breath-work, meditation, visualization, and prayer repeated at regular intervals daily.

Diaphragmatic breathing is a pattern of breathing that promotes deep relaxation and body cleansing. It is based on breathing slowly and deeply, causing an expansion of the abdomen on the inhale, and a falling in of the abdomen on the exhale. This allows the diaphragm to expand to its full capacity as one inhales, which gives a gentle massage and increased blood circulation to the liver. The liver is the body's main organ of detoxification. Diaphragmatic breathing permits increased oxygen to be absorbed from the lungs and distributed to the cells via the blood. Cancer does not thrive in a well-oxygenated environment. Long, deep breathing also promotes muscle relaxation and encourages release of stored emotions. This practice restores health to the pineal, pituitary, and thymus glands, coordinating the whole glandular system and strengthening immunity. It tends to activate the parasympathetic nervous system, which promotes many healing responses in the body and mind. The following series of diaphragmatic breathing exercises is effective in inducing a state of relaxation. It helps to normalize ultradian rhythms, stimulate the pineal and pituitary glands, cause increased release of melatonin, integrate the hemispheres of the brain, balance the sympathetic and parasympathetic nervous systems, and create integration between both sides of your body. This 'script' can be read slowly onto a tape and listened to at home or you can use the form at the back of the book to order the tape.

1) Sit in a quiet room where you will not be disturbed. You may sit on a chair or pillow, or cross-legged. (*Pause*). Maintain a receptive and reverential attitude for healing, putting any worries or preoccupations aside.

2) Close your eyes, then gently focus them up to a point midway between the eyebrows. Be aware of your spine, keeping it straight. Visualize a glowing silvery light radiating upwards through your spine. Strengthen this image with each long breath. Now take your right hand and block your right nostril with your thumb by pressing it against the side of your nostril, having the other fingers pointing up straight. Begin slow, long, deep breathing through the left nostril only. As you inhale, allow the belly to expand completely. Then let the breath slowly fill the lower, middle, and upper part of the lungs. As you exhale, empty the air from the top of the lungs downward, drawing the belly in towards the spine as you complete the exhale. Again inhale deeply, letting the lower abdomen expand with the breath, then filling the lower, middle and upper lungs. Exhale from the top of the lungs downward, drawing the navel to the spine as you complete the exhale. Allow each breath to become longer and deeper than the one before it. Feel each breath as it fills the body with energy, imagining each of your cells vibrating with renewed vitality. Continue for a few more minutes on your own. If your mind becomes preoccupied with thoughts, then bring your awareness to the sound of the breath as it comes in ... and goes out. Listen to the breath as though you are listening to the waves of the ocean slowly coming in and going out. Watch your thoughts as though from a distance without involving yourself with them or giving them energy. Keep your awareness on the focus of the eyes upwards between the eyebrows and on the feeling and sound of the breath. Now gently inhale and straighten your spine. Hold your breath for a few seconds. Exhale. (Total is 3 minutes of left nostril breathing.)

3) Relax your right hand on your knee and bring your left hand up to block the left nostril by placing your thumb against the side of the nostril. Begin slow, long, deep breathing through the right nostril. As you inhale feel the lower abdomen expanding completely and then let the breath fill the lower, middle and upper lungs. Exhale in reverse, drawing the navel towards the spine as you complete the exhale. Notice each breath becoming longer and deeper than the one before it. Imagine you can feel the energy of the breath permeating the whole of the body, bringing vitality to each cell. Notice where you experience tension within your body and release some of it with each exhale. (*Pause*) Relax your shoulders ... neck ... jaw ... and forehead. Listen to the sound of the breath and allow it to fill your awareness rather than giving energy to your

thoughts. Feel the breath as it fills the lungs. Keep your awareness on the sensations within your body. Continue slow, long deep breathing. Now inhale deeply, straighten your spine and hold your breath for a few seconds. Exhale and relax your left hand down on to your knee. (Total 3 minutes of right nostril breathing.)

4) Raise your right hand and block the right nostril with your thumb. Inhale very slowly through the left nostril. Use your little finger to block off the left nostril as you exhale through the right nostril. Continue to inhale through the left … and exhale through the right. Inhale left … exhale right. Feel the abdomen fill as you inhale. Let it fall gently as you exhale. Keep your eyes gazing up between the eyebrows. Listen to the sound of the breath as though it is an ocean wave coming in … and going out. Allow the energy of the breath to fill the whole body, going particularly to those places that need healing. Relax any areas of tension. Let tension dissolve with each exhale. Now inhale deeply, straighten your spine, and hold your breath for a few seconds. Exhale and relax your hand down on your knee. (Total 3 minutes of alternate nostril breathing.)

5) Raise your left hand and block the left nostril with your thumb. Inhale slowly through the right nostril. Use your little finger to block the right nostril as you exhale through the left. Continue with slow, long deep breathing, inhaling through the right nostril … exhaling through the left. Listen to the sensations within your body. Relax any tension wherever you experience it. Expand the abdomen fully with the inhale, let it fall gently with the exhale. Keep your mind focused on the feeling and sound of the breath rather than becoming distracted by thoughts. Enjoy this long deep breathing for a little longer. Imagine that the breath is your nourishment, totally filling the whole body, healing any areas of weakness or disharmony. Now inhale, straighten your spine, and hold your breath for a few seconds. Exhale and relax your arm down. Keep your eyes closed and be still for a few seconds as you experience the benefits of this relaxation. (Total 3 minutes of alternate nostril breathing.)

Summary:
3 minutes left nostril breathing
3 minutes right nostril breathing
3 minutes inhale left, exhale right
3 minutes inhale right, exhale left
slow your breath down to 3–5 breaths per minute

Kundalini Yoga Exercises for Balancing the Pineal Gland

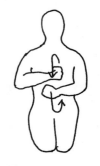

The following exercises are used in Kundalini Yoga to balance the pineal gland. They can be done anytime, alone or in sequence, but may be more effective if practiced before bed. As far as I know, they have not yet been subjected to clinical research but come from a yogic tradition which has existed for thousands of years.

1) Sit on your heels. If you are flexible enough, bring the heels to the sides of the buttocks with the knees spread apart, so your buttocks rest on the floor. This is called celibate pose. Place your thumbs on the mounds beneath the little fingers of each hand and close the fingers over the thumbs in a fist. Place the fists in front of your chest and rotate them rapidly around each other, making circles away from the body. Keep your eyes open, gazing down steadily at your rotating hands. Move them as fast as possible, so your hands become a blur. Continue for 1 1/2 minutes.[147]

2) Sit cross-legged. Place the left hand at the heart center in the center of the chest, between your breasts, with the palm facing up and the little finger against your chest. Extend your right arm and hand 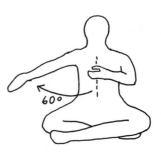 out in front of you parallel to the ground and out to the side at a 60 degree angle from the center of your body, with the palm facing down. Begin breath of fire from your navel for up to 7 minutes. Then inhale, hold your breath, and consciously squeeze all the muscles in your body. Exhale. Inhale deeply and hold the breath, spreading your fingers wide apart. Squeeze and tighten your whole body. Exhale. Inhale and squeeze again. Exhale and relax. Repeat this exercise the next day, using the opposite arm. Continue daily, for no more than 7 minutes at a time, using alternate arms each day.[148] Breath of fire is a breathing practice where you inhale, expanding the navel area and exhale,

is to pull the diaphragm down to increase the expansion of your lungs. The breathing is through your nose, working up to 2–3 breaths per second after accomplishing the rhythm. The inhale should equal the exhale in strength and intensity. Breath of fire acts to detoxify the blood, oxygenate the tissues, improve circulation of blood in the liver, strengthen the nervous system, and improve immunity.

▶ **Action for Prevention:** Practice the Alternate Nostril Series or Kundalini Yoga Exercises for increasing melatonin at least once daily, one hour before bedtime. If you are able to, practice it at another time in the day as well, perhaps upon rising. If you have breast cancer, practice this or other breathing or meditative exercises up to five times daily at two-hour intervals to increase melatonin levels and normalize

cell division. Combine these breathing breaks with the practice of visualization and prayer discussed in subsequent chapters to create a program that suits you. ◀

Summary

See Appendix 1: How to Manage Your Estrogen for a summary of the estrogen pathway. There are many interacting hormonal links to breast cancer and numerous ways that we can achieve hormonal balance to decrease risk through lifestyle and dietary changes and naturopathic support. The need to do so is even more pressing when we consider the impact our increasingly toxic environment has on our endocrine system — and thus our breast health.

Further Reading

Austin, S. and Cathy Hitchcock. *Breast Cancer: What You Should Know (But May Not Be Told) About Prevention, Diagnosis and Treatment.* Rocklin, CA: Prima Publishing, 1994.

Love, S. *Dr. Susan Love's Breast Book.* New York, NY: Addison-Wesley Publishing Co., 1995.

Rossi, Ernest. *The Psychobiology of Mind-Body Healing.* New York, NY: W.W. Norton, 1986.

Rossi, Ernest. *The 20 Minute Break.* Los Angeles, CA: Jeremy P. Tarcher Inc., 1991.

Singh, R. *Self-Healing: Powerful Techniques.* London, ON: Health Psychology Associates, 1997.

Weed, S. *Breast Cancer? Breast Health!.* Woodstock, NY: Ash Tree Publishing, 1996.

References

1. Cos S., E.J. Sanchez-Barcelo. Melatonin inhibition of MCF-7 human breast-cancer cells growth: influence of cell proliferation rate. *Cancer Lett*, 1995;Jul 13(2):207-12.
2. Aeron Laboratory estrogen profile information sheet, 1999.
3. Meyer, F., et al. Endogenous sex hormones, prolactin, and breast cancer in premenopausal women. *J Natl Cancer Inst*, 1986 Sep;77(3):613-6.
4. Katzenellenbogen, B.S. Biology and receptor interactions of estriol and estriol derivatives in vitro and in vivo. *J Steroid Biochem*, 1984, Apr;20(4B):1033-7.
5. Follingstead, A.H., Estriol: The forgotten estrogen? *JAMA*, Jan. 2, 1978; 239,1:29-30.
6. Lee, John R. *What Your Doctor May Not Tell You About Menopause.* New York, NY: Warner Books Inc., 1996:209.
7. Fractionated Estrogen, 1998. Handout from Meridian Valley Clinical Laboratory.
8. Zumoff, B. Hormone profiles in hormone-dependent cancers. *Cancer Res*, 1975;35:3365.
9. Lemon, H.M. Pathophysiologic considerations in the treatment of menopausal patients with oestrogens: the role of oestriol in the prevention of mammary carcinoma. *Acta Endocrinol (Copenh)*, 1980;233:S17-S27.
10. Longcope, C. Estriol production and metabolism in normal women. *J Steroid Biochemistry*, 1984;20:959-962.
11. Dewaillly, E, et al. Could the rising levels of estrogen receptors in breast cancer be due to estrogenic pollutants? *Journal of the National Cancer Institute*, 1997;89(12):888.
12. Davis, D. L. & H. Bradlow. Can environmental estrogens cause breast cancer? *Scientific American*, Oct. 1995:168.
13. Ho, GH, XW Luo, CY Ji, EH Ng. Urinary 2/16 alpha-hydroxyestrone ratio: correlation with a serum insulin-like growth factor binding protein-3 and a potential marker of breast cancer risk. *Annual Acad Med Singapore*, 1998. Mar;27(2):294-99.
14. Schneider, J., D. Kinne, A. Fracchia, et al. *Proceedings of the National Academy of Sciences*, 1982;79:3047-51.
15. Michnovicz, J. *How to Reduce Your Risk of Breast Cancer.* New York, NY: Warner Books, 1994:82.

16. Davis, D. L. & H. Bradlow. Can environmental estrogens cause breast cancer? *Scientific American*, Oct. 1995:168.

17. Pizzorno, J., and M. Murray. *A Textbook of Natural Medicine.* Seattle, WA:John Bastyr College Publications,1987: IV-2 Immune Support.

18. Davis, D.L., & H. Bradlow. Can environmental estrogens cause breast cancer? *Scientific American*, Oct. 1995:168.

19. Gorbach, S. Estrogens, breast cancer and intestinal flora. *Rev Infect Dis 6* (Suppl I), 1984:S85.

20. Goldin, B. Estrogen excretion patterns and plasma levels in vegetarian and omnivorous women. *N Engl J Med* 1982;307:1542.

21. Goldin, B. Estrogen excretion patterns and plasma levels in vegetarian and omnivorous women. *N Engl J Med* 1982;307:1542.

22. Goldin, B. Estrogen excretion patterns and plasma levels in vegetarian and omnivorous women. *N Engl J Med* 1982;307:1542.

23. Cohen, L.A., et al. Wheat bran and psyllium diets: Effects on N-methylnitrosoura-induced mammary tumorigenesis in F344 rats. *J Natl Cancer Inst.* 1996 Jul;88(13):899-907.

24. Waalaszek, Z., et al. Dietary glucarate as anti-promoter of 7,12-dimethylben(a)anthracene-induced mammary tumorigenesis. *Carcinogenesis.* 1986 Sep;7(9):1463-66.

25. Personal communication from Hope Nemiroff regarding an unpublished Sloan-Kettering study.

26. Lemon, H.M. Pathophysiologic consideration in the treatment of menopausal patients with oestrogens; the role of oestriol in the prevention of mammary carcinoma. *Acta Endocrinol(Copenh)*, 1980;233:S17-S27.

27. Head, K. Estriol: Safety and efficacy. *Alternative Medicine Review.* 1998;3(2):101-13.

28. Pratt, J.H., C. Longcope. Estriol production rates and breast cancer. *J Clin Endocrinol Metab*, 1978;46:44-47.

29. Lemon, H.M. et al. Reduced estriol excretion in patients with breast cancer prior to endocrine therapy. *JAMA*, April 21,1978;249(16):1638-41.

30. Ungar, Susan. What about estriol? *Menopause News*, March/April 1998 Vol.8 Issue 2, Madison Pharmacy Associates Inc.

31. More about that 1 in 8 breast cancer statistic, *Health Facts*, May, 1993.

32. Clavel-Chapelon, F., G. Launoy, A. Auquier et al. Reproductive factors and breast cancer risk. Effect of age at diagnosis. *Ann Epidemiol,* 1995;5:315-20.

33. Kagawa, Y. Impact of westernization on the nutrition of the Japanese: Changes in physique, cancer, longevity and centenarians. *Prev Med J*, 1978;7:205.

34. Frommer, D. Changing age of menopause. *Br Med J*, 1964;2:349.

35. Armstrong, B. Diet and reproductive hormones: a study of vegetarian and non-vegetarian post-menopausal women. *JNCI*, 1981;67:761.

36. Staszewski, J. Age at menarche and breast cancer. *J Natl Cancer Inst*, 1971;47:935.

37. Trichopoulos, D. Menopause and breast cancer risk. *J Natl Cancer Inst*, 1972;48:605.

38. National Research Council. *Biomarkers in Reproductive Toxicology.* Washington, DC: National Academy of Sciences, 1991.

39. *Rachel's Environment and Health Weekly.* Environment Research Foundation, Oct. 2, 1997, #566.

40. Herman-Giddens, M., et al. Secondary sexual characteristics and menses in young girls seen in office practice: A study from the pediatric research in office settings network. *Pediatrics*, 1997;99(4):505-12.

41. MacMahon, B, D. Trichopoulos, D. Brown et al. Age at menarche, urine estrogens and breast cancer risk. *Int J Cancer*, 1982;30:427-31.

42. Stoll, B.A. Western diet, early puberty, and breast cancer risk. *Breast Cancer Research and Treatment*, 1998;49:187-93.

43. Apter, F., M. Reinila, R. Vikho. Some endocrine characteristics of early menarche, a risk factor for breast cancer, are preserved into adulthood. *Int J Cancer*, 1989;44:783-87.

44. Boyce, Nell. Growing up too soon. *New Scientist*, Aug. 2, 1997:5.

45. Apter, D, I. Sipila. Development of children and adolescents; physiological, pathophysiological and therapeutic aspects. *Curr Opin Obstet Gynec*, 1993;51:764-73.

46. Stoll, B.A. et al. Does early physical maturity increase breast cancer risk? *Acta Oncologica*, 1994;33(2); 171-76.

47. Apter, D. Hormonal events during female puberty in relation to breast cancer risk. *European Journal of Cancer*, 1996;5(6):476-82.

48. Brown, H. The other reward of exercise. *Health*, July, 1994.

49. Whelan, E. Menstruation and reproductive history study. *American Journal of Epidemiology*, December 15, 1994.

50. Pill ups cancer risk in young women. *Science News*, June 10, 1995.

51. Oral contraceptive use and breast cancer risk in young women. *Lancet*, 1989:973-82.

52. Rinzler, C. *Estrogen and Breast Cancer: A Warning to Women.* Macmillan.1993.

53. Stanford, J. & D. Thomas. Exogenous estrogens and breast cancer. *Epidemiological Reviews*, 1993;15(1):98-105.

54. Beral, V., D. Bull, R. Doll, T. Key, R. Peto, G. Reeves. Breast cancer and hormone replacement therapy: collaborative reanalysis of data from 51 epidemiological studies of 52,705 women with breast cancer and 108,411 women without breast cancer. *Lancet*, 1997;350:1047-58, 1042-1043.

55. Stabiner, Karen. What price pregnancy? *Good Housekeeping*, July, 1998:100-03.

56. *National Women's Health Network News*, May/June 1990.

57. Colborn, Theo, D. Dumanoski, J. Peterson Myers. *Our Stolen Future.* New York, NY: Penguin, 1996:65.

58. Ekbom, A., D. Trichopoulous, et al. Evidence of prenatal influences on breast cancer risk. *Lancet*, 1992;340:1015-18.

59. Hsieh, C., S. Lan, A. Ekbom, E. Petridou, and H. Adami. (1992) Twin membership and breast cancer risk. *American Journal of Epidemiology*, 136:1321-26.

60. Colborn, Theo, D. Dumanoski, J. Peterson Myers. *Our Stolen Future*. New York, NY: Penguin, 1996:75-80.

61. Setchell, K., L. Zimmer-Nchemias, J. Cai, J. Heubi. Exposure of infants to phyto-oestrogens from soy-based infant formula. *Lancet*, July 5, 1997;350:23-27.

62. Cowan, L.D., L. Gordis, J. A. Tonasia, and G,S, Jones. Breast cancer incidence in women with a history of progesterone deficiency. *American Journal of Epidemiology*, 1981;114:209-17.

63. Lee, John R. *What Your Doctor May Not Tell You About Menopause*. New York, NY: Time Warner, Inc., 1996:323.

64. Foster, W.G., et al. Hexachlorobenzene (HCB) suppresses circulating progesterone concentrations during the luteal phase in the cynomolgus monkey. *J Appl Toxicol*, 1992;12:13-17.

65. Bergkvist, L., H.-O. Adami, I. Persson, R. Hoover, and C. Schairer. The risk of breast cancer after estrogen and estrogen-progestin replacement. *New England Journal of Medicine*, 1989;321:293-97.

66. Jato, I. Neoadjuvant progesterone therapy for primary breast cancer: rationale for clinical trial. *Clinical Therapies*, 1997;19(1):56-61, discussion 2-3.

67. Formby, B., T.S. Wiley. Bcl-2, survivin, and variant CD44 v7-v10 are downregulated and p53 is upregulated in breast cancer cells by progesterone: inhibition of cell growth and induction of apoptosis. *Mol Cell Biochem*, 1999 Dec;202(1-2):53-61.

68. Wiebe, J.P. et al. The 4-pregnene and 5alpha-pregnane progesterone metabolites formed in nontumorous and tumorous breast tissue have opposite effects on breast proliferation and adhesion. *Cancer Research*, 2000 Feb 15;60(4):936-43.

69. Personal communication with Gottfried Kellerman of DiagnosTech International Inc., Jan. 2000.

70. Zava, D., C. Dullbaum, M. Blen. Estrogen and progestin bioactivity of foods, herbs and spices. *Biol Med*, 1998;217(3):369-78.

71. Holmes, P. *The Energetics of Western Herbs*. Vol. II. 2nd. ed. Berkeley, CA: NatTrop Publishing, 1993:753.

72. Erichsen-Brown, C. *Medicinal and Other Uses of North American Plants: A Historical Survey with Special References to the Eastern Indian Tribes*. New York, NY: Dover Publications, Inc., 1995.

73. Zava, D., C. Dullbaum, M. Blen. Estrogen and progestin bioactivity of foods, herbs and spices. *Biol Med*, 1998;217(3):369-78.

74. Reichert, R., Comparing Vitex and vitamin B6 for PMS. *Quarterly Review of Natural Medicine*, 1998;19-20

75. Weed, Susun. *Menopausal Years - The Wise Woman Way*. Woodstock, NY: Ash Tree Publishing, 1992:107-08.

76. Nutrition Research News. *Nutrition Science News*. 1997;2(8):410.

77. Reichert, R., Comparing Vitex and vitamin B6 for PMS. *Quarterly Review of Natural Medicine*. 1998;19-20

78. Carr, C. Keep your (hormonal) balance. *Conscious Choice: The Journal of Ecology and Natural Living*, 1998;11(2):55.

79. Kamada et al. Effect of dietary selenium supplementaion on the plasma progesterone concentration in cows. *Journal of Veterinary Medicine and Science*, 1998;60(1):133-35.

80. Brun, J., B. Claustrat, M. David. Urinary melatonin, LH, oestradiol, progesterone excretion during the menstrual cycle or in women taking oral contraceptives. *Acta Endocrinol (Copenh)*, 1987, Sept;116(1):145-9.

81. Tetau, Max. Folliculinum and the premenstrual syndrome. *Dolisos Newsletter*, #10.

82. McMichael-Phillips, D.F., et al. Effects of soy supplementation on epithelial proliferation in the histologically normal human breast. *American Journal of Clinical Nutrition*. 1998;68(6 Suppl):1431S-1435S.

83. Meyer, F., et al. Endogenous sex hormones, prolactin, and breast cancer in premenopausal women. *J Natl Cancer Inst*, 1986 Sep;77(3):613-16.

84. Meyer, F., et al. Endogenous sex hormones, prolactin, and mammographic features of breast tissue in premenopausal women. *J Natl Cancer Inst*, 1986 Sep;77(3):617-20.

85. Zumoff, B. Hormonal profiles in women with breast cancer. *Obstet Gynecol Clin North Am*, 1994 Dec;21(4):751-72.

86. Kleinberg, D.L., W. Ruan, V. Catanese et al. Non-lactogenic effects of growth hormone on growth and IGF-1 messenger mRNA of rat mammary gland. *Endocrinology*, 1990;126:3274-76.

87. Darendeliler, F., P.C. Hindmarsh, M.A. Preece. Growth hormone increases rate of pubertal maturation. *Acta Endocrinol*, 1990;122:414-16.

88. Sharara, F.J., L.C. Giudice. Role of growth hormone in ovarian physiology and onset of puberty. *J Soc Gyne Invest*, 1997;4:2-7.

89. The Doctor's Medical Library. Wilson's Reverse T3 Dominance Syndrome. http://www.medicallibrary.net/sites/-wilson's-syndrome.html. Jan. 15, 1999.

90. Diogo, A., C. Merluza, B. Janczak. Thyroid function and breast cancer. Toronto, ON: *Canadian College of Naturopathic Medicine*, April, 1999.

91. Lee, J. *What Your Doctor May Not Tell You About Menopause*. New York, NY: Warner Books, 1996,146-47.

92. Rose, D.P. Plasma triiodothyronine concentrations and breast cancer. *Cancer*, 1979;43(4):1434-38.

93. Rasmussen, B., et al. Thyroid function in patients with breast cancer. *Eur J Cancer Clin Oncol*, 1986;22(3):301-07.

94. Lemaire, M., L. Baugnet-Mahieu. Thyroid function in women with breast cancer. *Eur J Cancer Clin Oncol*, 1986;22(3):301-07.

95. Kohrle, J. The trace element selenium and the thyroid gland. *Biochimie*, 1999, May;81(5):527-33.

96. Gerson, Max. *A Cancer Therapy: Results of Fifty Cases*. 3rd ed. Del Mar, CA: Totality Books, 1977:100

97. Holmes, P. *The Energetics of Western Herbs*. Vol. I. 2nd. ed. Berkeley, CA: NatTrop Publishing, 1993: 389-414.

98. Colborn, Theo, D. Dumanoski, J. Peterson Myers. *Our Stolen Future.* New York, NY: Penguin, 1996:75-80, 188.

99. Colborn, Theo, D. Dumanoski, J. Peterson Myers. *Our Stolen Future.* New York, NY: Penguin, 1996:75-80, 188.

100. Colborn, Theo, D. Dumanoski, J. Peterson Myers. *Our Stolen Future.* New York, NY: Penguin, 1996:75-80, 154.

101. Aziz, Laurel. The endpoint. *Equinox.* 1998; April/May:53.

102. Capen, C.C. Mechanisms of chemical injury to the thyroid gland. *Prog Clin Biol Res.* 1994;387:173-91.

103. Arnot, Bob. *The Breast Cancer Prevention Diet.* New York, NY: Little, Brown and Co., 1998:96.

104. Stoll, B.A. Western nutrition and the insulin resistance syndrome. *Eur J Clin Nutr*, 1999;Feb;53(2):83-7.

105. Bereket, A., C.H. Lang, T.A. Wilson. Alterations in the growth hormone-insulin-like growth factor axis in insulin dependent diabetes mellitus. *Hormon Metab Res*, 1999,Feb-Mar;31(2-3):172-81.

106. Shim M., P. Cohen. IGFs and human cancer: Implications regarding the risk of growth hormone therapy. *Hormone Research*, 1999, Nov;51 Suppl S3:42-51.

107. Clarke, R.B. et al. Type 1 IGF receptor gene expression in normal breast tissue treated with oestrogen and progesterone. *Br J Cancer*, 1997;75:251-57.

108. Stoll, B.A. Western diet, early puberty, and breast cancer risk. *Breast Cancer Research and Treatment.* 1998;49:187-93.

109. Macaulay, V.M. Insulin like growth factor and cancer. *Br J Cancer*, 1992;65:311-20.

110. Westley, B.R., F.E. May. Role of IGF in steroid-modulated proliferation. *J Ster Biochem Mol Biol.* 1994; 51:1-9.

111. Vadgama, J.V., Y. Yu, G. Datta, H. Khan, R. Chillar. Plasma insulin-like growth factor-1 and serum IGF-binding protein 3 can be associated with the progression of breast cancer, and predict the risk of recurrence and the probability of survival in African-American and Hispanic women. *Oncology*, 1999, Nov;57(4):330-40.

112. Oh, Y. IGFBPs and neoplastic models. New concepts for roles of IGFBPs in regulation of cancer cell growth. *Endocrine*, 1997, Aug;7(1):111-13.

113. Yu, H., J. Berkel. Do insulin-like growth factors mediate the effect of alcohol on breast cancer risk? *Med Hypotheses*, 1999;Jun;52(6):491-96.

114. Demori, I., C. Bottazzi, E. Fugassa. Tri-iodothyronine increases insulin-like growth factor binding protein-2 expression in cultured hepatocytes from hypothyroid rats. *J Endocrinol.* 1999;161(3):465-74.

115. Hankinson, S. et al. Circulating concentrations of insulin-like growth factor-1 and risk of breast cancer. *Lancet*, 1998;351:1393-96.

116. Gupta, D., R. Attanasio & R. Reiter. (Eds.) *The Pineal Gland and Cancer.* Tubingen, Germany: Muller and Bass, 1988.

117. Hajdu, S., R. Porro, P. Lieberman & F. Foote. Degeneration of the pineal gland of patients with cancer. *Cancer*, 1972;29:706-09.

118. Lissoni, P., S. Crispino, S. Barni et al. Pineal gland and tumour cell kinetics: serum labelling rate in breast cancer. *Oncology*, 1990;47:3:275-77.

119. Lissoni, P. et al. Melatonin as a modulator of cancer endocrine therapy. *Front Horm Res.* 1997;23:132-36.

120. Coss, G. Influence of melatonin on invasive and metastatic properties of MCF-7 human breast cancer cells. *Cancer Research*, 1998;58(19):4383-90.

121. Bartsch, C., H. Bartsch, U. Fuchs, et al. Stage-dependent depression of melatonin in patients with primary breast cancer. *Cancer*, 1989;64:426-33.

122. Lissoni, P. et al. Clinical study of melatonin in untreatable advanced cancer patients. *Tumouri*, 1987;73: 475.

123. Lissoni, P., S. Barni, S. Meregalli et al. Modulation of cancer endocrine therapy by melatonin: A phase II study of tamoxifen plus melatonin in metastatic breast cancer patients progression under tamoxifen alone. *Br. J. Cancer*, 1995;71:854-56.

124. Bartsch, H., C. Bartsch. Effect of melatonin on experimental tumours under different photoperiods and times of administration. *J. Neural. Transm*, 1981;52:269-79.

125. Murphy, C., L. Tettamanti Ratvay. Melatonin reduces breast cancer risk. Toronto, ON: *Canadian College of Naturopathic Medicine*, April 2000:3

126. Bartsch, C., H. Bartsch. The link between the pineal gland and cancer: an interaction involving chronobiological mechanisms. In Halberg, F. et al. *Chronobiological Approach to Social Medicine.* Rome,Italy: Istitiuto Italiano di Medicina Sociale, 1984:105-26.

127. MacPhee, A., F. Cole, F. Rice. The effect of melatonin on steroidogenesis by the human ovary in vitro. *J Clin Endocrin Metab*, 1975;40:688-96.

128. Wetterberg, L., J. Arendt, L. Paunier et al. Human serum melatonin changes during the menstrual cycle. *J Clin Endocrin Metab*, 1976;42:185-88.

129. Blask, D., S. Wilson, F. Zalatan. Physiological melatonin inhibition of human breast cancer cell growth in vitro: Evidence for a glutathione-mediated pathway. *Cancer Res*, 1997;57:1909-14.

130. Tamarkin, L., C.J. Baird, O. Almeida. Melatonin: A coordinating signal for mammalian reproduction? *Science*, 1985;227:714-20.

131. Singh, R. *Self-Healing: Powerful Techniques.* London, ON: Health Psychology Associates, 1997:29-30.

132. Singh, R., *Self-Healing: Powerful Techniques.* London, ON: Health Psychology Associates, 1997: 27.

133. Marz, Russell B. *Medical Nutrition from Marz.* Portland, OR: Omni-Press, 1997:96.

134. Pennington, Jean. *Food Values of Portions Commonly Used.* 15th edition. New York, NY: HarperPerennial, 1989: 219-57.

135. Dubbels, R. et al. Melatonin in edible plants identified by radioimmunoassay and by high performance liquid chromatography-mass spectrometry. *J. Pineal Research*, 1995;18:28-31.

136. Singh, R. *Self-Healing: Powerful Techniques*. London, ON: Health Psychology Associates, 1997.

137. Murch, S, C. Simmons, P. Saxena. Melatonin in feverfew and other medicinal plants. *The Lancet*, 350, Nov. 29,1997:1598-99.

138. Singh, R. *Self-Healing: Powerful Techniques*. London, ON: Health Psychology Associates, 1997:5.

139. Laakso, M.L. et al. Twenty-four hour patterns of pineal melatonin and pituitary and plasma prolactin in male rats under "natural" and artificial lighting conditions. *Neuroendocrinology*, 1988 Sep;48(3):308-13.

140. Carr, D.B., Reppert, S.M. et al. Plasma melatonin increases during exercise in women. *J Clin Endocrinol Metab*, 1981 Jul;53(1): 224-25.

141. Rossi, E. *The Psychobiology of Mind-Body Healing*. New York, NY: W.W. Norton, 1986.

142. Shannahoff-Khalsa, D.S., M.R. Boyle, M.E. Buebel. The effects of unilateral forced nostril breathing on cognition. *Int J Neurosci*, 1991;Apr;57(3-4):239-49.

143. Werntz, D.A., R.G, Bickford, D. Shannahoff-Khalsa. Selective hemispheric stimulation by unilateral forced nostril breathing. *Hum Neurobiol*, 1987;6(3):165-71.

144. Massion, A.O., et al. Meditation, melatonin and breast/prostate cancer: hypothesis and preliminary data. *Med Hypothesis*, 1995 Jan;44 (1):39-46.

145. Used with permission from the United Nations Environment Programme, United Nations, New York, NY.

146. Bhajan, Yogi. *Sadhana Guidelines for Kundalini Yoga Daily Practise*. Los Angeles, CA: Kundalini Research Institute, 1996. This series of exercises is adapted from the Basic Breath Series on p. 81.

147. Bhajan, Yogi. *Healing through Kundalini: Specific Applications*. Compiled by Vikram Kaur Khalsa and Alice Clagett. Eugene, OR, p.46. This exercise was derived from a yoga set given at a Winter Solstice celebration in Florida in the early 1980s.

148. Bhajan, Yogi. *The Science of Keeping Up, Vol.II, No. 2*. January, 1996:8. The exercise was taught by Yogi Bhajan in Los Angeles on April 7, 1995 as a 7 minute meditation for the pituitary and pineal.

CHAPTER

4

Environmental Impact on Breast Health

Exercises

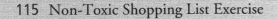

Contents

Margaret Mead once declared, "Never doubt that a small group of thoughtful citizens can change the world. Indeed, it's the only thing that ever has." We need such small groups to counteract the impact of radiation, electricity, petrochemicals, chlorinated chemicals, and formaldehyde on our environment — and on ourselves.

Radiation

Radiation contributes significantly to breast cancer development. Breast tissue is sensitive to radiation, particularly during the childbearing years; in fact, the breasts are the body tissue most sensitive to the cancer-causing effects of radiation.[1] The effects of radiation are cumulative and may manifest as cancer for at least 40 years after exposure. Possible sources of radiation include nuclear fallout from weapons testing, fission materials from nuclear power plants, leaking radioactive disposal sites, flying at high altitudes, mammograms and x-rays. Even the lowest level of radiation can cause cancer in susceptible individuals. There is no level that is safe.[2] Every exposure to radiation carries increased risk and higher levels of radiation cause higher incidences of cancer. Younger people are more sensitive to radiation and are more likely to die of cancer because of it. Radiation exerts a greater effect when absorbed into the developing breasts of young women 8–20 years old. When a woman receives significant radiation before the age of 20, she is more likely to be diagnosed with breast cancer before the age of 35.[3]

Nuclear Testing and Generation

When the U.S. government tested nuclear weapons in the 1950s, they put the American population at risk. When Dr Carl Johnson compared cancer incidence in women, he found that those living in the fallout path from the Nevada test site had double the incidence of breast cancer after the testing (between 1967–1975) as compared to before the testing (1951).[4] Exposure to radiation acts synergistically with environmental estrogens to increase risk significantly.[5,6,7,8] In Russia in the 1940s and '50s, nearly 500 nuclear tests were carried out in the area of present day Kazakstan. As many as 150 were above ground. The Soviet military deliberately used villagers as guinea pigs to test the potential impact of nuclear war. More than 1.2 million people were adversely affected by the testing and the horror continues in the gene pool of its survivors. In 1997, nearly 500 out of every 1,000 babies born in the city of Semipalatinsk had some form of birth defect or health problem, and 47 of them died. Birth defects have gone up four times in the last four years. Horribly deformed children are abandoned by parents unable to cope. One fetus had only one eye in the center of its forehead; another was born with four arms and four legs, but died shortly after birth. In some areas infant mortality has grown fivefold since 1950. Ninety percent of the people living near the test site suffer from immune deficiency, many of them afflicted with tuberculosis, cancer or blood diseases. Mental disability and suicide are common. The area is close to economic collapse.[9] This is the legacy of nuclear testing.

When the Three Mile Island reactor began to leak radiation, breast cancer rates increased in five counties adjacent to it with the incidence seven times higher than rates in similar rural areas.[10] San Francisco area white women have one of the highest breast cancer rates in the world: breast cancer activists in the area believe that their increased susceptibility to the disease is linked to leakage from radioactive material at the Livermore National Laboratory nuclear site, which is situated close to earthquake fault lines.[11] Breast cancer rates are high in the Great Lakes region, possibly due to the combination of proximity to nuclear reactors and abundance of hormone-disrupting chemicals. Greenpeace maintains that between 1972 and 1991 more than 29 trillion picocuries (equal to the radiation released from two Three Mile Island disasters) of radioactive elements were released into the Great Lakes ecosystem.[12]

In 1991, the U.S. used depleted uranium, or DU, a toxic nuclear waste material, to coat missiles and bullets used in Operation Desert Storm during the Gulf War. Approximately 630,000 pounds of DU were fired in the gulf in 1991. Since the Gulf War, Iraq has had a sixfold increase in cancers, possibly linked to the use of DU. There has been a particularly high increase in childhood leukemias. Depleted uranium bursts into flames once it hits its target and spreads radioactive dust in its wake. The dust remains radioactive for 4,500 million years. Because of the prevailing north-south winds, this radioactive dust is being blown into Saudi Arabia and Kuwait where there are also rises in cancer incidence. In time, it will make its way around the globe. Depleted uranium is now recycled and used in weapons manufacturing by at least 14 countries, including Britain, France, Russia, Greece, Turkey, Israel, Saudi Arabia, Kuwait, Egypt, and Pakistan.[13]

The Deloro mine site, near Marmora, Ontario, is one of the worst disaster areas in the province, if not in North America. When the United States was first developing the atomic bomb, American officials had the excess waste dumped at the Canadian site. Canadian waste from the Eldorado Nuclear uranium refinery in Port Hope, Ontario was also shipped there. For 50 years an insecticide manufacturer used the site, leaving behind tons of deadly arsenic. This mix of toxic waste is poisoning the Moira River, which runs through the area to neighboring communities, into Lake Ontario and down the St Lawrence River to the Atlantic Ocean.[14] No doubt many countries in the world could name similar sites on their own soil, most of them kept shrouded in secrecy and denial. It is our collective task to name these sites and demand clean-up to the best of our abilities.

One of the ways to assess exposure to radiation is by measuring strontium-90 in the baby teeth of children. The "Tooth Fairy Project" has been doing that for children in the U.S. and Canada. Their findings indicate that children whose teeth contain a lot of radioactive material live in areas with high breast cancer rates. Children born after 1990 show some of the highest levels of radioactive materials since the early 1960s when atomic bombs were tested in the atmosphere. Children who live downwind from nuclear power reactors in the path of their 'plumes' of radiation have more radioactive material in their teeth. Some of these children are exhibiting a higher-than-normal rate of rhabdomyosarcoma, a rare form of bone cancer. Vegetables grown in these areas and dairy products also are more radioactive than normal.[15] The Tooth Fairy Project needs thousands of teeth from the U.S.A. and Canada to make their study complete. Anyone interested in sending baby teeth to the Tooth Fairy Project can visit the web site www.radiation.org for instructions.

Frequent Flying

Frequent flying is a source of excess radiation that may increase breast cancer risk. Indeed, there is an observed increased incidence of breast cancer in flight attendants.[16] If we are at high risk for breast cancer, we should limit the number of times we fly annually to less than three. A jet flight of six hours exposes us to 5 millirads of radiation (a chest x-ray exposes us to 16 millirads).

X-rays and Mammograms

We cannot ignore the radiation that women receive during mammograms as a contributing cause of breast cancer. The smallest dose of radiation from a single screening mammogram is 340 millirads, and usually four mammograms are done to complete a series. Mammography is especially risky for younger women, since it can take up to 40 or more years for a cancer to appear after radiation exposure. Although useful as a diagnostic procedure, mammography will also cause death because of its use. It is a very difficult issue. Until other diagnostic tests are accessible, mammography will continue to be used. For some women, it will detect cancer at an earlier stage so that treatment is more effective. For others, it will be one more onslaught to already vulnerable breasts that may tip the scales towards cancer. On the one hand, a Canadian study of almost 90,000 women aged 40–49 at 15 hospitals across Canada found a 30–50% increase in deaths from breast cancer among women over 40 who had annual mammograms versus those who were given only physical exams.[17] On the other hand, women between the ages of 50 and 69 benefit from regular mammograms with a 29% reduction in mortality compared to those who do not receive mammograms.[18] So what are we to do?

Sea vegetables offer us significant protection against radiation. They contain sodium alginate, which binds radioactive isotopes in the small intestine to form an insoluble salt which is then excreted. Two tablespoons daily can be considered a maintenance dose, while four times that amount can be used during or after direct exposure to radiation.[19] Sea vegetables include kelp, nori, wakame, hiziki, arame, kombu, and dulse. Those of us who live near nuclear reactors can be diligent about including sea vegetables in our diets and taking antioxidants regularly such as vitamins A, C, E, alpha lipoic acid, and the minerals zinc and selenium. Other foods that protect us from radiation are included in The Healthy Breast Diet chapter. These are cysteine-containing protein, beans and lentils, garlic, beets, whole grains, miso, powdered green supplements, orange vegetables, and flaxseed oil.

▶ **Action for Prevention:** We can insist that government and industry develop safe, renewable energy sources such as wind and solar power. We can reduce our energy consumption by building more energy-conserving homes and using fewer electrical devices. We can install our own wind and solar powered units wherever possible or buy power from those people who have done it for us. We can join a movement to ban all nuclear power and weapons testing, such as the Campaign for Nuclear Phaseout in Ottawa (tel. 613-789-3634). We can write to our politicians and object to the burning of plutonium fuel bundles at electrical generation sites such as the Bruce nuclear station on the shores of Lake Huron in southern Ontario.

Generally, pre-menopausal women should avoid mammograms unless a lump is present and breast cancer is suspected. A woman over age 50 with high risk factors should consider having a mammogram every one to two years but also listen to her intuition and her body's signals.

Thermography, the AMAS or Immunicon blood test, and the other diagnostic procedures described in Chapter 2 are useful alternatives to detect early cancers and pose no risk. We can protect ourselves somewhat from radiation by including the following foods in our diets: broccoli, cabbage, miso, vegetables high in carotenes (squash, carrots, yams, cantaloupe), burdock root, Reishi mushrooms, seaweed, lentils and other dried beans, and the trace mineral selenium (found in nettles, astragalus, kelp, burdock, and milk thistle seeds).[20] ◀

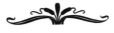

HOW DOES ONE WRITE ABOUT PLUTONIUM

plutonium sounds so innocent

like that soppy comic-book dog

but this is Pluto the God from Hell

coming soon

to a nuclear reactor near us

sniff only a little

of this alien green powder

and you die

these are leftovers

from the Cold War

coming here to chill us

I am not being melodramatic

I have read it

I have understood it

we have not been asked

we are betrayed

how dare they? how dare they?

Ontario Hydro is planning to burn uranium and plutonium fuel bundles at the Bruce Nuclear Plant by 2002. AECL claims that "public acceptance of burning plutonium is high in Canada." I don't remember being asked.

— Susan Gibson

Electricity and Electromagnetic Fields

Electricity and electromagnetic fields are linked to a higher incidence of breast cancer. Women who work in the electrical trade have a 38% greater risk of dying from breast cancer than other working women. The risk of female electrical engineers is 73% greater.[21,22] Shockingly, women who install, repair, or do line work with telephones have a risk 200 times more than average.[23] We are constantly bombarded with electromagnetic fields — house wiring, phone lines, computer terminals, TVs, refrigerators, hair dryers, electric blankets, clocks, ovens, and all electrical appliances are nagging sources, even the

little black boxes, or transformers, that come with your tape players, electric drills, etc. At a distance of two and one half feet from the source, electromagnetic fields are 80% less powerful. Computer video display monitors emit extremely low frequency magnetic fields that are probable human carcinogens. We should sit at least two feet away from the front of the monitor and stay at least four feet from the back or sides of another monitor. Proximity to video display monitors for prolonged periods during pregnancy has been associated with an increase in miscarriages. A newer threat to our health comes in the form of cell phones. Frequent use of cell phones has been linked to brain tumors.

Exposure to extra low frequency electromagnetic fields disturbs the normal growth pattern of cells by interfering with their hormonal, enzymatic, and chemical signals, causing DNA damage. These fields also reduce the production of melatonin by the pineal gland, which when deficient is linked to increased breast cancer. Sufficient melatonin acts to decrease the production of estrogen receptors, thus allowing lower levels of estrogen to get into the breast cell to initiate cancer. Long term exposure to power lines has also been linked to various cancers, including breast cancer, leukemia and childhood brain tumors.

▶ **Action for Prevention:** We can protect ourselves and our children by removing sources of extra low voltage electromagnetic fields from the bedroom, by moving our beds at least 2 1/2 feet away from electrical outlets, and by minimizing our proximity to them during the day. We and our children can stay the required distance from computer video display terminals (2 feet from the front; 4 feet from the sides), and minimize their use while pregnant (less than 20 hours per week). We can use less electricity and fewer of the modern electrical conveniences to conserve energy globally, decreasing our participation in the nuclear industry. (What can you live without? The dishwasher, the dryer, or the TV?) Turn off all electrical appliances when not in use. Buy a wind-up watch rather than one with a quartz crystal or battery — they too emit electromagnetic energy. Buy or rent a gauss meter and measure the electro-magnetic field emissions around your home. Keep work areas away from the place where electricity enters your home. Limit your use of cordless and cell phones to emergencies and brief conversations. ◀

Petrochemicals, Chlorinated Chemicals, and Formaldehyde

Petrochemicals, such as gasoline, kerosene, or those which include formaldehyde and benzene, also have been linked to breast cancer in animals.[24] Chlorinated chemicals are systematically added to gasoline and will produce dioxin when burned. Germany has banned the addition of such chlorinated chemicals to fuel in recognition of this health hazard. Other countries should do the same.

Products containing formaldehyde include adhesives, air deodorizers, antiperspirants, cellophane, concrete, cleaning solutions, contraceptive creams, cosmetics, detergents, disinfectants, dry-cleaning compounds, enamels,

To live content with small means,

to seek elegance rather than luxury,

and refinement rather than fashion,

to be worthy, not respectable, and wealthy, not rich,

to study hard, think quietly, talk gently, act frankly,

to listen to stars and birds, babes and sages,

with open heart,

to bear all cheerfully,

do all bravely,

await occasions,

hurry never —

in a word, to let the spiritual, unbidden and unconscious,

grow up through the common.

This is to be my symphony.

—William Ellery Channing

fabric finishes, fertilizers, finger paints, gas appliances, gelatin capsules, inks, insect repellent, urea formaldehyde insulation, carpets, laminating materials, lacquers, laundry starch, mouthwashes, nail polish, tempera paint, paper towels, particle board, perfume, pesticides, pharmaceuticals, photographic chemicals, photographic film, plaster, plastics, plywood, polyester fabric, rodent poison, shampoos, shoe polish, soaps, tobacco and tobacco smoke, toilet paper, toothpaste, wood stains, and preservatives.

▶ **Action for Prevention:** We can become aware of the products that contain formaldehyde and get them out of our homes as well as refrain from putting them on our bodies. Limit your exposure to petrochemicals, and insist that chlorine not be added to your fuel. Use your car less often, relying on public transportation, your bicycle, or your legs more often. Move your residence closer to your workplace or move more of your work into your home office. ◀

When despair for the world grows in me

and I wake in the night at the least sound

*in fear of what my life and
my children's lives may be,*

I go and lie down where the wood drake

*rests in his beauty on the water,
and the great heron feeds.*

I come into the peace of wild things

who do not tax their lives with forethought

of grief. I come into the presence of still water.

And I feel above me the day-blind stars

waiting with their light. For a time

I rest in the grace of the world, and am free.

— Wendell Berry

Organochlorines

Organochlorines are chemicals in which at least one atom of chlorine is bonded to a carbon molecule. Reacting chlorine gas with petroleum hydrocarbons produces many organochlorines. Today there are an estimated 11,000 different organochlorines being used, specifically in plastics, pesticides, solvents, dry cleaning agents, refrigerants, and other chemicals.[25]

Unfortunately, thousands more organochlorines are formed as by-products of chlorine-based industries. These include the bleaching of pulp for paper, the disinfecting of water, and the incinerating of waste containing chlorinated products. Chlorinated dioxin is one such by-product. Although chlorine is abundant in nature in its stable ionic form, the elemental chlorine that the chemical industry produces does not occur naturally. Industry first began producing organochlorines in the early 1900s; now about 40 million tons are manufactured yearly worldwide. No organochlorines are known to occur naturally in the tissues of humans, other mammals, or terrestrial vertebrates.

The pie chart below, reprinted by permission from Greenpeace, shows which substances contain organochlorines and in what proportions.

Perished

Organochlorines are problematic for several reasons. Use the acronym PERISHED to remember the first word of each of these reasons. Spread the word.

1) **Persistent.** They are stable molecules and resist breakdown in the environment for decades or centuries. Chloroform persists in the environment for over 1000 years before breaking down.

2) **Environmental loading.** Because they don't easily break down, organochlorines steadily accumulate in the global environment and are dispersed worldwide through air and water.

3) **Remain in our tissues for life.** Our bodies and the bodies of other species have not evolved ways of breaking them down and eliminating them. Therefore, they generally remain in our tissues for life unless specific, intensive methods are taken to eliminate them, such as periods of breast-feeding and intense use of saunas.

4) **Increasing concentration.** They concentrate in the fatty tissues of animals and humans and multiply in concentration as they move up the food chain. Meat, dairy, and fish eaters have higher body stores than vegetarians. Older animals and humans have higher concentrations than younger individuals.

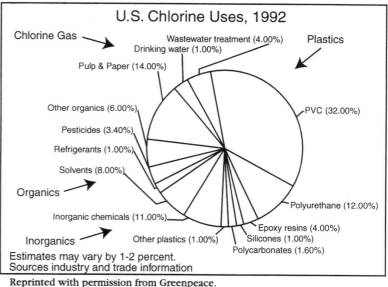

Reprinted with permission from Greenpeace.

5) **Subsequent generations.** They are able to cross the placental barrier, affecting the very sensitive fetus, and are mobilized from the body's fat stores into the breast milk of all mammals, including humans. The infants acquire a high concentration of environmental estrogens relative to their small body mass over a short period of time. Subsequent generations pass on higher and higher concentrations from prenatal exposure, breast-feeding, and lifetime exposure.

6) **Harmful.** They are highly toxic, causing such things as genetic mutations, cancer, hormonal imbalances, malformations of the reproductive organs, immune suppression, birth defects, neurotoxicity, learning disabilities and attention deficit disorders, infertility, impaired childhood development, and toxicity to the liver, kidney, skin, and brain. Even minute doses of many organochlorines can be extremely toxic. Natural estrogens exert their effects at low concentrations, measured in parts per trillion, which is 1000 times less than parts per billion. Organochlorines, acting as weak estrogens, are often present in breast milk, blood, and body fat in parts per billion or parts per million — 1000 or one million times more than the amount at which estrogen has an effect. And we have over a hundred in our systems acting synergistically, causing them to be more active than if they were present singly. Because they are persistent and our bodies cannot break them down, with time they accumulate in our tissues as well as in the environment. We are headed towards widespread infertility, hormonal imbalances, neurological disorders, cancer, birth defects, immune dysfunction, and the end of many wildlife species. Each of us must take immediate action to turn this trend around.

7) **Effects are synergistic.** A combination of only two different organochlorines together in minute doses has been found to be 1000 times more potent in affecting human estrogen receptors as either chemical alone. There is a synergistic interaction between environmental estrogens. Therefore, assessing the estrogenic activity from exposure to only one organochlorine is misleading. For example, dieldrin, endosulfan, or toxaphene by themselves only mildly stimulate growth of breast cancer cells in culture but showed greater than additive effects when given together.[26]

8) **Death to wildlife and humans.** They are harming wildlife and humans and threaten our survival. Combinations of two different PCBs at low concentrations were effective in reversing the sex of male turtle

When the animals come to us,

asking for our help,

will we know what they are saying?

When the plants speak to us

in their delicate, beautiful language,

will we be able to answer them?

When the planet herself

sings to us in our dreams,

will we be able to wake ourselves, and act?[37]

— Gary Lawless

eggs to become female.[27] Eagles and gulls which consume fish from the Great Lakes (contaminated with organochlorines) have a high rate of deformities, deaths of embryos, and exhibit abnormal nesting behavior. Eagles have been born with crossed beaks; female herring gulls have been found to share nests with other females.[28] Alligators hatched in Lake Apopka, Florida have abnormally small penises and altered hormone levels. In 1980 there was a massive pesticide spill in Lake Apopka.[29] Panthers living in areas of south central Florida in which soil or water contained high concentrations of heavy metals and organochlorines have a higher than normal number of males born with undescended testes.[30] There is a decrease in levels of male hormones in Dall's porpoises. Common seals and gray seals have increased sterility. Oysters taken from organochlorine contaminated water have shell deformities.[31] The population of beluga whales in the St Lawrence River is at risk. In 1994, autopsy reports on 24 stranded whales found 21 tumors in 12 specimens. Six of those tumors were cancerous. Cancers that are being found in the St Lawrence belugas include breast, ovarian, bladder, stomach, intestinal, and salivary gland. No cancers were found in their cousins living in the less polluted Arctic Ocean. The belugas are having trouble reproducing and high concentrations of PCBs, DDT, chlordane, and toxaphene were found dissolved in their fat.[32] The Environmental Health Committee of the Ontario College of Family Physicians warns that there is an increased risk of leukemia, brain cancer, and soft tissue sarcomas to children who have been exposed to herbicides and pesticides. Developmental problems such as poor co-ordination is occurring in children, along with smaller head size. There has been a drop in male fertility with a 50% reduction in sperm count since 1940.[33] In Europe, some organic farmers have over double the sperm count as non-organic farmers. Testicular cancer has more than tripled in the last 50 years in the United States and Europe[34] and cases of undescended testes in infant boys has doubled.[35,36]

Organochlorines and Breast Cancer

At least 16 organochlorines have been found to cause breast cancer in laboratory animals.[38] Some of these have already been restricted in Canada, such as DDT, aldrin, dieldrin, and chlordane — all pesticides. Other organochlorines found to be causative agents of breast cancer have not been restricted. These include PVC, or polyvinyl chloride, used in household plumbing, and polyvinylidene chloride, familiar to us as saran wrap. Methylene chloride, used in paint strippers, and dichlorobenzidines, used to produce dyes, are also still being produced. There is an established relationship between the levels of certain organochlorines found in a woman's blood, fat, or breast tissue and her risk of breast cancer. Studies have found that samples taken from breast cancer biopsies showed much higher levels of DDT, DDE, and PCBs than samples from benign breast lumps or from breast tissue in women without cancer.[39] A 1990 Finnish study found that the organochlorine beta-hexachlorocyclohexane (b-HCH) was 50% higher in cancerous tissue than in healthy breast tissue. When concentrations of b-HCH were as low as 100 parts per billion, women had a 10.5 times increased risk of developing breast cancer.[40,41] Women with the highest concentrations of specific organochlorine pesticides in their bodies have a risk of breast cancer 4 to 10 times higher than women with lower levels. At present they signify one of the greatest known risk factors linked with breast cancer.

Pesticides

Approximately 90% of all chemical pesticides use chlorine in their manufacturing process. The amounts and varieties of pesticides we use today are far greater than at any other time in history. Many foods have several pesticide residues on them: for example, the average Canadian peach has 31 pesticide residues. Although the amount of one pesticide residue may not be greater than the maximum allowable level, several pesticides from the same class acting at the same site in the body can have a toxic cumulative effect, particularly on children and the unborn.

We also are exposed to pesticides through our water supply. Groundwater in Canadian and American cities was found to have residues of 39 pesticides and their breakdown products. Spraying homes, lawns, roadways, golf courses, and agricultural crops causes the pesticides to leach through the soil and enter the groundwater.[42]

In 1998 world scientists were alerted to the fact that many pesticides and persistent environmental chemicals were ending up not in the areas where they were applied, but in the pristine mountainous areas of the world. Jules Blais, an assistant professor at the University of Ottawa, found high concentrations of pesticides and industrial chemicals in the alpine snow of the Rocky Mountains in British Columbia, at elevations of 3,100 meters above sea level. A phenomenon called 'cold condensation' sends the pollutants to the highest elevations with the most snowfall. Snowflakes are very efficient at extracting organic compounds from the air. The Columbia Icefields, Whistler, and Lake Louise have all been affected. Compounds that have been measured in disturbing quantities in these areas include lindane, endosulphan, chlordane, DDT, and PCBs. Higher amounts of lindane were found in the mountains than are found in the prairies where the insecticide is initially applied. Fish in alpine lakes are more contaminated than fish in subalpine lakes. Fish may be poisoning the birds and wildlife that feed upon them, such as osprey, otters, and eagles. Fresh water and well water in alpine locales may be unfit for animal and human consumption. The disappearance of frogs and salamanders from areas of high altitudes may also be linked to the high concentration of persistent organic pollutants in these areas. When the snow melts, these chemicals are released back into the environment. They hopscotch around the world, landing on different mountains each year.[43]

Currently Used Pesticides Linked with Breast Cancer

The following table, adapted from the *Journal of Pesticide Reform* (Spring 1996), show the pesticides currently in use, not yet banned, and their proven impact on breast health.

• Currently Used Pesticides Linked with Breast Cancer •

Name	Use	Comments
Atrazine	A weed killer widely used today on vegetable crops such as corn in Canada and the U.S. It is the most widely used pesticide in U.S. agriculture.	It promotes the formation of the 'bad' estrogen, 16 alpha-hydroxyestrone that has been linked to breast cancer. Caused breast cancer and disruption of menstrual cycles in one strain of rats and inhibits the metabolism of male hormones in other animal species. In northern Italy, a link has been made between atrazine use and ovarian cancer among women farmers. Because atrazine is widely used on corn, which is the staple in animal feed, we are consuming higher amounts of it when we eat corn-fed animals, such as meat, milk, poultry and eggs. Its use has been restricted in Germany and the Netherlands.
Cyanazine	A herbicide used mostly on corn. One of the top 5 most commonly used pesticides in the U.S. Production ceased in the U.S. Dec. 31, 1999 although its use will continue for 3 more years.	Caused significant increase in breast tumors in female rats.
1,3-dichloro-propene	Used as a soil fumigant, one of the top 10 pesticides used in the U.S.	Caused breast tumors in mice and rats.
Dichlorvos	An insecticide used in greenhouses, on fruits and vegetables and on livestock. It is used to make pet flea collars and fly strips.	Caused an increase in breast tumors in female rats.
Endosulfan	One of the most commonly used pesticides. Widely used on fruit and salad crops, found on apples, carrots, celery, cucumbers, head lettuce (not leaf lettuce), pears, peppers, plums, strawberries, and tomatoes.[44]	Causes breast cancer cells to increase in number in lab tests and promotes the formation of the C-16 "bad estrogen" linked to increased breast cancer risk.
Ethalfluralin	A herbicide used before planting soybeans, dry beans, and sunflower seeds.	Caused breast tumors in rats.
Ethylene oxide	A fumigant used on spices and to sterilize cosmetics and hospital equipment.	Increases breast tumors and several other cancers in female mice.
Etridiazole	A fungicide that is applied to soil and used to treat seeds.	When fed to rats there was an increase in breast tumors.
Methoxychlor	An insecticide related to DDT, used mostly on crops but also for household, garden, commercial, and industrial use.	Causes breast cancer cells to multiply in lab animals and causes changes to the ovaries in adult mice.
Oryzalin	An herbicide used on turf, almond orchards, and grape vineyards.	Caused increased breast tumors in female rats.
Prometon	An herbicide.	Causes breast tumors in rats.
Propazine	An herbicide used before planting sorghum and after planting carrots, celery and fennel.	Causes increased benign and malignant breast tumors in rats.
Simazine	An herbicide used on lawns, nut trees, corn production and fruit crops, specifically oranges, apples, plums, olives, cherries, peaches, cranberries, blueberries, strawberries, grapes, and pears.	Caused both breast and ovarian cancer in female rats.[45]
Terbuthylazine	A herbicide used to kill algae in ornamental ponds, fountains, and aquariums.	Caused increased breast tumors in female rats.
Terbutryn	A herbicide used before planting sorghum.	Increases malignant breast tumors in female rats.
Tribenuron methyl	An herbicide used in barley and wheat production.	Increases malignant breast tumors in female rats.

• Currently Used Pesticides Linked with Breast Cancer •

Name	Use	Comments
Lindane	Although banned from regular use in 1983, it is still allowed in lice shampoos for humans and flea dips for dogs. Some children use lice shampoos more than 20 times as well as apply insecticide sprays to the home. See alternatives on page 113.	Women whose breasts had the highest levels of lindane-like residues were 10 times more likely to have breast cancer than women with lower levels. Blood from women with breast cancer had 50% more of this pesticide residue than blood from women without breast cancer.[46,47,48]

Other pesticides that are known hormone disruptors include 2,4,5-T, 2,4-D, alachlor, aldicarb, amitrole, benomyl, beta-HCH, carbaryl, cypermethrin, DBCP, dicofol, esfenvalerate, ethylparathion, fenvalerate, h-epoxide, kelthane, kepone, malathion, mancozeb, maneb, methomyl, metiram, metribuzin, mirex, nitrofen, oxychlordane, permethrin, synthetic pyrethoids, trans-nonachlor, tributyltin oxide, trifluralin, vinclozolin, zineb, and ziram.[49]

Banned Pesticides: Aldrin and Dieldrin

Even though Dieldrin has been banned in the United States and Europe for many years, it persists in the environment and accumulates in our bodies. Aldrin was used as an insecticide on corn, citrus, cotton, and other crops. Banned in 1975, it was nevertheless allowed as a termite poison until 1987. It converts to dieldrin in soil and in our bodies. In humans, dieldrin suppresses the immune system and causes epileptic-like convulsions. In mice, aldrin and dieldrin cause malignant liver and lung tumors. Dieldrin is very persistent in the environment and has caused thinning of eggshells in bird populations and has been implicated in the decline of some wildlife species. In men, these two chemicals have been found to decrease sperm count and testosterone levels. In 1986, dieldrin was still found in cow's milk because the soil of hayfields sprayed a decade earlier remained contaminated. Dieldrin can travel in the atmosphere and has been found in arctic snow.

A 1998 study published in the *Lancet* that followed over 7,000 women for nearly 20 years found that women with the highest traces of dieldrin in their blood were twice as likely as women with the lowest levels to develop breast cancer.[50]

Banned Pesticides: Chlordane and Heptachlor

Chlordane and heptachlor were used agriculturally and as termite killers until 1988 and have been linked to leukemia and childhood cancer. Their effects on the nervous system include headaches, blurred vision, muscle twitching, convulsions, arrhythmia, and respiratory failure. They have been found to cause benign and malignant liver tumors in rats. They cross the placenta, contaminate breast milk and act as hormone disruptors linked to decreased fertility. Even now, despite their ban, residues of chlordane are found in oysters in the Gulf of Mexico and coastal North American whales. These two chemicals have been found in the fat of Arctic polar bears whose food source is contaminated seals. Arctic polar bears are having trouble reproducing and are creating offspring that demonstrate both male and female reproductive organs.

Banned Pesticides: DDT

DDT reached its peak usage in the U.S. in 1959 but was banned in the U.S. in 1972. It was routinely sprayed over rural and residential areas as an insecticide and is still present in our bodies. It was made into a paint that could be brushed on porches, window screens, and baseboards or added to the dry-cleaning process to mothproof woolen clothing and blankets. It was used to control mosquitoes, gypsy moths, and Dutch elm disease and was sprayed on fruit trees. Its use triggered population explosions of insects who became resistant to the drug or whose natural enemies were killed by it. It is a persistent chemical, found in soil, hazardous waste sites, and the tissues of most life forms. It is present in the deep basins of the Great Lakes. Global air currents carry it worldwide from countries where its use is still allowed, such as Mexico and India. It is still made in the United States and shipped overseas to be used on food crops in Third World countries and to combat malaria. It may come back to us on the food we import.

DDT is converted to DDE in our bodies. DDE and PCBs have been found in higher concentrations in breast tumors than in surrounding breast tissue. This is also true of lindane, heptachlor, and dieldrin. DDT has been linked to liver and pancreatic cancer as well as tumors of the lung, liver, and thyroid. DDE crosses the placenta to affect the fetus and is passed into breast milk. We ingest DDE when we consume milk, meat, eggs, and fish, as it is concentrated in animals higher up on the food chain. Although it was banned in 1959, it has a half-life in soil of 10–35 years, so we are still being exposed to it. DDE acts to block androgens (male sex hormones) by blocking their receptor sites. The consequences for men are lowered sperm counts, smaller testes, an increased incidence of testicular cancer, and more cases of undescended testes.

Our bodies cannot convert DDE into anything excretable. A 1993 study by Mary Wolff found that the blood from women with breast cancer contained 35% more DDE than the blood of healthy women, although a more recent study failed to show this correlation.

Banned Pesticides: Endrin

Endrin was used until 1986 as an insecticide and to control cutworms, voles, grasshoppers, and boring insects on sugarcane, tobacco, apples, and grain. It can be absorbed through inhalation, skin absorption, ingestion, and skin contact. It is thought to have caused birth defects such as cleft palate, webbed foot and fused ribs in animals. It is metabolized quickly and does not accumulate significantly in body fat. When it was used in the past it caused massive fish and bird die-off in rice fields and apple orchards. Its use on cotton fields and leakage from production plants wiped out brown pelican populations in Louisiana and Texas in the early 1960s.[51]

Banned Pesticides: Toxaphene

Toxaphene was used heavily as an insecticide on cotton fields in the United States until it was banned in 1982. Its half-life in soil may be up to 14 years. It still may be produced unintentionally today as a waste product from chlorine-based pulp mill bleaching. It lodges in fatty tissue and is very persistent. Its use caused die off of crappies, bass, and sunfish in southern U.S. streams and is linked to reproductive damage in seals. Concentrations found in the tissues of Arctic and Baltic salmon today are high enough to cause breast cancer cells to multiply in laboratory conditions.[52,53]

▶ **Action for Prevention:** Buy organic food and/or grow your own food if possible. Find a way to establish a community garden or greenhouse with like-minded people. Connect with local organic growers. Plant fruit and nut trees on your property. Peel your fruits and vegetables, especially if they have been waxed, or wash them with a vegetable wash or diluted vinegar to remove surface pesticide residues.

If you can't buy all organic food, the foods that contain the most pesticide residues in decreasing order among Canadian grown varieties, for example, are celery, carrots, apples, head lettuce, sweet peppers, fresh beans, leaf lettuce, strawberries, and blueberries. Imported foods highest in pesticide residues are red, bell, and green peppers, oranges, strawberries, spinach, green beans, grapes, head lettuce, pears, apples, tomatoes, cherries, peaches, Mexican cantaloupes, celery, apricots, and cucumbers. You can try to buy these organically grown, grow them yourself, or avoid them. To find out more about what pesticides and herbicides are in your foods and which foods are safest, view the web site www.foodnews.org. To help you to grow organic food, visit the web site www.organic-growers.com.

Talk or write to your local, provincial and municipal governments about banning pesticide use in public parks, playgrounds, and golf courses. Call your airline and request that they not spray the airplane with pesticides before takeoff, which most of them do. About 20 towns and villages, all in Quebec, have passed bylaws restricting pesticide spraying on private and public green spaces. The town of Hudson, Quebec, (population 5,000) takes 10–12 companies to court each year for illegal spraying. Its bylaw against pesticides was passed eight years ago.[54] We can learn from this small town and push for a moratorium on pesticide use in our own cities. It is much easier to win the battle against pesticides on the municipal level rather than the federal level, so start there. We can accomplish what Hudson has in our own communities.

Educate people about the hazards to children from pesticide use. If you are a medical doctor, call the Environmental Health Committee of the Ontario College of Family Physicians at (416) 867-9646 and request a copy of Pesticides and Human Health. Pass it on to your patients. Contact the World Wildlife Fund Canada (tel. 416-489-8800 or 800-26-PANDA, or fax. 416-489-3611) and ask for a number of free copies of "Reducing Your Risk from Pesticides" and circulate these among friends, neighbors, grocery stores, farmers, businesses, schools, hospitals, etc. For more information on pesticides and alternatives to pesticides, contact the Northwest Coalition for Alternatives to Pesticides in Eugene, OR (tel. 541-344-5044, fax. 541-344-6923, E-mail: info@pesticide.org, and web site www.efn.org/~ncap/). They publish the quarterly Journal of Pesticide Reform and supply fact sheets on pesticides and their alternatives. ◀

PVC (Polyvinyl Chloride) Plastics

PVC is responsible for the greatest production and use of chlorine, accounting for approximately one third of all organochlorine production. Over 20 million tons of PVC plastic or vinyl are manufactured each year and used in cars, children's toys, food containers, credit cards, raincoats, furniture, building supplies, water pipes, window frames, flooring, and even wall paper. Dioxins and phthalates are two groups of hormone-disrupting chemicals often added to PVC. Large quantities of dioxins are formed in the production, disposal, and combustion of PVC. PVC is often present with wood furniture, with steel in cars and with copper in cables. As these substances are recycled, dioxin is released into the environment. Dioxin is both carcinogenic and acts as a hormone disruptor. It is widely recognized as one of the most toxic chemicals ever made. The worst of the dioxins is called TCDD or 2,3,7,8-TCDD.[55] Phthalates are chemicals mixed in with PVC and added to plastics in general to soften them and increase their flexibility.

The Ontario Ministry of the Environment tested three major dumps in the Toronto area in 1994–1995 and found vinyl chloride and other volatile chemicals seeping into the air. The emissions were high enough to have the government freeze real estate development near the area. The emissions were caused by solvents and the decomposition of vinyl-chloride-containing plastics near the dump site.[56] There is no safe way to dispose of PVC plastic. Environmental groups such as Greenpeace are calling for phasing out its use.

Alternatives to PVC

Alternatives to most, if not all PVC products exist. PVC is not a necessity — we didn't need it until the chemical industry introduced it to us. Its convenience is not a valid reason to allow our very survival and the survival of wildlife to be threatened. There are readily available alternatives to PVC as shown on this list prepared by Greenpeace.

PVC Product	Healthy Alternative
Windows	wood (pine, larch, fir, spruce, beech), chlorine free plastics
Floorings	ceramic tiles, wood, parquetry, linoleum, rubber, stoneware tiles, cork, sisal hemp, terazzo, chlorine free plastic (polyolefine)
Walls	brickwork, pebble dash, wood, gypsum, plaster board
Wallpaper	uncoated paper (made from chlorine free recycled fibers), environmentally sound paints, paper wallpaper with protective coating on acrylate base, ceramic tiles
Facades, Curtain Walls	plaster, wood
Roll Joints, Hand Rails	wood, metal
Furniture	wood, metal, wicker
Blinds, Shutters	wood, textiles
Weather Stripping	natural rubber
Sewage Pipes	concrete, earthenware, stoneware, polyethylene (PE) and polypropylene pipes (PP)
Electrical Installations & Cables	chlorine free plastics like PE, special rubber
Packaging	minimize packaging, but when necessary, use cardboard, wood, glass, brown paper bags, waxed paper, and if plastic is necessary, use PE, PP. (We need to develop organic packaging as from hemp, straw, vegetable fibers etc. Wouldn't it be wonderful if all packaging could be composted to feed a garden or be used as mulch?)
Medical Products	switch from disposable (usually PVC) to reusable products; e.g., redden bottles, reusable scalpel handles, refillable glass bottles, and where disposable products are necessary, use chlorine free plastics such as PE for gloves, infusion bags, or use latex or natural rubber
Toys	wood, textiles[57]

▶ **Action for Prevention:** Avoid using PVC and plastics in general. PVC can be identified by a number 3 in the recycling symbol. If you are a retailer, you can choose not to stock PVC plastics and label your store PVC free — have a fact sheet available to consumers so they too can make healthy choices. As a consumer, encourage your retailers to phase out PVC; IKEA and The Body Shop have stopped selling products containing PVC. Make appointments with store managers and educate them about PVC. Discard your PVC blinds and any other sources you can change. Design and build a PVC free house. Talk to builders and carpenters about the health and environmental hazards of PVC. Do not buy plastic children's toys and call your credit card company to ask them to make the cards out of something other than PVC.

Bio-based polymers are made of natural raw materials, such as wood, cotton, horn or hardened protein, and raw rubber. One example is Biopol, made from chemicals produced by bacteria that have been feed sugar. These products degrade easily and can be composted. We need to investigate and develop their large-scale use.

Ask your supplement manufacturers to package your vitamins and herbs in glass rather than plastic bottles. Choose manufacturers that use glass. PVC is not part of a sustainable future for life on earth. ◀

Dioxins

Dioxins consist of a group of 75 chemicals that are produced during the manufacturing and combustion of other chlorine compounds. They are now widespread in our environment. The dioxin levels in the Great Lakes was zero in the 1920s but has steadily increased to be about 3200 parts per trillion today.[58]

TCDD, the most potent of the dioxins, blocks the male hormone testosterone. In adult males who were exposed to dioxins at work, there was a decrease in testosterone levels.[59] In animal studies, if just one dose of dioxin was given to a rat on a particular day of pregnancy, the male offspring had lowered levels of testosterone and a reduced sperm count. They also demonstrated more feminine sexual behavior. The effect on animals exposed in utero is permanent.

Dioxins are suspected as a causative factor in endometriosis — a painful, hormonally linked condition in women that can result in infertility and decreased quality of life. Monkeys exposed to dioxin at levels close to those found in human tissues developed an increased incidence of endometriosis.[60] Laboratory rats exposed to dioxin levels close to those encountered in our environment today gave birth to female offspring who suffered from decreased fertility and structural abnormalities of their reproductive systems.[61]

Hospital incinerators, ironically, are a major source of dioxin release. Many medical products are made out of PVC plastic, such as tubing systems, blood and infusion bags, gloves and packaging of hospital supplies. These products are routinely burned in hospital incinerators and dioxin is released into the surrounding communities. Recent public attention has caused some hospitals to switch to using plastic that is PVC free. Municipal, industrial and sewage sludge incinerators are also significant sources of dioxin release. Accidental fires are sources of dioxin release, since so much of the building industry uses PVC in its supplies. All buildings have a limited life span. What will happen to the PVC when the building is either torn down or burned? It will end up in landfill, poisoning the earth and water, or in incineration, poisoning the air.

The chemical facilities where PVC is made deliver very high releases of dioxin annually. A Greenpeace report suggests that Dow Chemical's facility in Edmonton, Alberta releases annual air emissions from its incinerator stacks that are much higher than allowable for the local population. Other sources of dioxin unrelated to PVC occur during the bleaching of pulp and paper, manufacture of chlorophenols, production of chlorine, magnesium and nickel smelting, and steel production.

Despite its ubiquitous presence in the environment, most human exposure to dioxin occurs through consumption of animal products in which the dioxin has become concentrated; primarily beef, fish, and dairy products. Dioxin is known to disrupt thyroid function in animals and newborns, resulting in low birth weight, hyperactivity, and learning and memory disorders. Is it any wonder so many children are on Ritalin? Not only are we undermining our fertility with estrogen mimickers, we are blocking male hormones and interfering with female hormones with dioxins. We pass dioxins on to our children in utero and through breast milk to compound the problem. At least ten dioxins have been found in human breast milk. We are interfering with our children's ability to learn and reproduce when we use PVC plastic and support the PVC industry.

▶ **Action for Prevention:** If there is a hospital near you, inquire as to whether its incinerator burns PVC plastic. Start or join a campaign to ban the production and incineration of PVC and chlorine based chemicals. Buy unbleached, chlorine-free paper products and ask your stores and photocopy shops to stock them for you. If there is a PVC manufacturer in your area, find out how much dioxin is released annually, and protest to local, provincial, state, and federal officials.

Although the number 3 in the recycling symbol can often identify PVC, not all plastics are labeled, making it difficult to know which ones contain PVC. Companies consider their formulas trade secrets and are not required to disclose whether they contain PVC or not. We can insist to government, retailers, and the plastic companies that they label their products "PVC free" or "Contains PVC" so that we can exercise our right to choose. Until then, refrain from buying plastics. Eliminate or limit your consumption of meat, fish, and dairy to reduce dioxin exposure. ◄

Phthalates

Phthalates are not organochlorines but are used in about 50% of all PVC products to soften them and add flexibility. They are an ingredient in plastic food wraps and packaging and are also utilized in paints, inks, and adhesives. We are also exposed to phthalates through our food and its packaging. Fatty foods, such as cheese and oils, are easily contaminated with phthalates and bisphenol-A when packaged in plastic. Phthalates may be present and can be absorbed from plastic baby bottles, nipples, and plastic 'soothers'. In the fall of 1998, some, but not all toys and soothers containing phthalates were removed from the shelves in Canadian stores. Through testing, the Danish and Dutch governments have found that these chemicals can be ingested from PVC toys during normal use; PVC toys have been taken off the shelves in Sweden, Spain, Italy, Argentina, Greece, Holland and Denmark.[62]

Phthalates are one of the most abundant environmental contaminants and are persistent, accumulating in living tissues. We store them in our fat and release them in breast milk. Several forms of phthalates have been found to be weakly estrogenic. When male rats were exposed to phthalates before and after birth, they had lower testicular weights and a reduced sperm count. Two types of phthalates, DEHP and DINP, have been found to cause cancer in animals.[63] Phthalates have been shown to be toxic to developing embryos, causing malformation and death. They also can lower progesterone levels,[64] potentially contributing to PMS symptoms, breast cysts, breast cancer, and miscarriages.

► **Action for Prevention:** For the sake of your children and future generations, avoid phthalates, which are added to PVC toys and are linked to cancer, kidney damage, and may interfere with your children's ability to reproduce. Urge your retailers not to sell PVC toys and pressure your municipal, provincial, state, and federal governments to ban the use of PVC plastic. Urge your daycares and schools to eliminate PVC and plastic toys in general. Tell your friends and relatives not to buy plastic toys for your children. Put pressure on toy manufacturing companies like Mattel, Hasbro, Playskool, Safety 1st, Gerber, and Disney to stop using PVC in their products. Explain to your children the hazards in their plastic toys in a way they can understand, and then discard them, replacing them with wood, cloth, or other natural fibers.

Buy oils or fatty foods in glass rather than plastic containers. Use waxed paper or butcher paper to wrap sandwiches and other foods in, and especially do not microwave food in plastic containers or plastic wrap. Use ceramic or glass containers instead. ◄

Bisphenol-A

Bisphenol-A is an ingredient in epoxy resins and polycarbonate plastics, which are hard plastics. Although it is not an organochlorine, it is an endocrine disruptor. It is used in formulas to seal cracks in water pipes, and in some dental materials designed to provide 'protection' against tooth decay and in the plastic fillings used to replace mercury amalgam fillings.

This hormone-disruptor is a breakdown product of polycarbonate, present in the plastic coating that manufacturers use to line metal cans. These coatings were added to prevent a metallic taste in the food. Plastic linings are present in 85% of food cans in the United States, and bisphenol-A was found to have leached into about half the canned foods that were tested. When analyzed, some cans contained 80 parts per billion of bisphenol A, which is 27 times more than researchers have demonstrated is enough to make breast cancer cells proliferate in the laboratory.[65] At these levels, we would expect a physiological effect in women's breasts from regular consumption of canned food or oily food in hard plastic containers containing Bisphenol-A. Some men in the plastics industry have developed enlarged breasts after inhaling the chemical in workplace dust over long periods of time.[66]

► **Action for Prevention:** If you consume canned foods, call the manufacturer to ask whether bisphenol-A, is used to line the can. If yes, express your concern about its capacity as a hormone disruptor and its impact on breast cancer. Stop using the cans. Buy food in glass jars or cans without the liners. Call the toll free numbers on the food packaging you buy and ask whether there are PVC, phthalates, nonylphenol ethoxylates, or bisphenol-A in any of it.

If your dentist suggests a new plastic coating for your children's teeth, ask her if she can guarantee in writing that it contains no bisphenol-A or other hormone disrupting chemical. Whenever possible, ask your dentist to use ceramic fillings on your teeth, and pressure the dental industry to test all their filling materials for estrogenic or carcinogenic activity before experimenting with them on children and the general public. Insist on mandatory release of names of ingredients used in dental fillings before you allow them into your mouth.

Contact the World Wildlife Fund (tel. 416-489-8800 or 800-26-PANDA or fax. 416-489-3611) and ask for a number of free copies of "Reducing Your Risk: A Guide to Avoiding Hormone-Disrupting Chemicals" and circulate these among friends, neighbors, businesses, schools, hospitals, etc. ◄

Nonylphenol Ethoxylates

Although they are not organochlorines, nonylphenol ethoxylates (NPEs) are hormone disrupting chemicals used in 11 industrial areas and in household and industrial soaps and detergents, natural and synthetic textile processing, plastic manufacturing, pulp and paper making, petroleum refineries, pesticides and for oil extraction. They are one of the ingredients used to make plastic soft, and readily leach out into fluids at room temperature. We may find them in our water bottles, fruit juice containers, and packaging of convenience food.

In the United Kingdom alone, 20,000 tons of nonylphenols are used annually. Approximately one third of this production ends up in rivers, lakes, and streams and eventually in drinking water. The United Kingdom National Rivers Authority has found nonylphenols present in some rivers in concentrations higher than 50 mcg per liter. Research has shown that maturing male fish

exposed to only modest amounts of nonylphenol (amounts that are present in their environments) have inhibited growth of their testicles.[67] The Paris Commission is an international body that sets standards for water quality. Their recommendation is that nonylphenols be phased out before the year 2000 because of their toxicity to aquatic life and their persistence in the environment.[68]

Wayne Fairchild, an eco-toxicologist with the Department of Fisheries and Oceans in Moncton, New Brunswick, believes that 4-NP, a commonly used nonylphenol ethoxylate, interferes with salmon's ability to find their way back home to spawn in streams. The chemical causes a mixed signal in the brains of young salmon that seems to stop their journey from the sea to the rivers where they would normally reproduce. It also disrupts the endocrine system of young salmon as they develop into adult fish.[69]

We should choose soaps and detergents, particularly liquid products, which the manufacturer guarantees do not contain NPEs. Usually there is a toll free number on product labels that can be used to find out this information. The following companies do not use nonylphenol oxalates in their detergents: Proctor and Gamble, Lever, Pond's, Tide, and Sunlight.[70]

► **Action for Prevention:** Use glass, ceramic, or stainless steel in containers for foods and beverages. Take cotton or hemp bags or cardboard boxes to the supermarket to load your groceries. Choose not to buy plastic packaging or containers. Call the companies whose products you buy and ask them to switch to non-toxic containers. Avoid industrial or

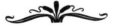

Until one is committed there is hesitancy, the chance to draw back, always ineffectiveness.

Concerning all acts of initiative (and creation) there is one elementary truth, the ignorance of

which kills countless ideas and splendid plans: that the moment one definitely commits oneself, then

Providence moves too. All sorts of things occur to help one that would never otherwise have occurred.

A whole stream of events issues from the decision, raising in one's favor all manner of unforeseen

incidents and meetings and material assistance, which no man could have dreamed would come his way.

Whatever you can do, or dream you can, begin it.

Boldness has genius, power and magic in it.

— Goethe

super-strength cleansers. Use environmentally friendly soaps such as those made by Nature Clean or create your own cleansers from the recipes at the end of this chapter. You can also often buy ecological cleansers in bulk at health food stores, recycling a glass or cardboard container. ◄

Other Organochlorines

PCBs (Polychlorinated Biphenyls)

Most industrialized countries stopped PCB production over 10 years ago, although their concentration in human tissues has not declined. This family of weak-acting chemical hormone disruptors contains 209 members. They were used on wood and plastic products to make them nonflammable and made stucco waterproof. They were used in paints, varnishes, inks, and pesticides. Two thirds of all the PCBs produced are still being used in transformers and electrical equipment and are subject to accidental release into the environment. They may be found in old fluorescent light fixtures, microscope oil, and hydraulic fluids. PCBs are persistent and may not degrade for decades or centuries. They are now present in the body fat of almost all living creatures. The most contaminated waters of the Northern Hemisphere are the Baltic Sea and the St. Lawrence River estuary.

The Inuit, who rely on seafood as a staple, have PCB levels of 4.1 parts per million, which is 5–10 times higher than the average Canadian's. Levels this high are linked to depressed immune systems, particularly a decline in the T-cells which would ordinarily keep cancer in check. People who eat fish regularly from the north shore of the St. Lawrence River in Quebec have a mean PCB level of 6 parts per million.[71]

Adult male harbor seals in the Strait of Georgia contain 21 ppm of PCBs, while seal pups from the Puget Sound area contain 17 ppm. These quantities cause immune deficiency in the seals, making them more vulnerable to infections and cancer. In 1988, 20,000 harbor seals in the North and Baltic Seas died of a viral infection, possibly so devastating because of the weakened immune systems of the seals due to PCB contamination. The phenomenon was referred to as the AIDS of the ocean.[72] When PCBs were present at 70 parts per million in their tissues, female seals developed suppressed immune systems and deformities of the uterus and fallopian tubes. In northern Norway, female polar bears carry as much as 90 parts per million of PCBs in their fat and are producing less than half of the expected number of offspring as in previous years.[73]

PCBs affect both thyroid and ovarian hormones. Interference with thyroid hormone during gestation may cause low birth weight, poor growth, hyperactivity, autoimmune diseases, immune suppression, and impaired learning and memory.[74]

In a recent study done by Dr Kristan Aronson of Toronto several PCBs were found to occur in higher amounts in the breast tumor biopsies of women with breast cancer as compared to biopsies from women with benign breast tumors. Women whose tumors had the highest amount of PCB105 were twice as likely to have breast cancer than women with lower amounts. The other PCBs associated with breast cancer were PCB118 and 156.[75]

A human baby breast-fed for six months receives five times the allowable daily limit of PCBs set by international health standards for a 150-lb adult.[76] A woman passes half of her lifetime accumulation of dioxins and PCBs on to her child when she nurses for just six months.[77] We need to sweat them out before we conceive.

► **Action for Prevention:** Avoid animal products, particularly if you hope to have children who are breast-fed. Detoxify regularly with saunas to eliminate PCBs through your sweat. Follow the sauna detoxification outlined in this book before conceiving. Take your children into the sauna with you once a week. ◄

CFCs (Chlorofluorocarbons)

Like DDT and PCBs, chlorofluorocarbons were considered extremely safe by their inventors. They were developed as a safer alternative to the toxic and flammable coolants used in refrigerators and were used for 40 years before James Lovelock, the scientist who developed the Gaia theory, discovered that CFCs were accumulating in the atmosphere. In 1974, two chemists, Sherwood Rowland and Mario Molina, published an article describing how CFCs attacked the ozone layer, making the earth more vulnerable to the sun's ultraviolet rays. CFCs had been used for 50 years before we were alerted to the fact that they had caused a huge ozone hole over Antarctica.

Perchloroethylene (PERC)

Perchloroethylene is used as a dry-cleaning solvent and is hazardous to workers and consumers because of its contribution to cancer and reproductive problems. It is commonly found as a contaminant in food and groundwater. Women who work in the dry cleaning industry have a greater risk of miscarriage.[78] PERC affects the pituitary gland, disturbing the hormones that regulate the menstrual cycle and pregnancy. Environment Canada and the U.S. Environmental Protection Agency are encouraging non-perc dry cleaning methods called Green Clean, which are already available in some cities.

▶ **Action for Prevention:** Talk to your dry cleaner about switching to 'Green Clean' methods and find out from Environment Canada or the USEPA if there is an outlet available in your city. Take the time to wash selected clothing by hand or buy clothes that don't need dry cleaning. ◀

2,4- dichlorophenoxyacetic acid (2,4 -D)

2,4-D was used in the Vietnam War to destroy the rain forest as a component of Agent Orange. It was introduced for agricultural use in the U.S. and Canada after that to control weeds and in the forests for shrub management. It became one of the most popular weed killers for lawns, gardens, and golf courses. It is marketed under the trade names Ded-Weed, Weedone, Plantgard, Lawn-Keep, and Demise. It is linked to a sixfold increased incidence of non-Hodgkin's lymphoma in humans. Dogs and pets also are at risk and the incidence of lymphoma doubles among pet dogs whose owners use lawn chemicals at least four times annually.[79] When pets and children run across sprayed lawns and then come into our homes, they bring with them traces of pesticides that find their way into our carpets, where they can accumulate over many years. Pesticide residues persist for longer periods indoors than outside, where they are washed away or broken down by sunlight, rain, and soil organisms. Infants and toddlers are exposed to significant amounts of pesticides from crawling on carpets and ingesting house dust. Children whose yards are treated with pesticides had a fourfold increase in soft tissue cancers over children living in homes that did not spray their lawns.[80] Brain tumors in children have been linked to increased use of pest-repellent strips, flea collars on pets, lice shampoos containing lindane, and weed killers on lawns.[81]

▶ **Action for Prevention:** Notice the number of residents in your area who use pesticides on their lawns and gracefully educate them about risks to their health. Minimize your use of carpeting in the home, using hardwood floors and natural fiber throw rugs instead. If you do have carpets, steam clean once or twice yearly with non-chlorinated cleansers. Insist on shoe removal in your home. Do not allow outdoor pets onto carpeted areas. ◀

Methyl Chloride

Methyl chloride causes mutations in bacteria and kidney cancer in mice. It is classified as a probable human carcinogen. In rats it causes birth defects and degeneration in male testicles. It is used in the manufacturing of silicone products, fuel additives, and herbicides. Hundreds of millions of pounds are produced in North America annually.

Chloroform

Chloroform was used in the past as an anesthetic because of its ability to alter brain function. It is classified as a probable human carcinogen and is now used as a solvent, fumigant, and as an ingredient in pesticides, synthetic dyes, and refrigerants. Trace amounts of it are formed when chlorine is added to drinking water, and it is prevalent in large dump sites. Although we excrete it from our bodies within 24 hours, we are constantly exposed to it through water, food, and inhalation. It takes over 1000 years to break down in the environment. According to the Commission for Environmental Cooperation, at least 4,625,354 kg of chloroform was released into the air, water, or soil in North America in 1996.[82]

Trichloroethylene (TCE)

TCE is used in industry to degrease metal parts and is one of the most common toxic substances at dump sites, from where it can trickle into groundwater. It is estimated to be in 34% of U.S. drinking water and traces are found in most processed foods.[83] It is also found in paint and spot removers, cosmetics and carpet cleaners. In the past, it was used as an obstetrical anesthetic, a grain fumigant, an ingredient in typewriter correction fluid, and as a coffee decaffeinater. Traces of it persist in the air that we breathe, especially if we live near a large dump site. In 1996, at least 10,472,026 kilograms of TCE were released into the air, water, and soil of North America.[84]

▶ **Action for Prevention:** Minimize your use of processed foods and stock your kitchen with what you need to cook from scratch. Filter your drinking water using a reverse osmosis or carbon filter. ◀

Disinfecting of Sewage, Drinking Water and Chlorinated Pools

When chlorine is combined with organic matter in sewage and water, hundreds of organochlorine by-products are formed. These damage the habitat of fish and marine animals living near sewage effluent, and damage us when we drink chlorinated water. Regular consumption of chlorinated water disrupts the healthy balance of organisms in our intestines, and has been linked with colon cancer; rectal cancer, bladder cancer, birth defects, and immune related disorders. The U.S. Environmental Protection Agency has identified at least two carcinogenic chemicals that are formed when chlorine in water reacts with organic material from decayed plants. These have been detected in significant amounts in 100 municipal water systems tested in 1995.[85]

Health Canada reported in its journal, *Chronic Diseases in Canada* (November 1998), that chlorinated water poses a risk to humans, particularly of bladder cancer. People who use chlorinated water for 35 years raise their cancer risk 1.5 times, and approximately 10–13 percent of bladder cancers in Ontario can be blamed on chlorinated water.[86]

Frequent use of chlorinated swimming pools also exposes us to chlorine toxicity. Other methods of water filtration and purification do exist, such as using ultraviolet light, ozone treatment, salination treatment for pools, and specialized filtration methods. These include reverse osmosis and charcoal or carbon filters. A public swimming pool in Vancouver uses ozonation as a purification method. The city of Montreal uses ozonation as a water purification treatment. So can we in our cities. Put pressure on your municipal governments.

Safer alternatives to using chlorine as a disinfectant are grapefruit seed extract and tea tree oil. Grapefruit seed extract has been used extensively throughout South America as an algaecide, bactericide, and fungicide rather than chlorine in hot tubs, jacuzzis, and swimming pools. The water clarity cannot be maintained as well with grapefruit seed extract in pools, and a combination of grapefruit seed extract and chlorine is sometimes used. The concentration of grapefruit seed extract needed to do the job of disinfecting is 10–15 drops per gallon of water. Grapefruit seed extract is a more powerful disinfectant than chlorine, tea tree oil, colloidal silver, and iodine.[87] Hospitals and clinics in the U.S. now use grapefruit seed extract in the laundry to ensure that the linen is fungi and bacteria free by adding 20–30 drops to the final rinse.[88]

▶ **Action for Prevention:** We can consider opting out of the toxic soup most cities call water by filtering stored rainwater, spring water, or groundwater from a drilled well. If this is not possible, then install a reverse osmosis or charcoal filter to your water supply and shower head. We can install composting toilets that recycle human waste and contribute nothing to global pollution. They also avoid the water wasting of flush toilets and the many chemicals used to clean up sewage. For information on composting toilets contact one of the following manufacturers: Sun-Mar Composting Toilets, Burlington, ON (tel. 905-332-1314); Storburn Pollution Free Toilet, Brantford, ON (tel. 800-876-2286); BioLet (tel. 800-6BIOLET); Envirolet Composting Toilet Systems, Scarborough, ON (tel. 800-387-5245); or Clivus Multrum (tel. 800-4CLIVUS).[89] We can insist upon safe, non-chlorine purification methods in our drinking water and swimming pools, such as ozonation and the use of grapefruit seed extract. ◀

The Pulp and Paper Industry

The pulp and paper industry releases thousands of kilograms of organochlorines into our rivers and lakes each year and is the largest North American discharger of organochlorine pollutants into water. Fish and wildlife downstream from pulp and paper mills are severely affected, with female fish taking on male characteristics, general increases in tumors, and decreased fertility. It is possible to use chlorine-free processes to make paper products. In Sweden and Finland, oxygen and hydrogen peroxide are used to bleach pulp for paper and diapers. The impetus for this transition came from the recognition and concern around organochlorine pollution in the Baltic Sea and aggressive regulations from government that forced industry to reduce and eliminate it. Pressure from the public and industry for access to chlorine-free paper will also cause the pulp and paper industry to switch to chlorine-free processing. Totally chlorine free (TCF) paper products are available from eco stores and progressive printers. Kinko's copy shops sell chlorine-free paper. In Ontario and British Columbia, for example, the government has proposed that pulp and paper mills stop using chlorine-based processing by the year 2002.

Be like a tree in pursuit of your cause.
Stand firm, grip hard, thrust upward, bend to
the winds of heaven, and learn tranquillity.[90]

Dedication to Richard St. Barbe Baker, Father of the Trees

▶ **Action for Prevention:** Buy totally chlorine free paper products (toilet paper, diapers, sanitary products, tampons, and paper packaging) or recycled paper that is chlorine free. Talk to your supermarket managers to have them stock these items, or buy them from ecological or health food stores. Use TCF paper for printing and photocopying. Recycle the paper products that you do use. ◀

Is There Any Place Safe to Live?

In North America, there are vast differences in the concentrations of toxins released from various states and provinces. Though environmental chemicals may be produced in one area, they are circulated widely, depending on water and wind currents. In the chart below

Highest Polluters					
Province/State	**# of Facilities**	**Total Releases and Transfers (kg)**	**Rank**	**Rank per Capita**	**Rank per km**
Texas	1,074	122,292,324	1	15	4
Ontario	733	68,763,262	2	31	16
Louisiana	269	67,921,157	3	59	40
Ohio	1,462	65,938,375	4	24	6
Pennsylvania	1,083	61,451,832	5	13	25
Michigan	795	50,084,864	6	7	8
Tennessee	574	46,502,196	7	23	22
Illinois	1,165	45,852,410	8	22	14
Indiana	936	45,448,692	9	25	18
Alabama	443	44,698,332	10	14	33
Lowest Polluters					
Province/State	**# of Facilities**	**Total Releases and Transfers (kg)**	**Rank**	**Rank per Capita**	**Rank per km**
D.C.	1	2	63	63	62
P.E.I.	2	17,553	62	62	58
*Hawaii	9	173,191	61	8	1
Vermont	32	310,375	60	57	61
Newfoundland	7	400,708	59	46	63
North Dakota	29	511,257	58	61	53
Virgin Islands	2	732,949	57	55	60
Saskatchewan	15	799,321	56	12	35
Alaska	8	1,039,945	55	1	37
* Hawaii is the highest polluter for its size, so it is not a safe place to live. It has a very high breast cancer incidence.					

are listed the top ten highest and lowest polluters without reference to wind and water patterns. The information is taken from *Taking Stock: North American Pollutant Releases and Transfers, 1996*, available from the Commission for Environmental Cooperation, Montreal, QC (tel. 514-350-4300 or fax. 514-350-4314) or from TRI in the United States (tel. 800-535-0202). If you want to find out what industries are releasing organochlorines and other carcinogens into your air, water, and soil, you will find it in this publication. You can then unite with other women in putting a stop to this production and release.

In the small town of Asbestos, Quebec, about 200 kilometers south of Montreal, preparations are underway to open the second largest magnesium processing plant in the world by the year 2000. According to a report by a Quebec environmental assessment panel, the plant will release 20 times the amount of dioxin that escapes annually from all the more than 40 pulp and paper mills in the province. The plant will create yearly 171 kg of PCBs, and 2100 kg of hexachlorobenzene. These three substances are on the list of 12 toxic chemicals that the United Nations is trying to ban by international agreement and they are all linked with breast cancer. Although an environmental assessment panel refused to issue a permit for Noranda Inc. to open the plant, the Quebec government reversed its decision in April 1998.[91] Our governments are not protecting us. Canada's Environment Minister recently announced at a United Nations meeting that Canada would eliminate the "dirty dozen" environmental contaminants; in the next breath, she admitted she would not intervene in the Noranda project. It is up to us to be vigilant in our communities and to demand action. We will not win the war against breast cancer if travesties like this continue to occur.

▶ **Action for Prevention:** If you live in a high polluting province or state, or close to an industry that releases any amount of organochlorines, put pressure on your municipal, provincial, state, or federal elected leaders to enforce regulations banning the production and release of organochlorines and other toxic chemicals. Put pressure on the industries themselves to stop production. Find out what quantities of environmental hormone disruptors are in your air and water supply and where they are coming from. In the United States, you can easily find out who is polluting in your area through visiting the web site www.scorecard.org/. A similar site is planned for Canada by the end of 2000 and can be accessed through www.net/cela/. Unite with other activist groups and use the many resources available, as listed in the resource directory at the back of this book.

There are three excellent films on the environmental links to breast cancer that you can show in your communities. One

---

We hear you, fellow-creatures.

We know we are wrecking the world and we are afraid.

What we have unleashed has such momentum now, we don't know how to turn it around.

Don't leave us alone, we need your help. You need us too for your own survival.

Are there powers there you can share with us?

"I, lichen, work slowly, very slowly. Time is my friend.

This is what I give you: patience for the long haul and perseverance."

"It is a dark time. As deep-diving trout I offer you my fearlessness of the dark."

"I, lion, give you my roar, the voice to speak out and be heard."

"I am caterpillar. The leaves I eat taste bitter now. But dimly I sense a great change coming.

What I offer you, humans, is my willingness to dissolve and transform.

I do that without knowing what the end-result will be, so I share with you my courage too."

— Joanna Macy

is called Exposure: Environmental Links to Breast Cancer and comes with an excellent resource guide and handbook to accompany the film. You can order it from Women's Network on Health and the Environment (517 College St., Ste 233, Toronto, ON, M6G 4A2, tel. 416-928-0880). Another is called Hormone Copy-Cats and can be ordered from the World Wildlife Fund Canada (90 Eglington Ave E, Ste 504, Toronto, ON, M4P 2Z7, tel. 416-489-8800 or 800-26-PANDA or fax. 416-489-3611). The third film is called Rachel's Daughters, a reference to Rachel Carson, founder of the environmental movement, which also comes with an excellent Community Action and Resource Guide, available from Light-Saraf Films (264 Arbor St, San Fransisco, CA 94131, tel. 415-469-0139). ◄

Rachel Carson Day (May 27)

Rachel Carson started the environmental movement with her book, *Silent Spring*, published in 1962. A marine biologist, ecologist, environmentalist, writer, and activist, Rachel was born on May 27, 1907 and died on April 14, 1964 from breast cancer. We can honor the spirit of Rachel and be fueled by her passion for the environment by celebrating Rachel Carson Day. Every year, on May 27, do what you can in your own corner of the world to preserve the safety and sanctity of the environment. Remove the toxins from your home. Reduce your use of plastic. Join other women and lobby against PVC, radiation, pesticides, dioxin, and chlorine. Stage a march for the environment. Create awareness for the environmental links to breast cancer every year on May 27. Be passionate, be active, be vocal, do it together. Do it for yourself; do it for your children and future generations; do it for wildlife; do it for the earth, air, and water; do it for Rachel — just do it.

You could, for example, write a letter or copy one of the samples on the following pages to your elected government officials. Send it to the mayor of your city, your provincial or state politicians, and federal government representatives.

Non-Toxic Body and Home Care Products

Clearly, there are an unprecedented number of chemicals used on the earth today which undermine our health, the health of future generations, and disturb the delicate planetary ecosystems of which we are a part. We can decrease our exposure to these chemicals by using non-toxic

alternatives and by encouraging others to do the same. The waters of the earth circulate in our arteries and veins; its soil becomes the nutritive base of our bodies. What we do to the earth, we do to ourselves. Please do not add toxic chemicals to this already impaired system.

Here are a few natural ways that we can support our planet as we are sustained by it.

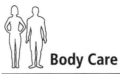

Body Care

Baby Oil

Ingredients: wheat germ oil, apricot kernel oil or sunflower, sweet almond oil, lavender.

Fill a 50 ml glass container half full with apricot kernel oil or sunflower oil, and half full with sweet almond oil. Add one capful of wheat germ oil. Add 3 drops of lavender.

Blush

Ingredients: glycerin, cornstarch, beet root powder, baking soda.

Add 50% glycerin (equal parts glycerin and water) to cornstarch in a saucer and make a thick paste. Slowly add beet root powder until you reach your desired color. Darken the color further with a bit of baking soda. Make the paste the same consistency as your brand name product; use a glass or ceramic container to store it in.

Contact Lens Solution

Ingredients: water, aluminum free salt.

Boil a cup of cold tap water in a glass saucepan. Add ¼ tsp. of aluminum free salt and return to a boil. Pour into a sterile jar and refrigerate. You can even freeze it.

Dandruff Relief

Ingredients: grain alcohol (or vodka), water, lavender, rosemary, eucalyptus.

After washing your hair, once your hair has dried, rub this healing lotion into your scalp: Fill a 50ml/2-oz container half full with grain alcohol (or vodka) and half full with water. Add 2 drops lavender, 1 drop rosemary and 2 drops eucalyptus. This quantity will be enough for a couple of applications.

Dental Floss

Ingredients: 2 or 4 pound monofilament fish line.

Floss your teeth with 2 or 4 lb nylon monofilament fish line, available at any hardware store. Double and twist it for extra strength and rinse it in water before you begin. Cut a month's supply at a time and keep them in a small paper bag in your bathroom cabinet.

Deodorant Body Splash

Ingredients: white or cider vinegar, water, lavender.

Fill a 50 ml glass container, ⅓ full with white or cider vinegar and ⅔ full with water. Add 5 drops of lavender. You can also add a capful of rose water.

Dry Skin/Eczema Healing Oil

Ingredients: sesame oil, olive oil, avocado oil, almond oil, vitamin E gelatin capsules, vitamin A capsules. This oil is based on a formula devised by Paavo Airola.

Pour 2 tbsp sesame oil, 1 tbsp olive oil, 2 tbsp avocado oil, and 2 tbsp almond oil in a small, dark glass jar or container. Take 10 vitamin E gelatin capsules (200 IU each) and 4 vitamin A gelatin capsules (25,000 units each) and puncture the capsules with needles or cut the ends with scissors and squeeze the contents into the bottle. Add a drop or two of your favorite essential oil to mask the aroma of the ingredients. Close the lid tightly and shake well. The best way to use this oil is at night before going to bed. After you wash your face, neck and hands take a few drops of the oil and massage into needed areas. The oil will be totally absorbed into the skin by morning.

Facial Oil

Ingredients: almond oil, vitamin E oil, lavender, geranium.

Fill a 50 ml container with cold pressed almond oil and 10 drops of vitamin E. If desired, add 10 drops of lavender and 10 drops of geranium. After washing your face, apply two to three drops of oil, lightly stroking it into your face. After a few minutes the oil should be absorbed. Blot any extra with a tissue.

Foot Powder

Ingredients: corn starch, peppermint oil, citricidal (grapefruit seed extract).

Rub 2 drops of peppermint oil and 3 drops of citricidal into 50 g/2 oz of cornstarch with your fingers. Keep in a jar (or a spice jar with a shaker cap). Apply after bathing or when feet are hot/sweaty.

Lice Killers

Use the following alternative to lindane-containing shampoos for lice:

Mix together the essential oils of:

Rosemary	20 drops
Geranium	10 drops
Lavender	20 drops
Eucalyptus	10 drops
Tea tree	20 drops

Add these to ½ cup of either olive oil or mustard oil and keep the mixture in a dark glass jar. Rub the blend into the scalp and leave it overnight with a towel wrapped around the head. Wash it out in the morning. Repeat one week later. Treat the whole family at the same time and wash bedding and hair brushes. Add a small amount of the oil (5 drops) to your shampoo each time you wash your hair until the infestation is over. Buy a LiceMeister comb (other combs won't work) and comb every family member's hair daily with it to remove the nits until no more are found. Check hair weekly for nits as long as there is an outbreak in the school. For more help, or to order the LiceMeister comb, call LiceBusters (416-410-LICE).

Massage Oil

Ingredients: vegetable oil, vitamin E oil.

Try vegetable oils like cold pressed almond, apricot kernel, sesame, sunflower, olive, or coconut oil. For 50 ml/2 oz of vegetable oil, add 5 drops of vitamin E. You can also add 5 to 20 drops of your favorite essential oils.

Powdered Deodorant

Ingredients: Corn starch or baking soda, lavender.

Stir 5 drops of lavender oil into ½ cup corn starch or baking soda and store in a glass, opaque, airtight container. Use a soft cloth, such as velvet or cotton flannel, to dust your underarms.

Shampoo

Ingredients: Borax liquid soap, citric acid crystals.

A few squirts of borax liquid soap, described above, serves as a great shampoo. The only thing you'll need to get used to is that the soap doesn't lather. After shampooing with borax liquid, use ¼ tsp citric acid crystals (not ascorbic) in a pint container of water to return your scalp to its natural acidity level.

Skin Disinfectant

Ingredients: tea tree oil or citricidal, water.

For cleaning cuts and wounds add 5 drops of tea tree oil or citricidal to a small bowl of cooled, boiled water. Swab the wounded area using cotton wool or a gauze cloth.

Soap

"Soapworks" makes totally natural soaps. Some good soap choices are: evening primrose, chamomile, oatmeal, or goatmilk. These soaps are available at health food stores.

Toothbrushing

Ingredients: baking soda, food grade hydrogen peroxide.

Brush your teeth with a pinch of baking soda dissolved in a glass with some water. If you have plastic, not metal, fillings dilute food grade hydrogen peroxide with equal parts water and store in a glass bottle. Brushing with this solution will help to whiten your teeth within 6 months.

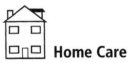

Home Care

Carpet Cleaner

Ingredients: borax powder, grain alcohol, boric acid, citricidal, white vinegar.

You can rent a machine to wash your carpet, but instead of the soap they suggest use ⅓ cup borax powder in the wash water and ¼ cup grain alcohol, 2 tsp boric acid, 20 drops citricidal, and ¼ cup white vinegar in the rinse water.

Clean Air

Ingredients: citricidal or tea tree oil, water.

Use 5 drops of citricidal or 10 drops of tea tree oil in 1–2 l of water in humidifiers and air conditioners to disinfect the air and deter mold growth.

Diaper Cleaner

Ingredients: citricidal or tea tree oil, water, borax powder, washing soda.

To clean and disinfect diapers, add 10 drops of citricidal or up to 50 drops of tea tree oil to ½ l of warm water and let soak for a ½ hour; otherwise, add the same amount to a liter of water and pour into the washing machine along with the laundry detergent mixture below.

Dish Soap

Ingredients: borax powder, washing soda.

Use equal parts borax powder and washing soda to clean your dishes. For dishes that aren't greasy, just wash them with running water.

Dishwasher Soap

Ingredients: borax powder, vinegar.

Use 2 tsp borax powder pre-dissolved in water. If you use too much, it will leave a film on the dishes. You can also use vinegar in the rinse cycle.

Disinfectant

Ingredients: citricidal or tea tree oil, water.

To control bacteria, fungi and mold, add 20 drops of citricidal or up to 50 drops of tea tree oil to a bucket of water and stir well. Use this solution for mopping or wiping floors, counters, sinks, bathroom tiles, shower stalls and toilets. Put 5 drops of citricidal into a spray bottle with water and spray bathroom tiles and shower stalls to discourage mold growth.

Drain Cleaner

Ingredients: plunger, baking soda, vinegar.

First use a plunger if the sink is backed up. Push down and release a few times to dislodge debris.

Pour ½ cup of baking soda and ½ cup of vinegar over the drain. Let it set for one hour, then run hot water to clear. Never pour liquid grease down the drain. Always use a drain sieve.

Dry Cleaning

Instead of dry cleaning, find a Green Clean outlet near you. They use safe water based alternatives to toxic chemicals. Ask your local dry cleaner to switch to Green Clean. The use of the organochlorine perchloroethylene ("perc") in dry cleaning impairs the health of workers and nearby residents.

Floor Cleaner

Ingredients: washing soda, borax powder, white vinegar.

Use washing soda with a bit of borax to deter insects (except ants). Use white vinegar in your rinse water for a natural shine and to deter ants.

Floor Wax

Ingredients: beeswax, linseed oil.

Mix beeswax and linseed oil, testing on a patch of floor to confirm desired proportions.

Furniture Polish

Ingredients: olive oil.

Use filtered water to dampen a cloth and place a few drops of olive oil on the cloth.

Hot Tubs, Jacuzzis, Swimming Pools

Ingredients: citricidal (grapefruit seed extract).

Use 10–15 drops of citricidal per gallon of water to disinfect hot tubs, jacuzzis, and swimming pools.

Insect Killer

Ingredients: boric acid.

Throw liberal amounts of boric acid (not borax) behind your stove, refrigerator, and under your carpets. Keep it away from food and out of children's reach.

Kitchen/Bathroom Cleanser

Ingredients: borax powder, washing soda.

Use ¼ cup borax with ¼ cup of washing soda and a minimum of water to clean in the kitchen and bathroom. You can use dry washing soda to scour.

Laundry Detergent

Ingredients: borax powder, washing soda.

Use a ½ cup of borax powder per load of laundry, or combine with washing soda for extra cleaning power. For getting out stubborn stains, try rubbing with bar soap first and/or rub with grain alcohol, vinegar, or baking soda.

Liquid Soap

Ingredients: borax powder, or vegetable oil-based liquid soap.

Use a funnel to put ⅛ cup borax powder in a 1 gallon jug. Fill the jug with cold tap water. Shake well and let it settle. After a few minutes pour off the clear liquid into dispensers for use as liquid soap. Alternatively, use vegetable oil based liquid soap.

Moth Balls

Ingredients: cedar chips, lavender flowers and oil.

Make up sachets with cedar chips sprinkled with lavender oil and flowers. Make the scent just strong enough to fill the storage area. If the closet is one you open often, you may have to refresh the oil every two months.

Oven Cleaner

Ingredients: baking soda, pure soap, lemon juice.

Scrub with baking soda on its own or mix 1 cup of pure soap, ½ cup lemon juice with one gallon of water, and scrub. Rinse with clean water.

Smells

Ingredients: dried herbs, coarse corn meal.

Basement, pet, carpet smells … try dry herbs such as thyme, lavender, tansy, rosemary etc. strewn around the floor and swept up again after a few days. This absorbs odor and repels insects. You can also mix coarse corn meal with a few drops of essential oil, sprinkle it on the carpets, and vacuum it up after a few hours. This combination is good for upholstery, too, though not good for ingestion by children and pets.

Toilet Bowl Cleaner

Ingredients: borax powder, lemon juice or vinegar, vitamin C capsules.

Pour 1 cup borax powder into toilet bowl and let sit overnight. Scrub with a brush and flush. For faster action, add ¼ cup lemon juice or vinegar to the borax. Wait a few hours before scrubbing. Alternatively, open two 1000 mg vitamin C capsules and drop them into the bowl, letting them sit overnight. Scrub with a brush and flush.

Window Cleaner

Ingredients: vinegar, newspaper.

Mix 2 tbsp vinegar in one liter of water in a spray bottle. Clean your windows using newspapers.

Non-Toxic Shopping List Exercise

You should be able to find these natural and organic products and ingredients for the specified purposes in supermarkets, health food stores, hardware stores, and ecological supply stores. Add them to your shopping list.

❏ Almond Oil, cold pressed : dry skin blend, facial oil

❏ Aluminum-free salt: contact lens solution

❏ Apricot Kernel Oil or Sunflower Oil: baby oil

❏ Avocado Oil: dry skin blend

❏ Beet Root Powder: blush

❏ Beeswax: floor wax

❏ Borax Powder : carpet cleaner, diaper cleaner, dish soap, dishwasher soap, floor cleaner, laundry detergent, liquid soap, toilet bowl cleaner

❏ Boric Acid: carpet cleaner, insect killer

❏ Cedar Chips: moth balls

❏ Citric Acid Crystals: shampoo

❏ Citricidal Drops (Grapefruit seed extract): disinfectant, hot tubs

❏ Essential Oils : lice killers

❏ Eucalyptus: dandruff relief

❏ Glycerin: blush

❏ Lavender: baby oil, dandruff relief, deodorant body splash, facial oil

❏ Lavender Flowers and Oil: moth balls, powdered deodorant

❏ Linseed Oil: floor wax

❏ Geranium: facial oil

❏ Hydrogen Peroxide (food grade): toothbrushing

❏ Monofilament Fish Line (2 or 4 lb): dental floss

❏ Peppermint: foot powder

❏ Rose Water: deodorant body splash

❏ Rosemary: dandruff relief

❏ Sesame Oil: dry skin blend

❏ "Soapworks" Soap

❏ Tea Tree Oil: clean air, diaper cleaner, disinfectant, skin disinfectant

❏ Vitamin A (gelatin capsules): dry skin blend

❏ Vitamin C (capsules): toilet bowl cleaner

❏ Vitamin E (oil): facial oil, massage oil

❏ Vitamin E (gelatin capsules): dry skin blend

❏ Vegetable Oils (almond/apricot kernel/sesame/sunflower/olive/coconut oil): massage oil

❏ Washing Soda: diaper cleaner, dish soap, floor cleaner, laundry detergent

❏ Wheat Germ Oil: baby oil

Great Spirit, whose dry lands thirst, help us to find the way to refresh your lands.

We pray for your power to refresh your lands.

Great Spirit, whose waters are choked with debris and pollution, help us to find the way to cleanse your waters.

We pray for your knowledge to find the way to cleanse the waters.

Great Spirit, whose beautiful earth grows ugly with misuse, help us to find the way to restore beauty to your handiwork.

We pray for your strength to restore the beauty of your handiwork.

Great Spirit, whose creatures are being destroyed, help us to find a way to replenish them.

We pray for your power to replenish the earth.

Great Spirit, whose gifts to us are being lost in selfishness and corruption, help us to find the way to restore our humanity.

We pray for your wisdom to find the way to restore our humanity.

— United Nations Environmental Sabbath Program

May 27, Year

Minister of Agriculture   or   Secretary
House of Commons   Agriculture, Nutrition and Forestry
Ottawa, ON K1A 0A6   Committee
                                                         United States Senate
                                                         Washington, DC 20510

Dear Minister,   or   Dear Secretary,

I am extremely concerned about the amount of pesticides used on the food that we eat. These pesticides end up in the groundwater and persist in the soil for many years. Many of them act as hormone disruptors linked to breast cancer and are eroding our ability to reproduce. Please tell me what steps you are making to ensure the following:

1) that the following pesticides be banned, as they are implicated in breast cancer: atrazine, cyanazine, dichlorvos, endosulfan, ethalfluralin, ethylene oxide, etridiazole, methoychlor, oryzalin, prometon, propazine, simazine, terbuthylazine, terbutyn, tribenuron methyl;

2) that organically grown food is more readily available all across the nation;

3) that the government encourage organic farmers through subsidies and educate all farmers in organic farming methods;

Sincerely,

Your address:

May 27, Year

Minister of Health (or)	or	Secretary
Minister of the Environment		Environment and Public Works Committee
House of Commons		United States Senate
Ottawa, ON K1A 0A6		Washington, DC 20510

Dear Minister,   Dear Secretary

As a woman and as a citizen I am extremely concerned about the government's lack of resolve in enforcing environmental regulations. I insist upon immediate action in the following areas:

1) that there is an immediate ban on the production and use of organochlorines, which are causative factors in the breast cancer epidemic, and are disturbing the reproductive ability of humans, birds, fish, turtles, whales, seals, polar bears, otters, and many life forms. These chemicals are extremely toxic and extremely stable. Some do not break down for over a thousand years. The planet cannot sustain their use any longer. We must achieve zero discharge of persistent toxic substances as described by the International Joint Commission on Great Lakes Water Quality. Why has the government not acted on these recommendations?

2) that PVC plastic is speedily phased out before the year 2001, as it has been in Sweden, and is replaced with readily available alternatives. These alternatives should be labeled PVC free.

3) that there be a strictly enforced ban on the incineration of PVC plastic, especially by hospitals. Dioxin is one of the deadliest chemicals known, and is released through the production and burning of PVC plastic. The government must maintain a regulatory body that mandates strict enforcement of standards and severe penalties for polluters.

4) that the following pesticides be banned, as they are implicated in breast cancer: atrazine, cyanazine, dichlorvos, endosulfan, ethalfluralin, ethylene oxide, etridiazole, methoxychlor, oryzalin, prometon, propazine, simazine, terbuthylazine, terbutyn, tribenuron methyl; and that there be programs in place that encourage farmers to reduce pesticides and grow organic food.

5) that there be a ban on the production and use of alkylphenols (present in some industrial detergents) and phthalates (used in the manufacturing of plastics). Both of these chemical groups are hormone disruptors and are found throughout the environment.

6) that industry must prove its products are safe through thorough testing before they are allowed on the market or in our bodies. It has taken 40 years to realize that the organochlorines are hormone disruptors, yet still they are in widespread use. The companies that make chemicals must be required to first test them thoroughly before they experiment on humans and wildlife. The testing must be done by a scientific lab without a vested interest in the industry. Industry and government must operate on the Precautionary Principle, which dictates that indication of harm, rather than proof of harm, is enough to restrict usage of toxic substances. It is possible to phase out production of organochlorines. Alternatives exist now for all major uses of chlorine including bleaches, disinfectants, plastics, pesticides, solvents, and refrigerants. We have an obligation to protect life and thousands of years of evolution. The onus must be placed on the chemical industry to prove that its products are safe rather than on us to prove that they are not.

Please let me know what specific progress you are making in each of these areas.

Sincerely,

Your address:

Summary

Once we know the sources of environmental toxins, we can set to work minimizing risk from our surroundings and cleansing our bodies from both externally and internally generated toxins.

I have come to terms with the future.

From this day onward I will walk easy on the earth.

Plant trees. Kill no living things. Live in harmony

with all creatures. I will restore the earth where I am.

Use no more of its resources than I need.

And listen, listen to what it is telling me.

— M.J. Slim Hooey

Further Reading

Berthold-Bond, Annie. Clean & Green: *The Complete Guide to Non-Toxic and Environmentally Safe Housekeeping.* Woodstock, NY: Ceres Press, 1994.

Clark, Hulda. *The Cure for All Diseases: 100 Case Histories,* San Diego, CA: Promotion Publishers, 1995.

Colborn, Theo, D. Dumanoski, J. Peterson Myers. *Our Stolen Future.* New York, NY: Penguin, 1996.

Dadd, Debra Lynn. *The Nontoxic Home: Protecting Yourself and Your Family from Everyday Toxics and Health Hazards.* Los Angeles, CA: J.P. Tharcher, 1986.

Dunford, Randy. *Clean Your House Safely & Effectively Without Harmful Chemicals,* McKinney, TX: Magni Group, Inc., 1993.

Epstein, S. and D. Steinman. *The Breast Cancer Prevention Program.* New York, NY: Macmillan, 1997.

Steingraber, Sandra. *Living Downstream: An Ecologist Looks at Cancer and the Environment.* Reading, MA: Addison-Wesley Publishing Co. Ltd., 1997.

References

1. Gregg, E. Radiation risks with diagnostic x-rays. *Radiology,* 1977; 123:447.
2. Clorfene-Casten, Liane. *Breast Cancer: Poisons, Profits and Prevention.* Monroe, ME: Common Courage Press, 1996:62.
3. Gofman, Johnl. *Preventing Breast Cancer: The Story of a Major, Proven, Preventable Cause of This Disease.* 2nd. ed. San Francisco, CA: Committee for Nuclear Responsibility, 1996.
4. Reported in *JAMA,* 1984.
5. John, E. and J. Kelsey. Radiation and other environmental exposures and breast cancer. *Epidemiologic Reviews,* 1993;15(1):157-61.
6. Harris, J., M. Lippman, et al. Breast cancer. *New England Journal of Medicine,* 1992;327:319-28.
7. Kelsey, J. and M. Gammon. The epidemiology of breast cancer. *CA: A Cancer Journal for Clinicians,* 1991;41:146-65.
8. Epstein, S. Europe's worries about U.S. meat should be our worry, too. *Los Angeles Times,* January 30,1989; (A11).
9. *Living at Ground Zero.* Toronto Star, Sunday, Jan. 10, 1999;(B1-2).
10. Clorfene-Casten, Liane. *Breast Cancer: Poisons, Profits and Prevention.* Monroe, ME: Common Courage Press, 1996:70.

11. Clorfene-Casten, Liane. *Breast Cancer: Poisons, Profits and Prevention*. Monroe, ME: Common Courage Press, 1996:72.

12. Greenpeace. Nuclear power, human health and the environment: Breast cancer warning in the Great Lakes region. Toronto, ON: Greenpeace International, 1995.

13. Lansberg, Michele. U.S. war toxins blamed for rise in Iraqi cancers. *The Toronto Star*, Sat., Nov. 21, 1998;(L1).

14. Baldwin, D. Former mine site dumping ground for U.S. atomic waste in the 40's. *The Toronto Star*, April 20, 1998.

15. Spears, Tom. Radioactive baby teeth flag cancer rate. *Ottawa Citizen*, July 25, 1999:(A1).

16. Stewart, T., and N. Stewart. Breast cancer in female flight attendants. *Lancet*,1995:Nov.25;346:1379.

17. Clorfene-Casten, Liane. *Breast Cancer: Poisons, Profits and Prevention*. Monroe, ME: Common Courage Press, 1996:107.

18. Nystrom, Lennarth, et al. Breast cancer screening with mammography: Overview of Swedish randomized trials, *Lancet*;1993:Apr 17;341(8851):973-978.

19. Chitale, Angeli. Breast cancer and the effects of radiation: What you can do to protect yourself from radiation-induced damage. Toronto, ON: Canadian College of Naturopathic Medicine, May, 1999:6.

20. Weed, Susun. *Breast Cancer? Breast Health!* Woodstock, NY: Ash Tree Publishing, 1996:211-12.

21. Electromagnetic Fields and Male Breast Cancer, *The Lancet*, December, 1990:336.

22. Health Report, *Time*, June 27, 1994.

23. Fackelmann, K. Do EMFs Pose Breast Cancer Risk?. *Science News*, June 18, 1994:388.

24. Weed, S. *Breast Cancer? Breast Health!* Woodstock, NY: Ash Tree Publishing, 1996:19.

25. Greenpeace, Death in Small Doses: *The Effects of Organochlorines on Aquatic Ecosystems*. 1992.

26. Arnold, S., D. Klotz, B. Collins, P. Vonier, L. Guillette Jr., J. Mclachlan. Synergistic activation of estrogen receptor with combinations of environmental chemicals. *Science*, Vol. 272, June 7, 1996:1489-91.

27. Colborn, Theo, D. Dumanoski, J. Peterson Myers. *Our Stolen Future*. New York, NY:Penguin, 1996:152.

28. Davis, Devra Lee, H.L. Bradlow. Can environmental estrogens cause breast cancer? *Scientific American*, Oct. 1995:172.

29. Davis, Devra Lee, H.L. Bradlow. Can environmental estrogens cause breast cancer? *Scientific American*, Oct. 1995:172.

30. Davis, Devra Lee, H.L. Bradlow. Can environmental estrogens cause breast cancer? *Scientific American*, Oct. 1995:172.

31. Davis, Devra Lee, H.L. Bradlow. Can environmental estrogens cause breast cancer? *Scientific American*, Oct. 1995:172.

32. Steingraber, Sandra. *Living Downstream: An Ecologist Looks at Cancer and the Environment*. Reading, MA: Addison-Wesley Publishing Co. Inc., 1997:133.

33. Sharpe, R., N. Skakkeback. 1993. Are oestrogens involved in falling male sperm counts and disorders of the male reproductive tract? *Lancet*, 341:1392-95.

34. Lee, John. *What Your Doctor May Not Tell You About Menopause*. New York, NY: Warner Books, 1996:55-56.

35. Chilvers, C. et al. Apparent doubling of frequency of undescended testis in England and Wales in 1962-81. *Lancet*, 1984:330-32.

36. Hutson, J. et al. Hormonal control of testicular descent and the cause of cryptorchidism. *Reproduction, Fertility and Development*, 1994;6:151-56.

37. Lawless, Gary. *First Sight of Land*. Nobleton, ME: Blackberry Books, 1990.

38. Davis, Devra Lee, H.L. Bradlow. Can environmental estrogens cause breast cancer? *Scientific American*, Oct. 1995;273(4):166-72.

39. Wasserman, M. et al. Organochlorine compounds in neoplastic and adjacent apparently normal tissue. *Bulletin of Environmental Contamination and Toxicology*, 1976:15:478-84.

40. Mussalo-Rauhamaa, H.E. et al. Occurrence of b-hexachlorocyclohexane in breast cancer patients. *Cancer*, 1990:66:2124-28.

41. Bishop, J., S. Ho, H. Hutchinson, L. Young. Organochlorines and their link to breast cancer. Toronto, ON:. *Canadian College of Naturopathic Medicine*, April, 1999.

42. Environmental Health Committee Newsletter for Family Physicians. *Pesticides and Human Health*. Toronto, ON: Environmental Health Committee of the Ontario College of Family Physicians, ND.

43. Nikiforuk, Andrew. Rocky Mountain Blight. *The Globe and Mail*, Saturday, Oct. 17, 1998:D5.

44. Neidert, E., P. Saschenbrecker. Occurrence of pesticide residues in selected agricultural food commodities available in Canada. *Journal of AOAC International*, 1996;79(2):549-66.

45. Steingraber, Sandra. *Living Downstream: An Ecologist Looks at Cancer and the Environment*. Reading, MA: Addison-Wesley Publishing Co. Inc.,1997:161-62.

46. Mussalo-Rauhamaa et al., Occurrence of beta-Hexachlorocyclohexane in breast cancer patients. *Cancer*, 1990;66:2124-28.

47. This list of pesticides is adapted from "Currently used pesticides linked with breast cancer" by Carolyn Cox, *Journal of Pesticide Reform*, Spring, 1996;16, 1.

48. A handout from WEDO of the same title as above

49. List of known and suspected hormone disruptors. World Wildlife Fund. www.wwfcanada.org/hormone-disruptors/list.htm.

50. Hoyer, A.P., P. Grandjean, T. Jorgensen, J. Brock, H. Hartvig. Organochlorine exposure and risk of breast cancer. *Lancet*, 1998;352, Dec.5:1816-20.

51. Greenpeace. *"Dirty Dozen" Chemical Profiles*. Toronto, ON: Greenpeace Canada, 1995.

52. Soto, A.M. et al. The pesticides endosulphan, toxaphene and dieldrin have estrogenic effects on human estrogen-sensitive cells. *EHP*, 1994;102:380-83.

53. Passivirta, J. et al. Chloroterpenes and other organochlorines in Baltic, Finnish and Arctic wildlife. *Chemosphere*, 1991;22:47-55.

54. Sarick, Lila. To spray or not to spray? – that is the question. *The Globe and Mail*, Sat. Aug. 29, 1998:A10.

55. Rice, Bonnie for Greenpeace. *Polyvinyl Chloride (PVC) Plastic: Primary Contributor to the Global Dioxin Crisis*. October 1995.

56. Mittelstaedt, Martin. Environmentalists urge testing of air near garbage dumps. *The Globe and Mail*, Sat., Nov. 28, 1998:A9.

57. This list is taken from a Greenpeace Report, *Taking Back Our Stolen Future: Hormone disruption and PVC plastic*, April 1996.

58. Greenpeace, Death in Small Doses: *The Effects of Organochlorines on Aquatic Ecosystems*. 1992.

59. Greenpeace, *Taking Back Our Stolen Future*. April, 1996:15.

60. Rier, S.E., D.C. Martin, J.L. Becker. Endometriosis in rhesus monkeys (Macaca mulatta) following chronic exposure to 2,3,7,8-tetrachlordibenzo-p-dioxin. *Fundamental and Applied Toxicology.* 1993;21:433-41.

61. Greenpeace. *Poisoning the Future: Impact of Endocrine Disrupting Chemicals on Wildlife and Human Health*. October 1997:23.

62. From a Greenpeace handout, *Which of these toys contain hazardous chemicals?*

63. Vinyl toys contain chemical that causes liver damage in rats. *The Globe and Mail*, Sat., Nov.14, 1998.

64. Ema, M., R. Kurasoka, H. Amano, Y. Ogawa. Comparative developmental toxicity of n-butyl benzyl phthalate and di-n-butylphthalate in rats. *Arch Environ Contam Toxicol.*1995;28:233.

65. Colborn, Theo, D. Dumanoski, J. Peterson Myers. *Our Stolen Future*. New York, NY: Penguin, 1996:136.

66. Davis, Devra Lee, H. Bradlow. Can environmental estrogens cause breast cancer? *Scientific American*, Oct. 1995:166-72.

67. Colborn, Theo, D. Dumanoski, J. Peterson Myers. *Our Stolen Future*. New York, NY:Penguin, 1996:134.

68. Waters, Jane. Taking back our stolen future, *Int'l J. Alternative & Complementary Medicine*, 1996;14 (12);19, 22-23.

69. Soap compound may be linked to salmon deaths. *The Toronto Star*, Dec. 23, 1998:A27.

70. World Wildlife Fund news release, "Lab analysis reveals hormone-disrupting chemicals in everyday household soaps", Feb. 11, 1997, and personal communication with Julia Langar.

70. Spears, Tom. Cancers may come out of the tap. *Owen Sound Sun Times*, Nov. 24, 1998:1.

71. Isabella, Judith. Getting too close to seal level. *The Globe and Mail*, Saturday, Oct.3, 1998:D5.

72. Isabella, Judith. Getting too close to seal level. *The Globe and Mail*, Saturday, Oct.3, 1998:D5.

73. Colborn, Theo, D. Dumanoski, J. Peterson Myers. *Our Stolen Future*. New York, Penguin, 1996. p.88.

74. Greenpeace. *Taking Back Our Stolen Future: Hormone Disruption and PVC Plastic*. 1996. p.15.

75. Aronson, Kristan. Breast cancer risk and organochlorines. Presentation at the World Conference on Breast Cancer in Ottawa, Ontario, July 28, 1999.

76. Colborn, Theo, D. Dumanoski, J. Peterson Myers. *Our Stolen Future*. New York, Penguin, 1996. p 107.

77. Greenpeace. *Poisoning the Future: Impact of Endocrine Disrupting Chemicals on Wildlife and Human Health*. October 1997. p.13.

78. Greenpeace. *Poisoning the Future: Impact of Endocrine Disrupting Chemicals on Wildlife and Human Health*. October 1997. p.23

79. Steingraber, Sandra. *Living Downstream*: An Ecologist Looks at Cancer and the Environment. Addison-Wesley Publishing Co. Inc., Reading, Mass. 1997. p. 52-53.

80. Leiss, J.K. & D. Savitz, Home pesticide use and childhood cancer: A case-controlled study, *AJPH*, 1993; 85:249-252.

81. Davis, J.R. et al. Family pesticide use and childhood brain cancer, *Archives of Environmental Contamination and Toxicity*, 1993;24:87-92.

82. Commission for Environmental Cooperation. *Taking Stock: North American Pollutant Releases and Transfers*. Communications and Public Outreach Department of the CEC Secretariat, Montreal, Quebec. 1999. p.67.

83. TCE: ATSDR, *Case Studies in Environmental Medicine: Trichloroethylene Toxicity*. Atlanta, Ga.: ATSDR, 1992.

84. Commission for Environmental Cooperation. Taking Stock: *North American Pollutant Releases and Transfers*. Communications and Public Outreach Department of the CEC Secretariat, Montreal, Quebec. 1999. p.67.

85. Joseph, B. Breast Health. *Vegetarian Times*, July 1997: 83-90.

86. Spears, Tom. Cancers may come out of the tap. *Owen Sound Sun Times*, Nov. 24, 1998:1.

87. *GSE Report*, Vol.1, Issue 1, Praxus, Inc., Novato, CA. p.6.

88. *GSE Report*, Vol.1, Issue 1, Praxus, Inc., Novato, CA. p.10.

89. thanks to Joanne Leung from the Canadian College of Naturopathic Medicine for providing this information in her research paper on composting toilets. April 7, 1999.

90. dedication to Richard St. Barbe Baker, father of the trees. Original source unknown.

91. McAndrew, Brian. Quebec mine to spew toxic chemicals. *Toronto Star*, Wed., July 1, 1998.

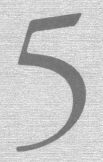
Detoxifying Our Bodies

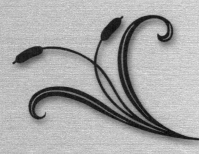

Exercises

Contents

Toxins are substances that are harmful to health. They may have their origin from outside the body (exotoxins) or within the body (endotoxins). When the body is unable to break down and eliminate a toxic overload, symptoms of illness may manifest. These could include headaches, joint pain, fatigue, irritability, depression, mental confusion, digestive disturbances, cardiovascular irregularities, flu-like symptoms, or allergic reactions such as hives, runny nose, sneezing, and coughing. Toxicity may also contribute to the presence of autoimmune diseases, rheumatoid arthritis, Alzheimer's disease, Parkinson's disease, and cancer. Most bodily ailments are due in some part to toxicity.

Toxins can do their damage in several ways. They combine with and destroy enzymes, can stagnate in tissues and interfere with circulation, causing high blood pressure, and can thicken the blood, resulting in decreased circulation and availability of nutrients to specific areas of the body. Toxins can block the transmission of nerve impulses, resulting in psychological disturbances. They can interact with hormones, causing disturbances in glandular balance. As health is impaired, there is first felt a general lowering of the body's vitality, decreased resistance to colds and flues, and irritability or depression. Over time the detoxification and eliminative organs become overwhelmed and disease results.

The journey toward wellness from most illness requires a process of detoxification, and regular detoxification is good prevention from all disease, including breast cancer.

Exotoxins and Endotoxins

Exotoxins come to us from the air we breathe, food we eat, water we drink, and drugs we use. These 'foreign' chemicals, known as xenobiotics, include pesticides, industrial chemicals, food additives, and other environmental pollutants, as well as toxic metals such as lead, cadmium, mercury, arsenic, and aluminum. They often act synergistically with one another in ways our bodies cannot manage. They have profound detrimental effects upon our immune, glandular, and nervous systems. The toxins specific to breast cancer include the environmental estrogens, synthetic estrogens, and many other chemicals.

Endotoxins are produced in the body and include the by-products of intestinal bacteria and yeast, as well as intermediary metabolites such as lactic acid, pyruvic acid, urea, and others. Too much of the body's own estradiol and the C-16 metabolite of estrogen break-down can be considered endotoxins.

We can also become sick from 'toxic' emotions, usually held in anger, grief, guilt, shame, fear, etc. These emotions leave an imprint on organs, glands, and tissues, mediated by biochemical pathways linked to the nervous system and brain. There are real links between our emotions and our physical bodies.

How We Detoxify

Who are the selfless unpaid workers in our bodies who clean up 24 hours of the day, every day? Here are the components of your personal clean-up crew.

The Moving Blood

Driven by the tireless rhythmic beating of the heart muscle (70 squeezes per minute), the blood carries food and oxygen to all parts of the body, and carries away cellular waste products, bringing them to the liver for detoxification and elimination. Without good circulation, toxins accumulate as they would in a stagnant pond, creating a kind of sludge in particular areas that becomes difficult to dislodge. People with cancer usually have high blood coagulability with increased 'stickiness' or blood viscosity. This interferes with circulation through the small capillaries and can more easily lead to the development of cancer and metastases. Exercise and alternating hot and cold showers are ways in which we can keep the heart muscle pumping strongly, allowing this river of blood to flow smoothly. Vitamin B3 opens up the capillaries to remove waste more efficiently for us. Certain Chinese herbs, such as salvia, sparganium, ligusticum, frankincense, paeonia, and myrrh are used to activate the blood and improve circulation.

The Lungs

The lungs handle about 20% of all body elimination. Each time we exhale, our lungs release toxic gases and the end products of cell metabolism. When we breathe slowly and deeply we aerate a greater volume of the lungs and so improve its cleansing ability. The quality of our breathing affects so many physical and mental processes — it should be one of the first things taught in grade school.

The Skin

The skin is the envelope that protects us, opening its pores to release toxins through perspiration. It handles about 10% of body elimination. The mechanism of sweating is one of the few ways we can eliminate toxins that reside in our fat cells. Stored in here are some of the environmental chemicals we have been accumulating since conception, which in sensitive persons may trigger symptoms of chronic fatigue or environmental illness. Ideally, we should sweat daily to maximize the skin's function as a detoxifying organ. Thus the importance of regular aerobic exercise, good hard physical labor, and frequent use of saunas or sweat lodges. Perspiration carries with it cellular and water-soluble toxins and toxic minerals.

The Digestive Organs

Many of the body wastes and poisons are organic in nature — they are still much like foods. The stomach and pancreas secrete their enzymes to break these down, and change them from threatening substances into harmless ones in the same way that they digest foods. The enzymes are capable of digesting and breaking down all foreign cells, including cancer cells. The acid in the stomach, as long as we have enough of it, is a deterrent to many organisms that otherwise might gain a foothold in our intestinal tracts.

The Liver

Acting as the main factory for breaking down, neutralizing, detoxifying, and removing chemicals, poisons, body wastes, and unused and undigested food surpluses, the liver deserves our unwavering gratitude. The liver handles about 40% of all the body's detoxification work. It cleverly makes bile which it uses to carry away all the harmful poisons and wastes. The bile passes through the bile ducts, into the intestines, and is eliminated with its accumulated gunk. We can use olive oil and herbs to produce and move the bile more efficiently, and foods, herbs, and nutritional supplements to help the liver in its awesome task. We can improve the circulation in the liver with deep breathing, expressing our emotions, yoga, and aerobic exercise.

The Intestines

After taking the good stuff and sending it off into the blood to nourish the rest of the body, the small intestine separates 'the clean from the unclean' and drives the unclean into the large intestine with its muscular movements. The large intestine retrieves whatever water and minerals it can and eliminates the rest through bowel movements. One bowel movement for every meal is the ideal for keeping the large intestine from backing up with waste. When was the last time you had three good bowel movements a day? Any excess waste will build up on the large intestine's walls, forming crusts and pockets of infection that feed hungry microorganisms waiting for a good dinner. There are over 400 different kinds of microorganisms in our large intestine, some beneficial and others harmful. We have more organisms in our intestines than we have cells in our bodies. Figure that one out. One third of our stools are composed of dead bacteria. We can help our large intestine with its elimination process by consuming a high fiber diet, encouraging bowel movements with herbal and fiber supplements and occasional enemas. We can walk and exercise regularly to stimulate its muscular movement. We can take probiotics or supplements that contain 'good' bacteria to keep our gut ecology healthy. We can avoid antibiotics that are like a pesticide spray to all the organisms in our intestines, disrupting the balance that protects us.

The Kidneys

Water-soluble toxins and minerals are eliminated through the body's great filter, the kidneys. The kidneys handle about 30% of the body's total elimination. They contain about one million tiny filtration units called nephrons, which collectively cleanse 180 liters of blood in 24 hours. This means that all of our blood is filtered through the kidneys 60 times per day! The surface area that the kidneys use to do their filtering of toxins is equal to the surface area of the skin on the rest of our bodies. We can help our kidneys immensely by drinking water free of chemicals and poisons and by using foods and herbs to make their job easier. We can maintain a low sodium/high potassium diet to make cellular detoxification and elimination through the kidneys more efficient.

The Thymus Gland

This is the main immune organ of the body, the general of the white blood cells. The thymus develops our resistance to bacteria, cancer, viruses, toxins, and allergens of all kinds and stimulates the production of white blood cells in the bone marrow. Located in the center of the chest, it trains white blood cells in their various tasks and then pushes them out to battle in the blood. Some of them take up residence in surveillance stations (lymph nodes) scattered through the body, like secret service agents. The thymus can control and turn up the volume on the elimination of wastes through the lymphatic system. It responds dramatically to our emotions and our will to live a purposeful life. It is further activated by melatonin and many vitamins, herbs, minerals, and nutritional substances. It shuts down when we are stressed and its soldiers then become fewer in number and less aggressive.

The White Blood Cells

Their function is to digest and break down all foreign elements, toxins, dead cells, wastes, bacteria, and impurities in the blood stream. They congregate in the lymphatic tissue, which includes the lymph nodes, spleen, thymus gland, and specialized clean-up sites in the liver and small intestine. The white blood cells are divided into specialized troops, each equipped with remarkable defence tactics used on our behalf against toxins. Many vitamins, minerals, and herbs can activate these troops to serve us better.

The Lymphatic System

This is the body's 'sewage' system, comprised of drainage pipes connecting every cell and all areas of the body. The lymphatic system drains toxins from all these corners. When overloaded, a multitude of filters come into play to prevent an excessive amount of toxins or waste from dumping into the bloodstream in quantities greater than the body can handle. These are the lymph nodes, small factories filled with eager, altruistic, cavalier types that defend our lives.

The Spleen

Lying behind and slightly below the stomach, the spleen is a fist-sized organ filled with devouring macrophages — white blood cells whose destiny is to digest bacteria, foreign particles, and old decrepit red blood cells whose time is up. The spleen is a powerful filter of blood poisons and can store blood for us to be released as we need it. It is also an effective blood rebuilder. We can strengthen the function of the spleen with herbal allies.

▶ **Action for Prevention:** To enhance detoxification generally, we should do the following daily: ensure 3 or 4 bowel movements through the use of fiber and enemas, drink at least two liters of water to flush the kidneys, take herbs or nutritional substances to cleanse the liver and kidneys, sweat through exercising and the use of saunas, use a skin brush to stimulate the lymphatic system and the skin, and practice breathing exercises to detoxify the lungs. ◀

Cleansing and Assisting the Liver

Because the liver is the chief detoxifying organ in the body, handling about 40% of the work, supporting the function of the liver helps to maintain good health generally and improve breast health. Cleansing the liver a few times a year can become a seasonal ritual.

The Functions of the Liver

Found beneath the diaphragm on the right side of the body, this large organ performs many major functions vital to good health.

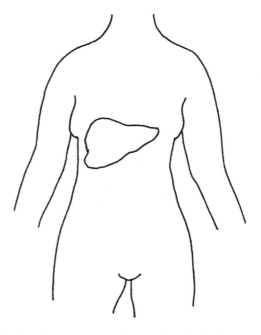

1) Breaks down proteins, fats, and carbohydrates, providing us with energy and nutrients.
2) Stores minerals, vitamins and sugars, to be used as needed by the body.

3) Filters the blood and helps to remove harmful chemicals (such as organochlorines) and bacteria.

4) Creates bile, which is stored in the gallbladder, and is used to break down fats and carry away toxins.

5) Helps to assimilate and store the fat-soluble vitamins A, E, D, K.

6) Acts as a reservoir for blood storage, and quickly releases it when needed.

7) Helps to make blood proteins, which maintain fluid balance.

8) Helps to maintain electrolyte and water balance.

9) Creates substances that function as part of the immune system, such as gamma globulin.

10) Breaks down and eliminates excess hormones.

11) Helps to regulate energy, moods, and emotions by controlling blood sugar and hormone levels.

The liver's ability to filter the blood to remove harmful chemicals and its ability to break down and eliminate excess hormones are two major functions we can improve to decrease the likelihood of breast cancer. If we were to regularly cleanse the liver (every three months) and continually assist it in the breakdown of excess estrogen, we could eliminate organochlorines and toxic chemicals before they become stored in our fat cells; and convert estrogen into its harmless forms (estriol and the C2 estrogen) so that it doesn't enter the breast cell to cause the growth of cancer. The frequency and duration of a liver cleanse depends upon our level of health, our exposure to environmental toxins, our emotional health, and our dietary history. (Much of the information in the next few pages is gleaned from *Foundations of Health: Healing with Foods and Herbs* by Christopher Hobbs who has done a wonderful job of organizing the different classes of foods and herbs that benefit the liver.)

The Liver's Detoxification Pathways

The liver uses two different biochemical processes to detoxify chemicals, hormones such as estrogen, pollutants, and toxins. These are termed Phase 1 and Phase 2 detoxification.

Phase 1 Detoxification: During the Phase 1 process, estradiol and estrone are broken down into the products C2 estrogen or 'good estrogen' and C16 estrogen, or 'bad estrogen', as well as to estriol. The C2 estrogen is harmless, whereas the C16 estrogen promotes breast cancer and is found in much higher levels in the blood of women with breast cancer. Estriol generally protects us from breast cancer when it binds to the estrogen receptor sites, preventing the stronger estrogens from doing so. If the liver were functioning better in its Phase 1 detoxification, the circulating levels of C16 estrogen, estradiol and estrone would be lower. The circulating levels of the C2 estrogen and estriol would be higher. Breast cancer would be less likely to occur.

Phase 1 detoxification of estrogen is hindered by substances that our bodies must also detoxify through this pathway. These include alcohol, toxins from cigarettes, barbituates, valium, antihistamines, sulfonamides, saturated fats, carbon tetrachloride, charcoal broiled meats, dioxin, exhaust fumes, pesticides, paint fumes, and methylxanthines which are found in caffeine, cola, chocolate, black tea, and coffee. For optimal Phase 1 detoxification and conversion of estrogen to the C2 form we should decrease our exposure to or ingestion of these substances.

▶ **Action for Prevention:** We can improve Phase 1 detoxification with the following nutrients:[1]

1) Niacin, riboflavin, copper, zinc, vitamin E, vitamin A, calcium, and magnesium are needed as cofactors in making Phase 1 enzymes.

2) Indole-3-carbinol from the raw brassicas, such as cabbage, broccoli, bok choy, and cauliflower, which promotes the conversion of estrone to the C2 estrogen, rather than the harmful C16 estrogen.

3) Isoflavones found in soy and limonene (present in oranges and tangerines).

4) Amino acids from protein, essential fatty acids, and complex carbohydrates in our diets.

5) The herbs *Schizandra chinensis, Curcuma longa,* milk thistle *(silybum marianum), Rosmarinus officinalis, Capsicum frutescens, Calendula officianalis, Solidago vigaurea* and *Sassafras albidum.* ◀

Phase 2 Detoxification: During Phase 2 detoxification, the estrogen breakdown products are bound to glucuronic acid which allows these metabolites to be carried out of the liver into the intestines. Other substances that must be metabolized through Phase 2 detoxification and interfere with the breakdown of estrogen include tartrazine dyes, non-steroidal anti-inflammatory drugs, the birth control pill, cigarettes, and phenobarbitol. A protein deficiency is also detrimental.

▶ **Action for Prevention:** We can improve Phase 2 detoxification with the following nutrients:

1) Cysteine (or NAC), methionine, choline, vitamins B6, B12, B5, and C, molybdenum, folic acid.

2) Foods from the brassica family, limonene, Omega 3 fatty acids (flaxseed oil and fish oils).

3) The herbs *Rosmarinus officinalis, Curcuma longa,* or turmeric. ◄

Other Liver Protectors

We can maximize the function of these detoxification pathways and improve liver function by including five classes of substances in our dietary and nutritional regimes: antioxidants, membrane stabilizers, choloretics, sulphur-contaning compounds, and enzyme assistants. It is primarily the sulphur-containing compounds that neutralize organochlorines and other hormone-mimickers, particularly the amino acids cysteine, methionine, and glutathione. Cysteine is very high in spirulina and soy foods, and moderately high in beans, sunflower seeds, and oatmeal. (See the list of sulphur-bearing proteins in chapter seven.)

Antioxidants

Antioxidants help to protect the cells of the liver and indeed all body cells from damage.

• Herbs: milk thistle, Chinese licorice, gingko, skullcap, Jerusalem artichoke, rosemary, bilberry, schizandra, eleuthero, chaparral, lemon balm, saffron, turmeric.

• Foods: cabbage, garlic, whole seeds, fruit, greens, red peppers, sprouts, spirulina, carrots.

• Vitamins: vitamins A, C, E.

• Minerals: zinc, selenium.

• Amino Acids: methionine, glutathione, cysteine.

• Flavonoids: catechin, quercetin, rutin, kaempferol, luteolin, pycnogenol and grape seed extract.

• Other: coenzyme Q10, alpha lipoic acid, melatonin.

Membrane Stabilizers

Membrane stabilizers protect the cell membrane from damage, making it less vulnerable to toxins.

• Herbs: milk thistle.

• Foods: cabbage, garlic, flaxseed oil, and seeds.

Choloretics

Choloretics move the bile out of the liver with the toxins in it to be eliminated.

• Herbs: globe artichoke, capillaris, garlic, chelidonium, burdock, barberry, blessed thistle, gentian, milk thistle, golden seal.

• Foods: olive oil.

Sulphur-Containing Compounds

These provide the building blocks for the liver's detoxification mechanisms.

• Herbs: milk thistle (St. Mary's thistle), dandelion.

• Foods: cabbage, cauliflower, Brussels sprouts, broccoli (brassica family), broccoli sprouts, onions, garlic, soy.

Enzyme Assistants

These help the liver enzymes work more efficiently.

• Herbs: schizandra, bupleurum, chelidonium, desmodium.

• Foods: brassica family, green vegetables, turmeric, ginger, garlic.

Liver Cleansers

In addition to these herbal and dietary liver protecting substances, the following help to cleanse toxins from the liver.

• Herbs: burdock, dandelion root, yellow dock, blue flag, Oregon grape root, phyllanthus, schizandra.

• Foods: apples, other juicy fruits, apple cider vinegar, lemon juice, grapefruit juice, garlic, beets, dandelion greens, turmeric powder.

Liver Builders

These substances help to rebuild the liver and supply the nutrients it needs to operate efficiently.

• Herbs: globe artichoke, milk thistle (St. Mary's thistle), butternut, oat, bupleurum, desmodium, phyllanthus.

• Foods: seeds (flax, sesame, sunflower, pumpkin), almonds, whole grains, vitamin B vitamin rich foods (wheat germ, nutritional yeast, royal jelly, bee pollen), beets, and other foods rich in iron.

Herbs for Liver Health

Many of the means of cleansing, protecting, and assisting the liver are herbal.

Milk Thistle (*Silybum marianum*)

The seeds of the milk thistle plant are used to benefit the liver and digestion. They are nutritious, slightly bitter as well as being sweet, and act to tonify the liver, spleen, and kidneys. They can be used for nine months or more at a time, followed by a two-week break. Historically, milk thistle has been used to cure jaundice, hepatitis, and cirrhosis of the liver. Flavonoids are present in milk thistle that bind to liver cell membranes and protect them from being injured by foreign chemicals, organochlorines, hormones, radiation, heavy metals, free radical damage, endo- and exotoxins. They protect the liver during chemotherapy and radiation and generally protect the cell membranes so that toxins can't get in. These flavonoids also enter liver cells to improve their ability to produce enzymes necessary for function and regeneration of the liver. Milk thistle can increase glutathione levels by 35%. This herb promotes the flow of bile so that toxins are quickly removed from the liver. It speeds up the liver's recovery from any injury and hastens the generation of new liver cells. It is also useful in stopping heavy menstrual bleeding. It is best taken on an empty stomach.

DOSAGE: Unstandardized liquid extract: 40 drops, 2–3× daily.
Tincture of fresh or dried seeds: 30–100 drops, 3× daily.
Powdered extract standardized to 10% silymarin: 100 mg, 2–3× daily.
Powdered extract standardized to 80% silymarin: 1–2 tablets daily.
CONTRAINDICATIONS: None known.

Schizandra

Schizandra berries contain vitamin C and vitamin E. It is an adaptogenic herb, meaning that it helps us adjust to stress in such ways as increasing endurance and regulating stomach acidity. It has been used in cases of hepatitis to normalize liver enzymes; it strongly regenerates a damaged liver. Schizandra exerts a stimulating effect on the cytochrome P450 system of the liver's Phase 1 detoxification pathway, which enhances our ability to break down toxins and estrogen. It improves energy levels and is a tonic to the eyes.

DOSAGE: 3–9 g, or 50–100 drops 3× daily.
CONTRAINDICATIONS: None known.

Dandelion Root (*Taraxicum officianalis*)

Dandelion root and leaves are often used to support the liver, kidneys, and breasts. The leaves are best eaten in spring and fall when the weather is cooler while the roots can be dug in the fall. They act to protect, heal and tonify the liver, decrease breast congestion, discourage cancer, improve digestion and appetite, cleanse the kidneys, stimulate weight loss by improving metabolism, and protect the immune system by increasing interferon production. They promote the flow of bile to relieve the liver of its toxins. Dandelion has demonstrated estrogen-lowering properties and both traditional use and modern research verify its ability to prevent and reverse breast cancer. It is commonly used in traditional Chinese medicine in

formulas for breast health. It has the ability to reduce lymphatic congestion and glandular swelling. It stimulates the activity of phagocytes. Its leaves are high in potassium, which makes it a good diuretic and cellular detoxifier.

Dandelion is ubiquitous. When we use pesticides to kill it, the leaves pop up again, undaunted, to remind us how much we need it to heal from the toxicity of pesticides. It is extremely loyal to humanity, though we seldom appreciate it. Make dandelion root and leaves a part of your life. Use the root in a tea, the leaves steamed, or in salads or juiced with fresh vegetables. It can and should be taken long term, but take a two- week break every three months if you are using it continuously.

DOSAGE: Cooked Greens: 1–2 cups
Dried Root Tea: 1–5 cups (simmer the root for 20 minutes, steep for 10; can be mixed with Chinese licorice)
Tincture: 15–50 drops, 3× daily.
CONTRAINDICATIONS: None known.

Bupleurum

The root of bupleurum has been used for over 2,000 years in Traditional Chinese Medicine to remove liver congestion, improve digestion, regulate the periods, and relax tension. It relieves the moodiness experienced by many women before their periods and alleviates depression. It helps to bring to the surface old emotions of sadness or anger that have been stored in the body's organs and tissues. It is used in formulas for hepatitis and liver cirrhosis. It increases the formation of bile, thus assisting the liver in digesting fats and removing toxins. It is one of the best herbs used for restoring the liver and its enzymes, harmonizing its function and protecting it against stress and damage from chemicals. It is the main ingredient in a commonly used Chinese patent herbal formula called Xiao Yao Wan, which is very helpful in alleviating premenstrual breast tenderness and fibrocystic breast disease.

DOSAGE: Tea: add 10 g of the herb to 12 oz of water. Simmer for 45 minutes, strain off the liquid into a glass jar, add 6 oz of fresh water, simmer another 20 minutes, strain and add to the first liquid and store in the refrigerator. Drink one cup twice daily, morning and evening, starting at a lower dosage and increasing to the full dosage.
Tincture: 20–30 drops, 3× daily.
CONTRAINDICATIONS: In large amounts it can cause nausea in some people; use cautiously with a persistent dry cough.

Globe Artichoke (*Cynara scolymus*)

Artichoke leaf and root are a tonic to the liver and digestion, activating bile production to help digest fats and remove toxins. Cynara decreases the fat and cholesterol content of the blood and encourages weight loss and removal of cellulite. It promotes urination and relieves edema, or water retention. It prevents the formation of gallstones. The bitter taste of artichoke also acts as an immune stimulant and activates the stomach to produce hydrochloric acid. A compound in this herb called cynarin enhances liver cell regeneration and protection and may slow down the aging process. Artichoke contains very high amounts of minerals, including iodine, potassium, magnesium, calcium, and trace minerals. It has substantial amounts of vitamins A, B1 and B2, and C. It is a fine herb to counter hypoglycemia and hypothyroidism.

It improves elimination by increasing the frequency of bowel movements, often healing cases of chronic constipation. The root is more stimulating to the liver than the leaf.

DOSAGE: Tincture: 20 drops, 3× daily.
CONTRAINDICATIONS: Use cautiously while breastfeeding, as it may clog up the milk ducts.

Celandine (*Chelidonium majus*)

The leaves and root of chelidonium promote the flow of bile and decrease liver congestion. Celandine is a healer for the gallbladder and stimulates the secretions of the pancreas to aid digestion. It improves elimination through increased bowel movements. It also stimulates the heart and circulation, improving the body's ability to deliver nutrients to the cells and remove toxins. Chelidonium decreases overall body toxicity and reduces edema. Another important attribute of this herb is its ability to reduce tumors, benign and malignant.

DOSAGE: Tincture: 12–50 drops, 3× daily.
Fresh juice: 2 tsp.
CONTAINDICATIONS: Do not use in pregnancy, as it is a uterine stimulant; if taken on its own, use for 2 weeks followed by a 4-day break.

Barberry (*Berberis vulgaris*)

The root of barberry helps to produce and activate the flow of bile in the liver. It is bile that carries away toxins after the liver has metabolized them. Barberry's bitter taste stimulates the production of hydrochloric acid in the stomach, which improves digestion. In combination with other herbs, it can be effective against intestinal parasites such as giardia and breaks up and moves out toxic intestinal accumulations. Along with acidophilus it helps to balance the intestinal flora and is an excellent herb for chronic candidiasis. It acts as an immune stimulant and is useful in cases of constipation. Barberry is one of the best herbs for such skin conditions as acne, psoriasis, eczema, and boils. It should be avoided in pregnancy and should not be used by itself for longer than three months at a time.

DOSAGE: Tincture: 20–40 drops, 2–3× daily.
Capsules: 2 capsules, 3× daily.
Powdered Extract: 100–200 mg, 2× daily
CONTRAINDICATIONS: Avoid in pregnancy; if using it on its own, take a break of two weeks after three months of use.

Liver Loving Formula for Healthy Breasts

Given this information about the various means of helping the liver, we can design a herbal liver formula that will help in the detoxification process and in the conversion of estradiol and estrone to the C2 estrogen and to estriol. There are many available commercially. Check the formulas and try to find one that has at least one herb from each of the above categories, or buy single tinctures of milk thistle, dandelion, and chelidonium and mix them together in equal proportions, or simply use milk thistle on its own. The freshness and potency of herbs is usually preserved better in tincture form rather than in capsule or tea. Always buy organic herbs.

Here is a formula I have designed that combines organic herbs from all of the above categories. You can use the order form at the back of the book to order it from me if you choose, or mix it up yourself from single tinctures.

25	parts milk thistle (Silybum marianum)
20	parts dandelion root (Taraxicum officianalis)
15	parts schizandra
15	parts bupleurum
10	parts globe artichoke (Cynara scolymus)
10	parts greater celandine (Chelidonium majus)
5	parts barberry (Berberis vulgaris)

DOSAGE: As prevention, 30–40 drops three times daily in a little water for six to eight weeks at a time, 1–4 times a year. For breast cancer recovery, take it consistently, stopping for one week every two months.
CONTRAINDICATIONS: If you are pregnant, omit chelidonium and barberry; increase dandelion and milk thistle.

Collectively, the herbs in this liver loving formula will help protect you from breast cancer by:

1) protecting the liver from the damaging effect of toxins so that it can do its job better;

2) breaking down and inactivating toxins generated from internal and external sources, including ones that might cause breast cancer;

3) decreasing estrogen levels so breast cells aren't stimulated to proliferate excessively;

4) improving thyroid function and supplying trace amounts of iodine;

5) improving circulation so that nutrients are delivered more efficiently where they are needed and wastes are removed;

6) improving elimination to decrease the accumulation of toxins in the body and the amount of circulating estrogen;

7) helping to release long held emotions of anger, grief, depression and frustration so that there is a more harmonious flow of energy within the body;

8) preventing and reversing tumor growth, both benign and malignant;

9) regenerating the cells of the liver;

10) eliminating yeast and parasites and helping to maintain healthy bowel flora;

11) increasing glutathione levels;

12) improving immunity;

13) improving digestion and absorption of minerals;

14) improving fat metabolism and helping to increase weight loss so our bodies will make less estrogen and be less prone to breast cancer;

15) relieving lymphatic congestion and swollen lymph nodes.

The Liver Flush

The liver flush is used to stimulate the liver to eliminate toxins, increase bile flow, and increase the circulation of blood in the liver, thereby improving overall liver function. It also helps to remove impurities from the blood and lymph.

1) Mix together freshly-squeezed citrus juices to make one cup of liquid. Use orange, grapefruit, lemon, and lime. It should taste sour. The sour taste activates the liver according to Traditional Chinese Medicine. Water it down to taste with pure spring, distilled, or filtered water.

2) Add 1–2 cloves of fresh garlic plus a small amount of fresh ginger juice or grated ginger. Both garlic and ginger protect the liver.

3) Mix in 1 tablespoon of high quality extra virgin olive oil from a metal or opaque glass container and blend the mixture together. Drink in the morning and wait one hour before eating anything else. Keep your diet simple the rest of the day, either eating mainly fresh fruits and vegetables or mung beans and rice cooked with vegetables, or brown rice and vegetables.

4) Follow the liver flush with two cups of a cleansing tea. Some of the herbs to look for in these preparations are fennel, burdock, dandelion, red clover, peppermint, nettles, fenugreek, and flax. To make your own cleansing tea mix:

    1 part fennel   ¼ part burdock
    1 part fenugreek   ¼ part licorice
    1 part flax

    Using 1 oz of the herbs to 20 ounces of water, simmer all the herbs for 20 minutes, then add 1 part peppermint. Let it steep for 10 more minutes. Drink two cups each morning after the liver flush.

5) Take a bowel cleansing formula which includes bentonite (or take 1 tbsp bentonite daily) at the same time as you do the liver flush as well as having 2–4 tablespoons of freshly ground flaxseeds daily. This will ensure that you eliminate the toxins released from the liver. Drink at least 2 liters of filtered water daily. You may use enemas to cleanse more quickly.

6) Continue for a cycle of 10 days. Stop for 3 days. Continue another 10 days if desired. Do it 1–4 times yearly.

7) If you have cancer, chronic disease or a serious health problem, do it under the supervision of someone experienced with detoxification regimens.

▶ **Action for Prevention:** Schedule a time to do a 10-day liver flush. If you can, do it within the next month. Prepare yourself physically and psychologically with relaxation and breathing exercises daily, a vegetarian diet, and consciously releasing negative thought patterns, old resentments, and anger.

Look at a calendar for the next year. Block in future 10-day periods when you will do the liver flush, up to four times per year. Block in the 6–8 week periods when you will take a liver loving herbal formula, overlapping it with the liver flush. You may choose to do it one to four times yearly, or continuously if you are recovering from breast cancer. ◀

Kundalini Yoga Exercises for the Liver

Practice the following exercises daily while you are cleansing your liver and at other times when your liver may need support. These five exercises are meant to be done together in sequence.

1) Sit cross-legged with a straight spine, your hands resting on your knees. Count to five mentally as you inhale. Exhale, to the count of 5. Hold the breath out for 15 seconds and pump your navel point in and out, rhythmically, using your abdominal muscles. Do it vigor-ously. This massages the liver and moves the liver blood. Continue the pattern of inhaling for five, exhaling for five, and holding and pumping for 15 seconds, for 5 minutes. Relax for 3 minutes.

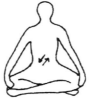

2) Lie on your back, with your legs straight and your ankles together. Keep your arms at your sides.

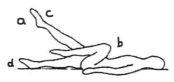

a) Inhale and raise both legs up to a 60 degree angle, holding the position and the breath for 15 seconds.
b) Exhale as you bring your knees to your chest, holding the breath out for 15 seconds.
c) Inhale, return the legs to an angle of 60 degrees, holding the breath in for 15 seconds.
d) Exhale and lower your legs back down to the floor, holding the breath out for 15 seconds.

Repeat this sequence 8 times. Do the best you can. Relax afterwards for 5 minutes and visualize your liver feeling energized and healed.

3) Sit on your right heel, with your left leg extended straight out behind you. Gently tilt your head back, gazing up at the ceiling. Bend your arms at the elbow and press your elbows against your sides with the palms facing forward. Hold the posture with long deep breathing into your belly,

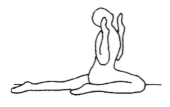

expanding the abdomen as you inhale and letting it contract as you exhale. Continue for from 2–5 minutes on this side. Change sides and continue for the same length of time on the second side.

4) Come lying on your back with your feet spread 3 feet apart and with your arms at your sides also about 3

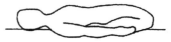

feet apart, palms facing up. Keep your arms and legs straight. Raise them 2 feet from the floor, still 3 feet apart. Hold the position with deep powerful breathing. Maintain the posture until you shake. Relax on your back for 3 minutes.

5) Sit on your heels or cross-legged, or with one foot on the opposite thigh (half-lotus). Gently lower yourself

down until you come lying on your back, still with your legs in the original position. Rest your arms at your sides. Hold it with slow, long deep breathing for 3 minutes. Relax on your back for 10 minutes.[2]

Add these two exercises to your daily routine.

1) Stand with your legs spread 2 feet apart and place your hands on your hips. Begin to roll the upper torso around on your hips, inhaling as you circle to the back and exhaling as you come round to the front, stretching forward. Breathe very deeply as you stretch in all directions in a circular motion. Continue for 2 minutes in one direction. Then reverse the direc-tion and continue another 2 minutes. This exercise gives the liver a good squeeze, improving its circulation and capacity to detoxify.

2) Cat stretch. Lie on your back with your arms straight out to the sides from your shoulders. Inhale your right knee into the chest and cross it over your body to

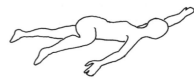

touch the ground to the left of you. Keep your shoulders and torso on the ground as much as possible. Exhale as you bring the knee back into the center and then straight out onto the ground. Reverse legs, inhaling the left knee into the chest, crossing it over the right side of the body, exhale as it comes on to the ground. Continue alternating legs for 3 minutes. This puts pressure on the liver, improving circulation and removing toxins.[3]

▶ **Action for Prevention:**

1) Food combining enhances digestion. Proteins and starches should be eaten at different meals. Avoid combining sweets and proteins. Regularly eat foods that assist the liver — beets, garlic, dandelion, cabbage and the other brassicas, turmeric, rosemary, seeds, lemon, grapefruit, apple cider vinegar. Use fresh organic vegetable juices regularly, such as a mixture of beet, carrot, celery and cabbage.

2) Reduce fat in your diet, eliminating saturated fats of animal origin. Have 2–6 tsp of unsaturated fat (such as flaxseed oil) daily. Reduce sugar in your diet. When eaten in refined form, sugar lowers the effectiveness of liver enzymes, decreases immunity. and favors the growth of yeast and parasites.

3) A weekly 'resting' of the digestive system will benefit the liver. Eat only when hungry, and not too close to bedtime, ideally before 6:00 p.m. Massage the liver daily.

4) Exercise daily, and use saunas regularly, as some toxins are only eliminated through perspiration.

5) Increase fiber and water intake to ensure at least two bowel movements daily.

6) Use the 'Lemon Aid' cleanse as described below or other cleansing diet as needed (early spring and fall are prime times).

7) Anger, anxiety, and other negative emotions can impede liver function. Be aware of your feelings and appropriately release emotions — exercise or find a good listener.

8) Vitamins C and E, beta-carotene, selenium, and zinc are antioxidants, protecting the liver. Take them regularly or obtain them through diet.

9) Recommended teas are dandelion, licorice, and ginger. Milk thistle rebuilds a damaged liver.

10) At least two times a year, take a herbal liver formula and go on a liver and bowel-cleansing program for 6–8 weeks. If you have breast cancer, do it continuously, with short breaks every 3 months. In this way, you will decrease the chemical load in the body and eliminate excess estrogen.

Once or twice a year do the liver flush. Consider using castor oil packs to detoxify your liver as well.

11) Cleanse the body of yeast and parasites twice yearly for at least 6 weeks at a time. ◀

Eliminating Parasites and Yeast

One of the impediments to optimal health is the presence of parasites and yeast within the body. A parasite is an organism that derives its food, nutrition, and shelter by living in or on another organism. It usually injures its host without contributing to its survival. There are over 130 types of parasites that can infect the human body. These include microscopic single-celled organisms (Protozoa); round, pin, and hookworms (Nematoda); tapeworms (Cestoda); flukes (Trematoda); and Spirochetes.

Many chronic health disorders stem from parasitic infection. These include chronic fatigue, hypoglycemia, hypothyroidism, hypoadrenalism, chronic respiratory infections, depression, low sex drive, endometriosis, constipation, diarrhea, irritable bowel syndrome, digestive complaints, food sensitivities, allergies, teeth grinding, joint and muscle aches, anemia, skin conditions, nervousness, sleep disturbances, immune dysfunction, arthritis, tumors and cancer. The body can become free of parasites through a multifaceted approach which includes taking substances that kill them, strengthening immunity, normalizing stomach acid and candida levels, modifying the diet, cleansing the intestines, recolonizing the gastrointestinal tract with friendly bacteria, and limiting contact with the parasites.

Factors Contributing to the Increase in Parasitic Infections

Several factors have contributed to the rising incidence of parasitic infection. With increasing international travel, many organisms endemic to certain areas are spread, and with increasing immigration, parasites are hitchhiking into other countries. These include malaria, roundworm, and giardia. The growing popularity of international cuisine, with exotic foods that are prepared raw or undercooked (fish, beef, and pork), can be a source of tapeworm infection; red snapper and Pacific salmon can be infested with anisakid worms which cause symptoms similar to Crohn's disease, stomach ulcers, and appendicitis. Water is still being contaminated by raw sewage. The increasing number of daycare centers spread diseases through direct contact with infected feces. There are 65 infectious diseases spread by dogs and 39 by cats. These include dog and cat roundworm, hookworm, and toxoplasmosis. Most house cats sleep with their owners. Generalized use of antibiotics kill the body's protective bacteria, upsetting the micro-ecosystem of the gastrointestinal tract and vagina. This often leads to yeast overgrowth and trichomoniasis. A yeast overgrowth can cause hydrochloric acid deficiency, leading to increased susceptibility to parasitic infection. Sexual freedom over the last 30 years has caused an increase in the number of sexual partners and practices, leading to the sexual transmission of Trichomonas vaginalis, Entamoeba histolytica, giardia, pinworms, and pork tapeworms. High stress lifestyles cause many people to eat quickly, without sufficient hydrochloric acid secretion from the stomach.

How Parasites Harm Us

Parasites destroy cells in the body faster than they can be regenerated, causing ulceration and perforation of various organs — such as the stomach, lungs, intestines, heart, and liver. When undigested food is released into the intestine, it seeps through its perforations into the lymphatic system, and the result is an increased allergic response. Food and environmental sensitivities and allergies are therefore often linked to the presence of parasites.

Parasites also irritate the tissues in which they are present, causing an inflammatory response. This can result in pain in joints and muscles or an increased susceptibility to infection in the lungs, sinuses, vagina, bladder, or any mucous membrane. They produce toxic substances that are poisonous to the host and difficult to get rid of. It is this metabolic waste that irritates the nervous system of the host, causing restlessness, irritability, teeth grinding, nervous habits, insomnia, and/or anxiety. In the body's efforts to eliminate parasites, it can produce elevated levels of eosinophils (white blood cells that fight microscopic invaders) which themselves can cause tissue damage, leading to pain and inflammation.

They can invade the skin, causing dermatitis, itching, psoriasis, eczema, hives, swellings, and rashes. Parasites can cause increased pressure in certain organs or tissues (brain, heart, lungs, spinal cord, eye, bones) due to the presence of parasitic cysts and can cause obstructions in the intestine and the pancreatic and bile ducts. The destroyed larva or parasitic eggs can clump together forming a tumor-like mass in the colon, lungs, liver, breast, peritoneum, or uterus.

Their presence activates the immune system, and over time lowers the body's defensive energy, allowing bacterial and viral infections to take hold. Depressed immunity also implies a lowered resistance to cancer.

Parasites need to eat and thereby rob us of many nutrients, (proteins, carbohydrates, fats, minerals, vitamins) causing anemia and fatigue. Roundworm and giardia interfere with vitamin A absorption, while hookworm causes iron deficiency. Fish tapeworms compete for vitamin B12 in the host. Drowsiness after meals can be a sign that parasites are present.

▶ **Action for Prevention:** It is much easier and cheaper to prevent parasites in the first place than it is to eliminate them. Our first method of contact with them is usually through the skin and mouth. The following guidelines will help to protect you and your children.

1) Always wash your hands before eating.

2) Wash your hands with soap and water after going to the bathroom, changing diapers, or handling pets.

3) Keep your fingernails short and use a nailbrush to scrub beneath them.

4) Wipe off the toilet seat before sitting on it or squat above the toilet. Wear rubber gloves while cleaning the bathroom. Clean bathrooms daily or at least twice weekly. Pinworm eggs and trichomonas can be found under toilet seats. Trichomonas can also be spread through mud and water baths and sauna benches.

5) Use sterilized lens preparations to clean contact lenses and remove them before swimming.

6) Don't walk barefoot in areas frequented by dogs, cats, raccoons, etc.

7) If you travel frequently, eat out regularly, have pets, or visit mountainous regions, have a complete parasite exam twice a year. Use a purged stool and rectal mucous exam to check for infection. Be aware that parasites don't always show up in a stool sample even when they are present.

8) Breast-feed your children as long as you can. Human milk has antibodies that protect against amoeba and giardia.

9) Keep young children away from puppies and kittens that have not been regularly dewormed. Prevent them from kissing house pets or being licked by them. Empty kitty litter boxes daily while wearing gloves. Disinfect litter boxes frequently with boiling water and grapefruit seed extract. If you are pregnant, wear disposable gloves and a mask while changing the litter box or have someone else do this task to avoid risk of toxoplasmosis. Keep children away from snails or have them wear gloves while playing with them. Be sure they wash thoroughly after contact with these and other animals. Freshwater snails are the intermediate host of schistosomiasis, a blood fluke. Keep

pets and their bowls out of the kitchen.

10) Do not allow children to eat dirt or play in areas where there are animal droppings. Encourage children to keep their fingers out of their mouths and not to bite their fingernails.

11) Damp mop or vacuum bedrooms and bathrooms weekly (don't sweep) to eliminate eggs that may be in dust. Keep bedrooms well aired.

12) Bathe or shower daily.

13) If pinworms are present, launder bedding and personal clothing daily, wear close-fitting underwear to bed, and don't share a bed with other family members.

14) Keep toothbrushes in closed containers to avoid exposure to bathroom dust.

15) Drink filtered water. Use reverse osmosis or carbon block filters. Always boil or filter water from rivers or streams to eliminate giardia.

16) If you eat fish, use varieties that are commercially blast-frozen. Cook until it is flaky and white. Bake at 400°F, eight to ten minutes per inch of thickness. Avoid sushi.

17) If you are a meat eater, cook at 325°F or higher and use a meat thermometer to check that the internal temperature is 170°F.

18) Avoid oral-anal sex to prevent transmission of trichomonas, pinworms, ascaris, giardia, strongyloides, and Entamoeba histolytica. Use condoms when engaging in sexual intercourse unless you know that your partner is free of parasites.

19) Wash your fruits and vegetables before eating them.

20) Avoid the use of antibiotics unless absolutely necessary. These disturb the ecology of organisms in the intestines and can cause an overgrowth of *Candida albicans* in the body which can damage the cells in the stomach that produce hydrochloric acid. Hydrochloric acid, when present in sufficient amounts, will kill most parasites when they enter the stomach so they cause no further damage. The gastric analysis test (available from HDC Corporation, 408-954-1909) can determine if enough stomach acid is present. Antibiotics also eliminate the bacteria that convert phytoestrogens into a usable weak estrogen. ◄

Natural Anti-Parasitic Substances

Certain foods have anti-parasitic properties. Pomegranate juice (four glasses daily) is effective against tapeworm. Papaya seeds are used in Mexico to eliminate parasites and can be added to salads. Finely ground pumpkin seeds (one-quarter cup) can be added to porridge or eaten on their own to eliminate many varieties of worms. They are also high in zinc, an immune-enhancing mineral, and magnesium, a relaxant. Two cloves of raw garlic daily help prevent roundworms, pinworms, tapeworms, and hookworms. Other foods with anti-parasitic properties are onions, carrot tops, radishes, kelp, raw cabbage, apple cider vinegar, ground almonds, pumpkin, calmyrna figs, cranberry juice, and sauerkraut. Add these foods to your diet unless otherwise contraindicated.

Herbs have long been used to eliminate parasites. Wormwood, black walnut, male fern, and cloves are an effective combination for treating roundworm, dog heartworm, hookworm, strongyloides, whipworm, pinworm, trichinella, tapeworm, and cryptosporidium. All kinds of tapeworm can also be treated with a combination of pumpkin seeds, garlic, crampbark, capsicum, and thyme, sold in a Hanna Kroeger formula called Rascal. Lung and blood flukes are eliminated with milkweed, pennyroyal, and black walnut. Liver flukes can be treated with goldenrod, goldenseal, and cloves. Spirochetes are killed with a combination of nettle, yerba santa, goldenrod, and monolaurin. Microscopic protozoa such as amoeba and giardia respond to grapefruit seed extract and cranberry juice. Herbs are best taken before meals and treatment is most effective if begun around the full moon when the parasites are most active. Continue for at least six weeks, then stop for two weeks, or until the next full moon. Several courses of treatment may be necessary.

Homeopathic remedies can also be used to rid the body of these unwelcome guests. Cina is best known for its effectiveness against pinworms. Chelidonium has been used for liver flukes. Unda #39 is effective against many intestinal parasites. Spigelia is an antiparasitic remedy. These and other homeopathic remedies are prescribed on the basis of symptoms as well as on which organisms are present. In the homeopathic literature, there are descriptions of cancer patients who have been given the cancer nosode scirrhinum and have responded by evacuating a clump of worms. There is a strong association between cancer and the presence of parasites. Remedies prescribed for the whole person have the effect of strengthening overall vitality, which in turn repels parasites.

► **Action for Prevention:** Because parasites are a prevalent health problem but are difficult to diagnose, it behooves each of us to do a routine parasite cleanse twice a year, during the time of the full moon, for a minimum of six weeks each time. A combination of wormwood, black walnut, cloves, male fern, goldenseal, grapefruit seed extract, and Unda #39, or Cina would tackle most varieties. We may have particular sensitivities to different products, so starting with a low dosage or testing energetically for compatibility is advised. ◄

Normalizing Stomach Acid

The acid in the stomach is usually a defence against parasites if there is enough of it. Many people have insufficient stomach acid, creating an overly alkaline condition in the body, which is conducive to parasites. The pH of the urine and saliva upon rising should be 6.4. Anything above 7.1 is an alkaline state; anything below 6.2 is too acidic. The pH of the stomach can be measured directly using the Gastro-test. It should be at 1–3. Hypochlorhydria, or low stomach acid, is evident when the pH measures 4–8. Signs and symptoms of hypochlorhydria include bloating, burning, and flatulence immediately after meals, fullness after eating, food allergies, nausea with taking supplements, anal itching, weak, peeling and cracked fingernails, iron deficiency, dilated capillaries in the cheeks, and undigested food in the stools. Stomach acid secretion decreases with age. Diseases associated with low stomach acid include asthma, diabetes, eczema, gallbladder disease, autoimmune disorders, hives, lupus, osteoporosis, psoriasis, rheumatoid arthritis, and hypo- and hyperthyroidism.

There are several ways to stimulate an increase in hydrochloric acid production. Specific herbs such as Indian long pepper (pippali), schizandra, wormwood, gentian, and goldenseal will do this. So will taking one tablespoon of lemon juice or apple cider vinegar in one cup of water a half hour before meals (the vinegar is contraindicated in people with candidiasis). Chinese herbs, acupuncture, kinesiology, specific yoga exercises, and homeopathic remedies can also normalize stomach acid. Folic acid and vitamin B6 assist in the production of stomach acid, and can be supplemented when it is deficient.

▶ **Action for Prevention:** Once a year, check your stomach acid through use of the Gastro test (available from HDC Corporation, 408-954-1909). Correct it with one of the available methods if it is low. ◀

Candidiasis

The overgrowth of *Candida albicans* in the body interferes with hydrochloric acid secretion in the stomach and often goes hand in hand with a parasitic condition. One of the secondary effects of candidiasis is an increase in gut permeability, which results in large molecules passing through the gut wall into the blood and lymph. The liver and the immune system are taxed in their attempts to rid the body of these substances, resulting in increased body toxicity, lowered immunity, and susceptibility to allergies.

Many herbal and nutritional products are available to bring down the levels of yeast in the body. These include grapefruit seed extract, taheebo or pau d'arco, capryllic acid, olive leaf, calcium undecylenate, oil of oregano, and garlic. Substances which help to heal the permeability of the intestinal lining include beta-carotene, glutamic acid, rice bran oil, flaxseed oil, slippery elm, comfrey, and cabbage.

▶ **Action for Prevention:** Once or twice yearly, do a Candida cleanse along with the parasite cleanse. Work with a practitioner to decide which supplements to use. Use the anti-yeast supplements for at least two months. Do it at the same time as you do the parasite cleanse. ◀

Cleansing the Colon

The colon, or large intestine, is our body's main route to eliminate waste. Over years of eating processed food, layers of dried mucus accumulate on the colon wall. This becomes a breeding ground for unhealthy bacteria, yeast, and parasites. We can remove this debris in a gentle manner with the use of fiber supplements and/or enemas. In order to eliminate parasites that may reside in the intestinal debris, we must cleanse the colon regularly. Nature has provided us with many substances to accomplish this.

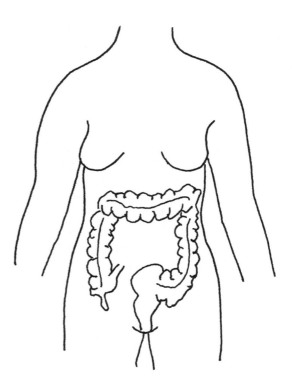

Fiber Supplements

Effective intestinal cleansers combine fiber to encourage bowel movements, absorbent compounds such as bentonite and pectin that attract toxins, and herbs that are soothing to the bowel lining. Intestinal cleansers may include oat bran, psyllium husks, guar gum, flaxseeds, bentonite clay, apple or citrus pectin, beet root, comfrey root, agar-agar, and papaya extract. In combination, these products act like a broom to sweep out the intestinal tract. The oatbran, psyllium, flaxseeds, and agar-agar are bulking agents that expand in the colon as they absorb water and help to peel away the layers of mucus, toxins, and old fecal matter. Occasionally, psyllium will cause abdominal bloating and discomfort to gluten-sensitive individuals. If you experience this, increase your water consumption so that you have at least two glasses with each dose of the fiber formula. If you continue to feel bloated, find a formula without psyllium or use a combination of freshly ground flaxseeds and bentonite. Apple and citrus pectin absorb toxins that can include chemicals, toxic metals, and waste produced by the body itself. Comfrey and beet root act as laxatives. These must all be taken with sufficient water for optimal effect.

Cleansing the intestines with these substances is a gentle process that should be continued for at least six weeks. Consider carrying out such a cleanse twice yearly on a regular basis and do it daily if you have been diagnosed with cancer or if you have a low C-2 estrogen to C-16 estrogen ratio.

▶ **Action for Prevention:** Cleanse your intestines with a fiber formula at least twice yearly for six weeks at a time, or use a fiber formula continuously, particularly if you have cancer. Use wheat bran and psyllium regularly, unless you are allergic or sensitive to them. Maintain a high fiber content in your diet, at least 30 g daily. Be sure to drink sufficient water, about two liters daily, while taking a fiber supplement. ◀

Enemas

Enemas and colonics are also methods to detoxify the bowel. They should not be overused. Different health practitioners may or may not recommend them. They are particularly useful when one must quickly remove toxins from the body, as is the case with cancer. Use them only under supervision with a naturopathic physician, herbalist, or holistic medical doctor.

Enemas are simple, painless, and immediate ways to remove toxins from both the bowel and the body. In removing toxins, you will generally feel more energetic and have fewer symptoms of pain. Think of using an enema if you have fewer than two bowel movements daily; you have been diagnosed with breast cancer and need to eliminate toxins quickly; you have symptoms of pain; you are experiencing a healing crisis, with uncomfortable symptoms such as joint pain, headaches, nausea, and fatigue.

There are several types of enemas. These include using distilled or spring water, herbal teas, cleansing juices, bentonite enemas, and coffee enemas.

Water Enemas

This is a basic enema, simply using water to dislodge and cleanse old fecal matter from the colon. Only distilled or spring water should be used. Avoid tap water, as the chlorine in it can combine with organic matter in the bowel to form chloroform. Chloroform is an organochlorine which may cause breast cancer and takes over one thousand years to break down in the environment.

Herbal Tea Enemas

Many herbal teas can soothe and detoxify the bowels and improve intestinal function in general. If the intestines are spastic or irritated, then chamomile, peppermint, comfrey, or licorice can be made into a tea and used in an enema. Fenugreek is a useful herb to dissolve mucus and encrustations in the bowel lining. To stimulate the liver while cleansing the colon, combine burdock root, red clover, yellow dock, and peppermint in equal proportions.[4] To soothe the intestinal wall while cleansing the liver and colon, dandelion root (35%), chicory root (30%), licorice root (10%) and marshmallow root (25%) can be mixed to make an enema. For a sluggish colon and a stronger cleanse, cascara bark (10%), dandelion root (40%), fennel (30%), and ginger (20%) can be combined.[5]

To make these teas alone or in combination, roots, barks, and stems are simmered for 20 minutes, then allowed to cool for 10 minutes before straining and using the tea. When using leaves and flowers, simmer for five minutes, turn off the heat, and let it steep for 10 minutes. Start with one part herbs to five parts of water, weight to volume. Therefore, one ounce of herbs would be added to five ounces of water to make the tea. Then approximately one half cup of tea is used per quart of distilled or spring water to make the enema. Some people may be able to use a full cup.

Cleansing Juice Enemas

Juice enemas act as a source of nutrients to the body as well as assisting with detoxification. The nutrients are delivered through the bowel wall to the liver. Aloe vera juice can be used to soothe intestinal cramping and helps to heal the mucous membrane lining of the bowel when it is inflamed. Use one tablespoon per quart (four cups) of water. Lemon juice is cleansing and alkalinizing, useful when the body is overly acidic. Use the juice of one lemon in four cups of water. Wheat grass juice is alkalinizing and high in minerals that help to feed the liver. Use two tablespoons per quart of water. This may be the enema of choice for cases of weakness and debility, particularly when digestion and absorption are poor. The Ayurvedic herb amla can be used in a retention enema for improving energy, for detoxifying the liver, and for its anti-oxidant properties.

Bentonite Enemas

Bentonite is a form of volcanic ash, with no chemical action or toxic side effect. It has a negative charge, and is able to strongly attract toxins, which are usually positively charged atoms. It has the ability to absorb and carry away 200 hundred times its own weight in toxins. Bentonite enemas are efficient at removing mucus and fecal matter attached to the colon wall. Use two tablespoons of bentonite per quart of water.

The Coffee Enema

A coffee enema should be performed only under the supervision of a naturopathic doctor or other health professional. Some professionals may or may not recommend them. An integral part of the Gerson program, they are included here as an option to quickly cleanse the colon and liver. Dr Sherry Rogers also recommends coffee enemas and discusses them in her book, *Wellness Against All Odds*.[6]

A coffee enema helps to detoxify the liver. The caffeine acts as an herbal stimulant, which goes directly to the liver through a circulatory route from the sigmoid colon called the entero-hepatic circulation system. The caffeine is transported through the hemorrhoidal veins into the portal veins and into the liver. When performed properly, a coffee enema speeds up the emptying time of the bowel, removing toxins at a faster pace; empties the toxins that have accumulated in the bile ducts of the liver, allowing other bodily toxins to come in to be metabolized; stimulates the production of the enzyme glutathione-S-transferase which assists liver detoxification; and causes an increased flow of bile. Bile helps to dissolve and carry away the end products of liver detoxification through the bile ducts and into the intestines. A toxic liver will dump many of its toxins into the bile and eliminate them in a few minutes. This provides quick relief to an overburdened body and may reduce symptoms of ill health and

increase energy. The normal functions of the liver become impaired and inadequate when the body is burdened by excess toxicity during the disease process. The bile that is released from coffee enemas contains toxins as well as valuable mineral salts. The minerals need to be replaced through the generous use of organic vegetable juices, sea vegetables and sprouted seeds, a green powder supplement, or a mineral supplement.

When coffee enemas are begun, the poisons contained in the bile produce spasms in the duodenum and the small intestines. Some of this may overflow into the stomach, causing nausea or possibly vomiting of bile. Should this occur, peppermint tea will help to wash the bile from the stomach and bring relief.

Drinking a cup of coffee has a very different effect from using a coffee enema. Drinking coffee results in the following physiological effects: increased reflex response, increased or decreased blood pressure, increased heart rate, insomnia and heart palpitations, over-stimulation of the adrenal glands, irritation of the stomach and gastro-intestinal tract, fibrocystic breast disease, and a build-up of toxicity.

To prepare a coffee enema, add two to three tablespoons of organic, freshly ground, lightly roasted coffee beans to one quart (four cups) of distilled water. If you are particularly sensitive to coffee and become overstimulated from it, use the lesser amount. Caffeine is not detected in the blood after coffee enemas. Do not use instant, decaffeinated or stale coffee. Store ground coffee beans in the freezer to prevent rancidity if you are not using them all right away.

Make the coffee fresh for each enema. Use an enamel, glass, or stainless steel pot. Do not use aluminum, teflon, or iron pots. Let it boil for three minutes, then simmer for 20 minutes. Strain it and allow it to cool to the body's temperature (98.6°F), or until it feels comfortable to the touch.

CONTRAINDICATIONS: Do not use a coffee enema if you have gallstones; if you become dizzy, nauseous, or lightheaded, stop the enema process.

Giving Yourself an Enema

1) Pour the enema liquid into an enema bag connected to plastic or rubber tubing. Clamp the tube as you pour in the liquid. A fountain syringe is the best enema applicator. Lubricate the nozzle with food grade vegetable oil, such as sesame, almond, flaxseed, or olive oil. Hang the enema bag 1½ to 2 feet above the body. You can change the height to control the speed of intake

into the colon. Place a large towel or mat on the floor of the washroom or in a room close by.

2) Lie on the mat or towel on your right side, with both legs drawn into the abdomen. Alternatively, you can start the enema in a knee-to-chest position with your chest on the floor and your buttocks in the air. This position allows the force of gravity to aid the flow of water into the colon. You can also lie on your back with a pillow beneath your buttocks. Breathe deeply while you begin the enema. Slowly insert the nozzle several inches into the rectum using a rotating motion. If the tube is inserted too rapidly or forcefully it can cause kinking inside of the colon, which may cause discomfort. Release the clamp and let the coffee mixture flow in slowly.

3) If the solution comes into the colon too fast, lower the enema bag; if it comes in too slowly, raise the bag a little higher. If you experience cramping, then the solution is coming in too quickly. You can stop the flow by pinching the enema tube and then lowering the bag. Wait until the cramps have stopped before allowing the solution to flow again. It may take several minutes for the enema solution to enter the body. If it does not seem to flow freely, the enema tube may be twisted or kinked. Slowly pull it part of the way out and then insert it again until it has gone in several inches.

4) Retain the fluid for 10 to 12 minutes. Dr Gerson found that all the caffeine was absorbed from the fluid within 10 to 12 minutes. If you cannot hold all the fluid in the colon with one enema, repeat it two or more times in sequence, emptying the bowel in between.

5) While the solution is in the colon, it is helpful to change positions every few minutes. The sequence might be: 3 minutes right side, 3 minutes stomach, 3 minutes on your back, 3 minutes left side. This helps the enema solution reach all parts of the colon.

6) When the bile duct empties, you will hear or feel squirting beneath the right rib cage. This is a sign that you have succeeded in releasing toxins from the liver.

7) Sterilize the enema syringe after each use by boiling it or thoroughly cleansing it with soap and water and soaking it for 5 minutes in a solution of 2 cups water and 4 drops of tea tree oil or grapefruit seed extract.

Frequency of Enemas

The frequency of enemas is dependent upon one's symptoms. As a general detoxification, you might use two or three a week, one to three times a year. If you presently

have cancer of any sort, one or two coffee enemas can be used daily until the cancer retreats, as long as you are replacing the lost minerals with several glasses of organic vegetable juices daily. The usual frequency of coffee enemas is three times a week for several weeks while you are attempting to detoxify.

One of my teachers, Dr Leo Roy, used to remind us that when dealing with cancer patients, we had to encourage at least four bowel movements daily — one for each meal and at least one extra to help remove the body's toxic burden. This can be accomplished through high fiber diets, fiber supplementation as listed above, adequate water consumption (2 liters daily), daily exercise, the addition of two tablespoons of flaxseeds to the diet daily, laxative herbs, and enemas or colonics if necessary.

▶ **Action for Prevention:** Choose a time period in which you will cleanse the colon and decide which method you will use — either a fiber supplement or a series of enemas or colonics. Work with your health practitioner. Consider a six week period, twice yearly for the fiber supplement, or enemas three times a week, for several weeks at a time, one to three times per year. If you have cancer, more frequent enemas may be necessary. Mark these times in your yearly calendar and start as soon as possible. Do it under supervision of a health care practitioner familiar with detoxification regimens. ◀

Squatting

Another simple way to improve elimination is by squatting when you have your bowel movements. When you use a toilet in a sitting position a portion of the large intestine is closed off, making complete elimination difficult. If you squat right on the toilet seat, or place your feet on a small 10-inch-high stool as you have a bowel movement, elimination will be more efficient. Over time you will have less bowel toxicity.

▶ **Action for Prevention:** Squat on the toilet at home or use a small 10-inch stool to place your feet on while having a bowel movement. ◀

Bringing Back Friendly Bacteria

Functions of Intestinal Bacteria

While removing unhealthy bacteria, parasites, and yeast from our intestines, we may also remove 'good' bacteria and various nutrients necessary to maintain the health of this microscopic ecosystem. There are over 400 different types of bacteria that live in our intestines. A delicate balance between these flora needs to be maintained to create a healthy gut.

When these good bacteria are on friendly terms, they function to synthesize certain vitamins such as vitamin K, biotin, vitamin B12, folic acid, pantothenic acid, pyridoxine, riboflavin; to make nonessential amino acids and butyric acid; to make short chain fatty acids, some of which can reduce the growth of cancer cells; to break down environmental carcinogens and other toxins; to help to break down cholesterol, causing lower levels in the blood; to break down hormones, including estrogen, either to enhance absorption or elimination of estrogen; to stimulate immune function; to convert dietary flavonoids and phytoestrogens so the body can use them to protect us from cancer; to stimulate metabolic rate and help with weight loss or gain; to make 'natural' antibiotics that protect us from infections; and to maintain proper pH levels of the intestines, deterring infectious organisms. The intestinal flora is considered by some people to be a separate 'organ' in its own right because of the many functions it performs.

Parasites, use of antibiotics, the birth control pill, steroid based medications, chlorinated drinking water, excess sugar and sweets, an overly refined diet, lack of fiber, excess meat and fat, an excess of carbohydrates, stress, and eating too quickly without proper chewing are all factors that upset this balance and create a toxic bowel. For example, a specific bacteria called *Clostridia paraputreficum* makes up only .4–.8% of the intestinal flora. Clostridia has the noble task of converting the plant lignans to the weak estrogen, enterolactone, which protects us from breast cancer. When a broad spectrum antibiotic is used, this conversion is severely diminished or absent for as long as one is taking the antibiotic and can take up to 30 days to resume after discontinuation of the antibiotic. In some individuals it may take as little as five days to resume[7] — the individual variations are due to the composition of the intestinal flora. This conversion happens in the beginning of the large intestine.

Reintroducing Good Bacteria

The reintroduction of friendly bacteria into the intestines helps to create a healthy bowel. We can promote a healthy balance of intestinal flora by supplementing with 'good' bacteria, which prevent the colonization of our intestines by unhealthy bacteria, overabundant yeast, or parasites.

The healthy bacteria are best taken in capsule form and include *Lactobacillus acidophilus, Lactobacillus bifidus, Lactobacillus bulgarus, Bifidobacterium bifidus,* and

Streptococcus faeceum. The first two of these are most commonly used in probiotic formulas. They should be taken once or twice daily for a period of months. Keep them refrigerated after opening. When taken with a plant substance called FOS, or fructo-oligosaccharides, the growth of bifidobacterium in the intestines is enhanced tenfold. FOS acts as a growth medium for these and other bacteria and is present in the following foods: asparagus, Jerusalem artichoke, onion, burdock root, honey, rye, and Chinese chive.

DOSAGE: Two capsules daily between meals for a total of 6–10 billion organisms per day.

Food Sources: Organic yogurt, sauerkraut, kefir, olives, pickles, vinegar, tempeh, tamari, mochi.
CONTRAINDICATIONS: None.

▶ **Action for Prevention:** Supplement your diet with probiotic organisms including Lactobacillus acidophilus and Lactobacillus bifidus as well as the growth medium FOS. Include asparagus, onions, Jerusalem artichoke, and/or burdock root as a regular part of your diet. ◀

Digestive Enzymes

Enzymes are energized protein molecules that catalyze or initiate almost all biochemical reactions and cellular activities which occurs in our bodies. The human body contains more than 2,700 different types of enzymes. Our organs, tissues, and cells are created and maintained by metabolic enzymes. Hormones, minerals, and vitamins will work only when enzymes are present. An excess of vitamins and minerals can actually deplete enzymes, as they cause more of them to be used up. Digestion is entirely dependent on enzymes. They are the body's workhorses. The processes of growing, living, and dying are governed by an ordered, integrated sequence of enzymatic reactions. Our health is dependent upon our enzyme reserve. When enzymes are depleted, we age faster and are more prone to degenerative diseases, including cancer.

Enzymes are very specific in their activities. Deficiencies of single enzymes caused by a genetic defect such as occurs in muscular dystrophy can cause disease and death. Generally, enzymes transform a particular substance into a different substance by breaking or attaching molecular bonds, while they themselves remain unchanged. The names of all enzymes end with "-ase" while the first part of its name defines what it acts upon. For instance, the enzyme "lactase" helps to break down the milk sugar, lactose.

Type of Enzyme	What It Does
Metabolic Enzyme	Catalyzes chemical reactions within cells such as detoxification and energy production.
Digestive Enzyme	Secreted in the saliva, stomach, pancreas and small intestine to break down food so it can be absorbed into the blood.
Food Enzyme	Are naturally present in all raw foods and assist the body in breaking down the food itself. Chewing activates food enzymes, which pre-digest the food in the mouth and upper stomach, until the stomach acid inactivates them, usually 45–60 minutes later. They become active once again in the alkaline environment of the small intestine. When food is cooked above 118°F enzymes are destroyed and the assistance of food enzymes is lost, calling on more activity from the digestive enzymes.

There are three main groups of enzymes: metabolic, digestive, and food enzymes. They are summarized in the chart above.

We each have a limited supply of metabolic enzyme energy at birth. Enzymes are like the body's battery and must last a lifetime. The faster we use up our enzyme supply, the faster we age. The use of alcohol, drugs, stimulants, cooked food, and overeating causes us to use up enzymes. Therefore, as we age and have enzyme depletion, we have more trouble digesting foods and more chronic illness.

Our enzyme level is proportional to our energy level. With an abundance of enzymes we will have more energy. Enzymes enhance the utilization of vitamins and minerals, and we need much less of a particular nutrient when we take enzymes along with it. There is also a link between our enzyme reserve and the strength of our immune systems — the more enzymes we have, the stronger our immune systems will be. White blood cells themselves contain amylase, protease, and lipase — enzymes that help to break down carbohydrates, proteins, and fats. The white blood cells release these into the blood to act as scavengers on whatever debris needs to be digested in the blood. The same enzymes are found in the white blood cells as are found in the pancreas. After we eat cooked food, the white blood cell count increases, while when we eat raw food, it does not. This implies that cooked food results in toxicity in the blood, which the white blood cells must act upon, while raw food does not strain the white blood cells. Over time this results in immune weakness and susceptibility to cancer.

Enzymes and Cancer

Cancer cells use several self-defense mechanisms to elude detection from ever-watchful white blood cells whose job it is to seek and destroy them. They can mask their surface antigens (which the white blood cells would otherwise recognize) with a protective coat of fibrin; release the antigens into the blood to form immune complexes which act as a decoy to preoccupy and overwhelm the white blood cells; and change their appearance by turning the cell membrane inward disguising the cell surface antigens.[8] Systemic use of proteolytic enzymes (that digest protein) between meals works to eliminate the fibrin coat and activate the immune system.[9] Certain Chinese herbs such as *Sparganium, Taraxicum mongolicum, Curcuma zedoaria, Laminaria* and *Sargassum* can also be used to break down the fibrin coat. When the fibrin coat is removed, the cell surface antigens are exposed and can be targeted by the immune sytem. Removing the fibrin coat also makes the cancer cells less sticky and decreases their ability to attach to other cells in the body, preventing metastases.

Proteolytic enzymes used between meals have been found to decrease the circulating immune complexes produced by the cancer cells in a dose dependent manner.[10] Proteolytic enzymes can be taken every half hour between meals in extreme cases, or, alternatively, two or three times daily between meals. They should not be used if the stomach or intestinal tract is irritated or inflamed, as they may aggravate it further. Otherwise, look for an enzyme combination with high protease content (10XUSP at 500–1000 mg).

Conserving Enzymes

There are two ways to conserve enzymes: eat plenty of raw foods and foods high in enzymes, such as sprouts; and take supplemental enzymes before or between meals. Enzymes are destroyed at temperatures above 118°F. This means that baked goods, canned food, roasted cereals, pasteurized dairy products, cooked meat, etc. are devoid of enzymes. Whenever we cook our foods between 118–149°F (48–65°C) or higher we destroy enzymes. Prolonged heat at 118°F and short heat at 149°F kills enzymes. Heating at 140–176°F (60–80°C) for one-half hour completely kills any enzymes. Boiling, baking, and microwaving destroy enzymes.

When we eat mainly cooked food, the pancreas enlarges in its efforts to produce sufficient enzymes. Over time, the enlargement of the pancreas is followed by its exhaustion and degeneration. The more digestion that can occur before the food reaches the small intestine, the fewer digestive enzymes are needed from the pancreas and small intestine. This enzyme-sparing allows metabolic enzymes to be conserved through the whole body and used for tissue and organ repair, preserving health.

Ideally, to conserve enzymes, we should eat much of our food raw or lightly cooked. Some people suffer from abdominal pain or diarrhea with even a little raw food. In these cases, warm soups and stews cooked in a slow cooker are a good idea with supplemental enzymes taken before meals. For those looking to improve their health through an enzyme-rich diet, Ann Wigmore's book *The Hippocrates Diet and Health Program* discusses the value of eating sprouts and explains how to grow them.

My daughter does a science project each year for her class at school. This year she wanted to make a solar oven. We made it out of sheet metal and glass, taped together with aluminum foil duct tape, improvising on a plan from a library book. We insulated it and painted it black inside. On a sunny spring day in southern Ontario, the temperature in the oven was constant at about 175°F. We baked potatoes and muffins, although it took about eight hours. They tasted great! It is possible to cook our food at low temperatures without the use of electricity. And if the temperature is low enough, the enzymes will be conserved.

▶ **Action for Prevention:**

1) Include sprouts as a regular part of your diet because they are high in enzymes. For breast cancer prevention, some of the best sprouts to use are clover, broccoli, pea, green lentil, chickpea, mung bean, and sunflower. If you eat these at the beginning of a meal with salad, the increased enzymes will help to digest the rest of the meal.

2) Include fresh raw juices as part of your daily diet.

3) Consume at least 50%–80% of your food raw.

4) Cook food on low heat or for shorter periods. Soak beans and grains overnight to increase their enzyme content and decrease their cooking time. Use a slow cooker for bean and grain dishes and stir fry for short periods.

5) Use supplemental enzymes before meals to help digest your food and between meals to detoxify the blood and to break down the fibrin coat of cancer cells. If you have breast cancer, consider using proteolytic enzymes several times daily between meals. Supplement your diet with probiotic organisms including Lactobacillus acidophilus and Lactobacillus bifidus as well as the growth medium FOS. ◀

Kidney Cleansing

Our kidneys filter all of our blood 60 times a day, removing metabolic wastes and excreting them to the outside through urine. The kidneys also help to control the rate of red blood cell formation, regulate blood pressure, regulate the absorption of calcium, and regulate the volume, composition, and pH of body fluids.

The best way to assist our kidneys with detoxification is by drinking plentiful amounts of pure water, somewhere between two to three liters daily. Unfortunately, pure water is not easy to come by.

In the United States, one government report named 2,110 chemicals in drinking water. At least 35% of all public water supplies contain toxic or bacterial contaminants. In 1988, the Environmental Protection Agency found more than 60 pesticides contaminating groundwater in 30 states.[11] We are exposed to many carcinogens through our drinking water. Organochlorines, lead, aluminum, cadmium, fluoride, and other toxic minerals are often present. Bacteria, protozoa, and viruses also contaminate drinking water.

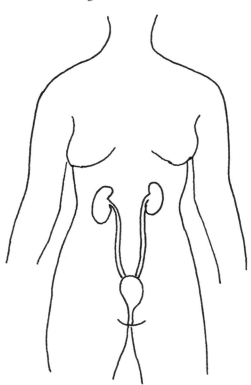

Water Filters

There are several kinds of filters that can be purchased for home use to remove most if not all water contaminants. The long-term answer is for us to not use toxic chemicals that will eventually contaminate the water supply. In the meantime, here is a brief description of various filters.

In summary, the best system is a reverse osmosis system with built in activated charcoal, if you can afford it. Otherwise, go with the activated carbon block filter without silver. Distillation does not remove the environmental chemicals. Carbon block does not remove many minerals, including aluminum and fluoride.

The following are some manufacturers who sell water filters in Canada:[12] Ametek (tel. 800-645-5427); Culligan (tel. 800-285-5442); Everpure (tel. 800-323-7873); Nimbus (tel. 888-829-4231); Ecowater (tel. 800-869-2837). You can contact the Water Quality Association (tel. 800-749-0234 or web site: http://www.wqa.org) to find out the validity of the claims made by specific manufacturers. The National Sanitation Foundation is an independent body that tests water filtration equipment to make sure they meet industry standards. You can obtain a list of approved products from them (tel. 800-673-8919 or web site http://www.nsf.org).

Type of Filter	How It Works	What It Removes
Screen Filters	A fine membrane removes bacteria from water.	bacteria
Activated carbon filters	Adsorbs contaminants, but bacteria can proliferate in poorly functioning carbon filters. They do a good job at removing organic chemicals but do not remove toxic minerals such as aluminum, cadmium, and copper. Some of these filters contain silver to discourage bacterial growth, which can enter the water at high levels. Avoid carbon filters with silver. Use a filter with a rated capacity for 2,000 gallons. Use a filter with a carbon block rather than powdered activated charcoal.	pesticides, radon, volatile organic chemicals
Reverse Osmosis Filters	Contain a membrane that removes contaminants and some minerals. They work slowly, producing only a few gallons of water a day, discarding about 90% of incoming water. Often they are combined with an activated carbon filter in one unit. Can cost several hundred dollars.	bacteria, organic matter, inorganic matter, pesticides, PCBs, lead, aluminum, nitrates, radium, uranium, fluoride
Distillation	Water is boiled, turned to steam, and collected as water again after passing through a series of baffles. Some chemicals have lower boiling points than water and will collect in the distilled end product. Some organisms are heat resistant and will not be killed by distillation. Minerals are removed from the water and over time mineral deficiencies may occur in the person who drinks it. The distillation process is slow and the water tastes flat.	some chemicals, most but not all organisms, minerals, fluoride
Ultraviolet Treatment	Ultraviolet rays change the molecular structure of bacteria and destroy their DNA. Some parasites and viruses are not affected, however.	bacteria

Bottled Water

Bottled water may be an option if it is stored in glass rather than plastic containers and if it is free of bacteria. Most companies will send you laboratory reports on their water quality if you ask.

▶ **Action for Prevention:** Drink 2–3 liters of filtered water daily, using a reverse osmosis or carbon block filter. Other choices for kidney cleansing are to add lemon juice to your water in the morning, use dandelion regularly (it's in the liver formula), drink green juices (including some parsley and watercress), and use beets regularly, which cleanse the kidneys and liver. ◀

Adjusting Acid and Alkaline Balance

Body fluids make up roughly 70% of our body weight and maintaining the pH (acid-alkaline balance) of these fluids is essential to life. Different tissues of the body vary in their pH, and will become more acid or alkaline in the body's efforts to maintain the blood at a constant pH of 7.35. A healthy person will have a urinary pH that averages between 6.4–7.2 (6.8 is ideal) and a salivary pH of 6.4–7.4. These can be measured easily with pH paper, also called hydrazine paper, which is usually available at drug stores and health food stores. It can be ordered from Micro Essential Laboratory in Brooklyn, New York.

The pH of the urine will fluctuate throughout the day. Usually it is more acid in the morning between 3:00 a.m. and 10:00 a.m. and more alkaline in the evening between 4:00 p.m. and 10:00 p.m. It typically becomes alkaline for two hours after eating.

If the pH of urine and saliva are characteristically outside of these ranges, our health is at risk. Certain minerals and vitamins are not absorbed or utilized beyond this range. Most cancer cells prefer an acid environment and may thrive when the body is too acidic. Bacteria, viruses, fungi, and parasites are more active when pH is unbalanced.[13] We need to maintain our urine and saliva in the proper pH range for good health. Enzymes and cellular metabolism works best in a precise pH range.

Acids are produced daily in the body and need to be neutralized. When carbohydrates, proteins, and fats are metabolized they produce inorganic acids. Proteins produce sulfuric and phosphoric acids while carbohydrates produce acetic and lactic acid. When we exercise, we also produce more lactic acid. When lactic acid and carbon dioxide combine with water, carbonic acid is formed. People with cancer who exercise vigorously need to take extra care in monitoring pH levels and neutralizing acids. All of these acids are toxic and can be eliminated through the kidney, large intestine, lungs, and skin. The body's built-in buffer system uses minerals to protect it from being overwhelmed with toxic acids. The alkaline minerals that neutralize acids are sodium, potassium, calcium, and magnesium. One of the reasons Dr Max Gerson gave potassium to all his cancer patients was to decrease acidity and encourage elimination of toxins through the kidney.

When the blood is burdened with excess acid, mild symptoms such as colds, headaches, sore throats, flus, aches and pains are likely to occur. The muscles and joints become stiff, energy levels drop, and we become irritable. Free radical damage occurs more readily, and antioxidants are used up faster. Vitamins and minerals from foods and supplements are less well absorbed, and enzyme function is impaired. When the extracellular fluid becomes acidic, symptoms such as excess mucus, chronic infections, gallstones, kidney stones, cysts, and benign tumors may occur.[14] When the acids accumulate even more, they can penetrate inside the cell and are believed to cause damage to the DNA, thus leading to cancer. The pH of most tumors is more acidic in comparison to the pH of normal tissue, and as tumors grow, their acidity increases.[15] There is poor removal of metabolic acids from cancer cells.[16] Thus one strategy for healing cancer is to alkalinize the pH of the body in general and of tumors specifically. Cesium and rubidium are very alkaline trace minerals that are used in treating malignant tumors by directly injecting them into the tumor site. Deep breathing, often an integral part of yoga and Qigong, helps the lungs release more carbon dioxide, which is an acid. Thus breathing exercises make us more alkaline.

We can balance excess acidity through our choice of foods and through using mineral supplements if needed, particularly potassium, calcium, and magnesium. Although sodium is alkaline, it tends to cause water retention and is not advisable to use other than as naturally occurs in food. When our urine has a pH that averages below 6.2, it means that fluids elsewhere in the body are too acidic and are being dumped in an effort for the body to become more alkaline. It also means that we have a shortage of alkaline minerals to neutralize the acids our bodies produce.

Foods affect our pH levels based on their mineral content. Those that have an abundance of the alkaline minerals will raise pH levels, while those that do not will lower it. (A pH above 7 is considered alkaline; below 7 is acid). Most proteins in food combine with sulfur and phosphorus, and when they are metabolized, by-products such as sulfuric and phosphoric acid are formed. Grains also contain sulfur and phosphorus. This explains why high protein foods and most grains are acid-forming. Fruits and vegetables, on the other hand, contain organic acids which become carbon dioxide and water when oxidized in the body. Their alkaline minerals remain in the blood to neutralize acids. Generally, we should attempt to choose about 80% of our foods from the alkaline group and only 20% from the acid group. This way we will easily eliminate toxic acids from the body on a regular basis. The following chart lists in descending order the acid and alkaline-forming foods, and includes activities that will affect pH. The foods at the top of the acid group are the most acid-forming. The foods at the beginning of the alkaline group are the most alkalinizing. Most of these foods are listed such that the more acid/alkaline forming the food is in each category, the higher on the list it will appear.

• Acid and Alkaline forming Foods (20% of Diet) and Activities •

ACID-FORMING FOODS (20% of diet) AND ACTIVITIES

ANIMAL	GRAINS	BEANS	OTHER	ACTIVITIES
dried squid	buckwheat	peanuts	beer	vigorous exercise:
dried fish	rice bran	coconut	liquor	jogging, rebounding,
egg yolk	oatmeal	cashews	sugar	dancing, sports
tuna	brown rice	Brazil nuts	honey	
octopus	pearl barley	pecans	maple syrup	hot showers or baths
chicken	buckwheat flour	walnuts	alcohol	shallow breathing
carp	white rice	black beans	wine	aging
oysters	white flour	chick peas	cranberry juice	
salmon	wheat gluten	fava beans	fried foods	
clam	bread	pinto beans	saturated fats	
scallops	cornmeal	lima beans	pesticides	
pork	millet	lentils	chemicals	
beef		peas	free radical damage	
cheese				
abalone				
shrimp				
butter				

ALKALINE-FORMING FOODS (80% of diet) AND ACTIVITIES

VEGETABLES	FRUITS	NUTS/BEANS	OTHER	ACTIVITIES
wakame	bananas	kidney beans	Greens +	sea salt baths
kombu	strawberries	soybeans	Pure Synergy	
ginger	orange juice	tempeh	Barley Green	gentle stretching:
raw rhubarb	grapefruit	almonds	spirulina	tai chi, yoga,
kelp	lemon	chestnuts	all sprouts	Qigong
Irish moss	apricots	adzuki beans	wheatgrass juice	
nori	apples	string beans	egg white	deep breathing
mustard greens	canteloupe	tofu	organic milk	massage
shitake mushrooms	cherries	flaxseeds	organic yogurt	meditation
maitake mushrooms	pineapple	sunflower seeds	apple cider vinegar	walking in the forest
reishi mushrooms	all berries	pumpkin seeds	Celtic sea salt	cold showers or baths
spinach	persimmons		antioxidants	
kale	pears		sodium bicarbonate	magnetic field
carrots	grape juice		stevia	therapy with negative
mushrooms	watermelon		good water	polarity magnets
potatoes			flaxseed oil	
burdock root				more dietary fiber
cabbage	**VEGETABLES**			
radish	*(continued)*			antioxidants
squash	Swiss chard			
bamboo shoots	pumpkin			enzymes
sweet potatoes	zucchini			
endive	cucumbers			
celery	tomatoes			
lettuce	eggplant			
broccoli	cauliflower			
turnip	asparagus			
dill pickles	avocado			
dulse	onions			

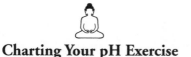

Charting Your pH Exercise

Testing Urinary pH

There are several systems that have been used to test urinary pH. Some practitioners recommend testing in the morning only, others several times throughout the day. As the pH will fluctuate depending on what and when you have eaten, what supplements you take and on your activities and stress levels, it makes the most sense to either collect all of your urine in a 24 hour period and measure its pH, or to take the pH each time you urinate in a 24 hour period and average it out. Do this once or twice a week until you have normalized the urinary pH to be between 6.4–7.2. Then check it once a month or so to keep it there.

If you choose to collect all your urine in a 24 hour period, store it in a glass jar and keep it in a brown paper bag in the refrigerator. Rip off a small piece of pH paper, dip it in the urine, and compare the color of the paper to the accompanying pH chart. Record the result.

If you choose to take the pH each time you urinate in a 24-hour period, hold a strip of paper in the stream of urine or urinate in a cup and take the pH afterward. Record the result of each urination in a 24-hour period and average them out. (Add them together and divide by the number of times you urinated). Record the final result. Use the chart below to monitor your urinary and salivary pH.

Testing Salivary pH

Moisten your tongue with saliva. Place the end of a strip of pH paper on the tongue until it is permeated with saliva. Allow the saliva to react on the pH paper for 30 seconds. Read the result by comparing the color of the pH paper to the color chart. Record the result using the table below. Continue for as long as it takes you to normalize the pH, testing once or twice a week until the salivary pH is between 6.4–7.4.

Acid Urine (below 6.4)

If the pH of the urine is characteristically below 6.4, you have excess acidity. This can be caused by overconsumption of acid-forming foods (meats, whole grains except millet, nuts and seeds, cranberries, tomatoes, corn, vinegar, oils), dehydration, overwork or exercise, aging, excess or deficiency of stomach acid, or deficiency of alkaline minerals (calcium, magnesium, sodium, potassium). Symptoms can include fatigue, irritability, ulcers, diverticulitis, tension in the neck and shoulders, rheumatoid and osteoarthritis, osteoporosis, vitamin D deficiency, and sinusitis.

To correct this, water intake should be increased to 2–3 liters daily. Eat more alkaline foods and eat fewer servings of protein and grains. Alkaline foods include green powdered supplements, vegetable juices, sea vegetables, fruit, most vegetables, kidney beans, soybeans, adzuki beans, tofu, yogurt, coconut, and millet. Grains are transformed into mildly alkalinizing foods by soaking them for 36 hours or more. Kelp tablets can be added to increase alkalinity. Emphasis should be placed on the

Date	Urinary pH	Salivary pH

daily practice of breathing exercises and relaxation, and supplementation of the alkaline minerals and digestive enzymes can be considered. The regular use of cold showers also alkalinizes the body.

Alkaline Urine (above 7.2)

If the pH of the urine is characteristically above 7.2, your body is too alkaline. This can be caused by insufficient protein, deficiency of hydrochloric acid, overwork, and degenerative disease. The body may be attempting to buffer an overly acid condition. If the pH commonly falls within this range, usually energy is deficient and anxiety is experienced. You may feel nervous, 'spaced out', and experience insomnia. Digestion and elimination become too slow with tendencies toward constipation, liver toxicity, and gallbladder stress. There is a decrease in the production of white blood cells causing increased infections. You may be prone to bacterial, yeast, fungal, and parasitic infections. Symptoms such as cystitis, headaches, muscle cramps, and anemia may be present. If there is a hydrochloric acid deficiency of the stomach, it will cause poor digestion of protein and poor absorption of minerals.

To remedy excess alkalinity, first check for hydrochloric acid deficiency using the Gastro-test. If it is low, use a herb like pippali, wormwood, gentian, or goldenseal before meals for six weeks to stimulate it, then recheck. If HCl is normal, use more acid-forming foods generally, such as flaxseed and olive oil, whole grains (especially buckwheat and oats), cranberry juice, prunes, plums, organic animal protein, lentils, cashews, and seeds. Intense exercise causes increased acidity, as will long hot baths or showers.

Alkaline Urine / Acid Saliva

When the urine is overly alkaline (above 7.2) and the saliva is overly acidic (below 6.4), you may be losing excessive amounts of potassium through the kidneys due to adrenal exhaustion. Part of the job of the adrenals is to retain potassium. Another cause of this pattern may be hydrochloric acid deficiency in the stomach.

Acid Saliva (below 6.4)

The normal range for salivary pH is between 6.4 and 7.4. When the saliva is acidic, it shows that the alkaline enzymes usually present in the mouth are deficient, probably due to a deficiency of the alkaline minerals that have been used up to buffer an overly acid state of the body. The most important of these minerals is calcium. Thus, an acid saliva pH suggests calcium deficiency. Other alkaline minerals include sodium, potassium, and magnesium.

When the salivary pH is too acidic, the deficiency of salivary alkaline enzymes will cause poor carbohydrate digestion. You will not obtain sufficient energy from food and the incompletely digested carbohydrates will lead to bowel toxicity, fatigue and allergies. There will likely be a significant amount of gas produced in the bowel. Often the excessive use of coffee, alcohol, drugs, and cigarettes will cause the saliva to become acidic.

Alkaline Saliva (above 7.4)

When the salivary pH is above 7.4 it may indicate either that there is too much bile being secreted from the liver, that there is insufficient hydrochloric acid, or that there is a protein deficiency.

▶ **Action for Prevention:** Monitor your urinary and salivary pH for several weeks and attempt to normalize it using the above guidelines. This will improve your absorption of minerals and relieve many symptoms related to pH imbalance. In general, your diet should consist of 80% alkaline-forming foods (sea vegetables, fruits, vegetables, millet, kidney beans, adzuki beans, tofu, flaxseed oil) and 20% acid-forming foods (grains, seeds and nuts, asparagus, cranberry, plums, prunes, lentils, animal protein). ◀

Sweating It Out

The skin is a major organ of detoxification and we release toxins through it when we sweat. Sweating can be induced by aerobic exercise or by saunas. Many cultures worldwide have used saunas or sweat lodges as regular tools for body cleansing and purification. Saunas have been used in Finland for over 1,000 years. The Romans, Greeks, Turks, Russians, and Japanese have their own variations on the sauna. Native Americans have utilized the sweat lodge as a healing and purification rite for equally as long. The Finns believed that the steam that rises from the stones of the sauna could drive diseases and evil humors out of the body and purify the mind and spirit. The sauna was viewed as the 'holy place' and sauna bathing was considered the 'medicine of the poor'.[17] Historically, the Finnish family enjoys a group sauna together once weekly, usually on Saturday. Often a bride and bridegroom will take a sauna together before their marriage ceremony. Sick people are taken to the sauna to heal, and many women give birth in the sauna. Old men and women are carried there to die. The Finns maximize detoxification while in the sauna by beating their skin with a birch branch whisk, increasing the circulation to the skin. There is a sauna for every five people in Finland today and 90% of the population over 80 years of age still takes a sauna regularly. The sauna occupies a primary place in Finnish culture.

I will never forget the feeling of elation I experienced after rushing over to the University of Toronto library one evening with a burning question in my mind. Were breast cancer rates lower in Finland than in surrounding Scandinavian countries? An hour later, I believed that they were and was thrilled about the possible benefits of saunas in preventing breast cancer. Finland had the lowest breast cancer rates of the Scandinavian countries, according to figures from 1979. The incidence was 39.9 per 100,000 women in Finland compared to Denmark's high incidence of 59.4. The incidence in the other Scandinavian countries were approximately as follows: Sweden, 54.9; Iceland, 54.2; and Norway, 47.4.[18] We need further studies that monitor women who take regular saunas to assess their breast cancer risk in comparison to women who don't take saunas.

We have all been exposed to environmental chemicals that increase breast cancer risk. As I was researching the environmental links to breast cancer, I became overwhelmed with the numbers of toxic chemicals that we are exposed to daily, the ease with which we pass those on to our children, and the difficulty with which we eliminate them from our bodies. It seemed to me that the environmental load was greater than our detoxification abilities and that we were destined for extinction within a few generations. Studies have shown that chemicals often linked with increased breast cancer risk are DDE and PCBs; with a fourfold increase in risk in women who have elevated serum levels of DDE and a doubling of risk when PCBs are higher than in normal controls.[19]

In recent years, the sauna has become recognized as one of the few methods to remove toxic chemicals from the body, particularly when they are stored in the fat cells. L. Ron Hubbard, father of the Scientology movement, pioneered its use for people with drug dependencies in 1977. He describes his method and its evolution in his book *Clear Body, Clear Mind.*[20] After his success, clinical ecologists began to use sauna therapy with individuals who have chemical sensitivities, chronic fatigue, environmental illness or who have been subjected to toxic chemical exposures. Substances that have been shown to be excreted through the skin during saunas are morphine, methadone, amphetamines, chlorinated pesticides, herbicides, and PCBs.[21]

A Vietnam War veteran who had been exposed to Agent Orange (dioxin) was placed on a 37-day protocol using exercise, vitamin and mineral supplements, and saunas. By the end of the treatments, a fat biopsy showed a 97% decrease in levels of PCBs and DDE.[22] Firemen exposed to PCBs from a transformer fire suffered memory impairment for stories, images, and numbers, attributed to the exposure. After undergoing a medically supervised diet, exercise, and sauna program, their mental function improved.[23] In his book *Diet for a Poisoned Planet*, David Steinman describes his experiences with sauna detoxification and outlines a home detoxification program that reduced his blood levels of DDT by 70%.[24] One clinic in Los Angeles called HealthMed has been able to remove over 90% of toxic chemicals from thousands of peoples' bodies through an exercise, sauna and supplement program based on Hubbard's work. A case report by Dr Krop, a clinical ecologist in Toronto, describes a similar successful protocol used for one woman with overexposure to solvents.[25]

I believe that it is essential that saunas become a regular part of our lifestyles if we are to protect ourselves and our children from breast cancer and other diseases related to chemical toxicity. These include hormonal imbalances, neurological ailments such as ADD, infertility, autoimmune and other immune-related diseases, environmental illness, and chronic fatigue syndrome, to name just a few. Many environmental chemicals are lipophilic, meaning they are attracted to fat, and so we store them in our fat cells. The skin accesses these fat stores through sweating. Better out through our sweat than into our children's mouths through breast milk. With the regular use of saunas, we can eliminate a good proportion of environmental toxins and hence reduce our risk of breast cancer. If you were to analyze blood, saliva, or fat samples before and after a sauna detoxification program to see how successful you had been at eliminating them, you might consider testing for the following chemicals: DDE; PCBs 105, 118, and 156; the pesticides, atrazine, endosulfan, methoxychlor and lindane; and bisphenol-A.

Some of the recognized health benefits of saunas are temporary relief from arthritic pain, relaxation of sore and tense muscles, and improved flexibility. Group saunas provide great opportunities to share honest feelings, heal emotional wounds, relax, and create friendships.

The Sauna Detoxification Program

During sauna detoxification patients are supervised for several hours daily over a three-week period as they participate in a program as follows.

1) The participant should be neither hungry nor have just eaten.

2) Niacin is taken as per the supplement schedule before exercising, usually beginning at 100 mg daily. Sensitive or smaller individuals may need to start with less. The daily dose of niacin is taken all at once at this time.

3) The participant begins with 20–30 minutes of exercise in the form of rebounding, running, or using a treadmill to stimulate the circulation of blood and lymph and to move the blood deeper into the tissues from where it can draw out toxic residues. Aerobic exercise causes the cell waste to be carried out quickly and efficiently. This is then followed immediately by time in the sauna to sweat out toxins. Aerobic exercise should be practiced daily once the program has begun, always immediately before the sauna for 20–30 minutes. The patient then goes immediately into the sauna after the aerobic exercise, accompanied by a partner or group. The partner is there for safety's sake, as a person undergoing sauna detoxification may experience unpleasant symptoms as chemical toxins are released. A towel is placed underneath one's whole body to avoid perspiring on the wooden seats. The next two to four and one half hours[26] are spent in the sauna, interrupted by short periods of cool showers every 15–30 minutes. Hubbard had participants stay in for four hours daily; Dr Krop had them do four sittings of 15–20 minutes each for five consecutive days, then off for two, for a total of 21 sauna days. Then the patient continues on their own twice weekly for two more weeks.

4) It may take a few days, weeks, or months to work up to the five-hour schedule. The daily saunas are continued for approximately three weeks, with a supplement schedule to go along with it. Sweating should be profuse while in the sauna. If the participant feels too warm or as though they are going to faint, they are advised to leave the sauna and have a cool shower and then return. The sauna partner ensures that the participant does not fall asleep in the sauna as salt or potassium deficiency could occur while asleep. Salt and potassium are lost through sweating and can be replaced with an electrolyte drink or tablets. Symptoms of salt or potassium depletion might include extreme tiredness or weakness, headache, muscle cramps, clammy skin, nausea, dizziness, vomiting, and fainting. Should any of these symptoms occur, salt tablets and potassium gluconate tablets are on hand, located just outside of the sauna or specific foods or teas containing sodium and potassium, such as miso soup and bananas.

5) Water or vegetable broth jugs are taken into the sauna or left just outside. If suddenly the body stops sweating and the skin becomes hot and dry while in the sauna, this may be a sign of heat stroke. Treatment for heat stroke is to cool off with a lukewarm or cool shower and take fluids, salt, and potassium. Water is drunk liberally (8–12 glasses daily) while in the sauna to replace what is lost through sweating.

6) The temperature in the sauna is maintained at 65°C to 71°C or 149–160°F. A dry sauna is more effective than a wet sauna, although either can be used.

7) The participant maintains her regular diet with added fresh fruits and vegetables, juiced or raw, while undergoing sauna detoxification. She waits one hour after eating before going into the sauna, or two hours after a large meal. Digestion requires a lot of blood, and the sauna brings the blood to the skin as a coolant. The blood cannot be effectively used for both at the same time. Alcohol and drugs are avoided during sauna detoxification.

8) Supplemental niacin is the key ingredient in sauna therapy. Niacin increases peripheral circulation and mobilizes chemicals from fatty tissue. Administration of niacin will cause flushing of the skin with a burning sensation within several hours. This can be alarming for some people unless they know to expect it. Initially, participants are given 50–100 mg of niacin daily until they have a flushing reaction. When the reaction is not evident after the niacin, the dosage is increased incrementally in 100 mg units, usually proceeding to between 2,000 and 4,000 mg daily by the end of the third week. At 1,000 mg, most patients increase the niacin in 500 mg increments rather than 100 mg units. Any dose above 2,000 mg must be monitored with liver function tests, as niacin may injure the liver in high doses. Niacin decreases blood pressure and lowers cholesterol levels. Sauna therapy is complete when there is no more flushing after any amount of niacin. This usually occurs after two to three weeks on the program.

9) Other vitamins, minerals, and oils are taken along with the niacin and increased proportionately to it. Calcium and magnesium are taken in a 2:1 ratio as a drink with apple cider vinegar to improve its absorption. Vitamin C is taken at 1,000 mg daily initially and increased incrementally to 6,000 mg daily as niacin is increased. A vitamin B complex is increased incrementally with the niacin to help prevent other B vitamin deficiencies and improve liver detoxification.

A multivitamin and mineral supplement is taken to provide the remaining nutrients. The chart on page 157 summarizes vitamin and mineral intake at the beginning and by the end of the program, after step-wise increments. These values are taken primarily from Hubbard's book *Clear Body, Clear Mind.*

10) Quality oils are taken varying between two tablespoons to one half cup of oil daily. The higher amount is needed for people who are overweight. Hubbard used a combination of soy, walnut, peanut, and safflower oil along with one to two tablespoons of lecithin daily. Krop used corn, olive, flaxseed, and evening primrose oil with 2–3 tsp of activated charcoal given daily to prevent the re-absorption of chemicals mobilized from fat. For breast cancer prevention, flaxseed and extra virgin olive oil with added lecithin and activated charcoal or 1 tbsp bentonite plus a fiber formula may be more appropriate. Many people are allergic to peanuts and corn, and the Omega 6 fatty acids in evening primrose oil can increase tumor growth, while the Omega 3 fatty acids in flaxseed oil shrinks tumors. Oils are cold-pressed and kept refrigerated. If the sweat becomes oily during the sauna, the oil intake is reduced.

11) The participant is advised to have sufficient rest while on the program, that is eight hours of sleep daily. The program works best when done at the same time daily.

As a less drastic alternative, Steinman recommends a home detox program that involves using saunas two to four consecutive days in a week for several months with two or three 20–30 minute sessions in the sauna each of those days.[27]

I believe the sauna therapy would be more effective if some of the liver and intestinal cleansers in this book were taken simultaneously, for example, The Liver Loving Formula, NAC, a fiber formula containing bentonite, guar gum, apple pectin, and citrus pectin, as well as a probiotic formula.

CONTRAINDICATIONS: Don't do sauna detoxification if you are pregnant or breast-feeding. You will pass on the toxins to your child. If you have heart, kidney, or liver disease, consult with a medical doctor before beginning the program and do it with medical supervision. Do not do the program without supervision if you are anemic, or if you have sutures from a surgery.

▶ **Action for Prevention:**

1) Encourage the building of saunas in our communities, or build our own.

2) Undergo a medically supervised three-week sauna detoxification program every one to five years, the frequency depending upon our toxin exposure, age, and general health. This would be a wonderful ritual for women to do together in their efforts to prevent breast cancer, connect with each other, and to feel better generally.

3) Develop the ritual of the family sauna, having a weekly sauna with our partners and children. In this way we will release toxins regularly, not giving them time to build up to high levels. If we don't have a family, then we can find a group of sauna-lovers to sweat with regularly.

4) Before getting married, spend at least a few days sweating it out and considers doing the full sauna detoxification program together, especially if the couple intends to have children in the future.

5) At least three months before you conceive, do the full sauna detoxification program. Toxins continue to be released for several months after the therapy is completed, so do the cleansing well in advance of conception. ◀

Building a Sauna

Supervised sauna programs are available from some clinical ecologists, from some Scientology centers (800-561-5808 in Canada or 800-367-8788 in the United States) and from HealthMed centers in Los Angeles (213-653-0837) and Sacramento (916-924-8060. They will soon be available at the Canadian College of Naturopathic Medicine in Toronto (see Resource Directory). Two excellent books on building your own saunas are *The Sauna* by Rob Roy and *The Art of Sauna Building* by Bert Olavi Jalasjaa of Finland, sold by Key Industries International (256 King St. N, Box 38051, Waterloo, ON N2J 2Y2).

In Northern Ontario, Finnish communities have established public as well as private saunas. One well-known public sauna exists in Thunder Bay, designed by architect Kal Kangas. The Kangas sauna is unique for its skylights, and special attention has been given to air circulation so that old air is continuously removed as fresh air is vented in. For a copy of this plan, contact Kal Kangas (807-623-1021). Perhaps it will inspire you to build your own sauna.

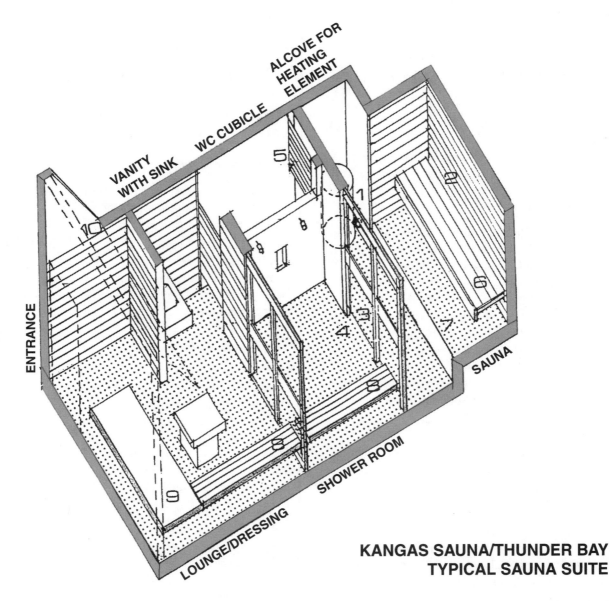

**KANGAS SAUNA/THUNDER BAY
TYPICAL SAUNA SUITE**

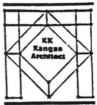

ARCHITECT NOT RESPONSIBLE
FOR UNAUTHORIZED USE OF
INFORMATION ON THIS PAGE

1. Sauna heating element c/w fresh air intake near floor level.
   *(Fresh air intake away from parking lots and building exhausts)

2. Heated air rises

3. Used air flows downward

4. Door and sidelight undercut to allow used air to be exhausted away from Sauna

5. Fan to exhaust all used air in Sauna suite

6. Sauna bench from untreated pine or obeche. (No vertical supports to floor)

7. Raised concrete floor to minimize non-useful room volume under bench

8. Bench from pine or obeche. (No vertical supports to floor)

9. Resting surface with mattress

10. Continuous skylight allowing natural light and sunlight to enter Sauna suite

A Cleansing Diet

Part of any detoxification regime is a fast or cleansing diet. At times fasting can be used to give the digestive system a rest and detoxify more thoroughly. Commonly done at the change of seasons for several days, annual fasting is a good health practice for most people. Do not fast if you are underweight, or if you have cancer. In these cases you will need quality nutrients from food to help you rebuild your body or you can use the Mung Bean and Rice diet below.

The Lemon Aid Cleanse

The 'Lemon Aid' Cleanse is designed to eliminate toxins and congestion while revitalizing the body. It can be used as a seasonal tune-up for women without breast cancer. If continued for from 3–10 days, it usually does not cause a significant lack of physical energy. Because of its simplicity, it is easy to follow at home, work, or while traveling. This cleanse may be done one or more times a year. It gives the digestive system a rest so that enzymes can be used for detoxification and cellular repair. Use it with medical or naturopathic supervision. The major part of the cleanse is to drink the following mixture:

2	tablespoons of the juice from *freshly* squeezed lemons or limes
1	teaspoon of maple syrup
1/10	teaspoon of cayenne pepper (more if desired)

Take this mixture and put it in 8 to 10 ounces of filtered or spring water, warm or cold. The lemons or limes should be fresh and organically grown if possible. The maple syrup should be B or C grade, since these are higher in mineral content. It may be easier to make up a day's supply at one time. Do this using:

2	cups of the juice from freshly squeezed lemons;
¾–1	cup of maple syrup (B or C grade);
1	or more teaspoons of cayenne pepper.

Of this mixture, take 3 tablespoons per 8 to 10 ounce glass. If you are at work or traveling, you can carry enough of this in a thermos. Drink between 6 to 12 glasses daily (more if desired). If you also want to lose weight, keep it close to 6 glasses daily.

During the cleanse, keep your bowels moving by taking a fiber supplement containing at least some of the following: psyllium seed powder, oatbran, apple pectin, guar gum, and bentonite. If you do not have one to two bowel movements daily using the fiber formula, then consider an enema. If your energy lags, add 2 to 4 tablespoons of a greens supplement like Greens + to water and drink once to three times daily. You can also consider drinking fresh carrot, beet, and cabbage juice 2–3 times daily during this fast.

To end the cleanse, drink a vegetable broth soup, sipping it slowly. The following day include more food in the form of steamed vegetables, fruits, sprouts, or salads.

Alkaline Vegetable Mineral Broth

Ingredients: 2 cups each of carrot tops (leaves) and potato peels (¼ inch thick), beet tops, fresh parsley (1 cup if dehydrated), and 3 cups of celery stalks and leaves.

Cover with distilled or filtered water and simmer for 20 minutes. Strain, keep the broth, and discard the vegetables. You can add garlic, onions, or other vegetables to the above if you wish. Add miso or Bragg's liquid aminos in the last few minutes for flavoring. Drink hot or cold.

Mung Beans and Rice

This is a wonderful predigested food, fine for those with chronic illness or cancer. It is easy on the digestive system, healthy for the liver, nourishing as well as cleansing. It is useful to eat this as a dietary mainstay with the addition of sprouts, raw fruits, and vegetables. It can be eaten for 40 days at a time one or more times a year as a cleanse rather than fasting. The recipe comes from Yogi Bhajan,[28] with my additions of dulse powder and Bragg's liquid aminos.

1	cup mung beans
1	cup basmati rice
9	cups water
4–6	cups chopped carrots, celery, broccoli, cauliflower, or other vegetables
2	onions, chopped
⅓	cup minced ginger root
3–5	cloves minced garlic
1½	tsp turmeric
½	tsp pepper
1	heaping tsp garam masala (optional)
1	tsp crushed red chiles (optional)
1	tbsp sweet basil
2	bay leaves
	seeds of 5 cardamon pods
	dulse powder or liquid Bragg's to taste

Soak beans overnight. Rinse. Bring water to a boil, add beans, and let boil over medium heat. Prepare vegetables. Sauté onions, garlic, and ginger in a little water plus olive

• Supplemental Schedule for Sauna Therapy •

NUTRIENT	BEGINNING THERAPY	ENDING THERAPY
Niacin	50–100 mg	2,000–4,000 mg
Vitamin A	5,000–10,000 IU	50,000 IU
Vitamin D	400 IU	2,000 IU
Vitamin C	1,000 mg	6,000 mg
Vitamin E	800 IU	2,400 IU
Vitamin B complex	100 mg	300 mg
Calcium	500–1,000 mg	2,500–3,000 mg
Magnesium	250–500 mg	1250–1500 mg
Iron	18–36 mg	90–108 mg
Zinc	15–30 mg	75–90 mg
Manganese	4–8 mg	20–24 mg
Copper	2–4 mg	10–12 mg
Potassium	45–90 mg	225–270 mg
Iodine	.225–.450 mg	1.125–1.350 mg
Cal-Mag Formula: mix together 1 tbsp. calcium gluconate ½ tsp. magnesium carbonate 1 tbsp. apple cider vinegar ½ cup boiling water ½ cup cold water or take calcium-magnesium tablets with apple cider vinegar.	1½ glasses	2–3 glasses`

oil until brown. When the beans have begun to split, add turmeric, bay leaves, pepper, and garam masala. Add rice. Add a little more water if necessary. Add vegetables, red chiles, and basil and cook, stirring frequently, until the rice and vegetables are cooked. It should have a thick, slightly soupy consistency. Add dulse powder and Bragg's to taste. Serve with a dash of lemon juice.

▶ **Action for Prevention:** Consider a cleansing diet or fast one or more times a year for several days if you do not have cancer. Consider the Mung Beans and Rice Diet if you have cancer. ◀

Homeopathic Formulas

There is a line of German homeopathic formulas that have been used for the last 15 years to assist in detoxification. The Phonix brand has three formulas — C-23, C-26 and C-3 — that are each used in sequence for

three days for a minimum of 45 days. Together they address detoxification through the liver, kidneys, and lymphatic system. When these were used for two months, three individuals were able to reduce their blood levels of PCPs by 78%. These can be ordered by health professionals from Bona Dea in Waterloo, Ontario (tel. 519-886-4200 or fax. 519-886-6735).

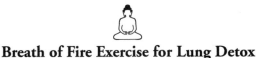

Breath of Fire Exercise for Lung Detox

The lungs release toxic gases and the end products of cell metabolism. We can improve the detoxifying ability of our lungs and alkalinize the body with regular long deep breathing and some specialized breathing exercises, one of which is called 'breath of fire'.[29] Here's how to do it:

Sit cross-legged or in a chair and raise your arms up to a 60-degree angle from the horizontal, forming a 'V' above your head. Curl your fingers into the palms making a fist, but keep the thumbs pointing up straight and pull them back slightly. Close your eyes and look up between your eyebrows, holding your gaze there.

Begin breath of fire. Inhale as the belly comes out; exhale as you bring it in, keeping up an even rhythm with the belly pumping in and out. The inhale should equal the exhale in strength and intensity. Once you have the rhythm, speed up your breathing so that you are doing 2–3 breaths per second. Continue for 1–3 minutes. After a while, you can increase the time gradually to 11 minutes daily. This practice will improve your energy levels, bring in more oxygen, strengthen your nerves, detoxify your lungs, and decrease susceptibility to cancer.

Kundalini Yoga Exercises for Whole Body Cleansing

1) Sit cross-legged and extend your arms out to the sides parallel to the ground with your elbows straight.

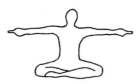

Make your hands into fists with the middle finger extended. Begin to circle your arms in small backward circles, keeping your arms straight. Continue for 3–5 minutes and then increase the speed, making the circles wider. Continue for 2 more minutes. This exercise helps to develop mental calmness and circulates the lymphatic fluid.

2) Remain cross-legged and interlace your fingers behind your neck, pulling your elbows back. Moving from right to left, rotate your torso around on your hips in a deep circular motion. Inhale as you push your chest

forward and rotate to the front; exhale as you slump your lower spine down and rotate to the back. Close your eyes and focus them up between your eyebrows as you move. Continue for 3 minutes. This exercise

acts as a gentle massage to the abdominal organs and improves digestion.

3) Sitting cross-legged, place the thumb of each hand on the pad at the base of the little finger. Stretch your arms out parallel to the ground with your palms facing down. Inhale as you raise the left arm up to an

angle of 60 degrees and exhale as you raise the right arm up to 60 degrees while the opposite arm comes down to touch the ground. Continue fairly rapidly with a powerful breath creating a seesawing motion with your arms. This exercise expands the aura and builds your power of projection.

4) Come into a kneeling position with the knees shoulder width apart. There is a difficult and an easy version of this exercise. **Difficult:** Arch the upper body backwards and hold on to your heels allowing the head to fall back as far as is comfortable. (This is known as camel pose.) Inhale as you push the pelvis

up keeping your elbows straight; exhale as you bend your elbows and lower your torso. Continue with a rhythmic movement coordinated with the breath. **Easy:** If this is too much of a stretch for you, then place your hands on the ground behind you and let your head drop back. Inhale as you lift the pelvis up off the buttocks; exhale as you bend your elbows and lower the pelvis. Continue going up and down for 2–3 minutes. This exercise strengthens the lower back and opens the meridians in the front of the body.

5) From the previous posture, come forward bringing the forehead to touch the ground and stretch the arms out in front of you with the palms flat together.

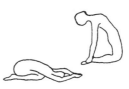

Inhale back into camel pose or the easy version of the previous exercise; exhale bringing the forehead to the ground and the palms together in front. Continue with a rhythmic movement and a deep breath for 2 minutes.

6) Sit cross-legged with the arms out to your sides parallel to the ground. Curl your fingers into fists with the thumbs pointing up. Inhale as you twist the

head, torso and arms to the left; exhale as you twist them to the right. Continue for 2 minutes. This exercise balances the electromagnetic field, circulates the lymphatic fluid, opens the heart chakra, and releases tension in the shoulders.

7) Come sitting on your heels with your palms resting on your thighs. Sit with a straight spine. Inhale, hold

the breath and pump the stomach in and out as many times as possible. Exhale, hold the breath out and continue to pump for as long as you can hold the breath out. Continue for 3 minutes. This exercise strengthens digestion and liver function and balances the reproductive organs.

8) Remain sitting on your heels with your palms on your thighs. Moving from right to left, rotate the spine.

Inhale as you come to the front, exhale as you go round the back. Keep the head more or less in the center as you push the chest out on the inhale and slump the lower spine to the back on the exhale. Continue one minute in each direction. This exercise relaxes the spine and massages the abdominal organs.

9) Sit on your heels. Make your hands into fists with the thumbs inside. Inhale and stretch the left arm forward, opening the fingers as though you are grabbing your future. Exhale and pull it back, closing your

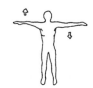

fist as you bring it to the chest. Do the same with the right arm. Continue alternating the arms, inhaling as each arm goes forward, exhaling as it is brought back. Continue with a powerful breath for 3 minutes. This exercise is a powerful lymphatic cleanser for the breast area and helps to direct your will.

10) Stand up with your feet close together. Hold your arms out to the sides parallel to the ground with the palms facing the floor. Inhale slowly as you lift the left

arm up bringing the elbow next to your ear, while simultaneously bringing the right arm down to your side. Exhale as the left arm comes down and the right arm is brought next to your ear. Continue with a very slow meditative breath for 5 minutes. This exercise works to balance the body's electromagnetic field.

11) Sit down with the left leg extended out in front. Bend the right leg, placing the sole of the right foot against the inner left thigh with the heel next to the groin. Reach forward keeping the left knee straight and place your hands on the knee, shin, ankle or grab your toes — wherever you can reach without bending the knee. Slowly stretch forward from your lower

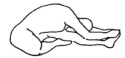

back and bring your chest down toward your knee while breathing slowly and deeply. Continue to stretch forward as you relax into the posture. Hold for 2 minutes, then switch sides. This exercise stretches the kidney, liver and spleen meridians, which govern the reproductive organs. It also stretches and strengthens the lower back and the sciatic nerve.

12) Sit cross-legged and interlace your fingers behind your back with the index fingers outstretched and together. Bend forward and raise your arms up as high as possible. Inhale and stretch up; exhale bend

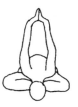

forward to the right knee. Inhale up; exhale down to the left knee, raising the arms as you come down. Inhale up; exhale down to the center. Continue the movement … right … left … center for 3 minutes. Relax on your back for 10 minutes. This exercise releases tension in the upper back and across the chest and helps to open the heart chakra.[30]

Summary

If we routinely detoxify each year, we can decrease our body's toxic load and improve our vitality and health. Detoxification used to be a regular part of the change of seasons in people and cultures that lived closer to nature than most of us do now. Many people choose to do a cleanse at the change of seasons, in the spring and/or the fall. Continue your cleanse for from 6–8 weeks or more, if needed. Write these dates into your calendar so that you can prepare for them. During this time you will want to take a liver cleansing formula such as the Liver Loving Formula, herbal or homeopathic products to eliminate excess yeast and parasites, a fiber formula to act as a colon cleanser, and good bacteria. Drink at least eight glasses of water daily while doing the cleanse. You will be more successful if you do it under the supervision of a naturopathic doctor. Practise the exercises for cleansing the lymphatic system from the next chapter to optimize the effect of your program.

Further Reading

Gittleman, Ann Louise. *Guess What Came for Dinner?* Garden City Park, NY: Avery, 1993.

Kroeger, Hanna. *Parasites: The Enemy Within.* Boulder, CO: Hannah Kroeger Publications, 1991.

Hobbs, C. *Foundations of Health: Healing with Herbs and Foods.* Capitola, CA: Botanica Press, 1992.

Krohn, Jacqueline, Frances Taylor, MA, and Jinger Prosser, LMT. *Natural Detoxification: The Complete Guide to Clearing Your Body of Toxins.* Point Roberts, WA: Hartley and Marks Publishers Inc., 1996.

Roy, Rob. *The Sauna.* White River Junction, VT: Chelsea Green Publishing Company, 1996.

Santillo, Humbart. *Food Enzymes: The Missing Link to Radiant Health.* Prescott, AZ: Hohm Press, 1993.

Steinman, D. *Diet for a Poisoned Planet.* New York, NY: Crown Publishing, 1990.

References

1. Bearss, C., B. Hairey, S. Woodsworth, J. Cidadao, A. Price. Breast cancer research project: Estrogen metabolism. Toronto, ON: *Canadian College of Naturopathic Medicine*, April, 1999.
2. From the teachings of Yogi Bhajan, from a very early kundalini yoga manual.
3. Bhajan, Yogi. *Kundalini Yoga for Youth and Joy,* Exercise Set for the Liver Colon and Stomach. Eugene, OR: 3HO Transcripts, 1983:14-17.
4. From a handout called *Detoxify for All You're Worth,* by Dr Leo Roy.
5. Hobbs, C. *Foundations of Health: Healing with Herbs and Foods.* Capitola, CA: Botanica Press, 1992: 158.
6. Rogers, S. *Wellness Against All Odds.* Syracuse, NY: Prestige Publishing, 1994.
7. Borriello, S.P., K. Setchell, M. Axelson, A.M. Lawson. Production and metabolism of lignans by the human faecal flora. *Journal of Applied Bacteriology,* 1985;58,37-43
8. Gignac, Tara. The use of digestive enzymes in cancer therapy. Toronto, ON: Canadian College of Naturopathic Medicine, April 2000:2.
9. Cichoke, A. The effect of systemic enzyme therapy on cancer cells and the immune system. *Townsend Letter for Doctors and Patients.* Nov 1995:30-32

10. Cichoke, A. The effect of systemic enzyme therapy on cancer cells and the immune system. *Townsend Letter for Doctors and Patients*. Nov 1995:31

11. Steinman, D. *Diet for a Poisoned Planet*. New York, NY: Crown Publishing, 1990:203.

12. Lad, A. The joy of water filters. Toronto, ON: *Canadian College of Naturopathic Medicine*, April, 1999.

13. Johnson, Jan. *Metabolic Balancing Organizational Workbook* (based on the teachings of Dr. Revici).

14. Compan, E., L. Lau, J. Prentice. The relationship between pH and our susceptibility to cancer. Toronto, ON: *Canadian College of Naturopathic Medicine*, April 2000.

15. Vaupel, P. et al. Blood flow, oxygen and nutrient supply, and the metabolic microenvironment of human tumors: A review. *Cancer Research*, 1989;49(23):6449-65.

16. Lee, A.H., I.F. Tannock. Homogeneity of intracellular pH and of mechanisms that regulate intracellular pH in populations of cultured cells. *Cancer Research*, 1998;1(9):1901-08.

17. Perasalo, J. The traditional use of sauna for hygiene and health in Finland. *Annals of Clinical Research*. 1988:20(4):220-23.

18. Moller Jensen, O, B. et al. *Atlas of Cancer Incidence in the Nordic Countries*. Helsinki, Finland: Nordic Cancer Union, 1988.

19. Wolf, M.S. et al. Blood levels of organochloride residues and risk of breast cancer. *Journal of National Cancer Institute*, 1993:85:648-652.

20. Hubbard, L. R. *Clear Body, Clear Mind*. Copenhagen, Denmark: New Era Publications Int., 1990.

21. Roehm, D.C. Effect of a clearing program of sauna baths and megavitamins on adipose DDE and PCBs and on clearing of symptoms of Agent orange (dioxin) toxicity. *Clinical Research*, 1983:31:243.

22. Roehm, D.C. Effect of a clearing program of sauna baths and megavitamins on adipose DDE and PCBs and on clearing of symptoms of Agent orange (dioxin) toxicity. *Clinical Research*, 1983:31:243.

23. Kilburn, K.H., R.H. Warsaw, M.G. Shields. Neurobehavioral dysfunction in firemen exposed to polychlorinated biphenyls (PCBs): possible improvement after detoxification. *Arch Environ Health*, 1989, Nov-Dec;44(6):345-50.

24. Steinman, D. *Diet for a Poisoned Planet*. New York, NY: Crown Publishing, 1990:300-06.

25. Krop, J. Chemical sensitivity after intoxication at work with solvents: response to sauna therapy. *Journal of Alternative and Complementary Medicine*, 1998;4 (1):77-86.

26. Ahuja, M., V. Comeau, M. Garieri, V. Lurie, C. Pustowka, K. Stauffert, B. Steels, C. Tibelius, S. Tripodi, F. Tutt. Sauna as a method of detoxification in the prevention and treatment of breast cancer. Toronto, ON: *Canadian College of Naturopathic Medicine*, April, 1999.

27. Steinman, D. *Diet for a Poisoned Planet*. New York, NY: Crown Publishing, 1990:304-06.

28. Bhajan, Yogi. *Foods for Health and Healing*. Berkeley/Pomona, CA: Spiritual Community/KRI Publications, 1983:114.

29. Bhajan, Yogi. *Sadhana Guidelines for Kundalini Yoga Daily Practise*. Los Angeles, CA: Kundalini Research Institute, 1996:30.

30. Bhajan, Yogi. *The Kundalini Yoga Manual*. Claremont, CA: KRI Publications, 1976:30-34.

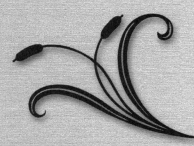

Activating the Lymphatic and Immune Systems

Exercises

Contents

Your immune system is your body's defense system. Its fundamental role is to protect the life of the body by distinguishing 'self' from 'non-self' and recognizing what needs to be destroyed (a cancer cell, virus, bacteria, environmental toxin, internal toxin). The stronger your immune system is, the more resistant to breast cancer you will be. Its function is intimately connected to what you think and feel. (What is truly you and what is not you and what do you need to destroy in your life?) Emotions of faith, hope, joy, and a fighting spirit enhance immune function, while depression, lack of purpose, and repressed anger deplete it. If we define self as the "unique qualities and soul direction of an individual in relationship to the universal energy field," then the immune system is a powerful barometer for how connected we are to our life's meaning and purpose. Though we can have a well-paying job, status in our communities, a busy schedule, and outward success, our immune systems will let us know when we are not living our truth. We may become ill. Illness is the messenger, the catalyst for change.

The lymphatic system is intimately connected with the circulatory and immune systems. It consists of a network of tubes and cleansing stations that move body fluids and debris away from the spaces between cells. The fluid is cleansed by different types of white blood cells housed in lymph nodes (the cleansing stations) and then is returned to the bloodstream to be recycled. (Not so different from our water treatment plants. Ideally the dirty water from our homes goes to a water treatment plant where it is cleansed and then is returned to us as clean water). The job of lymphatic fluid, or lymph, is to carry proteins, foreign particles, bacteria, viruses, and wandering cancer cells away from the fluid that bathes the body's cells. The lymphatic fluid with its debris is drawn into a thin fabric of very small tubules that empty into larger tubes called lymphatic vessels. The health of the lymph system is closely connected to the power of our immune systems in preventing breast cancer.

Low Immunity

There are many factors which negatively affect our immune status. Many of these we can change, some we cannot. Below is a list of factors that lower immunity. Circle the ones that apply to you and make efforts to change those that you can. These categories and examples have been derived in part from Luc De Schepper's book *Peak Immunity*.[1]

Hereditary Factors

Immunity may be lower and thus the risk of cancer higher when there is a family history of one or more of the following diseases:

Hypothyroidism	Rheumatoid Arthritis	Scleroderma
Cancer	Manic-depression	Hashimoto's Disease
Hypoglycemia	Allergies	
Diabetes mellitus	Lupus	

Personality Factors

The immune system may be weaker in those with the following personality traits:

Obsessive about exercise	Dominating	Competitive	Inability to relax
Nervous	Insecure	Impatient	Lives in the past
Easily frustrated	Overly pleasing	Easily angered	Aggressive
Overly analytical	Passive	Non-assertive	

Stress Factors

The following stress factors may tax the immune system:

History of child abuse	Divorce or separation	Jail term	Difficult mortgage
Family conflict	Unwanted pregnancy	Marital conflict	Change in residence
Alcoholic parents	Sexual difficulties	Job loss	Job conflict
Death of a loved one	Personal injury	Empty retirement	

Nutritional Factors

These nutritional patterns result in lowered immunity:

Addiction to sugar or chocolate	Irregular eating habits	Consume coffee regularly
Overconsumption of bread	Eat beef or pork regularly	Lack of whole grains
Overeating white flour products	Consume alcohol regularly	Consume fried foods
Skipping breakfast	Rarely eating fruit	Presence of food allergies
Canned rather than fresh foods	Drink soft drinks regularly	Drug or tobacco addiction

Chemical Factors

These chemical factors around your home lower immunity:

Aluminum pots or pans	Gas stoves	Teflon pots and pans
Ammonia cleansers	Hair sprays	Turpentine, paint fumes
Fluoridated and chlorinated water	Kerosene	Newspaper print
Dyes	Paint lacquer	Nail polish
Pesticides	Tobacco smoke	Formaldehyde
Exposure to insecticides	Recycled air	Underground parking
Ceilings containing asbestos	Exposure to electromagnetic radiation from copy machines	Exposure to X-rays or computers

Health Factors

The following health factors result in lowered immunity:

History of past surgeries	Recurrent infections — more than 6 in a year
Past use of chemotherapy or radiation	Sensitivity to ragweed or leaf mold
History of antibiotic use	Past history of cortisone use
History of use of the birth control pill	Environmental sensitivities

The Lymphatic System and Breast Health

The lymphatic vessels are a one-way transport system that can easily get clogged up when there is an excess of debris and not enough movement through the cleansing stations. (Sort of like a long line-up of cars waiting at a car wash.) This is when you notice that you have a swollen lymph node. There is more debris in the lymph node than the white blood cells can handle at that particular time. The debris is most often linked to a bacterial or viral infection, the presence of toxins, or cancer.

The axillary (underarm) lymph nodes are strategically placed close to our breasts. As long as our breasts and armpits move, we will circulate the lymphatic fluid around them so that effective cleansing can occur.

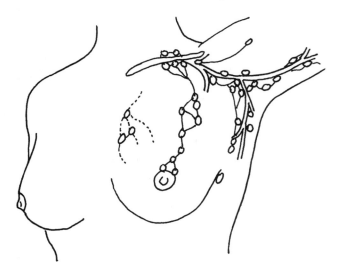

Wearing a bra for long periods of time or wearing a tight bra restricts lymphatic circulation in the breast area and can impair our ability to cleanse the breasts, indirectly promoting breast cancer.

What makes the lymphatic fluid move so that there is not a back up of debris and fluid? Muscular exercise and deep breathing. Lymphatic fluid is pumped by the contraction of skeletal muscle and pressure changes due to the action of breathing. Therefore, regular exercise and deep breathing are essential for great lymphatic circulation. If you do both at the same time plus jump up and down on a rebounder while waving your arms around, you pump that fluid big time. The more efficiently your lymphatic fluid circulates, the less cellular debris you have, the quicker your white blood cells can get to work on bacteria, viruses, and cancer cells in the lymph nodes, and the healthier you and your breasts will be. We want

the white blood cells housed in the lymph nodes to be real warriors — alert, quick, devouring, efficient, co-operative.

The lymphatic system is comprised of the lymph nodes, spleen, tonsils, and thymus gland.

Lymph Nodes

These are small round capsules that contain well-trained armies of white blood cells. The white blood cells include phagocytes which ingest and destroy bacteria, foreign particles, and worn out cells from the lymph, as well as T-Lymphocytes which co-ordinate attacks on viruses and cancer cells and B-Lymphocytes which make antibodies. The lymph nodes act as processing factories for cellular debris, including environmental toxins, toxins produced by the body, bacteria, viruses, dead tissue cells, and cancer cells. The lymph nodes are like islands along the rivers of the lymphatic vessels draining all the major areas of the body. Although they exist throughout the body, lymph

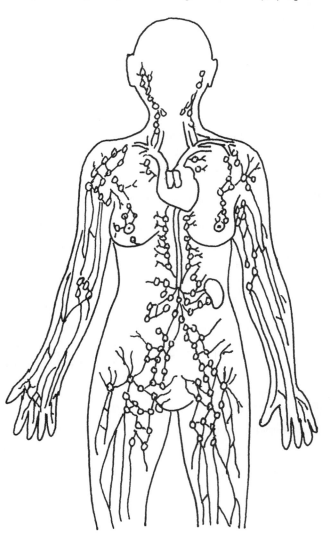

nodes are clustered in a few key spots such as the groin, underarm, and neck where we easily recognize them when they are swollen and overworked.

Spleen

You will find your spleen beneath the diaphragm and behind your stomach, on the left side of your abdomen.

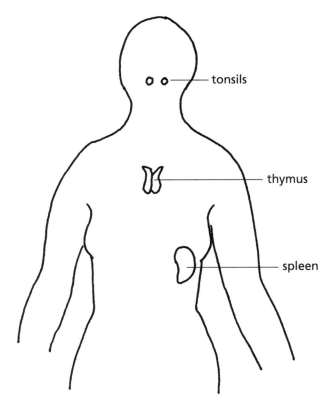

The spleen has two different kinds of tissue in it, known as white pulp and red pulp. The white pulp contains large numbers of white blood cells. The red pulp contains red blood cells, white blood cells, and macrophages. Macrophages engulf and destroy bacteria and foreign particles they find in the blood as it circulates through the spleen. The spleen has the capacity to store a lot of blood, and as it does this, the macrophages can get to work gobbling up what shouldn't be in the blood, defending the body from infection. An initiate in the mysteries of blood, the spleen plays a central role in the formation of blood, the storage of blood, and the filtration of blood.

▶ **Action for Prevention:** You can support the activity of your spleen through lifestyle, diet, and herbs.

1) Like the rest of the lymphatic and immune systems, the function of the spleen and its white blood cells is compromised by stress, and periods of relaxation are essential.

2) In Traditional Chinese Medicine, sugar and excessive sweets are recognized as harming the spleen; therefore, you should limit your sweet intake to occasional use.

3) You can use the herbs burdock root, goldenseal, echinacea, astragalus, and codonopsis to nourish the spleen when necessary. ◀

Tonsils

If you have managed to keep them, your tonsils can be seen on either side in the back of your throat. They are composed of masses of lymphatic tissue, filled with macrophages that protect you from bacteria roaming around in your eustachian tubes, mouth, and throat.

Thymus Gland

Tap the upper part of your sternum, or breast bone. Your thymus gland is under here. Think of the thymus gland as a teaching station where some of the white blood cells (the T-lymphocytes) are educated and taught to cooperate in coordinated attacks against viruses and cancer cells. The warriors that the thymus breeds are there to protect your life — hence they are fueled by your own self-love. If they don't get the message that you are worth it and you have something to live for, they will be less committed to your defense. The thymus gland speaks to your T cells from its central command station, sending a hormone into the blood to activate them when their energy is flagging.

▶ **Action for Prevention:** You can support the work of your thymus gland with nutritional supplements, herbs, and exercises.

1) You can use the antioxidant nutrients alpha lipoic acid, vitamins A, C, E, zinc, selenium, melatonin to protect the thymus from shrinking when you are under stress as well as vitamins B6 and B12.

2) Since the thymus secretes its hormones under parasympathetic stimulation when you are relaxed, you can develop a meditation practice and find ways to take 20-minute relaxation breaks regularly.

3) Bovine thymus extract and homeopathic thymuline 9CH have a modulating and strengthening effect on the gland and can be taken as directed by a naturopath or holistic doctor.

4) The following herbs can be used to improve thymic function: echinacea, licorice, European mistletoe, astragalus, maitake and shitake mushrooms, and reishi.

5) Exercises that involve coordinated arm and leg movements on alternate sides strengthen the thymus — you can swing your arms as you walk and avoid carrying heavy bags on one side, and can march, swim, and do yoga. ◄

Specialized Cells of Your Immune System

Complement System

The complement system is composed of proteins manufactured by the liver and spleen. These orchestrated proteins are able to destroy cancer cells, viruses, bacteria and immune complexes. The complement system is enhanced by herbs containing inulin which include echinacea, burdock root and dandelion root.

White Blood Cells

Macrophage
This cell type is able to engulf and digest debris that enters the bloodstream. When it encounters a foreign organism, it summons helper T-cells to the scene.

Helper T-cell
This cell type identifies the foreign substance or 'enemy' and rushes to the spleen and lymph nodes where it stimulates the production of other cells to fight the infection.

Killer T-cell
This cell type is recruited and activated by the helper T-cell and specializes in killing cells of the body that have been invaded by foreign organisms, as well as cancer cells.

B Cell
These cells are housed in the spleen or the lymph nodes and are activated to replicate by the helper T cell. They produce potent chemical weapons called antibodies that are protein molecules. The B cell rushes to the infection site with its antibodies and either neutralizes the enemy or marks it for attack by other cells or chemicals.

Suppressor T-Cell
This T cell is able to slow down or stop the activity of B cells and other T cells, playing an important role in calling off the attack once an infection has been conquered.

Memory Cell
This type of cell is generated during an initial infection and may circulate in the blood or lymph for years, allowing the body to respond more quickly to future infections.

Drawing the Components of Your Immune System Exercise

Use a large paper and drawing materials and draw a picture of your body. Inside of it draw the components of your immune system as vividly and actively as you are able to. Include in your drawing the thymus gland, spleen, lymph nodes (cervical, underarm, groin), liver, bone marrow, and draw the macrophages in the intestines, liver, spleen, lungs, lymph nodes, nervous system, and bone marrow. If you are taking any supplements to stimulate immunity or improve lymphatic circulation, draw them in as well, choosing symbols to represent them. If you are in a group, talk about the drawings once they are finished

Techniques that Assist Lymphatic Circulation

Good lymphatic circulation is an essential component of breast health and a way to speed up the inactivation of viruses, bacteria, toxins, and cancer cells. Five practices that will improve your lymphatic circulation are dry brush massage, contrast showers, rebounding, exercise, and going braless.

Dry Brush Massage

This simple technique is inexpensive and easy to do. Dry brush massage stimulates the lymphatic system to expel toxins through the skin. About one third of all body impurities are eliminated through the skin. This equals more than one pound of waste disposal every day. Dry brush massage helps to remove debris in the pores of the skin and dead skin cells. If skin pores remained clogged, the body removes its waste less efficiently and the burden is increased on other detoxifying organs. The body 'breathes' through the skin as well as the lungs, with oxygen being absorbed through its pores and carbon dioxide released. By dry brushing, dead layers of skin are removed and pores go unclogged. Blood circulation is increased to the internal organs as well as the skin, which promotes oxygenation and healing. The detoxification qualities of the skin remain intact and well functioning. Hormone and oil-producing glands are stimulated. Nerve endings stimulated in the skin help to maintain the health of the entire nervous system. The body's natural defenses against the common cold are assisted, especially when used with the hot-cold shower technique. Muscle tone is assisted and fat deposits are more evenly spread.

▶ **Action for Prevention:**

1) Buy a long handled, natural bristle brush, with a brush pad about the size of your own hand. If you can't find a natural bristle brush, you can substitute a natural plant fiber vegetable brush, a bath glove made of twisted hog's hair, or a loofah mitt

2) Start with the soles of your feet. Brush in a circular motion as you move up your body, feet to legs, hands to arms, back to abdomen, and chest to neck. The face and inner thighs are sensitive areas and can be avoided. Brush with as much pressure as is comfortably possible until your skin feels pleasantly warm (this is usually about five to 10 minutes). The massage is best performed when you rise in the morning and before you go to bed at night.

3) You can increase the cleansing qualities of a dry brush massage if you follow it with an alternating hot-cold shower (hot for three minutes, cold for 30 seconds), repeating the hot-cold pattern three times.

4) Make sure that you wash your brush every two weeks with soap and water to remove the debris that may have moved from your skin to your brush, and then dry it in a warm place. Use a separate brush for each family member. The scalp is not ignored, as increased blood flow to it will help keep your hair healthy and growing. Irritated portions of your skin are avoided so as not to damage them. Increased blood flow to the surrounding areas will assist in its healing. ◀

Hydrotherapy and Contrast Showers

Hydrotherapy involves the use of water applications in healing. Alternating hot and cold showers improve blood circulation, increase cellular oxidation, enhance immunity, strengthen the nervous system, and flush cellular toxins into the blood.

When we shower in hot water for less than five minutes, it has a stimulating effect on our circulation. Similarly, when we have a cold shower for less than one minute, we stimulate blood flow and metabolism. Cold applications first constrict and then later dilate blood vessels. By finishing with a short cold shower, we cause the following physiological effects: increased oxygen absorption; increased carbon dioxide excretion; increased nitrogen absorption and excretion; increased tissue tone; increased white blood cell count and thus improved immunity; increased red blood cell count; decreased blood glucose; heightened metabolism.

One of the factors that promotes tumor growth is poor microcirculation in the area where the tumor develops. Contrast showers are excellent ways to improve the micro-circulation, bringing nutrients to the cells and removing waste more efficiently. The supplements you take will nourish your body better if you use contrast showers. To some degree, healing is proportional to improved blood flow.

To use the principles of hydrotherapy, stand in the shower (after dry brush massage) and shower following this sequence: 1–3 minutes hot, 30 seconds cold. Repeat 3 times. As you shower, tap the sternum with your fingertips for a minute to stimulate the thymus gland. Lovingly touch your breasts with your hands, giving them a gentle massage. Rub your whole body briskly as you shower. Always finish with cold. Rub yourself down with a towel when you finish.

▶ **Action for Prevention:** Have a contrasting shower at least once daily, preferably in the morning as you begin your day. If you are recovering from any illness, consider having an additional one before bed. ◀

Exercise

It is primarily muscular movement that causes the lymphatic fluid to flow efficiently to the cleansing stations known as the lymph nodes. In the lymph nodes the white blood cells work away at keeping your body free of bacteria, viruses, toxins, and cancer cells. It is movement of the arms, armpits, and chest that assists lymphatic cleansing of the breasts. Exercises such as skipping, tennis, racquetball, swimming (in non-chlorinated water), rowing, window washing, drumming, jumping jacks, wood chopping, marching, and walking while swinging your arms are extremely beneficial on a daily basis. Women who exercise at least four hours a week in their leisure time and are active in their jobs have a lower risk of breast cancer. Regular exercise enhances the metabolism of estrogen.

One form of such exercise is rebounding. A rebounder is the equivalent of a small trampoline. Jumping on a rebounder greatly improves the circulation of lymphatic fluid within the body as muscular contractions push the fluid through the lymphatic vessels. When the muscular contraction is used in combination with deep breathing, lymphatic circulation is enhanced even more. This improves the body's cancer-fighting ability. Some of the additional benefits of rebounding include gentle massage of the internal organs, including the liver and colon;

increased oxygenation on a cellular level; improved muscle tone; improved digestion, elimination, and body detoxification; easier weight management through calorie expenditure; increased energy; improvement in cardiovascular health; stress reduction and release; and an increase in strength, stamina, balance, and agility.

Rebounding for 10 minutes has the aerobic effect equivalent to playing tennis for 40 minutes or jogging for 30 minutes. The lungs increase their efficiency and process more air, increasing the oxygen uptake of the blood. The heart muscle grows stronger and pumps more blood with each stroke, reducing the number of heartbeats necessary per minute. This allows the heart to last longer simply because it works less. The aerobic effect of rebounding also increases the size and number of blood vessels in the body. There is a greater total blood volume and increased ability to bring oxygen to all body cells. Cancer cells do not thrive in a well-oxygenated environment.

Any tendency to constipation is usually relieved by rebounding regularly because this exercise improves the peristaltic action of the intestines. Simply by improving bowel movements, we can lessen our risk of breast cancer by eliminating more toxins and estrogen from the colon. If you have any weakness in your bladder you may want to wear a small menstrual pad while rebounding to catch any urine that is released while jumping.

Rebounding Exercise

Place an image on the wall that you face while rebounding that will act as a centering device for you. Gaze at it as you rebound. It can be a mandala, a family photograph, a symbol of something that represents all you have to live for, or a picture that symbolizes health or brings tranquillity, such as a nature scene. Choose it carefully for it will help to activate your immune system as you exercise.

Each of the exercises below can be done anywhere from 30 seconds to 3 minutes, making your rebounding workout approximately 7 minutes to 45 minutes long. Do what you are able to depending upon your age, fitness level, and endurance. Start with a shorter time and slowly increase it. It is best to rebound once or twice daily.

1) Jump straight up and down and circle the arms in a backward direction as though swimming the backstroke. Complete one backward circle of the arms for every two jumps. Then speed it up so that you complete one arm rotation per jump. Move the armpits as you jump. Then reverse the movement, rotating the arms simultaneously to the front. Imagine that you are releasing any grief, anger or unresolved emotion from the past as you move the arms backwards. Imagine that you are moving to the future that is calling you as you roll the arms forwards.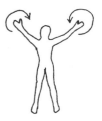

2) Jump straight up and down and alternate rotating the left arm and then the right arm to the back, as though doing the back crawl in swimming. As you do it, imagine that you are unwinding and releasing the past. Then reverse the movement, rotating the arms to the front as though doing the front crawl. Imagine that you are progressing towards your ideal future securely with each movement. You can make the journey towards your goals and ideals.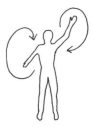

3) On the first jump clap the hands out in front of the body. On the next jump clap the hands behind the body. Continue alternating clapping in front and back. Clap for the life you have lived and the life you have yet to live.

4) Inhale as you raise the left knee up and lift the left arm above your head. Exhale on the next jump and raise your right knee up as you raise the right arm above your head. Lift the knees high. If this is too strenuous for you then include an extra jump between the raising of the knee and arm. If the breathing is difficult, coordinate the movements with a long deep breath.

5) Inhale as you raise the left knee up and the right arm high above your head. Exhale and jump with both feet on the rebounder and the arms at your sides. Then inhale as you raise the right knee up high and lift the left arm above your head. Exhale as you bring both feet down with the arms at your sides. Continue this pattern.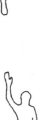

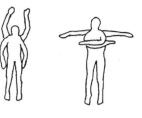

6) Jump up and down and circle the hands in front of the breasts with the palms facing forward. The left palm rotates counter-clockwise while the right palm rotates in a clockwise direction. Touch the tips of the thumbs as both hands come towards the center. As you do it imagine that you are washing any toxins or cancer cells out of your breasts and direct positive energy towards them.

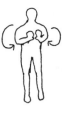

7) Jump straight up and down and alternate swinging both arms in front of the body to the left. On the next jump, swing them to the right. Inhale as you swing to the left, exhale to the right. Continue one minute. Then as you swing your arms to the left twist your hips to the right so your feet land pointing to the right. On the next jump swing your arms in front of the body to the right as you twist your hips to the left and land with both feet pointing to the left. Continue alternating the twist, coordinating it with the breath.

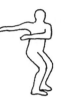

8) Jump up and down and swing the left arm out to the left side at shoulder height as you tap the sternum firmly between the breasts with the fingertips of your right hand. On the next jump swing the right arm out to the right side at shoulder height and tap the sternum firmly between the breasts with the fingertips of your left hand. Alternate swinging one arm out to the side while the other hand taps the area of the thymus gland between the breasts. Imagine that you are programming your thymus gland for super immunity.

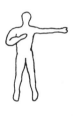

9) Jumping jacks. Inhale as you clap the hands above the head and spread the feet apart on the rebounder, exhale as you bring the arms down to the sides and bring the feet together. Continue this pattern. Do 26 jumping jacks or continue for 30 seconds to 3 minutes.

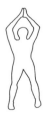

10) On the first jump swing the arms out to the sides at shoulder height and stretch the feet apart. On the next jump cross the arms straight out in front of the heart, pointing them in front of the body while the feet cross one in front of the other.

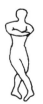

Alternate which foot or arm is in front with each movement. Continue crisscrossing the arms and legs with each jump.

11) As you jump, inhale and throw both arms up and behind your shoulders, exhale as they come down to your sides. Then inhale as you criss-cross them in front of your chest, exhale as they swing out to the sides. Continue this pattern alternating the criss-crosses each time. Coordinate the movement of the arms with jumping. Breathe powerfully in and out through your nose as you jump. Imagine that you are breathing in healing energy and embracing yourself as the arms cross in front, and releasing any toxins (physical or emotional) as you throw your arms behind your shoulders.

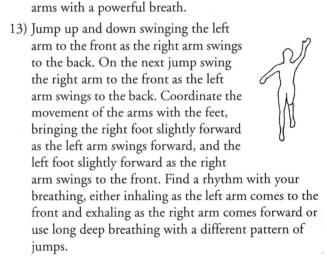

12) Inhale the left hand forward from the shoulder and open your fingers as you stretch the arm to the front; bend your elbow and pull the arm back as you close the hand into a fist. The fist should touch the side of your chest and the elbow is bent behind you. Then exhale as you stretch the left arm forward from the shoulder, opening the fingers as though you are reaching to grab your future and your health (or whatever it is that you most want in your life); then pull the elbow back and make your hand into a fist. Continue alternating the movement of the arms with a powerful breath.

13) Jump up and down swinging the left arm to the front as the right arm swings to the back. On the next jump swing the right arm to the front as the left arm swings to the back. Coordinate the movement of the arms with the feet, bringing the right foot slightly forward as the left arm swings forward, and the left foot slightly forward as the right arm swings to the front. Find a rhythm with your breathing, either inhaling as the left arm comes to the front and exhaling as the right arm comes forward or use long deep breathing with a different pattern of jumps.

14) As you jump on the right foot, raise the left leg out to the side and lift both arms out to the sides at shoulder height. On the next jump, have your arms at your sides and jump with both feet. On the third jump, raise the right leg out to the side as you jump on the left foot while simultaneously lifting both arms out to the sides at shoulder height. On the fourth jump, have your arms by your sides as you land on both feet. Continue this four-part sequence.

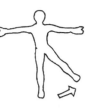

▶ **Action for Prevention:** Rebound 5–30 minutes once or twice daily while listening to your favorite music. ◀

Going Braless

Many types of bra restrict the movement of the breasts and impede lymphatic circulation. In their book *Dressed to Kill*, Singer and Grismaijer found that women who develop breast cancer usually wear their bras more than 12 hours per day and may wear them to bed. They found a 21-fold greater chance of developing breast cancer in women who wear their bras more than 12 hours daily and a 113-fold increase in breast cancer incidence among women who wore their bras all the time. On the other hand, women who wore their bras less than 12 hours daily had a 19-fold protection from breast cancer compared with the general population of women. They judged that red marks on the skin from a tight-fitting bra might indicate restricted lymphatic circulation. Breast cancer incidence is much lower in cultures where women go braless.[2] Although wearing a bra probably does not cause breast cancer, it may undermine the efforts of our lymphatic system to cleanse environmental toxins and cancer cells out of the breast area. If you have large breasts and need to wear a bra, take it off when you get home and make sure it isn't too tight.

▶ **Action for Prevention:** Choose a bra that is cotton, has no underwires, allows the breasts to move a little, and wear it less than 12 hours daily, or go braless. Don't wear your bra to bed. ◀

The Lymph Flush

This program came to me from a breast cancer survivor. It has been used by practitioners and cancer patients for many years to flush the lymphatic system and works well for lymphedema. The cleanse lasts for three days.

You will need to juice 6 lemons, 6 grapefruits, and 12 oranges each day. Pour the juice in a glass gallon container and fill the remainder of the container with pure water. On the first day of the flush, take 1 tbsp of epsom salts in ½ glass of water. Repeat this two more times at ½ hour intervals for a total of three repetitions. After the third glass of epsom salts and water, begin to drink the juice. Eat no other food for the three days, excepting an orange if you are hungry. On the fourth day, begin to eat lightly – vegetable broth soups, fruit, salads. Eat normally after that.

▶ **Action for Prevention:** Use the lymph flush when you feel sensitivity or swelling in your lymph nodes or with lymphedema. ◀

Kundalini Yoga Exercise for the Lymphatic System and Healthy Breasts

This set of five exercises can be practiced daily (or at least four times weekly) to improve the lymphatic circulation to the breast area. As you do them, visualize your lymphatic and immune systems powerfully cleansing and protecting your breasts.

1) Sit in a chair or cross-legged and extend the arms out parallel to the ground with the elbows straight. Make the hands into fists with the middle finger extended. Begin circling the arms backwards. The movement should be tight and powerful. Continue for 3 minutes and then increase the speed for 1 more minute.

2) Sit cross-legged and join the hands in Venus lock (interlaced) behind the head. Like a grinding wheel, roll the total spine around on the hips in a counter-clockwise rotation by working the abdomen. Roll down to the bottom and around in a deep circular movement. Continue for 3 minutes.

3) Sit cross-legged and place your thumbs on the pads at the base of your little fingers. Extend your arms out parallel to the ground with the palms facing down. Alternately begin to raise one arm up to 60 degrees while the other arm goes down 60 degrees. Continue the motion quickly

and powerfully for 3 minutes. Inhale as the left arm comes up; exhale as the right arm comes up.

4) Still in a cross-legged position sit with the arms parallel to the ground. Curl your fingers into fists, with the thumbs pointing up. Twist from side to side. Inhale as you twist to the left, exhale as you twist to the right. Continue for 1–2 minutes.

5) Sit on your heels. Make the hands into fists with the thumbs inside. Powerfully pull one arm back while the other extends forward. As each arm is extended its full length, the fingers open up as if they were grab-

bing something. They close quickly and then pull very powerfully toward the body. Inhale as each arm comes forward; exhale as you pull it back. Imagine you are pulling your future to you. Reach and grab it. Breathe powerfully in and out through your nose.

This is a composite group of exercises I have chosen specifically for breast health, taken from the teachings of Yogi Bhajan.

Western Herbs for Improving Lymphatic and Immune Function

Another way to improve lymphatic function and activate immunity is through the use of herbs. The following Western herbs have been used singly or in formulas for lymphatic circulation and cleansing, and for breast health. Ayurvedic and Chinese herbs and herbal formulas have similar applications. Calcium, iodine, and magnesium are additional minerals that help to resolve lymphatic congestion. They are found in high amounts in almonds and sea vegetables such as kelp, arame, hijiki, and dulse.

Burdock Root (Arctium lappa)

Burdock has a special affinity for the kidneys, bladder, and liver. It promotes detoxification, clears dampness, dissolves deposits and removes lymphatic congestion. It can help with breaking down tumors, including malignant breast tumors, and will help to prevent breast cancer. Burdock is able to clear internal heat and toxins, reducing infection, inflammation, and swelling. It is commonly used in chronic skin conditions. Burdock acts as a digestive tonic and promotes bile flow. The fresh root helps to remove heavy metals and chemicals and encourages the growth of beneficial intestinal bacteria. It is a tonic to the

immune system and is found in the Essiac formula developed by Rene Caisse, as well as the Hoxsey formula. It works well in combination with red clover and dandelion. Like dandelion, burdock is readily available, and its roots can be dug up in the fall.

DOSAGE: 25–100 drops tincture, 3× daily. It can be used for months or even years at a time.

CONTRAINDICATIONS: Do not use in pregnancy as it is a uterine stimulant. Begin with a low dosage otherwise, building up to a higher one if needed.

Marigold Flower (Calendula officinalis)

Marigold is a specific healer for the liver, heart, uterus, skin, veins, lymphatic, system, and blood. Like burdock, it clears heat and toxins, reduces infection and inflammation, relieves swelling and removes lymphatic congestion. Marigold helps in the treatment of bacterial, fungal, viral, and amoebic infections.

It has been used to reduce tumors, cysts, and cancer of the reproductive organs, breasts, and intestines. Marigold stimulates digestion and reduces liver congestion. Many practitioners recommend it before and after surgery because of its ability to promote tissue repair, decrease scarring and act as an antiseptic to the skin.

DOSAGE: 50–100 drops tincture, 3× daily.

CONTRAINDICATIONS: Do not use in pregnancy as it is a uterine stimulant.

Goldenseal Root (Hydrastis canadensis)

Goldenseal's action extends to the stomach, intestines, lung, heart, reproductive organs, bladder, kidneys, liver, and gallbladder. It acts to clear heat, dry up excess mucous, reduce infection and inflammation, and stop discharge while soothing mucous membranes. It is used in treating cirrhosis of the liver and gallstones. Goldenseal is one of the best herbal antibiotics, being effective against a wide array of bacteria, yeast, fungi, amoeba, and parasites while seemingly sparing normal intestinal flora. Like barberry, it is a very useful herb in treating chronic candidiasis. Goldenseal helps to shrink tumors of the reproductive organs, breasts, and stomach and will assist in decreasing breast pain and swelling.

As a digestive tonic it stimulates hydrochloric acid production, relieving appetite loss and fatigue. As an immune tonic, goldenseal improves the ability of macrophages to engulf and digest foreign particles and bacteria. It increases the blood supply to the spleen, enhancing the function of the white blood cells in defending us against bacteria, viruses, toxins, and cancer.

Because of its action on the spleen, it is a useful herb in treating mononucleosis and chronic Epstein Barr infections. Goldenseal will often help to lower a fever because of its action on the immune system. As it is a strong acting herb, usually only small doses are needed.

DOSAGE: 7–40 drops tincture, 3× daily.

In a powdered solid extract with a 10 per cent berberine content, the dose is 250–500 mg, 3× daily.

If using goldenseal on its own or in combination with echinacea, use it for three weeks at a time, followed by a week-long break. It has a slight cumulative toxicity. If you are using it in a formula with several other herbs, it can be taken for several months at a time.

CONTRAINDICATIONS: Do not use in pregnancy, as it is a uterine stimulant. Do not use in persons with high blood pressure, as it will elevate it. If you experience nausea while taking goldenseal, reduce the dosage.

Echinacea Root (Echinacea augustifolia)

Echinacea has an affinity for the blood, lymph, skin, stomach, and urogenital organs. It is able to clear heat and toxins, reducing infection, fever, and inflammation. Echinacea helps to remove lymphatic congestion and reduce tumors, and has been used in anti-cancer formulas for many generations. As an immune stimulant, it raises the white blood cell count when taken in large doses, improves macrophage activity, and increases interferon. Interferon is a substance produced by cells that inhibits the replication of viruses. It can be used for short periods of time to deal with acute infections, or for up to three months as a detoxifying, cancer inhibiting herb.

DOSAGE: 25–50 drops tincture, 3× daily.

CONTRAINDICATIONS: In sensitive people it can sometimes cause dizziness, nausea, throat irritation, joint pain, and canker sores.

Walnut Leaf and Hull (Juglans regia)

Walnut leaf is a detoxifying herb that clears excess mucous and heat, reduces lymphatic congestion, and can reduce tumors. It helps to promote bowel movements and eliminate parasites, particularly tapeworm and roundworm. Walnut leaf acts to tonify the blood, is able to relieve weakness and fatigue, and strengthens the bones, tendons, skin, and hair.

DOSAGE: 25–50 drops tincture, 3× daily.

CONTRAINDICATIONS: Do not use if you have tinnitus, or ringing in your ears.

European Mistletoe (Viscum album)

European mistletoe has an affinity for the heart, uterus, kidneys, lungs, stomach, intestines, blood, and the nervous and muscular systems. As a heart tonic it is used for angina and hypertension. It promotes urination and detoxification, dissolves deposits, stimulates immunity, and reduces tumors (benign and malignant). It is a traditional remedy for all stages of cancer. In Germany in 1995, mistletoe was the most commonly prescribed biological medicine for cancer and was used in 80% of patients.[3] To be effective, mistletoe preparations should be made from the fresh green or freshly-dried plant.

Mistletoe is a mild herb and can be used for years. Do not use American mistletoe. It is a different plant and can be toxic. Mistletoe contains proteins called lectins, similar to proteins found in medicinal mushrooms, which exhibit anti-tumor action.[4] A 1990 study found that mistletoe lectins I, II, and III increased the production of tumor necrosis factor-alpha, a substance secreted by immune system cells that targets cancer cells. This lectin also increased the production of two other immune components, interleukin-1 and interleukin-6.[5] Mistletoe contains arginine, an amino acid that inhibits tumor growth and increases the activity of T Killer cells.

Iscador is a fermented preparation of the European mistletoe and comes from the Anthroposophical movement linked to Rudolph Steiner. In 1916 Steiner first suggested mistletoe for the treatment of cancer based on the unusual qualities of the plant. It is a bushy plant that grows on trees, particularly oak, with no real roots of its own, drawing off the water and mineral salts that it needs. It grows in any direction, sideways, upwards, or downwards, and is self-willed, seemingly unaffected by the earth or the sun.[6] These are qualities not unlike the nature of cancer.

Iscador is marketed by Weleda AG and is a combination of fermented mistletoe and homeopathic dosages of silver, copper, and mercury. It is widely used in Europe for the treatment of cancer and is claimed to strengthen immune function. When injected into rabbits, it caused an increase in natural killer cell activity, increased numbers of other white blood cells, and improved the scavenging ability of macrophages.[7] Iscador caused a 78% increase in the weight of the thymus gland in rats when they were injected with it daily for six days. It caused the thymus cells to be 29 times more responsive to a stimulant. In women with breast cancer, it caused a significant enhancement in the scavenger activity of white blood cells.

Iscador is generally used for 10–14 days prior to surgery to prevent metastatic spread of the cancer from the surgical procedure. It is used after surgery or radiation for several years to reduce the risk of recurrence. Some of its noted effects are reduction of pain, relief of tiredness and depression, improved sleep and appetite, weight gain, and an increase in red blood cell levels. Generally, it is injected at or near the tumor site, and typically a course of treatment would include 14 injections given in increasing concentration.[8] The herb can also be taken in tincture form.

DOSAGE: 25–75 drops tincture, 3× daily.

CONTRAINDICATIONS: Do not use in pregnancy, as it is a uterine stimulant. In high doses it can act as a sedative or irritate the gastrointestinal tract. If this occurs, decrease the dosage.

Poke Root (Phytolacca decandra)

Poke root acts upon the digestive, lymphatic, and musculoskeletal systems. It promotes detoxification, clears dampness and heat, reduces lymphatic congestion, and can shrink tumors. Poke root can reduce liver congestion and relieve constipation. It has a particular affinity for the breasts and reduces fibrocystic breast disease and breast swelling. It is excellent in homeopathic dosage for mastitis. Poke root is also an immune stimulant and is found in the Hoxsey formula. Eclectic physicians in the 1850s included poke root routinely in formulas for breast disease.

DOSAGE: 1 drop of tincture daily for 6 weeks; or 3 pellets of a 6X homeopathic potency once daily for 6 weeks; or 3–25 drops on its own or in combination with other herbs (such as are in the Hoxsey formula) for several weeks. Then break for a week. It is toxic in high doses and has a cumulative toxicity even in small doses.

CONTRAINDICATIONS: Do not use in pregnancy as it can cause fetal abnormalities.

Red Clover (Trifolium pratense)

Red clover is a specific healer for the skin, lungs, nerves, and bladder. It promotes detoxification and urination, clears dampness, and shrinks tumors, particularly of the breasts, skin, and ovaries. It is used for chronic bladder infections and for drying up vaginal discharge. It is commonly included in formulas for clearing the skin of acne and eczema. Red clover can help us detoxify from heavy metal poisoning. Containing significant amounts of phytoestrogens, red clover is a wonderful herb to include

in a breast cancer prevention formula. It is part of the Hoxsey formula and is included in FlorEssence, a variation of the Essiac formula made by Flora. It has a long history of use and outstanding reputation as an anticancer herb. Hundreds of cases of cancer remission have been documented after regular use of red clover.[9] Red clover must be taken for months to achieve its deep cleansing and tumor-reducing effects. The fresh flower tops can be added to juices or steeped to make tea.

DOSAGE: 20–100 drops tincture, 3× daily or several cups as a tea daily. Steep flower heads for 15 min.

CONTRAINDICATIONS: None.

Cleavers Herb (Galium aparine)

Cleavers has an affinity for the liver, bladder, prostate, blood, lymphatic system, and skin. It is a detoxifying herb that can relieve breast swelling, help to break down benign and malignant tumors, and remove lymphatic congestion. It also acts as a blood thinner and can dissolve clots. This blood thinning action makes it contraindicated before or after surgery, and it may increase menstrual flow. Cleavers relieves liver congestion. It is a cooling, refreshing herb and can be used to lower a fever. This is a very safe herb when indicated, and best results are gained from long term use. The herb is always used fresh and is never boiled.

DOSAGE: 2 tsp of juice, 3× daily; or 40–100 drops tincture, 3× daily.

CONTRAINDICATIONS: Do not use while you have excessive menstrual bleeding or for three days before or after surgery.

Wild Indigo Root (Baptisia tinctoriae)

I have been preoccupied with this herb since I found out that it had a very high content of genistein, the phytoestrogen also found in soy (see phytoestrogen chart in diet section). It was in a related species, *Baptisia australis*, that this was measured, but the genistein content is likely to be similar in this North American herb. Though not commonly recognized as a lymphatic herb, Baptisia does relieve lymphatic congestion and has been used for lymphedema and breast infections (mastitis). It clears heat and toxins, reduces infection, fever and inflammation, and helps to stop discharge. It moves the blood in the liver, which when stagnant can lead to breast cysts. Baptisia is a digestive tonic and stimulates bile flow, helping to pull toxins from the liver. It is a herb used for constipation and improving elimination. Wild indigo also promotes tissue repair, helping to stop decay, heal sores and ulcers, and has a history of use in malignant tumors of the breast. It is also an immune tonic, increasing white blood cell count and activity.[10] In short, Baptisia seems to address all the areas necessary to prevent and treat breast cancer. It is a strongly acting herb, so generally only lower doses are necessary. I would like to see more exploration of this herb in breast cancer prevention and treatment.

DOSAGE: 2–25 drops, 3× daily.

CONTRAINDICATIONS: It is toxic in high doses, so stay within the recommended amount. Discontinue if you experience vomiting, diarrhea or respiratory difficulties. Do not use if you have chronic loose stools.

Bloodroot (Sanguinaria canadensis)

Another herb which contains phytoestrogens, bloodroot has been shown to inhibit the proliferation of both estrogen receptor positive and estrogen receptor negative breast cancer cell lines in vitro as did mistletoe, mandrake, and juniper.[11] Historically, bloodroot has been used successfully in external salves to reduce and remove breast cancer tumors.[12] For more information on this technique, consult Ingrid Naiman's remarkable book, *Cancer Salves: A Botanical Approach to Treatment*. Internally in small doses, bloodroot stimulates digestion and improves circulation, while in large doses it can cause nausea and vomiting and acts as a sedative. Small doses improve liver and glandular function. In the past, bloodroot was often added to formulas to benefit the lungs – it is effective in treating acute and chronic bronchitis, pneumonia, asthma, croup, and laryngitis. Two of the active constituents in bloodroot that inhibit cancer cells are berberine (which is also contained in goldenseal) and sanguinarine. Bloodroot should be used cautiously. It is a potentially toxic herb and very large doses can cause death.

DOSAGE: 2–10 drops, 3× daily.

CONTRAINDICATIONS: Work with a naturopath or herbalist when using this herb; do not use in pregnancy or when breast-feeding.

Pau D'arco or Taheebo

The inner bark of this South American tree contains a plant chemical called lapachol, which has shown anticancer properties. It has demonstrated activity against solid tumors, leukemias, and several cancers, including breast cancer. Pau d'arco is commonly used to treat candidiasis, a systemic fungal infection which lowers immunity, and is effective against bacterial, fungal, viral, and parasitic infections. Taheebo detoxifies the body, particularly through its action on the kidneys and bladder. It is a very useful herb for chronic cystitis, or bladder infections. It can also be helpful in lessening arthritic symptoms. It builds the blood and promotes tissue repair, helping to heal skin ulcers, eczema, and psoriasis. Pau d'arco is very safe, easy to make as a tea, and readily available.

DOSAGE: 50–100 drops tincture, 3× daily; or 6–18 g in tea form 3× daily.

CONTRAINDICATIONS: None.

Carnivora (Venus-flytrap)

Carnivora is an extract of the entire Venus-flytrap (*Dionaea muscipula*) in a highly purified form. It has been used for many chronic diseases, including cancer and AIDS. In cancer it works to break down tumors by blocking the protein kinase enzymes in the cancer cell which are needed to make protein. Without protein, cancer cells die. Dr Helmut G. Keller, MD, of Germany discovered the plant and has been using it regularly with his patients. His product in capsule form is called Carnivora and is available from Carnivora Research Inc.(Santa Rosa, CA, fax.707-568-7468). www.carnivora.com).

DOSAGE: 1 capsule 3× daily, before meals.

Green Tea

Though not a Western herb, I include green tea in this section because it is readily available. Green tea contains polyphenols and epigallocatechin-3-gallate, which have been found to regulate cancer cell replication and induce programmed cell death (apoptosis). Green tea protects against all stages of cancer — initiation, promotion, and progression.[13] It has particular benefit in preventing rectal, colon, and stomach cancers, even when consumed only once weekly. Part of its protection lies in its ability to suppress new blood vessel growth to tumors.[14] Green and black tea are harvested from the same plant, *Camellia sinensis*, but their difference lies in the processing of the leaves. Green tea does contain caffeine, although less than coffee. Because caffeine can increase fibrocystic breast disease, use decaffeinated green tea. Be sure your green tea is organic.

DOSAGE: Two cups daily.

CONTRAINDICATIONS: Do not use in pregnancy if it contains caffeine. Use infrequently if you have fibrocystic breasts unless it is decaffeinated.

Western Herbal Formulas for Breast Health

The Hoxsey Formula

The Hoxsey formula was popularized by Harry Hoxsey, who operated a cancer clinic in Illinois and Texas. The story goes that Harry's grandfather raised horses in Kentucky in 1840, and one of his horses developed cancer. The horse grazed on specific plants in the corner of the pasture and was cured. His owner picked the plants that healed the horse and made them into a medicine that he used with other horses. He passed the recipe down to his son, John Hoxsey, who was a veterinarian. John began using it on neighbors with cancer with some success. He passed on the formula for this and other remedies to his 18-year-old son, Harry, before he died. Harry began treating people with cancer, opened a clinic or two, and wrote a book called You Don't Have to Die (1956). He claimed to cure internal cancers 25% of the time and maintained a 50–60% cure with breast cancer. He endured many court battles.

"It follows that if the constitution of body fluids can be normalized," Hoxsey argued, "and the original chemical balance in the body restored, the environment again will become unfavorable for the survival and reproduction of these cells, they will cease to multiply and eventually they will die. Then if the vital organs have not been too severely damaged by the malignancy (or surgery or radiation), the entire organism will recover normal health. … Cancer cannot be cured successfully as an isolated phenomena, unrelated to basic body processes. We attempt to get at the roots of the disorder, rather than deal merely with its end result."[15]

Here is his original formula.

16 oz Hoxsey Formula:

150 mg	KI (potassium iodine)
20 mg	Chinese licorice
20 mg	red clover
10 mg	burdock root
20 mg	stillingia root
10 mg	berberis root (berberis vulgaris or berberis aquifolium)
5 mg	cascara amarga or cascara sagrada
5 mg	prickly ash bark
20 mg	buckthorn bark
10 mg	poke root (phytolacca)

At different times in the history of the Hoxsey Formula cascara amarga became difficult to obtain and cascara sagrada was used in its place. Prickly ash bark and buckthorn bark were dropped from the formula.

Hoxsey's formula acts to assist digestion (berberis, burdock, prickly ash); detoxify the liver and kidneys (red clover, berberis, burdock); inhibit estradiol from binding to estrogen receptors on breast cells (licorice, red clover); improve elimination (cascara, berberis, buckthorn bark); act as an antiparasitic (berberis); encourage the growth of bifidobacterium in the large intestine and act as a deterrent to bacteria that may cause estrogen to be reabsorbed (burdock, berberis); cleanse the lymphatic system (burdock, red clover, poke root, stillingia); reduce tumors (burdock, red clover, poke, stillingia); normalize the thyroid (potassium iodide); and contains the two minerals that Dr Gerson also believed were invaluable in cancer treatment, potassium and iodide.

A variation of this formula is used today at the Bio-Medical Center in Tijuana, Mexico, run by Mildred Nelson, who has been there treating cancer patients since 1963. The current formula does not contain prickly ash or buckthorn and cascara sagrada is used instead of cascara amarga. Currently at the Bio-Medical Center the Hoxsey formula is administered in the following way: the diluted tonic is taken in ⅓ glass water, grape juice, milk, or herb tea, initially at 1 tsp, 4× daily. It is taken in this way for at least 5 years and then every spring and fall after that for 3–4 months. Some people are recommended to take larger amounts, depending on their condition.[16]

I have used the Hoxsey formula numerous times with women who have breast swelling, fibrocystic breast disease, lymph node swelling, and mastitis and am rarely disappointed in its effectiveness. It is one of the remedies I most often prescribe for women with breast cancer.

DOSAGE: 25–100 drops (¼–1 tsp) tincture after meals and at bedtime, mixed with ⅓ cup water. (Be prepared for its awful taste). Take the lesser amount as prevention and the higher amount if you are recovering from breast cancer. Tinctures are always more effective than capsules or tablets. This is available in tincture form from St. Francis Herbs as Red Clover Combination and by Gaia and HerbPharm as Red Clover Supreme or Hoxsey Formula.

CONTRAINDICATIONS: Do not take while pregnant or breast-feeding. Do not use if you have a hyperactive thyroid or experience disturbing symptoms with use. It can be toxic in high doses so use should be supervised by an herbalist or naturopathic doctor.

▶ **Action for Prevention:** As part of a breast cancer prevention program, consider taking the Hoxsey formula for three months once or twice a year, the frequency and dosage being dependent upon your risk factors. Take it continuously with short breaks every six weeks if you are recovering from breast cancer. ◀

Essiac

Another popular formula for preventing and treating breast cancer is a Native American tea called Essiac.

Renee Caisse was a Canadian nurse from Bracebridge, Ontario, born in 1888, who worked as head nurse at the Sisters of Providence Hospital in Haileybury, Ontario. While on duty one day, she received a recipe from an elderly patient who had been cured of breast cancer 30 years earlier by drinking a mixture of eight herbs given to her by an Ojibway medicine man. Soon afterwards Renee's aunt, Mireza Potvin, was diagnosed with stomach and liver cancer, and after exploratory surgery was told she had six months to live. Renee gave her the Ojibway formula daily and at the end of a year she recovered fully. She lived another 21 years. The original recipe contained eight herbs, which Renee eventually reduced to four. She administered these in tea form to cancer patients who came to her from all over Ontario and witnessed hundreds of remissions. Renee refused payment for her services, accepting instead donations of food, labor, hand-knit sweaters, and other voluntary contributions. She spent over 50 years selflessly tending to the sick and died at the age of 90, in 1978.

Essiac is available at most health food stores, manufactured by the Respirin Corporation or in a slightly different formula called FlorEssence by Flora. The latter formula includes red clover, which makes it an even better formula for breast cancer prevention. If you are interested, here is the Essiac formula for making a large quantity of this herbal remedy. New Action Products of Buffalo, New York (147 Ontario St., Buffalo, NY, 14207, tel: 716-873-3738, fax: 716-873-6621, web site http://napherbs.com) provides the herbs for making Essiac if you are unable to get them at a local supplier.

Dry Mix:

6½ cups	dry burdock root, cut
16 oz.	powdered green sheep sorrel
1 oz.	Turkish rhubarb root, powdered
4 oz.	slippery elm bark, powdered

Method:

Use one cup of dry herb mix to two gallons of pure spring water. This yields 13–15, 16-oz bottles. All utensils, pots, etc. must be cast iron or stainless steel.

1) Bring two gallons of pure spring water to a hard boil.

2) Add one cup of herb mix, hard boil for 10 minutes, stirring very often.

3) Turn off burner and cover and then let the mix sit over night (12 hours) and stir about ½ way, if possible.

4) In the morning sterilize 15, 16-oz amber-colored glass bottles. The herbs are light-sensitive and should be stored in the dark. To sterilize the bottles, put ½ inch of water in each bottle and set one inch of water in a large roasting pan. Put the pan and bottles in a 300°F oven for 40–60 minutes, until very hot.

5) When bottles are close to being sterilized, turn on the burner under the herbal liquid and just barely bring to a boil.

6) Let the herbs settle to the bottom for a few minutes.

7) Now you can fill the hot sterilized glass amber bottles. As you empty the hot water out of the bottles, you then fill them with the liquid herb mixture. Tighten the lids on the bottles as you fill them so that you get a good seal. Wipe the inside of the lids with liquor (vodka) prior to bottling. Let them set until cool. Then store in a dark cool place. Refrigerate once the bottle has been opened.

To make a smaller amount for one individual, use:

1⅝ cups	cut burdock root
4 oz	powdered sheep sorrel herb
1 oz	powdered slippery elm inner bark
¼ oz	powdered Turkish rhubarb root

Follow the above instructions using ½ gallon of water and ¼ cup of herb mix.

DOSAGE: Do not eat or drink anything for at least one hour after taking Essiac. Take 1–2 oz of Essiac with an equal amount of hot water, 1–3× daily or every second day at bedtime, on an empty stomach, two or three hours after supper. Sip it slowly over a four-minute period. Different sources have recommended different dosages, the usual being 2 oz, 2× daily mixed with an equal part of purified hot water, in the morning before breakfast and in the evening at least two hours after the evening meal. In late-stage cases of cancer, increase it to a total of 6 oz daily in three divided doses for at least 12 weeks before reducing it to the usual 4 oz dose.[17] For prevention, 1 oz daily or every other day may be sufficient. Always keep Essiac refrigerated after opening but never in the freezer.

CONTRAINDICATIONS: Do not use Essiac while pregnant or breast-feeding.

▶ **Action for Prevention:** As part of a breast cancer prevention program, consider alternating the Essiac formula with the Hoxsey formula or use The Healthy Breast Formula below. Take Essiac or FlorEssence for three months when you are not taking the Hoxsey formula, once or twice a year. If you are recovering from breast cancer, use both of them simultaneously. ◀

The Healthy Breast Formula

Women with a history of benign breast disease or at high risk for breast cancer may consider the following formula, which I have composed. It integrates some of the herbs in both the Hoxsey formula and Essiac with more of a focus on the breasts and lymphatic system. Use organically grown herbs in tincture form to make the following. You can order this formula using the form at the back of the book.

Other herbs that look promising in breast cancer prevention and treatment are bloodroot (Sanguinaria canadensis), mandrake and juniper. These were all found to inhibit the proliferation of both estrogen receptor positive and estrogen-receptor negative cell lines in vitro, with bloodroot having the strongest effect.[18] Follow the recommendations of a naturopathic doctor or a herbalist in using these or other formulas.

20	parts red clover	*Trifolium pratense* (fresh flower heads)
20	parts burdock root	*Arctium lappa* (dried root)
20	parts European mistletoe	*Viscum album* (twig and leaf, from the fresh green or freshly dried plant)
20	parts cleavers	*Galium aparine* (fresh herb)
10	parts calendula	*Calendula officinalis* (flower petals)
5	parts poke root	*Phytolacca decandra* (fresh root)
5	parts wild indigo root	*Baptisia tinctoriae* (root)
	potassium iodide (3% w/v)	

DOSAGE: 20–100 drops, 2–3× daily, ½ hour before or two hours after a meal. As prevention, take it for three months, once or twice a year. If you have breast cancer, use it continuously with week long breaks every four to six weeks. It can be used in conjunction with one of the immune-activating formulas described elsewhere in this book plus goldenseal and echinacea for a stronger immune boosting effect.

CONTRAINDICATIONS: Do not use in pregnancy or if breast-feeding. Do not use or use cautiously with hyperthyroidism

Ayurvedic Herbs

Amla (Indian Gooseberry)

Amla is one of the richest sources of vitamin C (with 3,000 mg per fruit) and other bioflavonoids in the vegetable kingdom. It is also an excellent antioxidant, increasing Superoxide Dismutase levels by 216%. This herb is one of the best ones to help us adapt to stress, with anti-fungal, anti-viral, anti-bacterial, anti-inflammatory, anti-mutagenic, and yeast inhibiting properties. As a restorative herb, it strengthens the teeth and bones, causes the growth of nails and hair, improves eyesight, and stops the bleeding of gums. Amla protects the liver, improves appetite, and regulates blood sugar. Amla forms the basis of the Ayurvedic tonic, Chyavan Prash.

DOSAGE: Use 1 tsp paste 3× daily; or 5 g of powder in water 2× daily as a tonic.

CONTRAINDICATIONS: Do not use with acute diarrhea or dysentery.

Ashwaganda

Another excellent Ayurvedic herb for helping us adapt to stress, ashwaganda is an immune enhancer which helps to shrink tumors, especially when it is injected directly into the tumor. It can kill some amoeba, bacteria, and fungi. Ashwaganda is prescribed for nervous exhaustion, debility, memory loss, muscular weakness, glandular swelling, fatigue, and insomnia. Its sedative action generates calmness and a restful sleep.

DOSAGE: 250–1000 mg 2–3× daily or 3000 mg at night for insomnia.

CONTRAINDICATIONS: Do not use if you are severely congested.

Chinese Herbs

Etiology of Breast Cancer in Chinese Medicine

In order to understand the use of Chinese herbs in breast cancer prevention and treatment, we must understand the etiology of breast cancer from an Oriental medical perspective. Breast cancer arises after a process caused primarily by the following. First, there is stagnation of energy in the liver. One of the functions of the liver in Oriental medicine is to circulate the body's energy, or qi, freely in all directions. This energy flow can be blocked by suppressed emotions – holding on to anger, anxiety, worry, a long period of depression or frustration, or grief. These emotions will interfere with the smooth flow of energy in the liver, causing a blockage. Other variables that contribute to liver stagnation include lack of exercise, shallow breathing, and excess consumption of unhealthy fats. Qi stagnation may manifest as irregular periods, premenstrual breast swelling and pain, breast cysts, irritability, fatigue, and depression. Qi stagnation is also often linked to a deficiency of yin or blood in the liver and kidney.

Second, there is stagnation of blood in the liver. As the liver energy does not circulate freely, the blood that the liver holds becomes stagnant, not moving as it should. Energy moves the blood. If the energy flow is disrupted, the blood flow is impaired. There will be reduced circulation to the breast area. In medical terms, the blood coagulates more easily than it should, or has increased viscosity.

Another contributing factor to breast disease is the accumulation of dampness or phlegm. Phlegm arises from qi stagnation affecting the function of the spleen. The role of the spleen in Chinese medicine is to transform and transport food and to regulate the body fluids. The disturbance in the liver will affect the spleen so that it is unable to perform these tasks effectively. A build-up of fluids will occur, which over time can form a soft mass or lump.

Eventually, the combination of qi stagnation and phlegm accumulation may cause the mass to become more firm. The presence of an actual toxin encourages the mass to become cancerous. The toxins may be internally or externally generated. Toxins can include but are not limited to environmental chemicals, pesticide residues, encrusted fecal matter, and excess estrogen.

After a period of time the stagnant qi turns into heat or 'fire' and becomes what is known as toxic heat. The toxic heat injures the blood and yin even further so that the mass hardens, leading to a cancerous tumor. A soft breast lump indicates the accumulation of phlegm, while a hard breast lump is indicative of blood stagnation or toxic heat. I find it interesting that thermography can pick up the presence of cancer from the increased heat in the area, generated by the higher vascular supply to a tumor.

Accordingly, cancer prevention in Chinese medicine consists of effective means to treat depression, anger, anxiety, grief, or other emotional factors that interfere with the circulation of energy; avoidance of substances that increase the production of phlegm (such as unhealthy fats, wheat, dairy, and sweets); improving circulation so that stagnation will be kept to a minimum and elimination of toxins. The components of The Healthy Breast Program address each of these aspects.

Chinese herbs are almost always used in formulas rather than alone. Many Chinese herbal formulas have been used safely and successfully for over a thousand years. Herbs used in formulas for breast cancer prevention or treatment are divided into several categories.

Herbs for Removing Toxins

Generally these help to remove toxic heat or fire and include *Sophora flavescens, Oldenlandria diffusae, Isatis tinctoria, Solanum, Wikstroemia, Lonicera japonica, Prunella vulgaris, Lithospermum erythrorhizon, Scutellaria baicalensis, Viola yedonensis, Curcuma aromatica,* oyster shell *Concha ostreae,* dandelion *Taraxicum mongolicum,* garlic *allium sativa,* and sea weeds such as kelp *Laminaria* and *Sargassum.*

Oldenlandria is able to increase the white blood cell count and improve the ability of macrophages to engulf and destroy toxins. It acts to shrink tumors, particularly in the upper body, and improves liver function.

Herbs for Removing the Accumulation of Phlegm (Soften Lumps)

These herbs help to break down the fibrous protein that protects a tumor so that the cells of the immune system can get at it. For soft masses or lumps, the following are used: *Semen Coicis lachryma jobi, Bulbus Fritillariae thunbergii, Chih-ko, Carapax amydae sinensis, Conchae ostreae, Sargassum, Thallus algae, Laminaria,* and *Curcuma aromatica.*

To break down hard, painless lumps, use: *Bombyx batryticatus, Pericarpum Citri reticulatae viride, Sparganium, Taraxicum mongolicum, Curcuma zedoaria, Semen Vaccariae segetalis,* and *Squama Manitis pentadactylae.*

Herbs to Activate the Blood

When the blood is less 'sticky' or has a lower viscosity, circulation is improved and cancer is less likely to develop. In order for cancer cells to metastasize, they need the help of 'sticky' materials in the blood to attach to other sites. Blood-activating herbs help to prevent this from occurring. Herbs that move the blood often also help to prevent scar tissue from forming after surgery and can reduce the side-effects of chemotherapy. They dilate the capillaries, improving the microcirculation to bring nutrition to cells and remove waste. Blood-activating herbs include *Radix Salvia miltiorrhizae, Sparganium simplex, Pangolin scales, Frankincense, Flos Carthamus tinctoria, Myrrh, Curcuma zedoaria, Ligusticum wallichii, Paeonia rubra,* and *Semen Persica.*

Salvia not only invigorates the blood but also circulates the liver energy. It dilates the capillaries, improving the microcirculation to bring nutrition to cells and remove waste, preventing tumor formation. It improves symptoms of angina, and can prevent heart attacks. It promotes the repair and regeneration of tissues.

Ligustrum helps to break up blood stagnation and remove symptoms of pain. It replenishes the vital essence of the liver and kidney and can be used to increase the white blood cell count, particularly in patients experiencing a low white blood cell count caused by chemotherapy and radiation.

Herbs to Protect from the Side Effects of Chemotherapy

Chemotherapy works by preventing the reproduction of cancer cells. The drugs that are used affect cancer cells more than normal cells because cancer cells reproduce faster. However, all of the body's cells are affected, especially those with a fast turnover time, such as the bone marrow stem cells that produce white blood cells, the lining of the stomach, and the hair follicles. Thus, a lowered white blood cell count, nausea, and hair loss are frequent side effects of chemotherapy as these cells are destroyed. Herbs can be administered that protect the body's cells from the effects of chemotherapy without protecting the cancer cells. The main herbs used to restore the white blood cells are *astragalus, ligustrum, ganoderma* (*reishi* mushroom) and *shitake* mushrooms. A herb used for restoring both the red and the white blood cell count is *millettia.* Deer antler is sometimes used for this purpose as well. Nausea can be counteracted by ginger, the medicinal mushroom called *hoelen (fu ling)* and the underground stem of *pinellia.* Collectively these three herbs will reduce nausea, vomiting, and diarrhea.

Herbs that Promote the Function of the Internal Organs

Tonic herbs that promote the function of the internal organs and rebuild the body after cancer therapies include *Adenophora, Astragalus, Codonopsis, Cordyceps, Coriolus, Ganoderma, Glehnia, Gynostemma, Jujube, Licorice, Ophiopoon, Royal Jelly,* and *Rehmannia.* Together they will improve energy and stamina and tonify the immune system.[19]

Astragalus is used as an energy, blood, and immune tonic. It has a special affinity for the lungs and spleen, protecting from infection and strengthening digestion. It revitalizes and increases stamina in a person when there is weakness and fatigue. Astragalus regulates fluids in the body, promoting urination when there is water retention and decreasing excess perspiration. It is very safe, with no known toxicity.

• Formulas for Liver Qi Stagnation, Obstruction & Breast Distension •

Item	Description
Formula	*Xiao Yao Wan*
Contains	Bupleurum, angelica sinensis, atractylodes, paeonia lactiflorae, poria cocos, glycyrrhizae uralensis, zinziber officianalis, herba menthae.
Action	Moves stagnant liver energy, strengthens the spleen, nourishes the blood.
Indication	For liver qi stagnation due to blood deficiency, irregular periods, breast swelling and tenderness, relaxes emotions.
Dosage	8 pills 3× daily. No contraindications.
Formula	*Clear the Moon* (manufactured by Three Treasures, similar to the formula Wen Dang Tang, and available from Jade Pharmacy)
Contains	Pinellia, citri reticulatae, citri reticulatae viride, caulis bambusae in taenium, aurantii aimmaturus, jujube, trichosanthis, poriae cocos, acori tatarinowii, polygalae, albizziae, cyperi, curcuma, salviae miltiorrhizae, tetrapanacis papyriferi, taraxicum, bulbus lilii, spica prunella, ziziphi spinosae, cyperi rotundi, glycyrrhizae uralensis.
Action	Moves liver qi, removes toxic heat, clears phlegm obstructing the chest.
Indication	PMS, swollen and tender breasts, benign breast lumps, fibrocystic breast disease, fibroadenoma, heaviness in the chest.

Codonopsis is used to activate the immune system and improve energy. It strengthens the lungs to resist infection. It is a tonic to the spleen, improving appetite. It increases the red blood cell count and hemoglobin levels, and builds stamina.

Chinese Herbal Formulas

Chinese herbal patent medicines have been developed to perform a combination of the above functions. An overview of formulas used in breast ailments and cancer prevention and treatment is given on pages 177, 179 and 181.[20] Please work with a practitioner of Traditional Chinese Medicine before using any of these formulas. The ITM formulas listed above can be ordered from ITM (tel. 503-233-4907); Jade Pharmacy formulas can be ordered from Jade (tel. 800-478-4325). The rest of the formulas are available at Chinese herbal stores or from Chinese medicine practitioners. Two Canadian wholesalers supplying health care professionals are T.C. Unicorn (tel. 416-285-5608) and Sun Ming Hong (tel. 416-979-9559).

Other Chinese Herbal Formulas

In his book, *Chinese Herbology,* Subhuti Dharmananda lists several other formulas for breast cancer prevention and treatment.

Dandelion and Vacarra Combination

15 g	dandelion
15 g	solanum
15 g	lithospermum
15 g	anteater scales
30 g	prunella
12 g	trichosanthes root
12 g	vaccaria
9 g	orange leaves
9 g	aurantium
9 g	pleione
9 g	fritillaria thunbergii

Lithospermum and Oyster Shell Combination

15 g	tang-kuei
15 g	peony
15 g	cnidium
20 g	oyster shell
15 g	lithospermum
10 g	astragalus
10 g	cimicifuga
8 g	lonicera
8 g	rhubarb
3 g	licorice

To make enough of the Dandelion and Vacarra and the Lithopermum and Oyster Shell combinations for one week, multiply the amounts by six and follow the directions as under the Immune Tonic tea below. Keep refrigerated in a glass jar. Consume ½ cup twice daily, one half hour before or two hours after a meal.

Echinacea and Goldenseal Combination

A formula containing these two herbs can be used for up to three weeks at a time to deal with an acute infection or for longer periods if dealing with cancer.

DOSAGE: 15–30 drops tincture, 3–5× daily. Use for 6 weeks on, one week off.

CONTRAINDICATIONS: Do not use goldenseal during pregnancy

Astragalus 10+ (Seven Forests)

This formula of astragalus, eleuthero, ganoderma, ophiopogon, ligustrum, Ho Shou Wu, cistanche, atractylodes, licorice, ginseng, schizandra, and morus fruit is fabulous for nourishing the blood and activating the immune system. It can be used over a long period of time, and improves chronic fatigue and general weakness

DOSAGE: 2–3 tablets, 3× daily.

CONTRAINDICATIONS: Do not use in pregnancy.

Ganoderma 18 (Seven Forests)

Comprised of ganoderma, astragalus, rehmannia, cistanche, peony, ligustrum, epimedium, dioscorea, Tang-Kuei, ophiopogon, atractylodes, Ho Shou Wu, lycium fruit, eucommia, ginseng, schizandra, licorice, and citrus, this formula enhances energy, nourishes the blood, and is useful for lowered immunity and general debility

DOSAGE: 2–3 tablets, 3× daily.

CONTRAINDICATIONS: Do not use in pregnancy.

Astragalus 10+ and Ganoderma 18 are available from Seven Forests Herbs and the Institute for Traditional Medicine (503-233-4907).

Immune Power Formula

The following formula is one that I have devised to strongly activate your immune system. You can order it from me as a tincture using the form at the back of the book.

40	parts astragalus
20	parts codonopsis
10	parts ganoderma
10	parts St. John's wort flowers
5	parts pau d'arco
5	parts ligustrum

• Formulas for Breast Swelling, Inflammation, or Abscesses •

Item	Description
Formula	*Ru He Nei Xiao Tang/Wan (Breast Kernel Inner-Dissolving Pill)*
Contains	Bupleurum, cyperi rotundi, citri reticulatae, curcuma, angelica sinensis, paeonia rubra, spica bulbus vulgaris, rhapontici seu echinops, fasciculus vascularis luffae, glycyrrhizae uralensis.
Action	Removes qi stagnation, blood stagnation and toxic heat.
Indication	For inflammatory swellings of the breasts which have become hot and painful.
Formula	*Xi Huang Wan (West Gallstone Pill)*
Contains	Calculus bovis, secretio moschus moschiferi, boswellia carterii:444, myrrh
Action	Reduces toxic swellings, detoxifies fire poisons, moves stagnant blood and accumulation of phlegm.
Indication	Breast abscesses due to heat and fire poisons, and accumulation of phlegm, breast cancer, carbuncles.
Dosage	1 vial 2× daily. Do not use in pregnancy.
Formula	*Ru Bi Xiao (Tablet for Breast Nodules)*
Contains	Laminaria, sargassum, prunella spica, moutan radicis, paeonia rubra, scrophularia, carthami tinctorii, notoginseng, taraxicum, spatholobi, cornu cervi parvum.
Action	Resolves and softens hard lumps and masses. Clears heat and promotes blood circulation.
Indication	Nodular breast masses, including gynecomastia and tuberculosis of the breast
Dosage	1.6 g 3× daily. Do not use in pregnancy.
Formula	*Gua Luo Xiao Yao San*
Contains	Trichosanthis, poriae cocos, curcuma, paeonia lactiflora, bupleurum, angelica sinensis, cyperi rotundi, glycyrrhiza uralensis, mentha haplocalycis, cornu cervi.
Action	Removes qi stagnation, dissolves lumps and opens the collateral meridians. Improves appetite and prevents weight loss.
Indication	Large, relatively soft breast lumps, phlegm accumulation in the breast collaterals.
Formula	*Niu Huang Xiao Yan Wan (Cow Gallstone Inflammation Eliminating Pill)*
Contains	Calculus bovis, concha margaritifera usta, trichosanthis, rhizome rhei, indigo pulverata levis, secretio bufonis, realgar.
Action	Clears heat and removes inflammation due to fire poison.
Indication	Mastitis or inflammation of the breast, tonsillitis, pharyngitis, throat swelling.
Dosage	10 pills 2–3× daily. Do not use in pregnancy or while nursing.
Formula	*Chuan Xin Lian Antiphlogistic Pills (Chuanxinlian kangyanpian)*
Contains	Andrographis leaf, taraxicum, isatis root.
Action	Eliminates toxic heat, cools the blood, resolves inflammation, soothes the throat.
Indication	Throat infection with swollen glands and fever, mastitis and breast abscesses.
Dosage	3 pills 3× daily for 1–2 days. No contraindications given.
Formula	*Lotus Kang Liu Wan (Lianhua kangliuwan)*
Contains	Selaginella doederleinii, schefflera arboricola, isatis, tribuili, prunella spica, boswellia carterii, commiphorra myrrh, moschus moschiferi.
Action	Anti-inflammatory and detoxifying.
Indication	Reduces pain, swelling and bruising, reduces abscesses and tumors.
Dosage	2 pills 3× daily with warm water. No contraindications given.

• Formulas for Breast Swelling, Inflammation, or Abscesses •

Item	Description
Formula	Chih-Ko/Curcuma Tablets (ITM Formula)
Contains	Citri aurantii, curcuma, myrrh, fritillariae thunbergii, lonicera japonicae, ostrea concha, sargassum, sparginium stoloniferum, curcuma zedoaria, isatis, sophora.
Action	Reduces and softens masses, resolves phlegm, moves stagnant blood, removes toxins.
Indication	For abscesses and tumors.
Formula	Gynostemma Tablets (ITM Formula)
Contains	Citri aurantii, curcuma tuber, gynostemma, ganoderma, oldenlandria, astragalus, ostrae concha, sargassum, sparganium, curcumae zedoaria, isatis, sophora.
Action	Enhances immune function, reduces masses, improves qi, resolves phlegm, softens hardness, disperses stagnant blood, removes toxins.
Indication	Reduces swelling, bruising, abscesses and tumors.
Formula	Blue Citrus Tablets (ITM Formula)
Contains	Spica prunellae, radix curcuma, ostrae concha, sparganium, isatis
Action	Reduces masses, softens hardness, moves stagnant blood, removes toxins.
Indication	Reduces swelling and bruising, reduces abscesses and tumors.
Formula	Strong Xiao Jin Tan (Qiangli Xiaojindan)
Contains	Liquidambir, aconitum, angelica sinensis, boswellia carterii, myrrh, lumbricus, excrementum pteropi, semen momordicae, dianthis chinensis.
Action	Reduces fever, inflammation, and pain.
Indication	Thyroid gland disorders, swollen lymph nodes, mastitis, reduces tumors.
Dosage	1–2 pills 2× daily. Do not take in pregnancy.
Formula	Special Cure for Hyperplasia of the Mammary Gland
Contains	Scrophularia, scutellaria barbatae, salvia miltiorrhizae, fritillaria, radix curcuma, tinosporae, oldenlandria.
Action	Moves liver stagnation, alleviates depression, dissolves masses, improves energy and moves the blood.
Indication	Breast swelling and pain, mastitis.
Dosage	4–7 tablets 3× daily after meals with boiled water. Prolonged use may cause minor indigestion, dry mouth and dry stools.
Formula	Xing Xiao Wan (Tumor Reversing Pill)
Action	Dissolves lumps and masses.
Indication	Breast lumps, abscesses and tumors.
Formula	Nei Xiao Luo Li Wan
Action	Dissolves lumps and masses.
Indication	Fibrocystic breast disease, fibroadenomas, breast cancer.
Dosage	8 pills 3× daily.
Formula	Wu Wei Qui Shi Wan (Dampness Eliminating Pill)
Action	Resolves dampness and promotes blood flow.
Indication	Breast distension, breast lumps and cancer, lymphedema.

• Formulas to Protect from the Side Effects of Chemotherapy and Strengthen Immunity •

Item	Description
Formula	*Ji Xue Teng Jin Gao Pian (Caulis Millettia Tablets)*
Contains	Millettia reticulata benth.
Action	Increases white blood cell count, builds the blood, relaxes tendons
Indication	For the side effects of chemotherapy and lowered immunity.
Dosage	4 tablets 3× daily. No contraindications known.
Formula	*Ling Zhi Feng Wang Jiang (Ganoderma-Royal Jelly Essence)*
Contains	Ganoderma, royal jelly, codonopsis, lycii chinensis.
Action	Tonic to strengthen energy and blood.
Indication	Helps prevent the fatigue and weight loss that occcurs with cancer and chemo.
Dosage	1 10cc vial of liquid to be taken daily in the morning. No contraindications.
Formula	*Paris-7 (ITM Formula)*
Contains	Isatis, scutellaria, oldenlandria, sophora.
Action	Removes heat and toxins and inhibits cancer.
Indication	For weakness and toxicity.
Formula	*Coriolus-3 (ITM Formula)*
Contains	Coriolus, ganoderma, cordyceps, sophora
Action	Improves immune response.
Indication	For weight loss and energy depletion.
Formula	*Astragalus/Oldenlandria Tea (ITM Formula)*
Contains	Astragalus, glycyrrhizae uralensis, oldenlandria, rehmannia glutinosa, caulis millettia, salvia miltiorrhizae.
Action	Improves immune response, promotes blood circulation, improves digestion.
Indication	For exhaustion, and weakness on exertion.
Formula	*Canelim Tablets (Ping Xiao Pian)*
Contains	Radix curcumae, abrimoniae, fructus aurantii
Action	Promotes blood circulation, alleviates pain, clears toxic heat and toxins, stimulates immunity, shrinks tumors, helps prolong life. This formula is used for prevention and treatment of breast cancer. Dissolves breast masses.
Indication	Active cancer with lowered immunity.
Dosage	4–8 tablets 3× daily.

5 parts schizandra
3 parts Ho Shou Wu
2 parts licorice

DOSAGE: Use 30 drops 2 times daily ½ hour before dinner and before bed.
CONTRAINDICATIONS: Do not use in pregnancy.

Immune Tonic Tea

This recipe uses Chinese herbs to strongly activate the immune system. The recipe will last for approximately one week if you drink one cup daily or several days if two cups are consumed daily.

48g astragalus (huang qi)
24g schizandra (wu wei zi)
24g white atractylodes (bai zhu)
24g codonopsis (dang shen)
24g ganoderma (reishi mushroom)

Soak the herbs in 13 cups of water for one hour. Bring to a boil, then simmer for one hour. Strain into a glass jar. Keep refrigerated. Drink one to two cups of tea daily, warmed, at least one half hour before or two hours after a meal. The above ingredients are enough for several days to one week of tea. Consider purchasing several bags at once from a Chinese herbal store.

Medicinal Mushrooms

Maitake (Grifola frondosa)

Maitake has been used as food in Japan for hundreds of years, in amounts up to several hundred grams daily, and is entirely safe. Compounds in Maitake mushrooms called Beta-glucans are able to shrink tumors and have a beneficial effect on the immune system by increasing macrophage activity.[21,22,23,24] The most important of these compounds is called the D-fraction constituent. There has been considerable evidence to support the use of Maitake in the healing of breast and prostate cancer. In a non-randomized clinical study of advanced stage (III–IV) breast cancer patients, tumor regression or significant symptom improvements were observed in 11 out of 15 women.[25] It also inhibits the formation of metastases.[26] Maitake lessens the side effects of chemotherapy, helping to decrease nausea, keep the white blood cell count high, and reduce pain. One manufacturer is Maitake Products, Inc. (www.maitake.com) who produces a Maitake D-fraction extract in liquid form. The dosage is 1 mg per kg of body weight per day, which for a 150 lb woman is 34–68 drops daily. Maitake mushrooms are delicious for eating and you can purchase kits to grow your own from Wylie Mycologicals (RR #1, Wiarton, ON NOH 2TO, tel. 519-534-1570, fax. 519-534-9045, E-mail: wylie@interlog.com).

Shitake (Lentinus edodes)

Shitake mushrooms have been well-studied since the 1960s and possess constituents that have anti-tumor properties and enhance immune function. They contain two compounds called lentinan and LEM which increase macrophage and natural killer cell activity as well as interferon levels. A derivative of lentinan has been used as an injectible anti-cancer drug in Asia. This mushroom also exerts anti-viral and anti-bacterial effects and reduces cholesterol. It has been used as a tonic for chronic fatigue syndrome.[27,28] Shitake mushrooms taste delicious and can be added to stir fries and soups or made into a spread for vegetables and sandwiches. They are a staple in the macrobiotic diet, which has long been used in cancer recovery. Have them several times a week. Shitake mushrooms are available in dried form in Chinese herbal stores and sometimes you can find them fresh in supermarkets. Shitake growing kits are available from Wylie Mycologicals in Canada and Fungi Perfecti in the United States (PO Box 7634, Olympia, WA 98507, tel. 800-780-9126 or 360-426-9292, fax. 360-426-9377, E-mail: mycomedia@aol.com, web site: http://www.fungi.com).

Reishi (Ganoderma lucidum)

Also known as the 'Mushroom of Immortality', Ganoderma has been consumed for almost 2,000 years in China. Its active constituents which help fight cancer are B-Glucans, Hetero-B-Glucans, and Ling Zhi-8 Protein. These act to shrink tumors, enhance the immune system by increasing T-cell function, strengthening stamina, and reducing cholesterol, and are anti-viral.[29] This mushroom also has anti-oxidant and anti-inflammatory properties and has been used effectively for arthritis. Reishi mushrooms increase the absorption of oxygen by the lungs and have a positive benefit to patients with chronic fatigue syndrome. They have very low toxicity even at very high dosages but should not be used during surgery as their vasodilation effect can result in excess bleeding. They should also be used cautiously in women with heavy menstruation. They are available dried in Chinese herbal stores and from Wylie Mycologicals and Fungi Perfecti.

Zhu ling (Polyporus umbellatus)

This mushroom contains a constituent called B-Glucan, which has anti-tumor and immune-enhancing properties.[30] Zhu Ling has also been shown to act as an antibiotic, anti-inflammatory, diuretic and liver protector. Studies in China have demonstrated that it helps the immune system improve after chemotherapy and radiation and decreases the recurrence of cancer.[31]

A combination of the above four mushrooms is available in tea form called "Olympic Rainforest Mushroom Tea" from Fungi Perfecti, A Canadian source for fresh shitake and maitake mushrooms and home growing kits is Wylie Mycologicals.

Royal Sun Agaricus (Agaricus blazei)

This mushroom has very strong anti-tumor properties and contains more B-glucans than most, if not all, other mushrooms. It is immune enhancing and has caused complete recovery in cancer infected laboratory animals.[32] It also acts as an anti-viral and reduces cholesterol levels. It is available in tincture form from Fungi Perfecti.

Turkey Tail (Trametes coriolus versicolor)

Compounds from this mushroom have been shown to inhibit the growth of cancer cells and to increase the immune system's number of natural killer cells, which directly target cancer cells.[33] It has been used clinically in the treatment of cervical, breast, colon, stomach and lung cancer. Breast cancer patients who were positive for the HLA B40 antigen derived the greatest benefit. Trametes is the source of the anticancer drug known as 'Krestin', which has been demonstrated to increase the disease-free survival rate of cancer patients in Asia.[34,35] Available in tincture form from Fungi Perfecti.

MGN-3

MGN-3 is an extract of the outer shell of rice bran combined with extracts from the following three mushrooms: Shitake, Kawaratake, and Suehirotake. This combination possesses anti-cancer properties that improve the ability of the T-killer cells to destroy cancer cells by increasing the number of explosive granules in the T-killer cells. MGN-3 increases the body's levels of interferon and tumor necrosis factors, both of which help to destroy cancer cells. In one study involving 24 cancer patients who took the product for two months, the T-killer cells became 27 times more effective at killing cancer cells after the two months than they had been prior to treatment.[36] Used with chemotherapy, MGN-3 lessens toxic side effects of the chemo and fortifies the white blood cells.

DOSAGE: 250–750 mg daily.
CONTRAINDICATIONS: Do not use if you are allergic to mushrooms.

▶ **Action for Prevention:** As prevention, consider using an immune activating formula or tea for 1–3 months per year, particularly during the winter, or whenever you are most prone to infections. If you are recovering from breast cancer, use one of the formulas or a similar formula continuously with short breaks every six weeks. Drink Pau d'arco tea and decaffeinated green tea regularly, and use Chyavan Prash. Use antioxidants, meditation, thymus extract, echinacea, licorice root, European mistletoe, astragalus, maitake, shitake, and reishi mushrooms and co-ordinated exercise to strengthen your thymus gland. ◀

Topical Treatments for Breast Cysts and Cancer

A naturopathic tradition has quietly survived over the last century that utilizes pastes, salves, and herbal oils to treat breast cysts and breast cancer topically. External applications for cancer have been practiced in many traditions and cultures for generations. Native Americans commonly used poultices of roasted red onion and bloodroot or goldenseal to destroy and remove tumors, and some of their practices were adopted by European medical doctors in the 18th century. Ingrid Naiman has revived this tradition with the publication of her book *Cancer Salves: A Botanical Approach to Treatment*. Please read her book before using the treatments below, so that you know what to expect, or link to her web site at www.cancer-salves.com. The formulas are meant to be used alongside internal treatments such as the previous herbal formulas and an anti-cancer diet. In the early part of this century, numerous physicians used these topical formulas in place of surgery. They found that their use resulted in next to no bleeding, very little scarring, and less trauma to the patient. Often tumors could be removed using this method within 5–21 days.

Dr Eli Jones' Paste No. 3 (1911)

4 drams solid (soft) extract sanguinaria (alcoholic)
12 drams zinc chloride
1 dram starch
2 drams red saunders

Use water to soften the paste or more pulverized sanguinaria to thicken it. Place adhesive strips around the affected area. Spread the paste onto a soft white cloth the size of the diseased area and tape it in place. Change the dressing every 24 hours and wash the surface with warm water between dressings. Continue these applications until the patient senses a heavy weight beneath the dressing. When this occurs, switch to using the poultice powder below.

Dr Eli Jones' Poultice Powder (1911)

Equal parts of:

> Pulverized flax seed
> Pulverized slippery elm
> Pulverized bayberry bark
> Pulverized lobelia seed

Instructions: Put 1–2 tsp of the powder into a container, add enough boiling water to make a poultice. Stir the mixture until the lumps disappear. Then spread onto a soft white cloth large enough to cover the growth and the inflammation around the growth. Change the poultice every two hours. After each change, bathe the skin around the growth with equal parts of distilled witch hazel and warm water. When the growth breaks loose and drops onto the poultice, examine the exposed tissue to see if it looks healthy. If not, continue with more poultices.

Dr Samuel Thompson's Anti-Cancer Paste (1769–1843)

> Red clover blossoms
> Water

Instructions: Harvest the clover blossoms in the morning before they are exposed to the sun. Boil the blossoms in water for one hour, using a double boiler to prevent burning. Remove the blossoms from the water using a strainer, and squeeze any remaining liquid out of them. Refill the top of the double boiler with fresh blossoms and boil again for one hour. Strain and press the flower heads to remove as much juice as possible. Then simmer the remaining liquid until it is the consistency of tar. Spread it on gauze and apply it directly over the tumor. Change the gauze and repeat the process daily.

Dr William Fox's Cancer Liniment (1904)

2 oz Blue flag tincture
1 oz Red clover tincture
1 oz Bloodroot tincture

Instructions: Mix thoroughly. Saturate a cotton cloth and place it over the affected area. Cover it with plastic and tape to retain moisture. Change the dressings twice per day.

Dr John Pattison's Enucleating Paste (1866)

Equal parts of:

> Goldenseal root
> Zinc chloride
> Flour
> Water

Instructions: Make a paste out of the ingredients. Apply daily to the affected area, covering the paste with a soft cotton cloth. Cover with plastic and surgical tape to retain moisture. Use cautiously, as it can irritate the skin.

Escharotic Black Salve

Equal parts:

> Bloodroot
> Galangal
> Zinc chloride
> Distilled water

Instructions: Make a paste out of the ingredients. Apply once or twice daily to the affected area, covering with gauze, plastic and surgical tape to retain moisture. Use cautiously, as it can irritate the skin.

Dr John Christopher's Poke Root Poultice for Breast Cancer (1909–1983)

> Fresh green poke root (phytolacca)
> Fluid extract of poke root
> Apple cider vinegar
> Bayberry root powder

Instructions: Grind enough fresh poke root for one application. Apply it to a piece of muslin or gauze, with a space for the nipple cut out of the gauze. Place the cloth on to the breast, then moisten it with the fluid extract of phytolacca. Cover it with plastic to keep in the moisture. Leave it on for three days and then apply a new poultice. Generally, in two weeks the breast will break out in pustular sores and in four weeks all hardness will be gone. After this occurs, wash the area with apple cider vinegar. Cover it with bayberry powder and let the whole breast surface dry. It should heal within 7–10 days.

Herbal Oils for Breast Health

A variety of infused oils can be used to maintain healthy breasts and to alleviate breast cysts. These infused oils are made from fresh plants, except for the calendula blossoms which are dried for two days first. To make an oil from blossoms (calendula, dandelion flower, red clover, St. John's wort) pick dry blossoms on a sunny day, making sure there is no moisture or dew on the flowers. Shade the blossoms from the sun after picking. Fill a dry, large-mouthed, dark glass jar almost full with blossoms. Pour extra virgin olive oil over them until all the flowers are completely covered, stirring with a stick to mix it in. Put a lid on the jar, label the lid with the date and name of the plant, and store it at room temperature. After six weeks, pour the oil through a cotton cheesecloth to remove the plant materials. Store the oil in a cool, dry place until you are ready to use it.

To make an oil from a root (poke root, dandelion root) harvest the roots of the plant in the spring or the fall, when the leaves are not actively growing or have fallen off. Carefully dig around the roots and lift them out, shaking off as much dirt as possible. Keep the top of the plant attached. Place them overnight in a shady spot with good ventilation, brushing off more dirt the following morning. Avoid washing the roots unless they were already wet. When dry, chop the roots into small pieces and put them in a dark glass jar with a wide mouth. Cover them with extra virgin olive oil, leaving extra oil on top. Cap and label the jar and strain it after six weeks. Store in a cool dry place until ready for use.

Calendula Blossom Oil

Regular use of calendula oil on the breasts will help to reduce breast cysts and prevent breast cancer. It is especially useful after breast surgery to prevent scarring, or to remove old scars and keloids.

Castor Oil

Castor oil at room temperature can be applied morning and night for several months to reduce breast cysts.

Dandelion Oil

Both the flower and the root of dandelion can be used in an oil to reduce breast cysts, clear long-held emotions and improve liver function.

Poke Root (Phytolacca) Oil

Poke root is one of the herbs most often recommended for breasts cysts and cancer prevention and treatment. The oil will help to decrease breast swelling and breast cysts. Apply the oil to the area around a lump, cover it with a cotton flannel cloth, and place a hot water bottle on top. Keep the application on for at least an hour. Repeat twice daily until the lump has disappeared. If there is no change after three months, discontinue use. Poke root should not be used continuously for months at a time, but can be used intermittently with other oils, such as red clover.

Red Clover Blossom Oil

Red clover blossom oil will help to remove breast lumps, discourages breast cancer, and improves lymphatic circulation. It can be used daily for breast self-massage.

St. John's Wort Oil

St. John's wort is known particularly for its ability to regenerate and repair the nerves and skin. It is useful after breast surgery (with calendula) to heal damaged tissue, relieve pain, and prevent lymphedema. It can be applied before and after radiation treatments to reduce damage to the skin and to relieve nerve and muscle pain.

Essential Oils

Several essential oils show promise in preventing or reversing breast cancer. A class of chemicals called monoterpenes is present in high amounts in palmarosa, lavender, orange, lemongrass, and geranium. There are three primary therapeutic monoterpenes – geraniol, limonene, and perillyl alcohol. Perillyl alcohol is five times stronger than limonene[37,38] and is found in particularly high concentrations in palmarosa. It is also found in peppermint, spearmint, cherries, celery seeds, and lavender.

Monoterpenes act to inhibit the formation of cholesterol, and potentially lower estrogen levels; improve the liver's ability to break down carcinogens by increasing the amount of liver enzymes, thus protecting the breasts from cellular damage; stimulate programmed cell death (apoptosis) in breast cancer cells; and selectively block the division and multiplication of cancer cells. Perillyl alcohol has been found to be protective against breast, ovarian, and prostate tumors.[39,40] Other oils which have been used for breast health include Roman chamomile, marjoram, carrot, parsley seed, cypress, and clary sage.[41]

Juniper has been found to prevent breast cells from

replicating in a laboratory setting. It is a detoxifier for the liver and kidneys and promotes the excretion of uric acid and toxins as well as decreasing fluid retention.

Rosemary is antifungal and antiparasitic and stimulates the liver's ability to manufacture the protective C-2 estrogen from estrone (rather than the harmful C-16 estrogen). It supports the nerves and is a hormone balancer.

Frankincense acts as an immune stimulant, and has been used historically for cancer and as an antidepressant.[42] The herb is used in Traditional Chinese Medicine to activate the blood, improving circulation and discouraging metastases.

We can combine some of the herbal oils with essential oils to make a blend that will be healing for the breasts. Generally, 10 drops of one or more of the essential oils are used in one ounce (30 ml) of carrier oil. If only a small amount is necessary, use 3–5 drops of essential oil in 5 ml (1 tsp) of base oil. Extra virgin olive oil is the best choice of carrier oil for breast health.

These would be my choice to include in an oil blend:

Healthy Breast Oil

Combine several of the following herbal oils, depending on availability:

> Phytolacca oil
> Calendula oil
> Dandelion oil
> Red clover oil

Add the essential oils of:

> Palmarosa
> Lavender
> Rosemary
> Juniper
> Frankincense
> Lemon
> Celery
> Orange (optional) or
> Lemongrass (optional)

Gently and lovingly apply the oil mixture to your breasts or body one or more times daily. If you have breast cancer, consider applying the oil several times daily to the tumor site. If using phytolacca oil, take a break from it for one week of each month. Phytolacca and calendula herbal oils can be ordered from St. Francis Herb Farm in Canada (1-800-219-6226) and from Avena Botanicals in the U.S. (207-594-0694, Web site: www.avenaherbs.com).

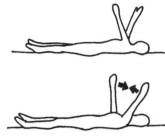

Kundalini Yoga Exercise for Circulating Energy and Lymph

1) Lie on your back. Connect the little finger and thumb of each hand and extend both arms up pointing towards the ceiling. Criss-cross your arms back and forth across your chest keeping the elbows straight and your hands pointing upward. Coordinate the breath with the movement. Continue for 2 minutes. This exercise circulates the lymphatic fluid in the armpits, helping to cleanse the breasts.

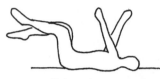

2) Stay in the same position as in #1, but pull your knees up, so your thighs are perpendicular to the ground and your calves are parallel to the ground. Criss-cross your ankles over one another as you simultaneously move the arms as in the first exercise. Alternate which ankle is on top with each repetition. Coordinate the movement with the breath. Continue for 2 minutes.

3) Remain lying on your back with your arms and legs relaxed and your head on the floor. Turn your head from side to side rapidly as you breathe long and deep. This exercise circulates the lymphatic fluid in the neck area and increases the circulation to the thyroid gland.

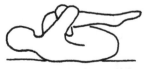

4) Lying on your back, bring your knees to your chest; wrap your arms around your knees and lift your head up so that your nose is between your knees. Hold the position and do breath of fire powerfully. Continue for 1 minute. This exercise improves the circulation to the thyroid gland.

5) Turn over on your stomach with your forehead on the ground and beat 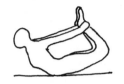 your buttocks with your fists. Continue for 2 minutes. This exercise stimulates acupuncture points on the buttocks which help keep the reproductive organs balanced. It improves the energy flow in the bladder meridian which benefits all your organs.

6) Lying on your stomach, reach back and take hold of your ankles and lift up the head, torso, and thighs as high as possible. (Bow pose). Hold this position with breath of fire. Continue for 2 minutes. This exercise opens the flow of energy through the meridians associated with the breasts — the liver, stomach, spleen and kidney. Consequently there is less stagnation in breast tissue.[43]

7) Come back into bow pose, as in exercise 6. Balance on your navel, lifting the torso and thighs off the ground. Begin rocking back and forth on your stomach.

Breath of fire is a breathing practice where you inhale, expanding the abdomen and exhale, pulling it in. This is done at a fairly rapid, even, rhythmic pace. The breathing is through your nose, working up to 2–3 breaths per second after accomplishing the rhythm. The inhale should equal the exhale in strength and intensity. Breath of fire acts to detoxify the blood, oxygenate the tissues, improve liver circulation, strengthen the nervous system, and improves immunity.

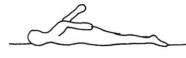

Kundalini Yoga Exercise for Internal Cleansing

1) Sit cross-legged. Keeping your arms close to your sides, bend your elbows so that the hands and fore-arms are pointing straight up and the palms are facing each other. 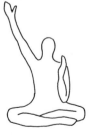 Strongly push one arm up and out at a 60-degree angle while the other arm remains bent. The bent arm should be firmly held, providing a solid balance for the extended arm. Then push out the bent arm while the extended arm returns to the balancing position close in to the side of the body. Push your arm out from the armpit, stretching your

armpit as you do so. The movement throughout the exercise should be vigorous and demanding. The exercise works to channel the energy flow in the spine to the rest of the body and to circulate the lymphatic fluid in the underarm area. Continue for up to 10 minutes.

2) Extend both arms up and out, creating a 'V' between your arms. Keep the elbows straight and criss-cross your arms in front of your face. Move very quickly with breath of fire. Continue for 1½ minutes.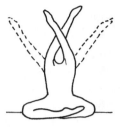

3) Extend both arms out in front of you with the palms facing up. Move them together as though you were splashing water up and over your head; then bring them back in front of you. Breathe powerfully through your mouth. Continue for 2½ minutes.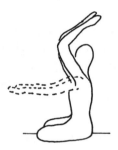

4) Lie on your back and inhale as you lift both legs up over your head, keeping your knees straight. 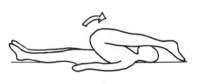 Bring them all the way behind you, touching your toes on the ground behind your head if you can. This is plow pose. Exhale as you return your legs to the floor. Continue alternating the back and forth movement for 2 minutes, breathing deeply into your belly as you do so.

5) Lie on your back with your hands beneath your neck. Spread your heels one foot apart. Begin 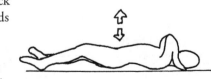 lifting the body off the ground from the hips without bending your knees. Jump the body up and down, keeping your heels and shoulders on the ground. Move vigorously for 3½ minutes.

6) Lying on your back, lift both legs up to a 90-degree angle from the ground and hold onto your toes, keeping your knees straight. If you can't reach your toes, hold onto the backs of your knees. Open 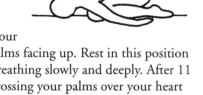 your mouth wide and breathe through your throat. Continue for 1 minute.

7) Sit on your heels and bring your forehead onto the floor in front of you. Rest your arms along your 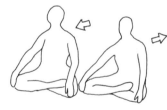 sides with your palms facing up. Rest in this position for 11 minutes, breathing slowly and deeply. After 11 minutes, sit up, crossing your palms over your heart center with the right hand over the left, and direct love and healing towards yourself for 5 minutes.[44]

Kundalini Yoga Exercise for Enhancing Immunity

1) Sit cross-legged; hold your ankles or shins with both hands. Inhale and flex the spine forward, exhale and flex it back, keeping the shoulders 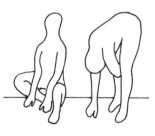 relaxed and the head straight. Breathe deeply in and out through your nose as you rhythmically inhale forward, exhale back. Continue 1–3 minutes.

2) Sit cross-legged, resting your hands on your knees. Begin rotating your waist from right to left, pressing the chest forward as you rotate to the front and slumping your lower spine down as you rotate to the back. Keep the head fairly stationary. Stretch your shoulders back as you rotate to the front and bring them forward as you rotate to the back. Inhale as you go around the front and exhale as you go around the back. This exercise acts as a gentle massage to the internal organs. Continue 1–3 minutes

3) Place your hands on your shoulders with your fingers in front, your thumbs behind. Inhale as you twist your head and torso to the left, exhale as you twist them to the right. Keep your elbows up at 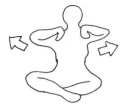 shoulder height. Lift up gently from your hips as you twist. Continue 1–3 minutes. Inhale to the center, pulling your elbows back slightly to open the chest. Exhale and relax your arms down.

4) Lie on your back. Inhale and raise the right leg to 90 degrees as you raise the left leg up to 45 degrees. Exhale as you lower both legs down together. Then inhale 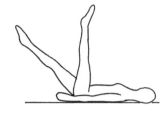 and raise the left leg up to 90 degrees as you raise the right leg to 45 degrees. Exhale as you lower both legs down together. Continue the sequence for 3–10 minutes depending on your fitness level.

5) Remaining on your back, extend your arms behind your head on the ground. Inhale as 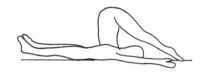 you raise your legs up over and behind your head, keeping the knees as straight as possible. If you are able to, touch the toes on the ground behind you. (This is called plow pose). Exhale as you lower the legs back down and come lying on your back. Continue at your own speed with a deep breath each time. If you are able to, complete 26 repetitions. Relax on your back for 2 minutes.

6) Squat down with the heels touching each other and off the ground and the fingertips on the ground between the knees. The knees are spread apart. Inhale as you lift the buttocks up 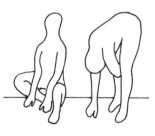 in the air and bring your head down between your knees; simultaneously touch your left hand to your heart (the right hand stays on the floor). Exhale as you come back into a squat, keeping both heels off the ground, and bringing the fingertips of both hands on the ground. The head comes facing forward as the buttocks come down. Inhale up again, this time

touching the right hand to your heart. Exhale down as both hands come down to the ground and the head faces forward. Continue the same sequence, counting up to 26 repetitions.

7) Come standing up. Extend the arms up straight with the elbows hugging your ears. Inhale in this position. Exhale as you bend forward touching your hands to the ground (or come as close as you can). Continue the sequence with deep breathing in and out through your nose for 26 repetitions.[45]

8) Sit with both legs stretched out in front of you. Keeping your knees straight, hold on to your legs wherever you can comfortably reach — either the knees, shins, ankles or toes. Inhale as you straighten your spine in the "up" position; exhale as you bend forward from your lower spine bringing your chest down towards your knees. On the forward bend, also rotate your head so that the forehead comes towards the knees during each rotation. Continue for 26 repetitions.

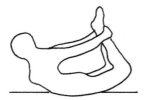

9) Lie on your stomach. Bend your knees and reach back, taking hold of your ankles. Inhale as you lift the torso, head and thighs off the ground. Exhale as you lower them down bringing your chin and thighs on to the ground. Repeat 26 times, inhaling as you lift up, exhaling as you relax down.

Summary

Your immune system is your body's defence system. Its fundamental role is to protect the life of the body by distinguishing 'self' from 'non-self' and recognizing what needs to be eliminated or destroyed (a cancer cell, virus, bacteria, environmental toxin, internal toxin). The stronger your immune system is, the more resistant to breast cancer you will be. Our immune systems resonate with the health of the planet. The planet is our collective body — if she is sick, so are we. She is in our blood, our bones, our muscles, our organs. When I had my first child, I felt the earth split as my daughter entered the world. I felt the oceans in my breasts as they filled with milk. I was initiated into the mysteries of the earth. I have not forgotten. She is my mother. I believe that as conscious women, we can and must act as the white blood cells of the planet. Our bodies' immune systems are not separate from the earth's self-protective functions. We have loaded our Earth matrix with debris of every description that does not belong in her body — nuclear fallout, plastics, plutonium, organochlorines, pesticides, chemical hormones, non-biodegradable landfill — just as we must recognize and rid our bodies of toxins, so must she. The earth is our body too. Our bodies arise from the 'mater' of the earth and to the earth they will return. There is no separation.

Mankind has become the cancer of the earth as cancer has become the scourge of twentieth-century humanity. Where are the white blood cells of the earth? We find them in the environmentalists, the activists, the educators, the naturopaths and herbalists, the organic gardeners, the builders of windmills and solar energy units, the clean-up crews of environmental disasters. We are the 'cure' for this cancer. I invite each of you to become one of the white blood cells of the earth as you activate your own immune systems. Answer this call to women to act against the breast cancer epidemic by using some of your renewed energy to participate in healing the planet. We need one another to survive. We are the guardians of life and growing things.

Further Reading

Boyle, W. & A. Saine. *Lectures in Naturopathic Hydrotherapy.* East Palestine, OH: Buckeye Naturopathic Press, 1988.

De Schepper, Luc. *Peak Immunity: How to Fight CEBV, Candida, Herpes Simplex Viruses and Other Immune-Suppressed Conditions and Win.* Van Nuys, CA: Le Fever Publications, 1989.

Dharmananda, Subhuti. *A Bag of Pearls.* Portland, OR: Institute for Traditional Medicine and Preventive Health Care, 1990.

Dharmananda, Subhuti. *Chinese Herbology.* Portland, OR: Institute for Traditional Medicine and Preventive Health Care, 1989.

Growing Gourmet and Medicinal Mushrooms. Berkeley, CA: Ten Speed Press, 1993.

Holmes, P. *The Energetics of Western Herbs.* Vol. I & II. 2nd ed. Berkeley, CA: NatTrop Publishing, 1993.

Naiman, Ingrid. *Cancer Salves: A Botanical Approach to Treatment.* Santa Fe, NM: Seventh Ray Press, 1999.

Singer, S. & S. Grismaijer. *Dressed to Kill: The Link Between Breast Cancer and Bras.* Garden City Park, NY: Avery Publishing Group, 1995.

Stamets, Paul. *MycoMedicinals: An Informational Booklet on Medicinal Mushrooms.* Olympia, WA: MycoMedia Publications, 1998. (Mr Paul Stamets, President, Fungi Perfecti, P.O. Box 7634, Olympia, WA 98507, tel. 800-780-9126 or 360-426-9292, fax. 360-426-9377, http://www.fungi.com)

Stamets, Paul. *The Mushroom Cultivator: A Practical Guide to Growing Mushrooms at Home,* Olympia, WA: Agarikon Press, 1983.

References

1. De Schepper, Luc. *Peak Immunity: How to Fight CEBV, Candida, Herpes Simplex Viruses and Other Immune-Suppressed Conditions and Win.* Van Nuys, CA: Le Fever Publications, 1989.
2. Singer, S. & S. Grismaijer. *Dressed to Kill: The Link Between Breast Cancer and Bras.* Garden City Park, NY: Avery Publishing Group, 1995.
3. Kloppenberg, R., et al. Heilpflanzen in der Krebsmedizin. Berlin, Germany: 1997.
4. Walters, R. *Options: The Alternative Cancer Therapy Book.* Garden City Park, NY: Avery Publishing Group, 1993.
5. Hajto, T. et al. Increased secretion of tumor necrosis factor-a, interleukin-1 and interleukin-6 from clinically applied mistletoe extract. *Cancer Research,* 1990 June;50(1):3322-26.
6. Leroy, R. *An Anthroposophical Approach to Cancer.* Spring Valley, NY: Mercury Press, 1982:44.
7. Moss, R. *Cancer Therapy: The Independent Consumer's Guide to Non-Toxic Treatment and Prevention.* New York, NY: Equinox Press, 1992:322.
8. Taddayoni, Dor. The use of mistletoe extract in cancer therapy. Toronto, ON: *Canadian College of Naturopathic Medicine,* April 2000:3.
9. Hartwell, J. Plants Used Against Cancer. *Lloydia;* 32(2) June 1968, 33(1); March 1970.
10. Holmes, P. *The Energetics of Western Herbs.* Vol.II. 2nd ed. Berkeley, CA: NatTrop Publishing, 1993:574-76.
11. Zava, D., C. Dullbaum, M. Blen. Estrogen and progestin bioactivity of foods, herbs and spices. *Biol Med,* 1998;217(3):369-78.
12. Naiman, Ingrid. *Cancer Salves: A Botanical Approach to Treatment.* Santa Fe, NM: Seventh Ray Press, 1999.
13. Ahmad, Nihal et al. Green tea constituent epigallocatechin-3-gallate and induction of apoptosis and cell cycle arrest in human carcinoma cells. *Journal of the National Cancer Institute,* 1997;89(24):1881-86.
14. Scientists learn how tea blocks cancer. *The Toronto Star,* Thursday, April 1, 1999:A14.
15. *Do You Have Cancer?* Patient pamphlet from Bio-Medical Center, Tijuana, Mexico.
16. Brinker, F. The Hoxsey treatment: cancer quackery or effective physiological adjuvant? *Journal of Naturopathic Medicine,* 1997;6(1):9-23.
17. Walker, Morton. The anticancer components in Essiac. *Townsend Letter for Doctors and Patients,* Dec. 1997:76-82.
18. Erichsen-Brown, C. *Medicinal and Other Uses of North American Plants: A Historical Survey with Special References to the Eastern Indian Tribes.* New York, NY: Dover Publications, Inc., 1995.
19. Dharmananda, Subhuti. Oriental Perspectives on Cancer and Its Treatment. *International Journal of Oriental Medicine,* Sept. 1997;22(3):119-28.

20. I owe the organization of these patent formulas to Timothy Mrazek, a third year student at the *Canadian College of Naturopathic Medicine*. His research paper was entitled "Treatment and Management of Breast Cancer with Chinese Herbal Medicine, with a focus on Chinese Patent Medicines," April, 1999.

21. Nanba, H., Maitake D-fraction: Healing and preventative potential for cancer. *Journal of Orthomolecular Medicine*, 1997;12:43-49.

22. Nanba, H., Activity of Maitake D-fraction to inhibit carcinogenesis and metastasis. *Annals of the New York Academy of Sciences*, 1995;768:243-45.

23. Nanba, H., Anti-tumor activity of orally administered D-fraction from Maitake Mushroom. *J. Naturopathic Med*, 1993;41:10-15.

24. Yamada,Y., H. Nanba, H. Kuroda. Antitumor effect of orally administered extracts from the fruitbody of Grifola frondosa (Maitake). *Chemotherapy* (Tokyo), 1990;38(8):790-96.

25. Nanba, H., Maitake D-fraction: Healing and preventative potential for cancer. *Journal of Orthomolecular Medicine*, 1997;12:43-49.

26. Activity of maitake D-fraction to inhibit carcinogenesis and metastasis. *Annals of the New York Academy of Sciences*, 1995;768:243-245.

27. Mizuno, T., H. Saito, T. Nishitoba, & H. Kawagishi, Antitumor active substances from mushrooms. *Food Reviews International*, 1995;111:23-61.

28. Stamets, P. & C. Dusty Wu Yao. MycoMedicinals: Information on medicinal mushrooms. *Townsend Letter for Doctors and Patients*, 1998;179:152-62.

29. Wang, S.Y., M.L. Hsu, C.H.Tzeng, S.S. Le, M.S. Shiao & C.K. Ho, The anti-tumor effect of *Ganoderma lucidum* is mediated by cytokines released from activated macrophages and T-lymphocytes. *International Journal of Cancer*, 1997;70(6):669-705.

30. Yang, D.A., S. Li, & X. Li, Prophylactic effects of Zhu LIng and BGG on postoperative recurrence of bladder cancer. *Chung-Hua-Wai-Ko-Tsa-Chih*, Jun 29 1994;(6):393-95,399.

31. Chang, H.M. & P.P. But. *Pharmacology and Applications of Chinese Materia Medica. Vol.1*. Singapore: World Scientific, 1986.

32. Ito, H., K. Shimura, H. Itoh, M. Kawade. Antitumor effects of a new polysaccharide-protein complex (ATOM) prepared from *Agaricus blazei* (Iwade strain 101) Himematsutake and its mechanisms in tumor-bearing mice. *Anticancer Research* Jan-Feb 1997;17(1A):277-84.

33. Ebina, T. & K. Murata. Antitumor effect of intratumoral administration of a Coriolus preparation, PSK: inhibition of tumor invasion in vitro. *Gan To Kagaku Ryoho* 1994;21:2241-43.

34. Sugimachi, K., Y. Maehara, M. Ogawa, T. Kakegawa and M. Tomita. Dose intensity of uracil and tegafur in postoperative chemotherapy for patients with poorly differentiated gastric cancer. *Cancer Chemotherapy and Pharmacology*, 1997;40(3):233-38.

35. Casura, L. "Mr. Medicinal Mushroom" An interview with mycologist Paul Stamets. *Townsend Letter for Doctors and Patients*, June 1998;(179):11-17,151-269.

36. Ghoneum, M. *Int J Immunotherapy*, 98;XIV(2):89-99.

37. Bardon, S., K. Picard, P. Martel. Monoterpenes inhibit cell growth, cell cycle progression and cyclin D1 gene expression in human breast cancer cell lines. *Nutr Cancer*, 1998;32(1):1-7.

38. Hang, J., M. Gould. Mammary carcinoma regression induced by perillyl alcohol, a hydroxylated analog of limonene. *Cancer Chemother Pharmacol*, 1994;34(6):477-83.

39. Jones, C. Lovely lavender holds compelling anticancer potential. *Herbs for Health*, 1998;Jan/Feb:17.

40. Ziegler, J. Raloxifene, retinoids and lavender: 'me too' tamoxifen alternatives under study. *Jour Nat Canc Inst*, 1996;88(16):1100-02.

41. Worwood, V. *The Fragrant Pharmacy: A Complete Guide to Aromatherapy and Essential Oils*. Toronto, ON: Bantam Books, 1990:328.

42. Essential Science Publishing. *People's Desk Reference for Essential Oils*. New York, NY: Essential Science Publishing, 1999:48

43. This set was sent to me by Nam Kaur Khalsa and was taught by Yogi Bhajan specifically for breast health at a birthday celebration for Sada Sat Singh in Los Angeles.

44. Adapted from a yoga set taught by Yogi Bhajan on Oct. 30, 1985 and published in *Physical Wisdom*, Los Angeles, CA: Kundalini Research Institute, 1997:8-9.

45. Khalsa, Gururattan K. *Transitions to a Heart-Centerd World through the Kundalini Yoga and Meditations of Yogi Bhajan*. San Diego, CA: Yoga Technology Press, 1988:73.

The Healthy Breast Diet

Exercises

Contents

In creating guidelines for a diet that protects us from breast cancer, I have considered many healing traditions. These include the macrobiotic diet as outlined by Michio Kushi, the Hippocrates health diet promoted by Ann Wigmore, the Gerson diet, the Hallelujah diet promoted by George Malkmus, Dr Joanna Budwig's use of flaxseed oil with sulphur-containing protein, food combining, an anti-Candida diet, rotation diets to improve immunity, and scientific research into the field of breast cancer. Although my recommendations are not true to any of the above traditions, they integrate some of their principles.

Each of us has a unique biochemistry, constitution, and dietary needs. In my naturopathic practice, I recognize that there is no one diet that suits all people. Some of us are fine as vegetarians; others seem to need animal protein now and then. Some individuals are reactive to carbohydrates, others to beans, tofu, or nuts and seeds. Raw food is easily digested by certain individuals but causes diarrhea or flatulence in others. Many of us gain weight easily and need to monitor our fat intake closely, while the lucky few may be able to feast on avocados with no weight gain. You know your body best and will be able to tell how it responds to a particular diet. Having said that, here is a breast cancer prevention diet. Adopt as much of it as agrees with you and listen to your body's needs if it doesn't. Work with a health professional to create a dietary program tailored for you using some or all of the recommendations below.

Organic Food

Eat organically grown food whenever possible, to be free of pesticides, herbicides, and organochlorines which can contribute to breast cancer. Organic foods have a much higher mineral content than non-organic foods. Cancer is partially a disease of mineral deficiency. One European study showed that organic farmers had over twice the sperm count as non-organic farmers. We can support planetary ecology through our food choices — the environmental toxins we use in food production are hurting wildlife, causing soil depletion, and contaminating our water and air globally.

▶ **Action for Prevention:** Call the makers of your favorite brands of foods and tell them you would like them to use organically grown crops in their products. Insist on an organic section in your local supermarket. Transform your lawn by growing your own vegetables in a front or backyard garden or push your city government into establishing community gardens. Many communities offer direct weekly deliveries from farms or organic food depots to your home. If you are so inclined, grow your own broccoli, red clover, alfalfa, and sunflower seed sprouts in your kitchen or grow lettuce in indoor window boxes. Investigate the principles of permaculture to transform our cities into green oases.[1] ◀

Vegetarianism

Consume a primarily vegetarian diet. Research shows that a vegetarian diet prevents 20–50% of all cancers.[2] The incidence of cancers of all types is 30–40% lower in Seventh Day Adventists, who are strict vegetarians.[3] The vitamins, minerals, fiber, and phytochemicals in vegetables offer significant protection from breast cancer, particularly when eaten raw. Eating lower on the food chain decreases the quantity of environmental chemicals that we ingest. The present trend to early onset of puberty in young girls can also be reversed when a vegetarian diet is eaten rather than the standard North American diet.[4]

Eat six to nine servings of fruits and/or vegetables daily, where one serving is equal to ½ cup of vegetables or one cup of salad or one large piece of fruit. A broad class of constituents known as phytochemicals work synergistically in fruits and vegetables to prevent breast cancer. Particularly good vegetable choices are those in the brassica family (see below), onions, garlic and leeks, sprouts, and sea vegetables. These should be consumed daily. Foods high in vitamin A are protective against breast cancer. These include orange fruits and vegetables and leafy greens. Women who eat only one serving of these daily have 25% more breast cancers than women who eat two servings daily. Other healing fruits, roots, and vegetables include cherries, apricots, asparagus, beets, carrots, celery, corn, cucumbers, figs, ginger, grapes, oranges, parsley, pineapple, potatoes, radishes, spinach, squash, strawberries, sweet potatoes, tomatoes, turnips, and watercress. Many fruits and vegetables are naturally high in anti-oxidants, which protect us from cancer.[5]

Cancer Fighting Phytochemicals

The following chart shows the 'phyto' or plant chemicals in common foods that are effective in fighting cancer.

Phytochemical	Effect	Food Sources
Allyl sulfides	Increases liver enzymes to detoxify carcinogens.	garlic, onions, leeks
Capsaicin	Prevents carcinogens from binding to DNA.	chili peppers
Carotenoids	Act as antioxidants that neutralize free radicals, enhance immunity, and high intake is associated with low cancer rates. They promote cell differentiation (cancer cells are non-differentiated).	parsley, carrots, spinach, kale, winter squash, apricots, cantaloupe, sweet potatoes
Polyphenols	Act as antioxidants; reduce damaging effects of nitrosamines. Kills human cancer cells.	broccoli, carrots, green tea, cucumbers, squash, mint, basil, citrus
Flavonoids	Prevents the attachment of cancer-causing hormones to cells by blocking receptor sites.	most fruits and vegetables, including parsley, carrots, citrus, broccoli, cabbage, cucumbers, squash, yams, eggplant, peppers, berries
Curcumin	Assists the liver in detoxifying carcinogens	turmeric
Isoflavones (genistein and daidzen)	Bind to the estrogen receptor so that harmful estrogens can't bind; block the formation of blood vessels to tumors, inhibit enzymes that might cause cancer; inhibits activation of breast cancer genes.	soybeans, tofu, miso, lentils, dried beans, split peas, garbanzo beans, green beans, green peas, mung bean sprouts, red clover sprouts (see chart on page 207)
Indoles	Induce protective enzymes, stimulate C-2 estrogen production. Decreases the estrogen that initiates breast cancer.	raw cabbage, broccoli, Brussels sprouts, kale, cauliflower, bok choy, kohlrabi, mustard, turnips
Isothiocyanates	Prevents DNA damage; blocks the production of tumors induced by environmental chemicals, act as antioxidants, assist liver detoxification.	mustard, horseradish, radishes, turnips, cabbage, broccoli, cauliflower, Brussels sprouts, kale, bok choy, watercress, garden sorrel
Limonoids	Induce protective enzymes in liver and intestines that fight cancer.	citrus fruits
Linolenic Acid	Regulates production of prostaglandins in cells.	flaxseeds and flaxseed oil
Lycopene	Protects from cell damage.	tomatoes, red grapefruit
Lutein	Protects against cell damage.	spinach, collard greens
Monoterpenes	Antioxidant properties, induce protective enzymes, inhibit cholesterol production in tumors, stimulate the destruction of breast cancer cells, inhibit growth of cancer cells.	cherries, lavender, parsley, carrots, broccoli, cabbage, cucumbers, yams, peppers, squash, basil, eggplant, mint, tomatoes, citrus
Phenolic Acids	Block the effects of free radicals; inhibit the formation of nitrosamine, a carcinogen.	berries, broccoli, grapes, citrus, parsley, peppers, soy, squash, tomatoes, grains
Plant Sterols	Prevent cells from becoming cancerous and lower fat levels in the body.	broccoli, cabbage, soy, peppers, whole grains
Protease Inhibitors	Block the activity of enzymes involved in the growth of tumors.	beans and soy products
Quinones	Neutralize carcinogens	rosemary, pau d'arco tea
Sulforaphane	Increases the ability of the liver's detoxifying enzymes to remove carcinogens. Acts as an antioxidant.	broccoli sprouts, broccoli, cauliflower, Brussels sprouts[6,7]

► **Action for Prevention:** Consume six to nine servings of vegetables and fruits daily. Follow a primarily vegetarian diet. ◄

Raw Foods

Eat foods rich in enzymes, namely raw fruits and vegetables, sprouted seeds and grains. Enzymes are destroyed at temperatures higher than 129°F or 50°C. Many vitamins are also destroyed through heating, as are the indoles in the brassica family of foods. Include at least 50–80% raw food, eaten at the beginning of each meal. When possible, cook the rest of your vegetables lightly, through steaming or the use of a slow-cooker. Consider the use of supplemental plant enzymes before meals if cooked food is the mainstay.

► **Action for Prevention:** Be sure that at least 50% of your vegetables are raw. Consume two salads daily at the beginning of your meals. If you cannot digest raw food, cook it lightly and use supplemental digestive enzymes. Use red clover, mung bean, and broccoli sprouts regularly. ◄

Beneficial Brassicas

Particularly potent healing vegetables include members of the brassica family, which are cabbage, broccoli, cauliflower, Brussels sprouts, bok choy, kale, kohlrabi, turnips, rutabagas, garden sorrel, radish, watercress, and collards. Experiments have shown that animals eating diets supplemented with vegetables from the brassica family develop far fewer breast tumors than animals that do not eat these vegetables.[8] A phytochemical in these called indole-3-carbinol enables the body to deactivate harmful estrogen more quickly, transforming it in the liver to a harmless form. Women who took pure indole-3-carbinol in supplement form for from one to 12 weeks doubled their production of C-2 estrogens (good estrogens) and reduced the amount of the cancer promoting C-16 estrogens (bad estrogens).[9] To prevent breast cancer, indole-3-carbinol should be taken in a dosage of 300 mg per day.[10] This is the equivalent to eating slightly less than ⅓ of a head of cabbage daily (which contains 400 mg of indole-3-carbinol). Indole-3-carbinol is present in cabbage juice as well as cabbage itself, so the simplest way to get our daily dose might be to juice ⅓ of a cabbage daily along with carrots and beets. To have the greatest effect, the brassicas should be eaten raw or only lightly steamed. Heavy cooking destroys indoles, negating their anti-cancer effect.

Two other compounds occurring in the brassicas are thiols and isothiocyanates, which are both sulfur-containing phytochemicals. Isothiocyanates help to prevent DNA damage and block the production of tumors induced by environmental chemicals. Sulforaphane is a particular isothiocyanate that increases the effectiveness of detoxification enzymes in the liver. It is highest in three-day-old broccoli sprouts.

For people with an underactive thyroid or goiter, caution is advised when consuming raw brassicas, although they are fine when cooked. In some people they may interfere with thyroid function. This is ameliorated in part by ingesting sea vegetables daily.

► **Action for Prevention:** Consume at least one half cup or about 14 oz of members of the brassica family daily.[11] Have coleslaw several times a week, add cabbage to salads, consume raw broccoli and cauliflower with hummus or other bean dips, and add broccoli sprouts to your main dishes and salads. Use fresh juices including cabbage, kale, bok choy, garden sorrel, watercress, or collards daily. Lightly steam kale, Brussels sprouts, and the other brassicas and have them as a side dish or mix them in a tofu stir-fry. Use the brassicas with seaweeds or dulse powder whenever possible. ◄

Sprouts and Cereal Grasses

Sprouts and cereal grasses are powerhouses of minerals, vitamins, and enzymes. Sprouts can be grown in your kitchen or purchased at supermarkets, while cereal grasses are present in many powdered green supplements, such as Greens+, Pure Synergy, and Barley Green, to name a few. All of these help to alkalinize the body, and are especially rich in beta-carotene. Toronto has a remarkable sprouting store called Super Sprouts (197 Spadina Ave, tel. 416-977-7796) where sprouts and seeds can be ordered regularly. Part of my vision for healthy cities includes greenhouse-sprouting depots every few blocks that supply sprouts to neighborhood homes.

Many sprouts contain significant amounts of phytoestrogens which protect us from breast cancer. These include mung bean, red clover, soybean, yellow pea, green lentil, chick pea, fenugreek, adzuki bean, alfalfa, and fava bean sprouts. Mung bean sprouts are highest with a 20-fold higher content of the phytoestrogen coumestrol than alfalfa sprouts. They also contain significant amounts of genistein and daidzen. Mung bean sprouts are a humble food. I have often overlooked them in supermarkets, as they lie heaped in bushel baskets in the produce section. They are inexpensive and versatile — you can use them in salads, stir-fries, mixed into bean and rice dishes, or juiced with vegetables. Clover sprouts contain high amounts of the phytoestrogens genistein and daidzen and are simple and inexpensive to grow at home.

Benefits of Broccoli Sprouts

Broccoli sprouts contain a constituent that is turned into a cancer-fighting agent called sulforaphane when the plant cells are crushed during chewing. Sulforaphane activates the liver's Phase 2 detoxifying enzymes, which protect us from environmental toxins. Three-day-old broccoli sprouts have the highest amount of sulforaphane in broccoli's growth cycle. The amount of sulforaphane available from only 5 g of three-day-old sprouts is equal to what we would get from 150 g of adult broccoli. Sulforaphane has been found to dramatically inhibit chemically induced cancers in rats.[12,13] We can provide ourselves with a natural form of chemotherapy by ingesting a few tablespoons of broccoli sprouts daily. We can even grow them in our kitchen laboratories! They have the spiciness of a radish and are delicious as a sandwich topping or mixed into a salad.

Seeds should be untreated with pesticides and organic. To sprout broccoli seeds, place 3 tsp of seeds in a glass jar with a wide mouth. Cover the seeds with one cup of distilled or filtered water and soak for 8–12 hours. Cover the mouth of the jar with a piece of cheesecloth or screen secured with a rubber band. Drain out the water and rinse the seeds again. Place the jar in a dish drainer upside down so the water can drain out. Rinse them three times daily, placing the jar upside down in the drainer after each rinse. Keep them near a light source to accelerate growth and increase chlorophyll. Eat after three days, or keep them refrigerated. Sulforaphane content diminishes each consecutive day after the third day of growth. You can prevent the growing sprouts from becoming moldy by using a wide mouth jar to increase air circulation, and by rinsing several times daily, being sure that they drain well. If need be, add a small amount of food grade hydrogen peroxide to the rinse water. Sprouts are more potent when consumed raw. Add them to soup, stir-fries, bean dishes, salads, and tofu dishes, have them on toast or use them in juices.

▶ **Action for Prevention:** Buy or grow your own mung bean, red clover, broccoli, sunflower, and alfalfa sprouts and consume them daily or several times weekly. Use them in salads, on top of bean dishes, added to stir fries, or mixed with vegetable juices. Aim for at least six cups weekly. Consume them at the beginning of the meal so that their enzyme power will assist in digesting your food. See the recipe section for details on growing various sprouts. For a great book on sprouts and sprouting, read *The Hippocrates Diet and Health Program* by Ann Wigmore. Consume 2 tsp twice daily of a cereal grass supplement, mixed in water or juice, such as Greens+ or Barley Green. ◀

Garlic, Onions, and Leeks

Garlic has been proven to inhibit the growth of breast cancer cells and helps prevent the initiation, promotion, and recurrence of many forms of cancer. Garlic is especially high in the trace minerals selenium and germanium, which reduce the risk of cancer.[14] It contains protective antioxidants, isoflavones, and allyl sulfides (see chart above). Garlic also shields us from many species of bacteria, fungi, parasites, and viruses especially when we consume at least 10 g or three cloves daily.[15] Garlic, onions and leeks contain sulfur bearing amino acids, which aid the liver in its detoxification pathways.

▶ **Action for Prevention:** Eat a raw onion and one to three cloves of garlic daily. Make potato leek soup when leeks are in season and freeze for year round use. ◀

Sea Vegetables

Eat sea vegetables daily. These include nori, arame, hijiki, kelp, dulse, and kombu. Sea vegetables offer some protection against radiation and breast cancer, are high in trace minerals, and are a very alkaline food.[16] They have long been used in Chinese medicine to dissolve tumors, particularly kelp. They contain substantial amounts of calcium and iron. They are also rich in iodine, an essential nutrient for the thyroid gland and one of the integral components of the Gerson therapy. Gerson believed that iodine inhibited the growth of cancerous tumors.[17] Ann Wigmore also included sea vegetables as part of the Hippocrates Health Diet for their high mineral content. With the farming methods used today, the soil and our foods are deficient in minerals such as iodine, zinc, and selenium. The Japanese, with their low rates of breast cancer, consume high amounts of tofu and sea vegetables.

Be patient and creative. For some people sea vegetables are an acquired taste. In our family, we frequently have a dulse shaker and a package of nori sheets on the table at dinner. We wrap the nori around rice or salad and sprinkle the dulse powder into soups and bean dishes. My six-year-old son loves to crumple up wakame and add it to his soup. Dried sea vegetables can be soaked in warm water for 10 to 20 minutes, rinsed to remove the salt, and then used in dishes. Aim for two tablespoons daily of sea vegetables, more if you have had higher radiation exposure. Use kelp tablets if you are not able to incorporate sea vegetables into your diet. Be cautious with sea vegetables if you have a hyperthyroid condition.

► **Action for Prevention:** A simple way to incorporate sea vegetables into your diet is by sprinkling dulse or kelp powder on your food and adding it to soups, juices, salad dressings, and bean dishes. Use it to replace salt. A side portion of soaked and drained hiziki or arame can become a regular part of your meals. Most children like to munch on nori sheets or dried dulse as snacks or have them with rice during mealtimes. Have two tablespoons of sea vegetables daily. ◄

Dandelion Root and Leaves

Get out there on your hands and knees and harvest dandelion greens in the spring and fall, and dig up the roots in the fall. Offer to harvest your neighbor's lawn, too, so they won't be inclined to spray. Dandelion root prevents and reverses breast cancer,[18] decreases estrogen levels, promotes bile flow, and reduces lymphatic congestion. In Chinese medicine, a relative of dandelion is used specifically to reduce hard breast nodules.[19]

The leaves are very high in vitamin A and minerals. Add them to salads and fresh juices, steam them and serve with lemon and flaxseed oil. Take them at the beginning of the meal to promote appetite and digestion. Make the root into a tea by boiling it with Chinese licorice. Use regularly in the spring and fall as foods and use in tincture form throughout the winter.

► **Action for Prevention:** Eat dandelion greens and root in season. ◄

Fresh Vegetable Juices

Drink freshly made vegetable juices daily. Juices supply vitamins, minerals, and phytochemicals that support good health. The Gerson Therapy Center in Baja, California, which regularly treats patients with advanced cancer, provides its residents with 13 glasses daily of various raw organic juices prepared hourly. They also serve three full vegetarian meals daily, freshly prepared from organically grown vegetables, fruits, and whole grains. Some vegetables that are particularly healthful juiced include carrot, beet, cabbage, parsley, watercress, asparagus, potato, tomato, bok choy, mustard greens, and kale. The staple for breast cancer prevention is two parts carrot, one part beet, and one part cabbage juice. Add the other vegetables for variety and as they are available. Dulse or kelp powder,

ground flaxseeds, citrus peels, garlic, ginger, and sprouts (broccoli, red clover, mung bean) can be added to vegetable juice combinations for greater benefit. Aim for two to three glasses of fresh juice daily as prevention, taken between meals or at the beginning of a meal. If you have breast cancer, include at least five glasses of fresh juice daily, using at least ⅓ of a cabbage throughout the day. When you drink several glasses of vegetable juice daily, your body will quickly detoxify, and must be supported in the cleansing process with the use of liver regenerating herbs and bowel cleansers or enemas. There are many kinds of juicers on the market today, the better ones being the Green Power, Green Life, Norwalk, and Champion juicers. The Green Power and Green Life juicers can be ordered from Teldon of Canada (800-663-2212).

► **Action for Prevention:** Consume freshly pressed vegetable juice two to five times daily, using carrot, beet, and cabbage as the base and adding other vegetables and sprouts for variety. ◄

Lycopene: Tomatoes, Grapefruit, Watermelon, Guava

Lycopene is a form of carotene and acts as a good antioxidant. Its structure gives a deep red color to the fruits and vegetables in which it is present, which include tomatoes, watermelon, pink grapefruit, guava, and rosehip. Tomatoes are by far the highest source, and approximately 85% of dietary lycopene comes from tomatoes and tomato products. Lycopene is more bio-available when tomatoes are heated and processed; there is five times more available lycopene in tomato sauces than in an equivalent amount of fresh tomatoes. Olive oil used in the cooking of tomatoes improves lycopene absorption. In the body, lycopene is found in the liver, breasts, prostate gland, colon, and skin. Studies have shown that it protects us from cancers of the breast, cervix, mouth, pharynx, esophagus, stomach, bladder, colon, and rectum.[20,21,22] The benefits of lycopene can be gained by drinking about two glasses of tomato juice daily.[23]

A little caution is necessary before we consume a lot of processed tomato products. People with arthritis may find that their joints are made worse by tomatoes. Tomatoes are slightly acidic, and may not be recommended for someone whose pH is already too acidic. The macrobiotic diet recommends avoidance of the nightshades, which include tomatoes. My suggestion would be to include tomatoes in your diet twice weekly generally, less often if you have arthritis, are overly acidic, or have an allergy to them. Lycopene is also available in supplement form, and the recommended daily dose is 15 mg.

▶ **Action for Prevention:** Consume tomatoes or tomato products regularly, at least twice weekly unless contraindicated by joint pain or allergy. ◀

Flavonoids and Limonene: Citrus Juices and Peel

A group of phytochemicals called flavonoids act as natural antioxidants and are widely distributed in plants. Citrus juices contain flavonoids that have been found to inhibit the growth and proliferation of breast cancer cells. The following chart outlines the effectiveness of citrus flavonoids in reducing breast cancer in animal studies.

Type of Citrus	Flavonoid	Effectiveness
Grapefruit	naringenin	effective
Oranges and lemons	hesperetin	more effective
Tangerines	tangeretin and nobiletin	most effective[24]

Citrus contains another phytochemical called limonene that inhibits breast cancer as well. Limonene is an oil that assists the liver in removing carcinogens and nourishes the production of digestive enzymes. It is found in highest amounts in the peels of citrus fruit, with the juice containing lesser amounts. Bitter orange peel has been used therapeutically in traditional Chinese medicine for hundreds of years. Limonene is also found in dill, lemon, caraway, and mint. Animal studies have shown that limonene can prevent breast cancer caused by environmental chemicals[25] and can shrink existing breast tumors. Ninety percent of tumors became smaller and the number of new tumors was reduced by 50% when animals were fed a diet containing 10% d-limonene.[26] A phytochemical closely related to limonene is perillyl alcohol, which is apparently over five times stronger that limonene in its action on breast tumors. It is found in high amounts in the essential oils of palmarosa, lavender and in cherries.

▶ **Action for Prevention:** Include freshly squeezed organic citrus juices in your diet regularly, or simply eat citrus several times a week, if not daily. Save the peels and as long as they are organic, grate a little over your salad or consume them in a tea daily. If you have a known allergy to citrus, avoid it. Drink mint tea regularly and make dill a familiar kitchen herb. Include organic cherries and cherry juice in your diet and use palmarosa and lavender oil on your skin. ◀

Fats

Over the last decade there has been much confusion about the role of fat in breast cancer risk. In the last several years, it has become clear that it is not so much the amount of fat that is the problem, but the kinds of fats used in our diets and the ratios that exist between them. Also of importance is the way in which they are both processed and packaged. We still do not know all the facts about fat and breast cancer, but approximate guidelines can be made based on what we do know.

Diets that recommend no fat will make us sick, for we cannot do without the two essential fatty acids: alpha-linolenic acid and linoleic acid. They are necessary for life and protect us from many illnesses. As a general rule, fats and oils should make up 15–20 % of our daily caloric intake,[27] with a higher ratio of Omega 3 to Omega 6 oil,[28,29] and some olive oil daily. Persons with cancer may need to take higher amounts of flaxseed oil until the cancer retreats.

Omega 3 fatty acids, found primarily in flaxseed oil, purslane, black currant seed oil, and cold water fish oils, protect us from breast cancer. The Omega 9 fatty acid, found in olive oil, is also protective. Omega 6 fatty acids, found in safflower, sunflower, borage, black currant seed, evening primrose oil, and other vegetable oils listed below, will promote an already existing breast cancer when they are used in excess without the balancing influence of Omega 3 fatty acids. Saturated fats found in meat, butter, animal products, coconut oil, and peanut oil increase breast cancer risk, as do hydrogenated and partially hydrogenated fats. All oils altered by processing are toxic. Processing includes hydrogenation, deep frying, refining, deodorizing, and exposure to light, heat, or oxygen during storage.

The Role of Essential Fatty Acids (alpha-linolenic acid and linoleic acid)

Our bodies cannot make essential fatty acids so we must get them from food sources. There are two essential fatty acids: these are alpha-linolenic acid, which belongs to the Omega 3 family; and linoleic acid, part of the Omega 6 family of oils. The best source of alpha-linolenic acid is flaxseed oil, but it is also found in hemp seed, pumpkin seed, soy bean, walnut, and dark green leaves. Linoleic acid is found in safflower, sunflower, hemp, soybean, walnut, pumpkin, sesame, and flax. Together these oils promote good health and help to prevent a wide variety of diseases. They maintain the integrity of the cell membrane so that it is less vulnerable to carcinogenic substances. They are the precursors for hormones and about 50 different chemical messengers called prostaglandins.

Prostaglandins are made by every one of our cells and progress down one of several pathways to either create disease or restore health. Prostaglandins regulate blood pressure and arterial function and play an important role in calcium and energy metabolism. They prevent inflammation and help to control arthritis. Certain prostaglandins inhibit cancer growth by regulating the rate of cell division and improving the function of the T-cells, the guardians of our immune systems.

Essential fatty acids are unique in that they attract oxygen, absorb sunlight, and carry a slight negative charge. Because of the negative charge, their molecules repel each other, causing them to spread out in a very thin layer over surfaces. This ability, called surface activity, allows them to carry toxic substances to the surface of the skin, intestinal tract, kidneys, or lungs where these substances can be eliminated. The negative charge allows them to bind to protein molecules. Essential fatty acids help transport oxygen from the air in the lungs to each cell membrane in the body, where the oxygen acts as a barrier to viruses, bacteria, parasites, and cancer.

Essential fatty acids also perform the following functions: they are able to increase the rate of metabolic reactions in the body when used in amounts higher than 15% of one's total calories, resulting in fat burn-off and weight loss; they are digested slowly and prevent hunger for as long as five to eight hours after a meal; they help transport excess cholesterol so that it does not clog the arteries; they help to generate the electrical currents that keep the heartbeat rhythmic; they are found around the DNA where they regulate chromosome stability, preventing damage from radiation and chemical toxicity; they are required in cell membrane formation; they are essential in the health of the immune system; they are required for brain development in infants and children and a deficiency during fetal development can result in permanent learning disabilities; and they can help to buffer excess acid in the body.

The integrity of essential fatty acids is easily destroyed by light, air, and heat. This is why the processing and packaging of them is so crucial. Refined vegetable oils are chemically changed and toxic. In their processing, they have been distilled at 300°F, bleached at 230°F, deodorized at 450°F, and preserved with chemicals. This processing alters the fat molecules, creating trans fatty acids which interfere with many bodily functions. Essential fatty acids should be packaged in opaque glass bottles

where there is no exposure to light, as light speeds up the reaction of the oil to air 1000 times, resulting in rancid oil. The processing should be done in an environment with no oxygen, as the oxygen breaks down the essential fatty acids, also causing rancid oil. Therefore, a usable oil will have to be pressed and packaged in the dark, with no oxygen, and stored in opaque glass containers, which exclude air and oxygen.

Fats to Avoid

It is too simplistic to tell women to avoid all fats as a method of preventing breast cancer, for there are fats that kill and fats that heal, as Udo Erasmus has described in his book of the same title.

Hydrogenated Fats

The process of hydrogenation, used in making margarine and vegetable shortening, can shift the shape of naturally occurring *cis* fatty acids, which are flexible and fluid at room temperature, into their *trans* forms, which are more solid. Hydrogenated fats containing trans fatty acids are toxic and increase breast cancer risk. Trans fatty acids interfere with immune function and contribute to poor health generally. Margarine contains 30–50% trans fatty acids. These are also present in potato chips, fried foods, French fries, and commercial baked goods, cookies, and crackers. The more trans fatty acids that are present in the diet, the more essential fatty acids are needed to repair the cellular damage they cause.

▶ **Action for Prevention:** Avoid all products that say "hydrogenated" or "partially hydrogenated" on their labels.[30] ◀

Saturated Fats

Saturated fats, found in red meat, milk, cheese, butter, vegetable shortening, palm and coconut oils, animal products and lard, are linked with a higher incidence of breast cancer. Saturated fats prevent the transport of glucose from the bloodstream into muscle cells, which causes blood sugar levels to rise. To compensate for this, the body makes more insulin, which increases breast cancer risk. Saturated fats interfere with the way our cells utilize oxygen. Cancer cells grow in environments where there is low oxygen.

Breast cancer is more prevalent in countries with a diet high in fat, such as Canada and the United States where most people derive 40% of their total calories from fat. The five-year survival rate of women with breast cancer in Tokyo, where dietary fat is reduced, is 15% greater than in Western countries.[31] When dietary fat is decreased, there is a subsequent decrease in circulating levels of estradiol and estrone.[32] Women who consume large amounts of beef and pork double or triple their risk of breast cancer.[33] These foods are also loaded with toxic chemicals and pesticide residues, since animals higher on the food chain accumulate these in their fat cells as they age. Although banned in Canada, DDT is found at low levels in fatty foods, especially dairy products.[34] Even organic animal products will have some environmental toxins, distributed to the water, soil, and plants from winds and rain. People whose diets contain meat and animal fat also excrete less of the protective phytoestrogens in their urine — either because their diets are lower in those protective foods or because meat and fat inhibit the bacterial conversion of the plant precursors to protective weak estrogens. This will increase breast cancer risk.

▶ **Action for Prevention:** Decrease saturated fat content to not more than 5 % of your caloric intake, or less than 7–10 g daily. ◀

An Excess of Omega 6 Fatty Acids

There are four types of Omega 6 fatty acids: linoleic acid (LA), gamma-linolenic acid (GLA), dihomogamma-linolenic acid (DGLA), and arachidonic acid (AA). Linoleic acid is found in safflower, sunflower, hemp, soybean, walnut, pumpkin, sesame, and flax. Gamma-linolenic acid is found in borage, black currant seed, and evening primrose oil. Dihomogamma-linolenic acid is found in mother's milk. Arachidonic acid is found in meats and other animal products.

We need some linoleic acid regularly, as our bodies do not make it and it is essential for health. Adding a small amount of sunflower seeds, sesame seeds, almonds, and pumpkin seeds to our diets supplies us with this oil, valuable protein, and minerals. Evening primrose oil containing GLA is very beneficial for many ailments, including fibrocystic breast disease, menopausal symptoms, eczema and learning disabilities.

Studies on rats suggest that Omega 6 oils inhibit breast cancer when used in amounts less than or equal to 1% of their diets. In higher amounts, they promote breast cancer when other causative factors are present.[35,36] If a tumor is present, they may encourage it to grow. In humans, all of the Omega 6 essential fatty acids may promote breast cancer and its metastasis when *used in excess without the balancing influence of Omega 3 oils and when they are improperly processed.* We don't know what the precise ratio of these oils should be, but Udo Erasmus recommends a 2:1 ratio of Omega 3 to Omega 6 essential fatty acids, present in his oil blend called 'Udo's Choice'. Omega 6

oils are commonly found in margarine, mayonnaise, and store bought salad dressings, and are added to packaged foods such as crackers. Their amounts have increased substantially in the North American diet in the last two decades, probably contributing to breast cancer incidence. One reason that Omega 6 fatty acids may be harmful in excess is that they are easily transformed into trans fatty acids through refinement and hydrogenation.

▶ **Action for Prevention:** Consume small amounts of Omega 6 oils in the form of raw unsalted nuts and seeds. These can include sunflower, sesame, pumpkin seeds, and almonds. Two tablespoons daily is a reasonable amount. Balance it with a higher amount of flaxseed oil. If you have cancer, do not use these seeds – take only flaxseeds and flaxseed oil until the cancer is gone. ◀

Fats to Use

Omega 3 (Flaxseed and Fish Oils)

Omega 3 fatty acids are divided into four subgroups: alpha-linolenic acid (LNA), stearidonic acid (SDA), eicosapentaenoic acid (EPA), and docosahexaenoic acid (DHA). Alpha-linolenic acid is the essential fatty acid found in flaxseeds, hemp seeds, pumpkin seeds, soy beans, walnuts, purslane and dark green leafy vegetables. Flaxseed is the finest of these, containing 57% of its oil as LNA. It also contains less than 20% Omega 6 oil as linoleic acid, the other essential fatty acid. Stearidonic acid is found in black currant seeds.

Eicosapentaenoic acid and docosahexaenoic acid are found in fish oils such as salmon, trout, white tuna, mackerel, sardines, cod liver oil, and herring oil. Because fish oils are often highly processed and can be contaminated with environmental pollutants, we should use them only if we are certain of their purity and quality.

Symptoms of Omega 3 fatty acid deficiency include growth retardation, poor vision, learning disabilities, tingling in the arms and legs, loss of motor coordination, defective glandular regulation, and behavioral problems. Omega 3 fats weaken the effect of estrogen on breast cells and balance the tumor-promoting effects of Omega 6 fatty acids when used in a ratio of approximately 2:1, Omega 3:Omega 6. The most benefit of the Omega 3 essential fatty acids is obtained when their amount is greater than the Omega 6, reducing both the progression and metastasis of breast cancer.[37,38]

In his book, *Fats that Heal, Fats that Kill,* Udo Erasmus states that flaxseed oil is the only oil recommended for cancer patients.[39] It helps to stop the initiation and retard the progress of breast cancer. It possesses anti-tumor qualities and is antimiotic (preventing cell division) and anti-viral. It has a toxic effect on cancer cells.[40] Flaxseed oil prevents cancer cells from sticking to other tissue cells, decreasing the likelihood of metastases.[41] Populations who consume higher amounts of Omega 3 fatty acids have lower breast cancer rates.[42,43] In studies on rats, Lilian Thompson and her co-workers from the University of Toronto found that flaxseed oil and flaxseeds reduced the growth of established tumors in late stage cancer.[44] Other studies have verified flaxseed oil's ability to suppress tumor growth.[45]

Flaxseed oil should never be used for cooking but can be used on food such as beans, grains, vegetables, and baked potatoes after they have been cooked. It can also be used on bread instead of butter. It should be used within six weeks of purchase and kept in the freezer (it will not freeze) or refrigerator between use. It is fine mixed with lemon as a salad dressing. If you dislike the taste of flaxseed oil, buy it in capsule form. Use vitamin E as a supplement to protect from oxidative damage when consuming essential fatty acids such as flaxseed oil. Vitamin B6 is required in essential fatty acid metabolism, along with other minerals and vitamins, and should be included in your diet or supplements in the dose of 50–200 mg per day.

In my family, we bring the flaxseed oil on to the table with dinner and frequently "pass the oil, please" from one person to the next. The five of us go through a bottle a week. Even my three-year-old won't start to eat his rice until it has flaxseed oil on it.

▶ **Action for Prevention:** If you are in good health, consume 1–2 tbsp of flaxseed oil daily, along with 2 tbsp of ground flaxseeds. If you have a degenerative condition, like arthritis, diabetes or cancer, take 3 to 5 tbsp of the oil daily with 2–4 tbsp of seeds. Individuals with cancer metastases can take 6 to 7 tbsp daily along with 6 to 7 tbsp of ground seeds daily. Six tablespoons of ground flaxseeds contain 2 tablespoons of oil. ◀

Omega 9 (Olive Oil)

The Omega 9 fatty acid (known as oleic acid) is found in olive oil. Olive oil, known as a monounsaturated fatty acid, provides protection against breast cancer. In Mediterranean countries where olive oil consumption is high, there are lower breast cancer rates than in Northern European countries.[46] Because olive oil promotes the flow of bile in the liver, and the bile carries toxins, it helps us detoxify the liver and gallbladder more efficiently. We can use extra virgin olive oil, purchased in a metal or opaque glass container, in moderation. It is best not to cook with olive oil, but to use it in salad dressings and on foods after they have been cooked, or on bread. One way to minimize the harm done to olive oil when it is cooked is to add 1–2 tablespoons of water to the pot before adding the oil. This will prevent the olive oil from getting too hot, as its temperature will not exceed that of the water. If the oil starts to sizzle and pop, it's too hot.

▶ **Action for Prevention:** Use a small amount of extra virgin olive oil daily. ◀

The Fat in Foods

The amount of fat a person should consume varies with age, weight, health, gender and level of physical activity, but generally an average man (25–49 years old) needs 30 g or less and an average woman (25–49 years old) needs 20 g or less. The ideal fats to use, in decreasing order, are flaxseed oil, extra virgin olive oil, nuts, and seeds. Avoid cooked oils, fried foods and hydrogenated or partially hydrogenated fats. Avoid or minimize saturated fat. The meat and dairy items in the chart are included for your interest only. They are not recommended. The following chart, compiled from information available from Health Canada, the Beef Information Centre, and various restaurants, lists the fat content, in grams, for popular foods. The asterisk * indicates only trace amounts.

Fruits and Vegetables

1 medium apple	*
1 medium banana	*
green salad	*
4 spears of asparagus	*
1 cup of green peas	*
1 cup of broccoli	*
1 baked potato	*
1 ear of fresh corn	*
1 sweet potato	1
1 slice of watermelon	2
5 olives	3
20 French fries, deep fried	16
1 California avocado	30

Dairy Products

1 cup of skim milk	*
of 1% milk	3
of 2% milk	5
of homogenized milk	9
2 cups of chocolate milk shake	12
½ cup of regular frozen yogurt	5

½ cup of 6% milk fat yogurt. 6
½ cup of 1.5% milk fat yogurt 2
½ cup of vanilla ice cream. 8
   of premium ice cream. 12
1 ounce of part-skim mozzarella 5
   of regular mozzarella. 7
   of cheddar 10
1 slice of processed cheddar. 10
1 ounce of ricotta 3
½ cup cottage cheese, 2 % milk fat 2.5
1 tbsp. regular cream cheese 5
1 tbsp. light cream cheese 1
1 cup ice cream with 10% milk fat 16
1 egg, boiled 6

Meats and Alternatives

Beef

3 ounces of inside round broiled 5
3 ounces of sirloin steak, broiled 9
   with fat rimmed 6
3 ounces of rib roast, trimmed 10
3 ounces lean ground, broiled 13

Chicken

3 ounces of breast, roasted. 7
   with skin removed 3
3 ounces of leg, skin removed 5
   breaded and fried 14

Pork

3 ounces of tenderloin, lean, broiled 4
3 ounces of center loin chop, trimmed and broiled 6
3 strips of side bacon, fried crisp 9

Fish

3 ounces of tuna, water-packed 1
   oil-packed 7
3 ounces of haddock, baked 1
   breaded and fried 7
3 ounces of sockeye salmon, baked 8

Processed Meats

1 ounce of turkey roll 2
   of regular ham 3
   of corned beef 6
1 ounce of summer sausage 9
1 wiener, beef or pork 11
1 wiener, chicken 7

Beans and Tofu

1 cup cooked kidney beans 1
1 cup cooked lentils 1

1 cup cooked split peas 1
1 cup cooked white beans 1
1 cup cooked chick peas 4
1 cup of baked beans with pork. 4
½ cup tofu, extra firm 14
1 tofu dog 1.5

Nuts and Seeds

½ cup nuts 35
½ cup pumpkin seeds 38
½ cup sunflower seeds 38
½ cup sesame seeds 38
1 tbsp. nut butter 8

Breads and Baked Goods

1 slice of whole wheat bread . . . . *
1 slice of white bread. . . . . *
4 soda crackers 1
1 bagel 2
1 medium bran muffin 4
2 small chocolate chip cookies. 6
1 croissant. 12
1 piece of apple pie 18

Cereals

¾ cup of bran flakes with raisins . . . . *
1 Shredded Wheat biscuit . . . . *
½ cup of instant oatmeal. 3
   ½ cup of plain toasted wheat germ 6
½ cup granola, homemade 17

Pasta and Rice

½ cup of long-grained cooked rice . . . . *
1 cup of spaghetti 1
   with ⅓ cup meat sauce. 5
¾ cup of macaroni and cheese. 13

Fats

1 teaspoon of margarine 4
1 teaspoon of butter 4
1 teaspoon of oil, all types 5

Fast Foods and Snacks

pretzels . . . . *
1 cup plain popcorn . . . . *
10 potato chips 1
1 doughnut, glazed 16
1 slice of pizza 16
1 beef burrito 19
6 Chicken McNuggets 20
poutine (20 fries with curds and sauce) 24
Big Mac 27

Calculating Your 15% Fat Allowance Exercise

To determine fat-gram allowance based on 15% of calories, multiply your average daily calorie intake by 0.15, then divide by 9 (since each gram of fat represents 9 calories). In the chart, find the average number of calories you eat in a day. Then look to see how many grams of fat should be your maximum intake to keep your daily fat calories at 15%. Consider flaxseed oil and flaxseeds as medicine and do not include them in your fat allowance.

Average Daily Calories	Allowable Fat (grams)
1200	20
1400	23
1600	27
1800	30
2000	33
2200	37

Fiber

High Fiber Diet

Women whose diets are high in fiber have 30% less risk of breast cancer than women who have very little fiber in their diets. Fiber is present in fruits and vegetables, legumes, grains, nuts, and seeds. East Africans, who have one of the lowest rates of breast cancer in the world, consume close to 40 g of fiber daily and eat no processed food. Their dietary staples include brown rice, potatoes, maize, and casaba.[47]

The outer fibrous coat of grains contains numerous vitamins, proteins, and minerals. We lose these when the grain is refined into flour. It is therefore much more beneficial to eat the whole grain rather than a refined flour product, such as bread, baked goods, or pasta. In your meal planning, use the cooked whole grains often and pasta and breads infrequently.

Fiber reduces the amount of circulating estrogen in the blood through at least six mechanisms and protects us in many other ways. Fiber reduces the recirculation of estrogen from the intestines to the liver and back into the bloodstream. Many plants and vegetables contain isoflavones and lignans which can be converted by bacteria in the bowel into weak estrogens that may compete with estradiol for receptor sites in breast tissue. A high fiber diet is less often associated with obesity, which tends to increase estrogen production by the body's fat cells. A high fiber diet usually has a lower content of fat and a higher content of antioxidant vitamins which may protect against breast cancer. Diets high in fiber and complex carbohydrates stabilizes blood sugar and improve insulin sensitivity, which is associated with a drop in circulating estrogen.[48] A high fiber diet modifies the composition of flora in the bowel to decrease the numbers of bacteria that can split the glucuronide conjugate, thus decreasing estrogen reabsorption.[49]

Other benefits of a high fiber diet are reduction of serum cholesterol. Women with high cholesterol are more prone to breast cancer. Fiber increases the feeling of fullness for a longer period, so there is less tendency to overeat. It reduces bacterial toxins and speeds up excretion of bile acids and toxins from the liver. Fiber speeds up elimination and decreases toxicity, while improving bowel disorders such as irritable bowel syndrome and colitis.

Types of Fiber

Fiber is divided into two types — soluble and insoluble fiber. We need them both. Studies show that the most protection is gained when we consume equally high amounts of psyllium (soluble fiber) and wheat bran (insoluble fiber) as opposed to either one by itself.[50,51] Together they decrease the enzyme beta glucuronidase, which is generated by intestinal bacteria and causes reabsorption of estrogen. One study compared the diets of 519 cases of confirmed breast cancer patients to the food intake of 1,182 women who had not developed breast cancer. Women with the highest fiber intake had a 30% risk reduction of breast cancer compared to those who consumed the lowest amount of fiber.[52]

Soluble fiber includes the following foods: bananas, oranges, apples, potatoes, cabbage, carrots, grapes, oatmeal, oatbran, sesame seeds, flaxseeds, psyllium seeds, and beans. Soluble fiber absorbs water and improves the motility of the bowel so that food moves more quickly through the intestinal tract. It also lowers cholesterol, triglycerides, and sugar levels in the blood.[53] Lower blood sugar levels are associated with decreased estrogen levels.

Insoluble fiber also improves the transit time required to move fecal matter through the colon, decreasing the likelihood of constipation. It absorbs little water. Insoluble fiber includes wheat bran, unpeeled apples and pears, tomatoes, strawberries, canned peas, raw carrots, bran cereals, whole grain breads, beets, eggplant, radishes, and potatoes.[54] Fiber is beneficial in that it encourages regular bowel movements. Regular elimination ensures that internally or externally generated toxins leave the body more quickly before being absorbed through the gut wall. Constipation increases breast cancer risk. One study has shown that women with two or less bowel movements per week had 4.5 times the risk of precancerous breast changes than other women who had bowel movements more than once daily.[55] Part of a breast cancer prevention program, therefore, includes encouraging at least two bowel movements daily, preferably three.

A high fiber diet also maintains the integrity of the intestinal flora, which is necessary for the health of the immune system. Specific intestinal bacteria (*Clostridia paraputreficum*) are necessary to convert the phytochemicals from soy and flaxseeds into weak estrogens that protect us from breast cancer.

You can incorporate a high fiber diet by eating a cooked cereal for breakfast such as oatmeal, quinoa, buckwheat, amaranth, rye flakes, 7 grain or millet meal with added wheat bran (which is better tolerated than wheat), and freshly ground flaxseeds. Wheat bran rather than oatbran has been found to be more beneficial in preventing breast cancer because it is highly insoluble and helps to draw estrogen bound to the glucuronide complex out of the body, preventing its release back into the bloodstream.[56] Wheat bran was found to significantly decrease the levels of estradiol and estrone circulating in the blood when used daily as part of the diet.[57] Oat bran did not.

Grains that can be included in lunch or dinner are brown or basmati rice, wild rice, millet, quinoa, buckwheat, barley, and kamut. Wheat (other than the bran) and corn are common food allergens, and should be used infrequently, perhaps once weekly, or not at all. Psyllium can be taken in powdered or capsule form for additional benefit and bowel cleansing. Beans are a wonderful source of fiber and can be consumed daily in soups, spreads, or with grain dishes. Fruit can be consumed by itself as an alternative to grain at breakfast, or as a snack between meals.

▶ **Action for Prevention:** Consume equal amounts of wheat bran (if tolerated) and psyllium daily, approximately one tablespoon of each. Eat 30 g of fiber daily, using beans, raw fruits and vegetables, and whole grains to do so. ◀

Beans

Beans are very high in fiber, particularly kidney beans. Dried beans, especially lentils, contain cancer-inhibiting enzymes that prevent the development and recurrence of breast cancer. Many beans contain phytoestrogens that are converted into active hormone-like compounds by bacteria in the colon, particularly fava beans, yellow peas, pinto beans, green lentils, garbanzo beans, black turtle beans, mung beans, adzuki beans, bush beans, navy beans, baby lima beans, black-eyed peas, and kidney beans. These competitively inhibit estradiol uptake by attaching to estrogen binding sites in breast tissue.[58] Diets high in soybeans, mung beans, and adzuki beans in Asian populations are associated with reduced cancer risks.[59]

▶ **Action for Prevention:** Consume 1–2 cups of beans daily, particularly soybeans, fava beans, yellow peas, pinto beans, green lentils, garbanzo beans, black turtle beans, mung beans, adzuki beans, bush beans, navy beans, baby lima beans, black-eyed peas, lentils, and kidney beans. ◀

Evaluating Fiber Content Exercise

Using the following chart, estimate what your daily fiber intake has been each day over the last three days. My average daily fiber intake is: _____ grams. How close do you come to 30 g?

Grams Fiber	Food Item
15 g	1 cup kidney beans
10 g	½ cup wheat or oat bran 1 cup split peas 1¼ cup lentils ¾ cup navy beans
5 g	½ cup cooked dried beans, peas or lentils 1 serving of a high fiber wheat bran cereal
2 g	1 serving of a fruit or vegetable 1 serving of any whole grain food 1 slice of whole grain bread ½ cup whole grain pasta ½ whole grain bagel 1 slice rye crisp bread ½ cup cooked brown rice
1 g	1 serving of refined grain

▶ **Action for Prevention:** Consume 30 g of fiber daily. This is equivalent to one serving of high fiber cereal, one cup of cooked beans, two pieces of whole grain bread, one serving of cooked whole grains such as brown rice, quinoa or millet and six servings of fruit or vegetables. Minimize flour products such as bread, baked goods, and pasta. Focus on whole grains instead. ◄

Phytoestrogens

Phytoestrogens are a varied group of substances with a chemical structure similar to estrogen. So far about 15 different phytoestrogens have been discovered in human urine. The two main classes of phytoestrogens are isoflavones and lignans. Isoflavones are found in soy products, some legumes and their sprouts, and several herbs. Lignans are highest in flaxseeds, pumpkin seeds, berries, some vegetables, and grains. Coumestrol is a less common phytoestrogen found in mung bean sprouts.

One of the effects of all phytoestrogens is to increase the production of SHBG (steroid hormone binding globulin), the transport system that carries estrogen in the blood before it attaches to a receptor. The more SHBG, the less estrogen is available.

Phytoestrogen Contents of Various Foods

The information in the chart on page 207 is derived from a study by the Finnish Medical Society called "Phytooestrogens and Western Disease, and "A Comparative Survey of Leguminous Plants as Sources of the Isoflavones, Genistein and Daidzen published in the *Journal of Alternative and Complementary Medicine.* The mean (ug/100g) isoflavonoid and lignan concentrations (after

removing the water content) of various foods is provided. These amounts will vary for each sample tested depending upon environmental conditions, soil quality, attack by pathogens, and genetic makeup.[60,61] (*Information on the coumestrol value of these sprouts was unavailable.)

If the chart on page 207 seems intimidating, focus on these "fabulous five" to get your fix of phytoestrogens.

Fabulous Five	Suggested Amounts
Flaxseeds, freshly ground	2–4 tablespoons daily
Tofu and soy products	½ cup tofu or 1½ cups soy milk daily
Raw pumpkin seeds	1–2 tablespoons daily
Clover sprouts	3 or more cups weekly
Mung bean sprouts	3 or more cups weekly

For about $2.00 a day, you can help protect yourself from breast cancer with these foods. Snack on pumpkin seeds, add them to salads or grind them with your flaxseeds and sprinkle over cereal. Find places to buy them fresh and keep them refrigerated until use. Experiment with growing the other sprouts high in phytoestrogens: pea, green lentil, chick pea, and adzuki bean sprouts. See the recipe section to learn how.

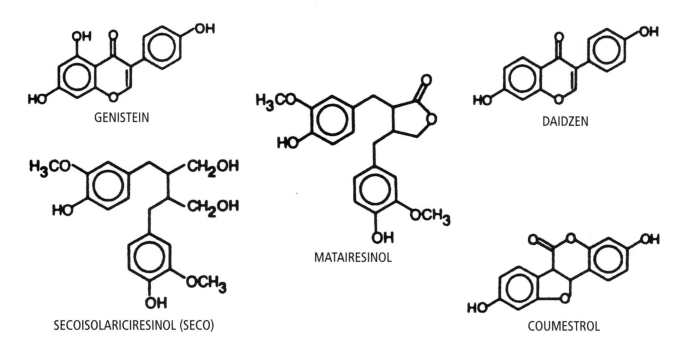

GENISTEIN

DAIDZEN

MATAIRESINOL

SECOISOLARICIRESINOL (SECO)

COUMESTROL

• Phytoestrogen Content of Various Foods •

Phytoestrogen	Isoflavones		Lignans		Coumestrol
Food Source	**Genestein**	**Daidzein**	**Seco**	**Mataresinol**	**Coumestrol**
Soybean Flour	96,900	67,400	130		
Kikkoman Firm Tofu	21,300	7,600			
Nasoya Soft Tofu	18,700	7,300			
Hatcho Miso	14,500	13,700			
Soy Milk	2,100	700			
Soybean Sprouts	4,290	6,270			low amount
Soybeans	241	376			
Flaxseeds			369,900	1087	
Clover Seeds	323	178	13	4	5
Clover Sprouts	11,000	7,360			high amount
Yellow Peas	458	4			
Yellow Pea Sprouts	6,150				*
Green Lentil Sprouts	3,340	1,650			*
Pinto Beans	223	232			*
Black Turtle Beans	451	4			
Small Lima Beans	401	4			
Large Lima Beans	344	3			
Red Lentils	250	52			
Adzuki Beans	212	46			
Adzuki Sprouts	1,300	910			*
Fava Beans	199	50			
Black-eyed Peas	233	3			
Wheat Bran	7	3	110		
Rye Meal			47	65	
Rye Bran			132	167	
Sunflower Seeds	14	8	610		
Oat Bran			24	155	
Chick Peas	76	11	8		5
Chick Pea Sprouts	4,610				*
Urid Dahl Beans	60	30	240	79.4	10
Mung Beans	365	10	172	0.25	2
Mung Bean Sprouts	1,902	745	468		1,032
Fenugreek Sprouts	910	2,310			*
Pumpkin Seeds			21,370		
Carrots	2	2	192	3	
Garlic	2	2	379	4	
Broccoli	7	5	414	23	
Cranberry			1,510		
Alfalfa Sprouts	730	720			51
Baptisia australis	35,070	3,400			
Glycyrrhiza sp.	5,190				
Japanese Green Tea			2,460		
Converted to:	Equol	daidzein	enterodiol	enterolactone	

Soy: Genistein and Daidzen

Soy products contain phytoestrogens which prevent the initiation, promotion, and recurrence of breast cancer. Along with flaxseeds, they can be thought of as a natural, non-toxic Tamoxifen. Two of the isoflavones found in soy are genistein and daidzen, of which genistein is the stronger phytoestrogen. Isoflavones act like weak estrogens (similar to the body's estriol) and bind to breast cell receptors so that the body's strong estrogens (estradiol and estrone) are blocked from doing so.[62] They are similar enough to estrogen that they can bind to the estrogen receptor on the breast cell but are too weak to activate the cellular DNA to initiate or promote breast cancer. They act paradoxically as anti-estrogens opposing the body's strong estrogens that might cause breast cancer, and as weak estrogens that have the ability to prevent osteoporosis. Soy products (particularly miso) protect cells from the cancer-promoting effects of radiation and chemicals.

Genistein is invaluable for its ability to help prevent and reverse breast cancer. It influences enzymes that regulate cell growth and division and has anti-oxidant properties.[63] Genistein inhibits platelet aggregation, which means that the blood is less 'sticky'. This improves circulation and oxygenation of tissues, protecting us from cancer, heart attacks and strokes. It lowers production of LH and FSH by the pituitary gland and decreases estrogen production by the ovaries in pre-menopausal women. Genistein induces apoptosis, or programmed cell death, which is a form of suicide by damaged or cancerous cells, and inhibits DNA topoisomerase II, helping to prevent cancer cells from multiplying. It also inhibits the formation of blood vessels that feed cancerous tumors (angiogenesis), helping to starve tumors of their blood supply. Genistein reduces the bioavailability of sex hormones, so that there is less circulating estradiol and estrone. It induces differentiation in cancer cells, which means they become more clearly defined, so that they are more similar to normal cells; and inhibits protein tyrosine kinases, which are enzymes that encourage the transformation of normal cells to cancer cells and increase their ability to multiply. Protein tyrosine kinases also activate breast cancer genes. Therefore genistein slows down or reverses the cancer process and deactivates breast cancer genes.

There is a lowered breast cancer risk in women who have high dietary intakes of the isoflavones genistein and daidzen, which intestinal bacteria convert to equol, and the lignans, secoisolariciresinol (SECO) and matairesinol,

which are converted to enterodiol and enterolactone, respectively. Enterodiol is then converted to enterolactone. Equol and enterolactone are able to bind to estrogen receptors and exhibit weak estrogenic activity while their precursors do not. Equol has a slightly higher protective effect than enterolactone as a phytoestrogen. Equol and enterolactone excretion in urine is significantly lower in women with breast cancer than in healthy women.[64] An Australian study found that women who excreted the highest amounts of equol had one quarter the breast cancer risk of women excreting the lowest levels of equol, while with enterolactone the risk reduction was one third.[65] Excretion is higher in vegetarians and highest in those who follow a macrobiotic diet. Those of us who consume a macrobiotic diet have approximately a tenfold higher excretion of dietary estrogens than those eating a typical North American diet.[66] A diet high in fat and meat significantly decreases equol production. Some people are unable to produce equol, despite soy consumption, or produce it in very low amounts.[67] This is most likely linked to the health of the intestinal flora, and an absence or deficiency in the bacteria that convert the isoflavones to equol and the lignans to enterodiol and enterolactone.

In Asian countries where breast cancer rates are at least two thirds lower than in Canada and the United States, the average consumption of soy products is 35–60 g per day. The urinary excretion of phytoestrogens in Japanese women, where breast cancer rates and menopausal symptoms are lower than in western women, is 20 to 30 times higher than in Finnish women.[68]

Of all foods, soy also has one of the highest amounts of the amino acid cysteine, which allows more glutathione to be manufactured in the liver and body. Glutathione is a great detoxifier and immune enhancer. Soy is able to protect us from cancer on various levels. Additional benefits of soy foods are its ability to lower cholesterol levels and to decrease the LDL:HDL ratio, which reduces our risk of heart disease.

The chart on page 209 outlines the soy protein content of common soy foods.

▶ **Action for Prevention:** Each day you should eat either ½ cup of firm tofu or tempeh, 1½ cups soy milk, ¼ cup soy nuts, or some combination of these, aiming for 35–60 g of soy protein daily.

Include miso in your diet several times a week, perhaps as miso soup. You may also supplement with quality soy protein powder, mixed with fruit to make a shake. Find soy products that are organic and non-genetically modified, since the common pesticides used on soy are ones that can promote breast cancer. Be sure your soy milk has no added oil or sugar.

Balance the high salt content of miso with high potassium foods eaten in the same day. If you have high blood pressure or kidney disease, have miso only once or twice per week. If you have a problem with candidiasis, avoid miso and minimize tofu until you clear the excess yeast from your body. The isoflavones in miso are more easily absorbed from the small intestine than those from other tofu products and lead to a higher urinary output of equol, meaning that miso exerts more activity as a weak estrogen than other soy products. This is because genistein and daidzen exist in miso in an unconjugated form, whereas they are conjugated and less bio-available in tofu, soy milk, and soybeans.[69] ◄

Soy Food	Soy Protein in Grams	Quantity Required
Miso	5.9	½ cup
Soy flour, defatted	47.0	½ cup
Soy protein powder	58.1	1 ounce
Soybeans, boiled	16.6	½ cup
Soybeans, dry-roasted	39.6	½ cup
Soy milk	5.6	1 cup
Tempeh	19.0	½ cup
Tofu, firm	15.6	½ cup
Tofu, silken	8.1	½ cup

Protection for Infants and Daughters before Puberty

Evidence suggests that short-term exposure to dietary isoflavones found in soy is especially beneficial for newborns and girls who have not yet reached puberty. This early exposure may increase the proportion of differentiated breast cells and decrease risk of breast cancer caused by carcinogens later in life. The diet of Japanese and Chinese women may confer part of its protective effect early in life.[70] We should introduce our children to moderate but not extreme amounts of soy products early in life, with higher amounts before and through puberty. There has been concern that infants exposed to a regular diet of soy milk and soy foods may be getting too much. However, a recent study found that although four-month-old infants were fed soy, there was an absence of equol in their urine. This means that they do not yet have the intestinal bacteria to convert genistein and daidzein to equol, so that the soy has a limited estrogenic action.[71] Pregnant women, on the other hand, would make this

conversion, and pass on the phytoestrogens to the fetus. Because soy products lengthen the menstrual cycle, they decrease fertility slightly. Therefore, we should be cautious about the amount of soy we consume while pregnant or when trying to conceive.[72]

► **Action for Prevention:** Be cautious about consuming high amounts of soy while pregnant or when trying to conceive. Give your children moderate amounts of soy early in life and higher amounts before and through puberty. ◄

Soy's Effect on the Menstrual Cycle

Breast cancer risk is in part linked to the total estrogen exposure and the cumulative number of menstrual cycles a woman experiences in her lifetime. Because of their higher consumption of soy foods, Japanese women have an average menstrual cycle length of 32 days as opposed to 28–29 days for North American women. In Japanese women, the follicular (pre-ovulation) phase of the menstrual cycle is longer than in Western women, resulting in reduced breast-cell division over their premenopausal years. As the length of the menstrual cycle increases, the duration of the follicular phase (pre-ovulation) increases, while the luteal phase (post-ovulation) decreases, causing less breast cell division over the premenopausal years.[73] Breast cells proliferate 2–3 times more rapidly in the luteal phase than in the follicular phase.

Thus, Japanese women have fewer menstrual cycles over their life span, have lower levels of estradiol overall, and are less likely to be diagnosed with breast cancer.

Soy Allergies and Thyroid Function

There are several reasons to be cautious when using soy products regularly. One of them is that soy is a relatively common food allergy. Dr Max Gerson asked his patients to avoid soy because many people had allergic reactions to it and because of its high oil content.[74] If you experience fatigue, bloating, and gas after eating soy, you may be sensitive to it or unable to digest it. We should avoid or limit our exposure to any foods to which we are sensitive or our immune systems will be affected adversely. If this is the case for you, avoid or limit your exposure to soy and use more beans, fish, or occasional servings of organic eggs, poultry and lamb as protein sources. Miso and tempeh are easier to digest and may be a better option for some individuals.

The second area of concern is that soy may have a negative impact on the thyroid gland. The phytoestrogens found in soy (genistein and daidzen) block an enzyme (thyroid peroxidase) that is responsible for attaching iodide ions to the amino acid tyrosine to form the thyroid hormones, T4 and T3. Instead, the iodide ions attach to either genistein or daidzen, causing a deficit of thyroid hormones.[75] When iodide is added to the diet along with soy, this effect on the thyroid is diminished substantially or eliminated.

Infants in particular, when fed soy formula without the addition of iodine or seaweeds, are more likely to develop autoimmune thyroid disease later in life.[76]

Alterations in thyroid function would result in a lowered basal body temperature and an elevation in TSH, the hormone from the pituitary that signals the thyroid to produce more hormones.

I believe that soy is an extremely beneficial food in breast cancer prevention and treatment, but it should be used judiciously with annual monitoring of thyroid function through blood tests and tracking body temperature. We must incorporate sea vegetables in our diets or take a kelp supplement regularly to offset the potential of soy and the raw brassicas for interfering with thyroid function. If soy formulas are given to infants, and the evidence suggests that they may protect infants from breast cancer later in life[77], then the formula should also contain small amounts of iodine or seaweed, such as kombu. The Edensoy brand of organic soy milk contains kombu.

Other Foods and Herbs with Genistein and Daidzen

Genistein and daidzen are found in the following foods in decreasing amounts: tofu, soy milk, miso, red clover sprouts, fava beans, Indian potato, yellow peas, pinto beans, green lentils, garbanzo beans, black turtle beans, mung beans and mung bean sprouts, adzuki beans, bush beans, navy beans, baby lima beans, black-eyed peas, and kidney beans. They are generally found in higher amounts in the sprouts and roots of legumes (particularly mung bean and red clover), being more concentrated in the root. We would do well to consume the living sprouts of these legumes on a regular basis.

Genistein is found in the following herbs in significant amounts: wild indigo, *Baptisia australis*, red clover, *Trifolium pratense*, licorice, *Glycyrrhiza glabra*, fenugreek, and alfalfa, being particularly high in *Baptisia australis*. Traditionally used to decrease liver stagnation, stimulate immunity and remove lymphatic congestion, *Baptisia* may become a staple ingredient in alternative breast cancer prevention and treatment. Red clover and licorice are

already commonly used. Phytoestrogens are also found in decreasing amounts in mandrake, *Podophylum peltatum*, bloodroot, *Sanguinaria canadensis*, thyme, *Thymus vulgaris*, yucca, turmeric, *Curcuma longa*, hops, *Humulus lupulus*, verbena, *Verbena hastata*, yellow dock, *Rumex crispus*, and sheep sorrel, *Rumex acetosella*.[78] Yellow dock and sheep sorrel are present in the Essiac formulas.

The highest source of genistein is the leaves of the plant *Psoralea corylifolia* or Indian breadroot. Although the roots and seeds are commonly used in Chinese medicine for skin diseases and as a tonic, the leaves of this plant can be quite toxic and carcinogenic.[79]

Bacteria, Antibiotics, and Phytoestrogens

We need the activity of certain intestinal bacteria to convert the isoflavones and lignans into weak estrogens. This conversion happens in the first part of the large intestine and is followed by recirculation of the weak estrogens from the large intestine to the liver. When we use antibiotics, the activity of the intestinal bacteria on the isoflavones and lignans is reduced or absent, sometimes for as long as one month after stopping antibiotic use.[80] If you are using antibiotics, your body is unable to convert the phytoestrogens into anything usable. *They will be ineffective in protecting you from breast cancer*. This is particularly important for women receiving chemotherapy for breast cancer who have also been prescribed antibiotics.

We can wonder if the higher incidence of breast cancer in North America and Northern Europe might also be linked in part to our overuse of antibiotics and the damaging effect that this has on intestinal flora. We have done to our bodies what we have done to the soil — used 'heroic' measures to conquer organisms while destroying the natural ecology that has existed in equilibrium through generations. We must replenish the balance of microorganisms in our intestines as we replenish the land upon which we grow our food. We can develop natural, less destructive means to control organisms in the fields and in our bodies without upsetting global and gut ecology.

▶ **Action for Prevention:** Use herbal medicines first before resorting to antibiotics when you need to fight an infection. Try to avoid antibiotics. If you must take them, use probiotics or 'good bacteria' while taking antibiotics and for a month afterward. Consider using immune enhancers such as astragalus, goldenseal and echinacea intermittently instead of antibiotics to protect from secondary infections. Generally avoid antibiotics unless absolutely necessary. ◀

Flaxseeds and Other High Lignan Foods

Lignans have been shown to have anti-viral, anti-bacterial, and anti-fungal properties. These properties help protect our digestive tracts from invading organisms and exert a sparing effect on our immune systems. Lignans also contain two phytoestrogens, known as secoisolariciresinol (SECO) and matairesinol. Like the isoflavones in soy, these are converted by intestinal bacteria to weak estrogens (enterodiol and enterolactone, respectively).[81] Enterodiol is converted by gut bacteria to enterolactone, which acts as the weak estrogen. Enterodiol and enterolactone have been found to stimulate the production of progesterone receptors, which would help to protect us from breast cancer.[82] Women with breast cancer excrete lower amounts of urinary lignans than healthy women.[83]

Vegetarians excrete more lignans than non-vegetarians, and vegetarian women who do not consume dairy or eggs excrete the most.[84] Flaxseeds contain hundreds of thousands more amounts of SECO than any other food studied so far. Ninety-five percent of the lignans are present in the fiber of the seeds, while less than 5% is present in flaxseed oil. Animal studies have shown that flaxseed was able to reduce the size of breast tumors by 67% when fed to animals with breast cancer, and was effective at preventing cancers induced by chemicals.[85] Lilian Thompson has found that women who used flaxseeds in their diets between the time of diagnosis and the time of surgery to remove a breast tumor were able to decrease their tumor size before the surgery.[86,87] Lignans are also found in smaller amounts in berries, fruit, legumes, pumpkin and sunflower seeds, some vegetables, and the outer bran of wheat, rye, and oats.

Flaxseeds boast a full complement of amino acids, being a complete protein. They act as a mild laxative and are high in fiber, soothing and healing the bowel wall as they encourage regular elimination. Flaxseed oil is extremely beneficial and protects us from all cancers, particularly when tumors have already been established. The Omega 3 essential fatty acid (alpha-linolenic) in the oil is the protective ingredient.

Flaxseeds also protect the heart, reduce LDL cholesterol, help insulin to control blood sugar more effectively in diabetics, and improve kidney function.

▶ **Action for Prevention:** Eat flaxseeds any way you can. Buy a small electric coffee grinder and add them ground to pancakes, muffins, cookies, breads, cereals, or even sprinkled in salad. Grind them daily so that the oil does not become rancid with storage. Freshly ground flaxseeds should be consumed within 15 minutes of grinding. Aim for two to four tablespoons (25–50 g) daily. If you have more than 2 tbsp. daily, you may need extra vitamin B6. They can also be mixed with juice. ◀

Mung Bean Sprouts and Coumestrol

Another lesser known phytoestrogen is coumestrol, which has a stronger estrogenic effect than the isoflavones and the lignans. Coumestrol is found in high amounts in mung bean sprouts, with lower amounts found in the sprouts of the following seeds: red clover, alfalfa, soybean, yellow pea, green lentil, chick pea, fenugreek, adzuki bean, and fava bean. Coumestrol is found in small amounts in the following legumes: chickpeas, urid dahl beans, and mung beans.

▶ **Action for Prevention:** Eat mung bean sprouts several times a week aiming for 3 cups weekly. Add them to salads, on top of bean dishes, mixed in juices, or munch them on their own. ◀

Protein

Not Too Much Protein

Protein should be sufficient but not excessive to prevent cancer in general, and needs to be combined with quality oils for optimum health. Although individual needs for protein may differ, the average adult requires approximately 30–60 g per day. More is required if you are very athletic or physically active, because exercise causes the body to use protein at a faster rate. High protein diets that encourage weight loss may promote cancer by causing excess acidity. Excess protein causes narrowing of the terminal capillaries, obstructing the transportation of oxygen, which then favors formation of cancer cell colonies. During the breakdown of amino acids in high protein diets by intestinal bacteria, toxins are produced in the colon, which are linked to increased cancer risk. High protein diets also cause more calcium to be lost, promoting osteoporosis. Adequate vegetarian protein would include 2 or 3 servings a day where one serving equals 1 cup of cooked legumes, ½ cup tofu, 2 tbsp nut butter or 3 tbsp of nuts or seeds. Legumes include kidney beans, soybeans, chickpeas, split peas, and lentils.

▶ **Action for Prevention:** Consume approximately 30–60 g of vegetarian protein daily. ◀

Sulphur-Bearing Protein in Combination with Flaxseed Oil

Sulphur-bearing amino acids include cysteine and methionine. Dr Joanna Budwig, who pioneered studies on fats and oils in the early 1950s, found that the combination of flaxseed oil with sulphur-containing protein prevented or helped to heal cancer. When sulphur-containing protein and Omega 3 oils are taken together, there is increased oxygen uptake in tissues. In order to prevent or reverse cancer, we need to increase tissue oxygenation. When protein is given to animals without quality oil, they die very quickly. Diets that are high carbohydrate and low in protein result in weight gain, as do diets that are high carbohydrate and high protein. When quality oils are added to the diet, better food utilization and energy production take place, and there is less weight gain. There is a synergistic effect between sulphur-containing protein and flaxseed oil that causes increased oxygen uptake.

Budwig analyzed blood from cancer patients and found they it lacked linoleic acid, which helps to form phospholipids that maintain the integrity of cell membranes. A deficiency of linoleic acid would prevent the formation of healthy cell membranes and cause incomplete cell division. She also found that cancer patients lacked lipoproteins, which contain linoleic acid combined with sulphur-rich protein. Their blood contained a yellow-green protein instead, which disappeared when she added linoleic acid and sulphur-rich protein. The red blood pigment, hemoglobin, appeared in its place. This explains why many cancer patients are anemic and lack oxygen and energy. Linoleic acid deficiency prevents hemoglobin from being made and the blood can't carry enough oxygen.

In practice, Budwig found that flaxseed oil (which contains alpha-linolenic and linoleic acid) combined with skim milk protein helped cancer patients. She claimed that linoleic acid reacts with sulphur-containing protein to form a new substance that is water-soluble and attracts oxygen from the air. Her mixture was 20 parts by weight skim milk protein, 8 parts flaxseed oil, and 5 parts milk to liquefy it.

The amino acids cysteine and methionine help to synthesize alpha lipoic acid from linoleic acid. Alpha lipoic acid is produced in high amounts by the liver and in lower amounts by every cell. It has the extraordinary ability to prevent damage to the cell at the genetic level. It is an excellent free radical scavenger and antioxidant, and enhances immune function by increasing the number of helper T-cells. It also decreases the toxic side effects of chemotherapy and regenerates the liver. By consuming foods high in the sulphur-bearing amino acids along with flaxseed oil, we maximize the amount of alpha lipoic acid our bodies produce and protect ourselves from breast cancer and many other ailments.

Because many of us are allergic to dairy, we can choose alternate sources of sulphur-containing protein, and combine them in our meals with flaxseed oil in approximately a 5:2 ratio. In foods cysteine is found in the form of cystine, which consists of two cysteine molecules joined together. The chart on page 214, derived from Jean Pennington's *Food Values of Portions Commonly Used*, lists foods that contain highest amounts of the sulphur-bearing amino acids, cystine and methionine.

▶ **Action for Prevention:** We should aim for 500 mg twice daily of sulphur-containing protein in combination with at least 2 tbsp of flaxseed oil daily. To prevent breast cancer, vegetarian sources are best, which include soy nuts, pumpkin seeds, sunflower seeds, oatmeal, beans, tofu and all soy products, broccoli, kale, kelp, and spirulina. Spirulina is an especially high source and is one of the main ingredients in Greens+. ◀

Low Sodium / High Potassium Foods

Sodium and potassium exist in a 'teetottering' balance in our bodies: sodium is present in the extracellular fluid, while potassium is found inside each of our cells. When one is low, the other will be high. If sodium levels are high, the body's cells swell and trap toxins. Gerson counseled his patients to restrict salt so that there would be less fluid retention and fewer toxins in the body generally. He believed that it was important to eliminate salt if one wanted to detoxify fully. One of the ways he encouraged elimination of sodium was through supplementation with potassium.[88] Potassium preserves alkalinity of the body fluids and encourages the kidneys to eliminate poisonous waste products. Excess use of salt will deplete potassium. Some foods with the best low sodium/high potassium ratios are navy beans, adzuki beans, caraway seeds, dark cherries, dried apricots, lentils, walnuts, oranges, almonds, apple, avocado, peaches, banana, grapefruit, pineapple, potatoes, soybeans, squash, tomatoes, sage, mint, and apple cider vinegar.[89] Walnuts, avocado, and almonds may be too high in fat for women who are overweight and should be used minimally in a breast cancer prevention program.

▶ **Action for Prevention:** Eat 3000–6000 mg of high potassium fruits and vegetables daily to help with cellular detoxification. ◀

• Foods That Contain Highest Amounts of the Sulphur-bearing Amino Acids, Cystine and Methionine •

Food	Cystine	Methionine	Total
Nuts and Seeds			
1 cup coconut milk	108	103	211
24 almonds	102	64	166
1 tbsp almond butter	43	28	71
47 pistachios (1 oz)	146	108	154
142 pumpkin seeds (1 oz)	85	156	241
½ cup dry roasted soy nuts	549	459	1008
1 oz sunflower seeds	128	140	268
Vegetables			
½ cup cooked broccoli	16	28	44
½ cup boiled Brussels sprouts	12	19	31
½ cup cabbage, shredded, raw	6	3	9
½ cup cabbage, boiled	14	8	22
½ cup chopped, boiled kale	16	12	28
Grains			
⅓ cup dry oatmeal	112	75	187
Beans			
1 cup boiled aduki beans	161	182	343
1 cup baked beans	157	218	375
1 cup black beans	165	229	394
1 cup pinto beans	152	212	364
1 cup chick peas	195	190	385
1 cup hummus	155	101	256
1 cup kidney beans	166	230	399
1 cup boiled lentils	234	152	386
1 cup boiled mung beans	125	170	295
1 cup boiled navy beans	173	238	411
Soy			
1 cup boiled soybeans	461	385	846
½ cup miso	131	206	337
½ cup tempeh	265	220	485
½ cup raw, firm tofu	275	255	530
1 cup defatted soy flour	757	634	1391
1 cup full fat soy flour	473	396	869

• Foods That Contain Highest Amounts of the Sulphur-bearing Amino Acids, Cystine and Methionine •

Food	Cystine	Methionine	Total
Dairy			
1 cup 1% fat cottage cheese	259	843	1102
8 oz 2% fat milk	75	204	279
1 large poached egg	144	195	339
1 duck egg	199	403	602
8 oz breast milk	48	48	96
Fish			
3 oz Atlantic cod	162	448	610
3 oz haddock	221	610	831
3 oz halibut	243	672	915
3 oz herring	210	580	790
3 oz lobster	196	490	686
3 oz mackerel	218	600	818
3 oz sockeye salmon	249	687	963
3 oz sardines	53	181	234
3 oz cooked shrimp	199	501	700
3 oz tuna (water packed)	269	745	1014
Meat			
99 g beef	167	441	608
99 g chicken	191	390	581
99 g lamb	207	471	678
99 g turkey	185	472	657
Other			
3.5 oz kelp	98	25	123
1 tsp barley, rye, or wheat grass	8	15	23
3.5 oz Spirulina	662	1149	1811

Potassium Content of Common Foods

The chart on page 217 outlines the potassium content of various foods. Review the chart and try to include at least 3000 mg of potassium in your daily diet. These values are taken from *Food Values of Portions Commonly Used* by Jean Pennington.

Shitake and Maitake Mushrooms

Shitake mushrooms are the top agricultural export of Japan. They have traditionally been used to treat cancer, rheumatoid arthritis, poor circulation, parasites, lack of stamina, and cerebral hemorrhage. Michio Kushi recommends shitake mushrooms as a regular part of a macrobiotic diet, and undoubtedly they account for part of the

• Potassium Content of Common Foods •

FOOD	QUANTITY	POTASSIUM CONTENT IN MG
JUICES		
Prune juice	8 oz	706
Carrot juice	6 oz	538
Orange juice	8 oz	436
Tomato juice	6 oz	400
Grapefruit juice	8 oz	400
Grape juice	8 oz	334
Pineapple juice	8 oz	334
Apple juice	8 oz	296
Apricot juice	8 oz	286
FRUIT		
Dried figs	10	1332
Papaya	1	780
Raisins	⅔ cup	746
Dried prunes	10	626
Canteloupe	1 cup pieces	494
Banana	1	451
Mango	1	322
Apricot	3	313
Kiwi	1	252
Orange	1	250
Pear	1	208
Apple	1	159
VEGETABLES		
Avocado	1	1097
Potato	1	844
Squash	½ cup	445
Sweet potato	1	397
Carrot	1 medium	233
BEANS		
Adzuki beans	1 cup	1224
White beans	1 cup	1003
Lima beans	1 cup	955
Tofu, raw, firm	½ cup	298
Soybeans	1 cup	886

• Potassium Content of Common Foods •

FOOD	QUANTITY	POTASSIUM CONTENT IN MG
BEANS (continued)		
Soymilk	1 cup	338
Soy meal, defatted	1 cup	3038
Black turtle beans	1 cup	801
Pinto beans	1 cup	800
Lentils	1 cup	731
Kidney beans	1 cup	714
Great northern beans	1 cup	692
Navy beans	1 cup	669
Black beans	1 cup	611
Mung beans	1 cup	536
Chick peas	1 cup	477
GRAINS		
Dark rye flower	1 cup	1101
Carob powder	1 cup	852
Pearl barley	1 cup	320

success that some macrobiotic practitioners have had in reversing cancer. Maitake mushrooms are also extremely beneficial for breast health and are delicious.

An experimental medicine called Lentinan has been made from shitake mushrooms and used in treating advanced cancer patients. It increases numbers of macrophages, T-killer cells and T-helper cells, and prolongs the lives of some cancer patients.[90] It improves the helper-suppressor ratio and significantly lowers the level of T-suppressor cells when used for four weeks duration. This effect is lost by eight weeks, implying that we should use shitake mushrooms for one month and then take a break before continuing their use. An extract of shitake has demonstrated ability to inhibit breast cancer in women.[91] When mice with breast cancer were given shitake extracts that composed 20% of their feed, there was a 78.6 tumor inhibition rate.[92] Other health benefits derived from intake of extracts of shitake include lowered cholesterol levels, improved liver function in patients with hepatitis B, and improvement of candidiasis symptoms in AIDS patients.

For health maintenance we can consume three to four mushrooms a day for a month at a time,[93] taking a break for a week and then including them in our diets again.

If this is unaffordable or impractical for you, try to include them in your diet at least twice weekly or use them in tea or tincture form. They are available fresh in some supermarkets and dried in Chinese herbal stores.

Last night's dinner at my house included shitake mushrooms freshly harvested from right beside the kitchen sink. (Where the clover and broccoli sprouts were growing last month.) My husband has become a kitchen mushroom farmer, and we delight in the marvelous fecundity of these delicacies as they magically appear out of 'the blob'. We've made a pact — I do the sprouts, he does the mushrooms.

Shitake and Maitake growing kits, tinctures and teas can be ordered from Fungi Perfecti (PO Box 7634, Olympia, WA 98507, tel. 800-780-9126 or 360-426-9292, fax. 360-426-9377, E-mail: mycomedia@aol.com., web site: http://www.fungi.com.) In Canada, fresh mushrooms and growing kits can be ordered from Wylie Mycologicals (RR#1 Wiarton, ON N0H 2T0, tel. 519-534-1570, fax. 519-534-9145, E-mail: wylie@interlog.com.)

▶ **Action for Prevention:** Eat shitake mushrooms daily (or at least twice weekly) for a month followed by a seven-day break. Buy them fresh, dried, or as a tea. Use them in stir-fries, sandwich spreads, casseroles, and soups. ◀

Your Kitchen Pharmacy

Turmeric

Turmeric powder has been traditionally used as a spice in East Indian cookery, and as a medicinal in Traditional Chinese Medicine as well as Ayurvedic medicine. It has antioxidant, anti-tumor and anti-inflammatory activity.[94] It stimulates bile production in the liver, improves the ability of liver enzymes to detoxify, relieves intestinal gas, is cleansing to the blood and skin, and may be helpful in treating epilepsy and arthritis. It has a cooling effect and breaks up stagnation in the liver.[95]

Curcumin, the main active ingredient in turmeric, is thought to prevent the formation of a blood supply to cancerous tumors so that they aren't able to grow.[96,97] Researchers have found that curcumin reduces the growth of both hormone-dependent and hormone-independent breast cancer cells, as well as cells that were resistant to chemotherapy.[98] Recently, it has been found that curcumin is helpful in protecting breast cells from the effects of cancer-inducing pesticides such as chlordane and endosulfan. We now know that there is a synergistic estrogenic effect arising from the use of a combination of pesticides, sometimes causing them to be a thousand times more toxic than if used individually.[99] Both curcumin and genistein (derived from soy) were able to reduce the proliferation of breast cancer cells caused by estrogenic pesticides or estradiol. When used together, curcumin and genistein were able to completely inhibit cell growth caused by the mixture of pesticides or estradiol. They demonstrated a synergistic action together greater than the sum of their actions individually.[100]

This is great news. We can protect ourselves to some degree from the harmful effects of pesticides by using a combination of turmeric and soy regularly in our diets.

▶ **Action for Prevention:** Have one teaspoon of turmeric powder daily, or supplement with curcumin. Sauté onions, ginger, and garlic in water and olive oil and add turmeric before adding other ingredients for a stir-fry. Use a little in a tofu sandwich spread and add it to soup and bean dishes or boil it with basmati rice. ◀

Rosemary and Sage

Rosemary and sage contain the essential oil eucalyptol, which helps to kill Candida albicans, bacteria, and worms. Rosemary stimulates digestion, promotes bile flow, and cleanses the liver and kidneys. Rosemary contains a phytochemical called a quinone that acts to neutralize carcinogens. It blocks the initiation of cancer, interfering with the transformation of normal cells to cancer cells. It is more effective if taken with oil. Add rosemary to your salad dressing.

An extract of rosemary leaves increased the 2-hydroxylation of estradiol and estrone by 150% in mice to form more of the 'good' C-2 estrogen and decreased the formation of the 'bad' C-16 estrogen by 50%. It also increased the linking of estradiol and estrone to form the glucuronide complex in the liver, allowing estrogen to be eliminated more effectively.[101]

A while ago I was able to buy a large potted rosemary plant which now resides on my front porch. I have developed the habit of snatching a few leaves before lunch and dinner and adding them to salads, tofu dishes, soups, etc. I have begun also to use the essential oil of rosemary in my bath and add it to almond oil as a skin moisturizer. Simple healing practices.

Sage is a glandular balancer and immune tonic but should be avoided while pregnant. When you heat these two herbs at 200°F for longer than 20 minutes, their potency is lost. Add them to your foods after they are cooked, just before eating.[102]

Thyme

Thyme stimulates digestion and relieves intestinal fermentation. It improves energy, restores the glandular and immune systems, and is a tonic to the nervous system. It helps to antidote toxins and clears parasites. Thyme is useful to combat bacterial, viral, and fungal infections, including candidiasis. It should not be used while pregnant or for those with a hyperactive thyroid.[103]

Ginger

Ginger is a digestive tonic, immune stimulant, tonic to the nervous system and aids detoxification of toxins. It should not be used in early pregnancy, during labor, or in someone with excessive internal heat.

▶ **Action for Prevention:** To improve digestion, maintain the health of the intestines and protect from parasites, use rosemary, sage, thyme and ginger regularly to season your foods. ◀

Rotate Your Foods

When we eat the same foods day after day we can develop sensitivities to them which may result in weakened immunity. Food sensitivities can manifest as headaches, chronic ear, eye, or throat infections, fatigue, digestive upsets, arthritis, allergies, asthma, persistent cough, chronic congestion, nausea, abdominal cramps, irritability, hyper-activity, insomnia, palpitations, eczema, itching skin, joint pain, edema, frequent urination, depression, and learning disabilities. The most common food sensitivities are to dairy, wheat, Brewer's and bakers yeast, eggs, sugar, peanuts, citrus, corn, and tomatoes. Many people react to foods that are healthy but which they have overused. An accurate test for food sensitivities is the ELISA blood test, which measures immunoglobulin response to specific foods. It can be ordered through your naturopathic or medical doctor from Immuno Laboratories (800-231-9197). Generally, a period of avoidance of from three to six months for the foods you are sensitive to plus a five-day rotation diet help to restore digestive and immune health.

▶ **Action for Prevention:** To follow a five-day rotation diet, prepare a diet plan where you attempt to eat a particular food only once every five days, with the exception of the 'fabulous five' phytoestrogens, the brassicas, flaxseed oil, and garlic. Eat these daily unless you have reason to believe that you are reacting negatively to them. Rotate your grains and beans. Tofu and soy products can also provoke sensitivities in some people. If you experience any of the above symptoms after ingesting frequent amounts of soy products, then decrease soy consumption to every four days rather than having it daily. Use some of the other foods and herbs containing phytoestrogens instead of relying on soy. Avoid known food sensitivities. ◀

Foods with a Low Glycemic Index

When we have higher amounts of insulin and IGF-1 in our blood, we are three to seven times more prone to breast cancer. Carbohydrates are broken down into glucose, a form of sugar that provides energy to our cells. Certain carbohydrates dramatically raise blood sugar levels after we eat them, which in turn elevates insulin levels. The degree to which a carbohydrate raises blood sugar two to three hours after eating is called its glycemic index and has been measured for different foods.

The pancreas secretes insulin into the blood in response to elevated blood glucose levels. Insulin's job is to move into the cell and facilitate the transport of glucose from the blood into the cell for energy production. The trace mineral chromium enhances insulin's ability to enter the cell. Insulin also helps to move other nutrients such as vitamins, minerals, and amino acids into the cell. A diet high in carbohydrates with a high glycemic index will cause consistently high blood levels of insulin (and IGF-1), which leads to increased fat deposition. Increased fat storage means increased estrogen, since fat cells help to make a particular form of estrogen. Together, the combination of estrogen and IGF-1 strongly promotes breast cancer.

If we consistently eat foods that trigger hypersecretion of insulin we may develop what is known as 'insulin resistance', whereby insulin does not enter the cell. This causes the pancreas to produce higher amounts of insulin, and insulin, glucose, vitamins, minerals, and amino acids will remain outside of our cells, rather than nourishing them. Eventually this can lead to diabetes. Weight loss, regular exercise, chromium, alpha lipoic acid, and flaxseed oil help to improve insulin resistance.

Some carbohydrates do not elevate blood sugar levels. Generally, we should eat carbohydrates with a low glycemic index and avoid or minimize those with a high glycemic index. If we do eat foods in the high category, by combining them with either fiber, healthy fats, or protein we will cause a less dramatic rise in blood sugar. Foods high in fat or protein don't cause elevations in blood sugar, and fiber slows down the rise in blood sugar levels. Fiber, quality oils, and protein also contribute to a feeling of satiety after eating, and decrease cravings and the tendency to overeat.

The chart on page 222 demonstrates the glycemic index of various foods. The numbers refer to how fast the carbohydrate of a particular food is converted to glucose and enters the bloodstream, and are compared to the action of glucose itself. On the scale, glucose equals 100, so anything above 100 raises blood sugar faster than glucose, and any food below 100 does it that much slower. The amount of food used for the test depends on its carbohydrate content – the quantity used contains 50 grams of carbohydrate.

These are relative numbers, based on averages. Since the glycemic index measures a physiological response, it will vary from person to person and the numbers tend to increase as we age. Most of these values are extrapolated from the book The G.I. Factor: *The Glycaemic Index Solution* by Dr Jennie Brand Miller, Kaye Foster-Powell and Dr Stephen Colagiuri.[104]

▶ **Action for Prevention:** Let most of your diet consist of foods with a low glycemic index. If you do consume foods from the high category, combine them with fiber, healthy oils such as flaxseed and olive oil, or protein. ◀

• The Glycemic Index of Various Foods •

Low Glycemic Index		Medium Glycemic Index		High Glycemic Index	
7–45		*46–60*		*61–115*	
Grains & Pasta					
Burgen Soy Lin Bread	19	Macaroni	46	Rye Bread	64
Pearl Barley	25	Linguini	46	Semolina Bread	64
Rice Bran	27	Bulgur	47	Couscous	65
Chick Pea Flour Chapati	27	Red River Cereal	49	Rolled Barley	66
Fettucine	32	Pumpernickel Bread	50	Crackers	67
Vermicelli	35	Cracked Barley	50	Gnocchi	67
Spaghetti	6	Special K	54	Taco Shells	68
Whole Rye	37	Corn	55	Cornmeal	69
Barley Kernel Bread	39	Brown Rice	55	Melba Toast	70
Wheat Bran	42	Oatbran	55	Cream of Wheat	70
Barley Chapati	43	Buckwheat	55	Shredded Wheat	70
		Linseed Rye Bread	55	White Flour Products	71
		Popcorn	55	English Muffins	71
		Muesli	56	Millet	71
		Wild Rice	57	White Bagels	72
		Pita Bread, White	57	Puffed Wheat	74
		White Rice	58	Cheerios	74
		Rice Vermicelli	58	Puffed Cereals	74
		Oatmeal	60	Rice Cakes	77
				Rice Krispies	82
				Corn Chips and Cornflakes	83
				Brown Rice Pasta	92
				French Baguette	95
Beans					
Chana Daal	18	Romano Beans	46	Broad Beans (fava)	79
Soybeans	17	Baked beans	48		
Red Lentils	25				
Kidney Beans	29				
Green Lentils	29				
Butter Beans	30				
Black Beans	31				
Chick Peas	33				
Navy Beans	38				
Mung Beans	38				
Pinto Beans	38				
Black-eyed Beans	41				

• The Glycemic Index of Various Foods •

Low Glycemic Index		Medium Glycemic Index		High Glycemic Index	
Protein					
Plain Yogurt	14			Ice Cream	61
Nuts	15				
Skim Milk	32				
Fruit					
Cherries	22	Canned Peaches	47	Raisins	64
Grapefruit	25	Orange Juice	52	Pineapple	66
Dried Apricot	31	Kiwi	53	Dried Fruit	70
Pear	37	Banana	54	Watermelon	72
Plum	38	Mango	56		
Apple	38	Blueberry	57		
Peach	42				
Orange	44				
Vegetables					
Peas	<15	Raw carrots	49	Beets	64
Green Beans	<15	Yams	51	Mashed Potatoes	70
Tomato	<15	Sweet Potatoes	54	Rutabaga	72
Brassica Family	<15	White Potatoes, Boiled	56	French Fries	75
Sea vegetables	<15			Pumpkin	75
Herbs	<15			Cooked Carrots	85
Powdered Greens	<15			Parsnips	98
Green Vegetables	<15				
Other					
Fructose	22	Lactose	46	Sucrose	65
Stevia N/A		Chocolate	49	Soft Drinks	68
Licorice Root N/A		Honey	58	Glucose	100
				Maltose	105
				Alcohol	>100

Foods to Avoid

In addition to the fats we should avoid in our diet, there are other food groups that should be consumed in small amounts, if at all.

Meat

Due to its high saturated fat content, presence of pesticides, organochlorines, antibiotics, and hormones, and slow transit time, which allows for more fermentation and putrefaction in the digestive tract, red meat should be avoided. Meat is difficult to digest and decreases the utilization of plant estrogens that might protect us from breast cancer. A high meat diet promotes the growth of a specific intestinal bacteria that causes more reabsorption of estrogen through the intestinal wall. Avoid beef, pork, ham, bacon, liver, and processed meats. A breast cancer prevention diet is a meatless diet. However, some women feel better when they consume meat, either because it suits their blood type or is helpful for hypoglycemic symptoms. If you are one of these women and don't feel well on a vegetarian diet, use organic poultry or lamb sparingly, perhaps once weekly. Use instead tofu, beans, sea vegetables, and a few nuts and seeds as protein sources.

Fish

Be cautious with fish. Although fish oils have been found to protect from breast cancer, fish act as reservoirs of toxic environmental chemicals that circulate on global air currents and fall into our rivers and oceans as rain. Organochlorines such as PCBs, lindane, DDT, and dioxins accumulate in the oil of fish from polluted ocean waters.[105] Dioxins, which are extremely carcinogenic, have been found in the bodies of fish at concentrations 159,000 times higher than the water they swim in.[106,107,108] Similarly, a 10,000 times greater concentration of PCBs is found in fish tissues than in their surrounding waters.[109] Fish breathe through their gills. With each flap of their gills, they filter the surrounding water and any toxic residues accumulate in their fat as they do so. We won't drink the water they swim in, so why would we eat the fish?

Children whose mothers consumed Lake Ontario fish only twice monthly while pregnant displayed learning disabilities and lower IQ levels than children whose mothers had not eaten the same fish.[110] Fish contain high amounts of PCBs, which interfere with thyroid function. These children had trouble with short and long term memory, and suffered with reading difficulties and attention deficit disorder. The most highly exposed children had a decrease of 6.2 IQ points, which was still present at age 11.[111] The wildlife that are most affected by hormone disrupting chemicals are ones that consume fish (polar bears, herring gulls, seals, otters, beluga whales) or fish themselves. The effects are particularly damaging to the native communities around the Great Lakes and coastal waters and the Inuit, who rely on fish as a dietary staple. More than ever, the indigenous peoples need their sweat lodges and saunas to prevent chemical toxicity in their children and subsequent generations. We all do.

In 1997, three times more salmon grown on fish farms were sold to Canadians than wild salmon. This means that most of the salmon we buy has been genetically manipulated, born in a plastic tray, vaccinated, often treated with antibiotics, fed a bright red dye and doused with pesticides before making it into our mouths. Fish don't come with labels so we are unsure if the ones we're eating are wild or farmed. Salmon farms wreak environmental havoc on nearby ocean beds and make it difficult for fisherman to eke a living when fish prices drop.[112]

Although fish have often been recommended as part of a breast cancer prevention diet due to their Omega-3 oils, I cannot include them here. Michio Kushi also advises avoidance of fish as part of a breast cancer prevention plan, unless there is a strong craving for them. Then he suggests a small amount of white-meat fish, no more than once weekly.[113] I leave it up to your discretion to use the following fish sparingly, if at all — salmon, haddock, trout, sardines, herring, and cod. Be cautious of eating fish if one day you hope to conceive. If you have breast cancer, do not eat fish.

▶ **Action for Prevention:** Avoid fish, unless you know it is not contaminated with chemicals, and then have it seldom. Eat fish no more than once weekly and only if you crave it. Try to find fish from clean waters. Use flaxseed oil to obtain Omega 3 fatty acids. If you have breast cancer, do not eat fish. ◀

Dairy

The dairy industry has succeeded in convincing most people that we cannot survive without milk products for their calcium value. Although dairy products are high in calcium, they come at a cost that is not worth the gain. Dairy products are reservoirs of environmental toxins, are difficult to digest, and many people's immune systems are stressed by them.

Cows are treated with hormones and antibiotics and are fed grains that may have been sprayed with pesticides. These accumulate in the fat of the cow over its life span and are discharged into its milk. We ingest these when we consume dairy products and accumulate them in our tissues over our life spans, passing them on to our children in utero and when we breast-feed. Animal studies have shown that environmental toxins from one mother will be passed on into the tissues of offspring five generations later. Thus there is a generational magnification of environmental toxins that will persist, leading to higher levels of breast cancer, hormonal disruption, and infertility in succeeding generations. The only way to stop this toxic magnification is through changing to a vegetarian diet, eating organic food, and reducing the load of environmental chemicals by decreasing their production and using saunas to detoxify regularly.

Cow's milk contains roughly four times as much calcium, three times as much protein, two thirds as much carbohydrate, and much more fat than human milk. These nutrients are important in these ratios for the development of a calf, not a human infant. Goat milk is closer to human milk in its composition. Cholesterol and fatty acids from dairy products build up in our organs and tissues, adding to heart disease, cancer, and other degenerative conditions.

The processing of milk products includes pasteurization, homogenization, and sterilization. These processes devitalize dairy products further, rob them of enzymes and make them even more difficult to digest. Many of us are deficient in lactase, the enzyme that digests lactose, or milk sugar. Our bodies can react to dairy products by producing excess mucus. Mucus tends to accumulate in particular areas and be linked to certain conditions: in the eustachian tubes it leads to chronic ear infections; in the sinuses, sinusitis; in the lungs it can result in asthma; and in the breasts, uterus or ovaries, it may cause tumor formation. Casein is a dairy protein often found in soy products that are meant to imitate dairy. Read labels and avoid casein as well. Substitute tofu, soy milk, almond milk, and rice milk for dairy products.

A 1979 study found that dairy products as a class increased the risk of breast cancer.[114] A large case-control study in France in 1986 found that women who ate cheese regularly had 50% more risk than women who didn't eat cheese and those who drank milk regularly had 80% higher risk.[115] More recently, two Harvard studies published in 1998 link consumption of milk from hormone treated cows to increased risk of breast cancer. The Physicians' Health Study and the Nurses' Health Study found that insulin-like growth factor 1 (IGF-1), a protein that is elevated in the milk of cows treated with bovine growth hormone, increases risk of both breast cancer and prostate cancer. We all have IGF-1 circulating naturally in our bodies but its levels are increased slightly by consuming hormone treated milk and carbohydrates with a high glycemic index. The Nurses' Health Study reported that pre-menopausal women with high levels of IGF-1 in their blood were seven times more likely to get breast cancer than women with low levels. The Physicians' Health Study found that men with the highest levels of IGF-1 in their blood were four times as likely to develop prostate cancer as men with the lowest levels. A 1995 study on rats published in the *Journal of Endocrinology* found that casein, a protein found in milk, slows down the breakdown of IGF-1, allowing it to circulate in blood at higher levels for longer periods of time.[116] It makes sense, then, to avoid hormone treated milk and products containing casein so that our levels of IGF-1 might be lower.

Women in their menopausal years are often given estrogen replacement therapy and are told to drink milk.

Both of these recommendations increase breast cancer risk. There is an alternative. Use sea vegetables, sesame seeds, almonds, kale, and parsley as calcium sources and take 1000–1500 mg of a calcium supplement daily to prevent osteoporosis. The calcium supplement should contain calcium, magnesium, vitamin D3, boron, molybdenum, vanadium, manganese, copper, zinc and vitamin K — some that have most of these include Bone-Up, Osteoprime and OSX by Genestra. Maintain a diet high in soy products, mung bean sprouts, and flaxseeds and low in sweets and salt with no animal protein, coffee. or carbonated beverages. The diet recommended in this book is also a diet to prevent osteoporosis and will help with menopausal symptoms. Walk an hour a day. By doing these things you will help to maintain your bone mass without endangering your breasts.

▶ **Action for Prevention:** Avoid or limit milk products and products that contain casein, such as soy cheese. ◀

Calcium Content of Various Foods

The calcium values shown in the chart on page 227 are derived from Jean A.T. Pennington's *Food Values of Portions Commonly Used*.

Sweets

When we consume sweets, a type of white blood cell called the phagocyte decreases its numbers within 30 minutes, and this decline lasts for over five hours, with a 50% reduction in phagocytes approximately two hours after ingestion. This leads to a poorly functioning immune system. This effect occurs after glucose, fructose, sucrose, honey, and orange juice.[117] Sweets will also promote an overgrowth of unwanted organisms in the intestinal tract, such as yeast and parasites. Included in the category of restricted sweets are soft drinks, juice-flavored drinks, powdered instant drinks, canned juices, candy, chocolate bars, granola bars, chocolate, donuts, and cookies.

Breast cancer susceptibility can be increased if soft drinks are consumed on a regular basis. After drinking soft drinks, there is a fast and dramatic increase in both glucose and insulin levels within the first hour. This response is more pronounced when body mass is lower, in children, for example. Increased insulin leads to higher circulating levels of IGF-1 which increase breast cancer risk sevenfold. Therefore, children who consume soft drinks regularly increase their breast cancer risk later in life.[118]

• Calcium Content of Various Foods •

Type of Food	Ca Content
Fish	
Sardines + bones	325 mg/ 3 oz
Pink salmon + bones	179 mg/ 3 oz
Chum, Coho salmon + bones	300 mg/ 4½ oz
Sockeye salmon + bones	300 mg/ 3½ oz
Chinook salmon + bones	300 mg/ 7 oz
Vegetables	
Broccoli, steamed	89 mg/ ½ cup
Chopped turnip greens, raw	53 mg/ ½ cup
Chopped turnip greens, boiled	99 mg/ ½ cup
Bok choy, raw, shredded	37 mg/ ½ cup
Bok choy, steamed	79 mg/ ½ cup
Rutabagas	100 mg/ 1 cup
Lambsquarters, steamed	232 mg/ ½ cup
Dandelion greens	150 mg/ 1 cup
Collards, boiled, chopped	148 mg/ 1 cup
Rhubarb	266 mg/ 1 cup
Long radish greens	60 mg/ ½ cup
Mustard greens, steamed	52 mg/ ½ cup
Parsley, chopped	39 mg/ ½ cup
Beet greens, steamed	82 mg/ ½ cup
Spinach, chopped, raw	28 mg/ ½ cup
Spinach, steamed	122 mg/ ½ cup
Watercress, chopped	20 mg/ ½ cup
Shepherd's purse	300 mg/ 100 g
Radish root, dried	400 mg/ 100 g
Collard greens	220 mg/ 1 cup
Kale leaves	210 mg/ 1 cup
Broccoli	150 mg/ 1 cup
Carbohydrates	
Millet	20 mg/ 3.5 oz
Enriched cornmeal	140 mg/ 1 cup
Carob flour	359 mg/ 1 cup
Soybean flour, defatted	241 mg/ 1 cup
Dark rye flour	69 mg/ 1 cup
Amaranth, boiled	138 mg/ ½ cup
Dairy Products	
Milk, 2%	297 mg/ 1 cup
Evaporated skim milk	344 mg/ ½ cup
Plain yogurt (2–4%)	396 mg/ 1 cup
Swiss cheese	272 mg/ 1 oz
Cheddar cheese	150 mg/ 1 oz
Blue cheese	300 mg/ 3½ oz
Cottage cheese	300 mg/ 1⅓ cups

Type of Food	Ca Content
Beans	
Kidney beans, boiled	50 mg/ 1 cup
Broad beans, boiled	62 mg/ 1 cup
Mung beans, boiled	55 mg/ 1 cup
Lentils, boiled	37 mg/ 1 cup
Black turtle beans, boiled	103 mg/ 1 cup
Black-eyed peas, boiled	130 mg/ 1 cup
Soybeans, boiled	175 mg/ 1 cup
Tofu, raw, firm	258 mg/ ½ cup
Miso	92 mg/ ½ cup
Adzuki beans, boiled	63 mg/ 1 cup
Great northern beans, boiled	121 mg/ 1 cup
White beans, boiled	161 mg/ 1 cup
Pinto beans, boiled	82 mg/ 1 cup
Navy beans, boiled	128 mg/ 1 cup
Chick peas, boiled	80 mg/ 1 cup
Hummus	124 mg/ 1 cup
Seeds and Nuts	
Sesame seeds	630 mg/ 100 g
Sunflower seeds	140 mg/ 100 g
Sweet almonds	282 mg/ 100 g
Almond butter	43 mg/ 1 tbsp.
Hazel nuts	186 mg/ 100 g
Brazil nuts	169 mg/ 100 g
Seaweeds	
Hijiki	300 mg/ 1 cup
Wakame	300 mg/ 1 cup
Kombu	800 mg/ 100 g
Arame	1170 mg/ 100 g
Agar-agar, dried	625 mg/ 3.5 oz
Irish moss, raw	100 mg/ 3.5 oz
Nori, raw	70 mg/ 3.5 oz
Kelp or kombu, raw	150 mg/ 1 tbsp
Fruits	
Papaya, raw, medium sized	72 mg
Figs, dried	269 mg/ 10 figs
Miscellaneous	
Blackstrap molasses	150 mg/ 1 tbsp
Soy milk (not Ca fortified)	50 mg/ 1 cup

Use instead fruit, stevia, small amounts of maple syrup and honey, frozen fruit desserts, and sugar-free natural fruit jams. Dilute your natural fruit juices with water.

▶ **Action for Prevention:** We should limit our sweets to a treat perhaps once weekly and otherwise use fruit to satisfy a sweet craving. Discourage a desire for sweets in your children by restricting their intake of processed sweets from infancy onward. If children are not given sweets, they often will not crave them as adults. ◀

White Flour Products

White flour robs the body of B vitamins and minerals, which are essential for healing. Refined flour is quickly converted into sugar in the blood, which raises insulin levels. Chronic high levels of insulin increase breast cancer risk and cause weight gain. A diet high in refined flour products can disturb the balance of bacteria within the large intestine that normally exerts an immune-enhancing and protective function.

▶ **Action for Prevention:** Avoid white flour products. Use instead whole grains and a limited amount of whole grain baked goods. ◀

Processed Food

Processed food is devoid of enzymes, vitamins and minerals, lacking in fiber, and often contains colorings and preservatives that are harmful to us. Plastic containers and cans in which processed food is packaged can also be hazardous to our health. Avoid processed food as much as possible. Buy simple ingredients and make your food from scratch.

▶ **Action for Prevention:** Avoid processed food and food packaged in plastic. ◀

Alcohol

Alcohol use causes a woman to be more susceptible to breast cancer. A weekly intake of four to seven drinks or more will increase risk. In one study, the risk increase was 250% for women who drank two or more drinks daily. Women who have even one drink a day have an 11% higher risk of breast cancer. Alcohol may interfere with the liver's ability to detoxify both chemicals and excess estrogen in the body.[119] Moderate consumption of alcohol increases the production of insulin-like growth factors by the liver, which promote the development and/or growth of breast cancer.[120]

▶ **Action for Prevention:** Drink less than two to three alcoholic beverages weekly, preferably drink none. ◀

Salt

Gerson believed that salt and excess sodium in general were a major cause of cancer. He theorized that chronic disease begins with a loss of potassium from cells followed by a flow of sodium and water into the cell. This causes a loss of electrical potential, poor enzyme formation, and decreased cellular oxidation. A low-salt diet withdraws water from the cells. A high potassium diet is beneficial. Potassium is a highly alkaline mineral that reduces acidity in the body. High potassium foods include sea vegetables, olives, almonds, prunes, figs, raisins, apples, apple cider vinegar, bananas, potatoes, legumes, beets, green leafy vegetables, sunflower seeds, yams, winter squash, pumpkin, and mint leaves.

▶ **Action for Prevention:** Avoid salt. ◀

Coffee

Coffee is an adrenal stimulant that causes a short-lived output of adrenal hormones followed by a depletion in them, creating the desire for another coffee. It is high in chemicals that have been used both in the growing and the processing of it. These burden the liver so that it is less able to detoxify both internally generated and external toxins. Use Greens + or an adrenal tonic to help kick the coffee addiction.

▶ **Action for Prevention:** Avoid coffee. ◀

The Healthy Breast Daily Diet

Here is the 'Healthy Breast Diet' I recommend, based on seven 'meals' each day.

On Rising	• green drink — either 1–3 tsp Greens +, Pure Synergy, Barley Green, spirulina or other green powder in water (or 1–3 oz of wheatgrass juice) — followed by two glasses filtered or spring water, with a little lemon or lime juice added plus a pinch of cayenne pepper
Breakfast	• 1 cup whole grain cereal (use barley, oatmeal, buckwheat, quinoa, millet meal, amaranth, brown rice) with 2–3 tbsp freshly ground flaxseeds, 1 tbsp wheat bran (if tolerated), small amount of stevia, honey or maple syrup if desired, plus ½–1 cup soy milk or fruit by itself
Snack	• 2 cups fresh vegetable juice, especially carrot, beet, and cabbage, with 1 tsp dulse or kelp powder or 1–2 pieces fruit, especially, cherries, apple, pear, banana, orange, grapefruit, tangerine, or berries • 2 glasses filtered or spring water or herbal tea (green tea, licorice, immune tonic tea, red clover, fenugreek, Pau d'arco, mint, dandelion, rosehip)
Lunch	• 1–2 cups salad with cabbage (eaten at the beginning of the meal so their enzymes will aid digestion) • ¾ cup vegetables (at least 50% raw, including ½ cup brassicas) • ½ cup mung bean, red clover, sunflower or broccoli sprouts (in salad or in bean and rice dish) • 1–2 tbsp. flaxseed oil, as salad dressing, and over beans and grain • ½–1 cup beans, with onion and garlic (hummus, bean dips, bean soup, or bean and grain dish) • ½–1 cup grain, preferably whole grain rather than flour products (rice, millet, barley, quinoa, buckwheat) • 3–4 shitake mushrooms
Snack	• 1–2 tbsp raw almonds, pumpkin seeds, soy nuts and/or sunflower seeds • 2 cups vegetable juice (especially carrot, beet, cabbage, dulse powder with added watercress, parsley, kale, mustard greens, garlic, ginger, sprouts, dandelion greens, or apple) • 2 glasses filtered or spring water or herbal tea, as above
Dinner	• green drink (as before breakfast, taken ½ hour before dinner) • 1 cup salad with fresh sprouts, onions and garlic, raw sunflower or pumpkin seeds, and grated citrus peel • ½ cup firm organic tofu or tempeh • ½–1 cup whole grains (wild rice, quinoa, millet, rice, barley, and buckwheat — omit this if you are food combining or wanting to lose weight) • ¾ cup vegetables, raw or lightly steamed • ½ cup red clover, sunflower, mung bean or broccoli sprouts • 2 tbsp sea vegetables (hiziki, arame, wakame, nori, dulse, kelp) • 1–2 tbsp flaxseed oil and 1 tablespoon olive oil as part of salad dressing or over grain or vegetables
Snack	• 2 glasses filtered or spring water or decaffeinated green tea • 1 cup Healthy Breast Drink (1 cup soy milk, 1 tsp. turmeric paste, optional banana, blended or warmed) • Note: One serving of fruits or vegetables is, for example, • 1 cup of raw leafy vegetables • ½ cup of other vegetables or fruit (cooked or raw) or ¾ cup vegetable or fruit juice • 1 medium apple, banana, or orange • ½ cup fruit or 2 tbsp dried fruit • Six servings in a day might include two pieces of fruit, one cup of salad, and one and a half cups of steamed or raw vegetables.

Developing a Dietary Routine Exercise

Use the chart on page 232 over the next two weeks as a tool to assess how well you are maintaining a breast health/cancer prevention diet. Aim for an increased number of check marks over time. Be patient. Change takes time. Some of us may be able to make a diet transition in a few weeks; others of us will do a little more each year. Respect your pace while making your best effort. If you are in a group, share your successes, difficulties and recipes with other women. Repeat this assessment every three months or more to help you stay on track.

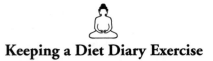

Keeping a Diet Diary Exercise

Record your weekly intake of food using the chart on page 232 to determine the approximate number of servings of fruits and vegetables, fiber, soy products, calories from fat, etc. you are consuming.

Summary

Eating a healthy diet is obviously a sensible way of preventing breast cancer, but often the food available to us is nutrient deficient because of demineralized soil and poor growing conditions. For this reason we need to consider supplementing our diet with vitamins, minerals, essential fatty acids, and other nutrients.

Further Reading

Arnot, Bob. *The Breast Cancer Prevention Diet*. New York, NY: Little, Brown and Co., 1998.

Erasmus, Udo. *Fats that Heal, Fats that Kill*. Burnaby, BC: Alive Books, 1993.

Gerson, Max. *A Cancer Therapy: Results of Fifty Cases*. 3rd ed. Del Mar, CA: Totality Books, 1977.

Joseph, Barbara. *My Healing from Breast Cancer*. New Canaan, CT: Keats Publishing, Inc., 1998.

Keuneke, Robin. *Total Breast Health*. New York, NY: Kensington Books, 1998.

Kushi, Michio. *The Cancer Prevention Diet*. New York, NY: St Martin's Press, 1993.

Wigmore, Ann. *The Hippocrates Diet and Health Program*. Garden City Park, NY: Avery, 1983.

• Dietary Routine Worksheet •

From (date)_____ to _____

Daily Food	Please Check Daily														
Vegetarian Diet															
Organic Food : fill in what %															
Raw Food : 50% or more															
Broccoli Sprouts (3× weekly)															
Mung Bean Sprouts (3× weekly)															
Red Clover Sprouts (3× weekly)															
Dandelion in season (3× weekly)															
Vegetable Juice: 2 or more c.															
Cabbage: ⅓, juiced or raw															
Tomato Products (2× weekly)															
Fruits: 2 or more															
Citrus Juice: organic (3× weekly)															
Vegetables: 4 or more servings															
Brassica Family: 1 cup															
Onion: 1															
Garlic: 2 cloves, raw is better															
Sea Vegetables: ⅓ cup															
Shitaki Mushrooms (2× weekly)															
Low Salt/High Potassium															
< 15 % saturated fat/ total cal.															
Flaxseed Oil: 2 or more tbsp															
Olive Oil for cooking, low heat															
Fiber: 30 g															
Whole Grains: 1 cup															
Beans: 1–2 cups daily															
Flaxseeds: 2–4 tbsp, ground															
Pumpkin Seeds: 2 tbsp, raw															
Wheat Bran: 1 tbsp															
Protein: 30–60 g daily															
Tofu: ½ cup															
Soy Milk: 1 cup															
Miso: 1 tbsp (3× weekly)															
Citrus Peel: 1 tsp organic grated															
Turmeric: 1–2 tsp powder															
Rosemary, Sage, Thyme, Ginger															
Water: 8 glasses filtered															
Alcoholic Drinks: < 2 /week															
Coffee: none															
Sugar: none															
Canned or Processed Food: none															
Dairy: none															

• Diet Diary •

	Monday	Tuesday	Wednesday	Thursday	Friday	Saturday	Sunday
Breakfast							
Snack							
Lunch							
Snack							
Dinner							
Snack							

References

1. Mollison, B. *Introduction to Permaculture.* Tyalgum, NSW, Australia: Tagari Publications, 1991.
2. Steimetz, K.A., J.D. Potter. Vegetables, fruit and cancer prevention: a review. *J Am Diet Assoc,* 1996;96:1027-39.
3. Phillips, R.L., Cancer among Seventh Day Adventists. *Journal of Environmental Pathology and Toxicology,* 1980;3:157-69.
4. Sanches, A., et al. A hypothesis on the etiological role of diet on age of menarche. *Medical Hypothesis,* 1981;7:1339-45.
5. Weed, Susun. *Breast Cancer/Breast Health!* Woodstock, NY: Ash Tree Publishing, 1996:46-52.
6. Zimmerman, M. Phytochemicals and disease prevention. *Alternative and Complementary Therapies,* Apr/May 1995;1(3)154-57.
7. Holzman, D. Nutritional chemoprevention: using food to fight cancer. *Alternative and Complementary Medicine,* Mar/Apr, 1996;2(2), 65-67.
8. Wattenberg, L.W. & W.D. Loub. 1978. Inhibition of polycyclic aromatic hydrocarbon-induced neoplasia by naturally occurring indoles. *Cancer Research,* 1978;38:1410-13.
9. Michnovicz, J.J. *How to Reduce Your Risk of Breast Cancer.* New York, NY: Warner Books, 1994:103.
10. Wong, GYC et al. A dose-ranging study of indole-3-carbinol for breast cancer prevention. Strang Cancer Prevention Center. *Breast Cancer Research and Treatment,* 1997;46(1):81.
11. Carper, Jean. *Food:Your Miracle Medicine.* New York, NY: Harper Collins, 1993:222.
12. Fahey, J.W., Y. Zhang, & P. Talalay. Broccoli sprouts: An exceptionally rich source of inducers of enzymes that protect against chemical carcinogens. *Proc. Natl. Acad. Sci.* USA., 1997; 94:10367-72.
13. Raloff, J., 1997. Anticancer agent sprouts up unexpectedly. *Science News,* 152:183.
14. Garlic fights nitrosamine formation…as do tomatoes and other produce. *Science News,* Feb. 1994, Vol. 145.
15. Galland, L. Intestinal toxicity: New approaches to an old problem. *Alternative and Complementary Therapies,* 1997;3(4):288-95.
16. Teas, J. The consumption of seaweed as a protective factor in the etiology of breast cancer, *Medical Hypotheses,* 1981;7:(5)601-13.
17. Gerson, M. *A Cancer Therapy: Results of Fifty Cases.* Del Mar, CA: Totality Books, 1977:205-06.
18. Weed, S. Breast Cancer? *Breast Health.,* Woodstock, NY: Ash Tree Publishing, 1996:272.
19. Bensky, Dan, A. Gamble. *Chinese Herbal Medicine Materia Medica.* Seattle, WA. Eastland Press Inc., 1986:129.
20. Balch, J.F. *The Super Anti-oxidants: Why they will change the face of healthcare in the 21ˢᵗ Century.* New York, NY: M. Evans & Co., Inc., 1998:129.
21. Kantesky, P.A., et al. Dietary intake and blood levels of lycopene: association with cervical dysplasia among non-Hispanic, black women. *Nutrition and Cancer,* 1998;31:31-40.
22. Sharoni, Y., et al. Effects of lycopene-enriched tomato oleoresin on 7,12-dimethyl-benz(a)anthracene-induced rat mammary tumors. *Cancer Detection and Prevention.* 1997;21(2):118-23.
23. Buckler, J., A.J. DeNault, V. Franc, T. Strukoff. Breast cancer treatment and prevention: limonene, lycopene and alpha-lipoic acid. Toronto, ON: *Canadian College of Naturopathic Medicine,* April, 1999.
24. Guthrie, N., K. Carroll. Inhibition of human breast cancer cell growth and metastasis in nude mice by citrus juices and their constituent flavonoids. In *Biological Oxidants and Antioxidants: Molecular Mechanisms and Health Effects.* Packer, L. and A. Ong, eds. Champaign, IL: AOCS Press, 1998:310-16.
25. Gould, M., et al. Limonene chemoprevention of mammary carcinoma induction following direct in situ transfer of v-Ha-ras. *Cancer Research,* 1994;54(13):3540-43.
26. Elegbede, J. Prospective roles of plant secondary metabolites in the treatment of mammary cancer. *Dissertation Abstracts International (Nutrition).* 1985;46:(6):1874.
27. Erasmus, Udo. *Fats that Heal, Fats that Kill.* Burnaby, BC: Alive Books, 1993:400.
28. Erasmus, Udo. *Fats that Heal, Fats that Kill.* Burnaby, BC: Alive Books, 1993:53.
29. Kohlmeier, L. Biomarkers of fatty acid exposure and breast cancer risk. *Am J Clin Nutr,* 1997;66(suppl): 1548S-56S.
30. Aziziyan, S., N. Rezvani, C. Radulovici, A. Nozari. Dietary fat and breast cancer prevention. Toronto, ON: *Canadian College of Naturopathic Medicine,* April, 1999.
31. Boyd, N. Nutrition and breast cancer. *Journal of the National Cancer Institute,* 1993;Jan.6;85(1):6-7.
32. Woods, M., et al. Hormone levels during dietary changes in pre-menopausal African-American women. *Journal of the National Cancer Institute.* 1996;Oct.2;88(19):1369-74.
33. Phillips, R.L., Role of life-style and dietary habits in risk of cancer among Seventh-Day Adventists. *Cancer Research,* 1975;35:3513.
34. McAndrew, Brian. Toxic chemical gets into fatty products. *The Toronto Star,* Wed., July 1, 1998.
35. Ip, Clement. Review of the effects of trans fatty acids, oleic acid, omega-3 polyunsaturated fatty acids. *Am J Clin Nut.* 1997:66(suppl):1523S-9S.
36. Bakker, N., P. Van't Veer, P. Zock. Adipose fatty acids and cancers of the breast, prostate and colon: an ecological study. *Breast Cancer,* 1997;72:587-91.
37. Cave, W. Omega three PUFAs in rodent models of breast cancer. *Breast Cancer Research and Treatment,* 1997:46:239-46.
38. Okuyama et al. Dietary fatty acids – the Omega 6/Omega 3 balance. *Progress in Lipid Research,* Dec. 1996;35(4):409-19.

39. Erasmus, Udo. *Fats that Heal, Fats that Kill.* Burnaby, BC: Alive Books, 1993:365.

40. Takeda, S. et al. Lipid peroxidation in human breast cancer cells in response to gamma-linolenic acid and iron. *Anticancer Research.* 1992;12:329-34.

41. Jiang, W., R. Bryce and R. Mansel. Gamma linolenic acid regulates gap junction communication in endothelial cells and their interaction with tumor cells. *Prostaglandins, Leukotrienes and Essential Fatty Acids*, 1997,56(4):307.

42. Bakker, N., P. Van't Veer and P. Zock. Adipose fatty acids and cancers of the breast, prostate and colon: An ecological study. *Breast Cancer*, 1997(72):587-91.

43. Fogg, J., D. Derbyshire, E. Bennett, M. Melanson. Essential fatty acids and their role in breast cancer prevention and treatment. Toronto, ON: *Canadian College of Naturopathic Medicine*, April, 1999.

44. Thompson, L. et al. Flaxseed and its lignan and oil components reduce mammary tumor growth at a late stage of carcinogenesis. *Carcinogenesis*, 1996:17(6):1373-76.

45. Abdi-Dezfuli, F. et al. Eicosapentaenoic acid and sulphur substituted fatty acid analogues inhibit the proliferation of human breast cancer cells in culture. *Breast Cancer Research and Treatment*, 1997;45:230.

46. Lipworth, L., et al. Olive oil and human cancer: An assessment of the evidence. *Preventive Medicine*, 1997;26:181-90.

47. Walker, M. Health enhancement with high fiber foods. *Townsend Letter for Doctors.* July, 1992:580-83.

48. Jibrin, Janis. The ultra diet for healthy breasts. *Prevention magazine*, Sept., 1996.p.65-71,148.

49. Gerber, M. Fiber and breast cancer: another piece of the puzzle - but still an incomplete picture. *Journal of the National Cancer Institute*, 1996;88:13,857-58.

50. Gerber, M. Fiber and breast cancer: another piece of the puzzle - but still an incomplete picture. *Journal of the National Cancer Institute*, 1996;88:858.

51. Cohen, L.A., et al. Wheat bran and psyllium diets: effects on N-methylnitrosoura-induced mammary tumorigenesis in F344 rats. *J Natl Cancer Inst*, 1996;Jul;88(13):899-907.

52. Rohan, T.E. et al. Dietary fiber, vitamins A, C, and E and the risk of breast cancer: A cohort study. *Cancer Causes and Control*, 1993;4:29-37.

53. Simone, C. Nutritional Medicine Today 1997 Conference – *Breast cancer nutritional and lifestyle modification to augment oncology care (audiotape).* Richmond Hill, ON: Audio Archives of Canada, 1997.

54. Koch-Kattenstroth, S. and E. Shoyama. Fiber and breast cancer. Toronto, ON: *Canadian College of Naturopathic Medicine*, April, 1999.

55. Petrakis, N.L. & E.B. King. 1981. Cytological abnormalities in nipple aspirates of breast fluid from women with severe constipation. *Lancet*, 1981;ii:1203-05.

56. Rose, D.P., M. Goldman, J.M. Connolly & L.E. Strong. High fiber diet reduces serum oestrogen concentrations in pre-menopausal women. *American Journal of Clinical Nutrition*, 1991;54:520-25.

57. Rose, D.P., M. Lubin and J. Connolly. Effects of diet supplementation with wheat bran on serum estrogen levels in the follicular and luteal phases of the menstrual cycle. *Nutrition*, 1997;13(6):535-39.

58. Carper, Jean. *The Food Pharmacy.* New York, NY: Bantam, 1988.

59. Kennedy, A. 1995. The evidence for soybean products as cancer preventive agents. *J Nutrition*, 125:733.

60. Kaufman, P., et al. A comparative survey of leguminous plants as sources of the isoflavones, genistein and daidzen: implications for human nutrition and health. *Journal of Alternative and Complementary Medicine*, 1997;3(1):10-11.

61. Adlercreutz, H., & W. Mazur. Phyto-oestrogens and western disease. The Finnish Medical Society DUODECIM, *Ann Med*, 1997;29:95-120.

62. Walker, Morton. Soybean isoflavones lower risk of degenerative diseases, *Townsend Letter for Doctors*, August/September, 1994.

63. Constantinou et al. *Cancer Res*, 1990;50:2618-24.

64. Ingram, D., K. Sanders, M. Kolybaba, D. Lopez. Case-control study of phytoestrogens and breast cancer. *Lancet*, 1997;350 Oct.4: 990-93.

65. Ingram, D., K. Sanders, M. Kolybaba, D. Lopez. Phyto-oestrogens and breast cancer. *Int Clin Nutr Rev*, 1998;18(1):35-36.

66. Adlercreutz, H., & W. Mazur. Phyto-oestrogens and western disease. The Finnish Medical Society DUODECIM, *Ann Med*, 1997;29,103.

67. Adlercreutz, H., & W. Mazur. Phyto-oestrogens and western disease. The Finnish Medical Society DUODECIM, *Ann Med* 29, 1997:95-120.

68. Wahlqvist, M. Phytoestrogens: Emerging multifaceted plant compounds. *Medical Journal of Australia*, 1997;Aug.4;167:119-20.

69. Cassidy, A., S. Bingham, & K. Setchell. Biological effects of isoflavones in young women: importance of the chemical composition of soyabean products. *British Journal of Nutrition*, 1995;74:587-601.

70. Colditz, G.A., A. Frazier. Models of breast cancer show that risk is set by events of early life: prevention efforts must switch focus. *Cancer Epidem Biomarker Prevent*, 1995;4:567.

71. Setchell, K.D.R., et al. Exposure of infants to phyto-estrogens from soy-based infant formulas. *The Lancet*, 1997;350:23-27.

72. High, C., K. Wolfe. Are soy products safe for infants and pregnant women? Toronto, ON: *Canadian College of Naturopathic Medicine*, April, 1999.

73. Lu, L.W., Anderson, K.E. et al. Effects of soy consumption for one month on steroid hormones in premenopausal women: implications for breast cancer risk reduction. *Cancer Epidemiol Biomarkers Prev.* 1996;5:63-70.

74. DeSimone, S., B. Finucan. Soy: Too good to be true. (Part 2 of 2). *Gerson Healing Newsletter Online*, March 11, 2000; http://gerson.org/healing/articles/nl_soytoogood.htm:3.

75. Divi, R.L., H.C. Chang, D.R. Doerge. Anti-thyroid isoflavones from soybean: isolation, characterization, and mechanisms of action. *Biochem Pharmacol*, 1997 Nov 15;54(10):1087-96.

76. Fort, P., N. Moses, M. Fasano, T. Goldberg, F. Lifshitz. Breast and soy-formula feedings in early infancy and the prevalence of autoimmune thyroid disease in children. *J Amer Coll Nutr*, 1990; Apr 9(2):164-67.

77. Setchell, K.D., L. Zimmer-Nechemias, J. Cai, J.E. Heubi. Isoflavone content of infant formulas and the metabolic fate of these phytoestrogens in early life. *Am J Clin Nutr*, 1998 Dec 68(6)Suppl:1453S-1461S.

78. Zava, D., M. Blen, G. Duwe. Estrogenic activity of natural and synthetic estrogens in human breast cancer cells in culture. *Environmental Health Perspectives*, April 1997;105(Sup.3): 637-45.

79. Kaufman, P., et al. A comparative survey of leguminous plants as sources of the isoflavones, genistein and daidzen: implications for human nutrition and health. *Journal of Alternative and Complementary Medicine*, 1997;3(1):7-12.

80. Adlercreutz, H. Evolution, nutrition, intestinal microflora, and prevention of cancer: A hypothesis. *Proc Soc Exp Biol Med*, 1998;217(3):241-46.

81. Thompson, L. and M. Serraino. Lignans in flaxseed and breast carcinogenesis. Toronto, ON: Dept. of Nutritional Sciences, Univ. of Toronto, 1989.

82. Setchell, K.D.R., H. Adlerkreutz. Mammalian lignans and phyto-estrogens:recent studies on their formation, metabolism and biological role in health and disease. In Rowland, I.R. (Ed.), *Role of the Gut Flora in Toxicity and Cancer*. London, UK1, Academic Press, 1998:315-75.

83. Adlercreutz, H., et al. Excretion of the lignans enterolactone and enterodiol and of equol in omnivorous and vegetarian post-menopausal women and in women with breast cancer. *Lancet*, 1982;ii:1295-99.

84. Adlercreutz, H., et al. Determination of urinary lignans and phytoestrogen metabolites, potential antiestrogens and anticarcinogens, in urine of women on various habitual diets. *J Steroid Biochem*, 1986;25:791-97.

85. Serraino, M., L. Thompson. The effect of flaxseed supplementation on the inhibition and promotional stages of mammary carcinogenesis. *Nutrition and Cancer*, 1992;17:153-59.

86. Thompson, Lilian. Antitumorigenic effect of a mammalian lignan precursor from flaxseed. *Nutrition and Cancer*, 1996;26(2):159-65.

87. Thompson, Lilian. Flaxseed and its lignan and oil components reduce mammary tumor growth at a late stage of carcinogenesis. *Carcinogenesis*, 1996;17(6):1373.

88. Gerson, M. *A Cancer Therapy: Results of Fifty Cases*. Del Mar, CA: Totality Books, 1977:163-66.

89. Pizzorno, J. & M. Murray. Sodium, potassium, calcium and phosphorus content of foods. *A Textbook of Natural Medicine*. Seattle, WA: John Bastyr College Publications, 1985:A:NKCPFd-1.

90. Inagawa, H., T. Nishizawa, K. Noguchi et al. Anti-tumor effect of lipopolysaccharide by intradermal administration as a novel drug delivery system. *Anticancer Res*, 1997;17:2153-58.

91. Wong, G.Y.C., M. Katare, M.P. Osborne, N.T. Telang. Preventive efficacy of *Lentinas elodes* mycelium extract (LEM) in human mammary carcinogenesis (abstr. 321). In *19th Annual San Antonio Breast Cancer Symposium*. [San Antonio, Texas] December 11-14, 1996, Program and Abstracts, 1996:265.

92. Nanba, H., K. Mori, T. Toyomasu, H. Kuroda. Antitumor action of shiitake (Lentinus elodes) fruit bodies orally administered to mice. *Chem Pharm Bull*, 1987;35:2453-58.

93. Jones, Kenneth. Shiitake: a major medicinal mushroom. *Alternative and Complementary Therapies*, Feb.,1998:55.

94. Sharma, O.P. *Biochem Pharmacol*, 1976;25:1811-12.

95. Bensky, D. & A. Gamble. *Chinese Herbal Medicine Materia Medica*. Seattle, WA: Eastland Press, 1986:390-91.

96. Thaloor, D., et al. Inhibition of angiogenic differentiation of human umbilical vein endothelial cells by curcumin. *Cell Growth and Differentiation*, 1998;9(4):305-12.

97. Hall, A. Curcuma longa – a therapeutic role in the fight against breast cancer. Toronto, ON: *Canadian College of Naturopathic Medicine*, April, 1999.

98. Mehta, K. et al. Antiproliferative effect of curcumin (diferuloylmethane) against human breast tumor cell lines. *Anti-Cancer Drugs*.1997;8(5):470-81.

99. Arnold, S.F., D.M. Klotz, B.M. Collins, P.M. Vonier, L.J. Guillette Jr., & J.A.McLachlan. *Science*, 1996;272,1489-92.

100. Verma, S.P., E. Salamone & B. Goldin. Curcumin and genistein, plant natural products, show synergistic inhibitory sffects on the growth of human breast cancer MCF-7 cells induced by estrogenic pesticides. *Biochem and Biophys Res Comm*, 1997;233:692-96.

101. Zhu, B.T., D.P. Loder, M.X. Cai, C.T. Huang, A.H. Conney. Dietary administratio of an extract from rosemary leaves enhances the liver microsomal metabolism of endogenous estrogens and decreases their uterotropic action in CD-1 mice. *Carcinogenesis*, Oct. 1998;19(10):1821-27.

102. Galland, L. Intestinal toxicity: New approaches to an old problem. *Alternative and Complementary Therapies*, Aug. 1997;3(4):288-95.

103. Holmes, P. *The Energetics of Western Herbs*.Vol. I. 2nd ed. Berkeley, CA: NatTrop Publishing, 1993:227-29.

104. Brand Miller, J., K. Foster-Powell, S. Colagiuri. *The G.I. Factor: The Glycaemic Index Solution*. Sydney, Australia: Hodder Headline Australian Pty Ltd., 1996.

105. Greenpeace. Chlorine Chemicals in Cod Liver Oil. London, England: Greenpeace Communications, 1995.

106. Clorfene-Casten, Liane. *Breast Cancer: Poisons, Profits and Prevention*. Monroe, ME: Common Courage Press, 1996:27.

107. Greenpeace. Death in Small Doses: The Effects of Organochlorines on Aquatic Ecosystems, 1992.

108. EPA. U.S. Environmental Protection Agency, National Dioxin Study Tier 4-Combustion Sources: Engineering Analysis Report, Washington, DC. U.S. EPA Office of Air Quality Planning and Standards, 1988.

109. HSDB. Hazardous Substances Databank, on line records for mirex, DDT, hexachlorobenzene, hexachlorobutadiene, trichloroethylene, hexachlorocyclopentadiene and vinyl chloride, Bethesda, MD. *National Library of Medicine*. June-July, 1991.

110. Jacobson, J.L. and S.W. Jacobson. Intellectual impairment in children exposed to polychlorinated biphenyls in utero. *New England Journal of Medicine*,1996;335(11):783.

111. Jacobson, J.L. and S.W. Jacobson. Intellectual impairment in children exposed to polychlorinated biphenyls in utero. *New England Journal of Medicine*, 1996;335(11):783.

112. Toughill, K. Disease fears spawn debate over fish farms. *The Toronto Star*, Sun., Nov.1, 1998:B1,3.

113. Kushi, Michio. *The Cancer Prevention Diet*. New York, NY: St Martin's Press, 1993:125

114. Gaskill, S.P., et al. Breast cancer diet and mortality in the United States. *Cancer Research*, 39:3628-37.

115. Le, M. G. et al. Consumption of dairy produce and alcohol in a case-control study of breast cancer. *Journal of the National Cancer Institute*, 77:633-36.

116. Gilbert, Susan. Fears over milk, long dismissed, still simmer. *The New York Times*, Tues., Jan.19, 1999:D7

117. Pizzorno, J. & M. Murray. Sodium, potassium, calcium and phosphorus content of foods. *A Textbook of Natural Medicine*. Seattle, WA: John Bastyr College Publications, 1985: IV:ImmSup.,3-4.

118. Janssens J.P., et al. Effects of soft drink and table beer consumption on insulin response in normal teenagers and carbohydrate drink in youngsters. *Eur J Cancer Prev*, 1999;Aug;8(4):289-95.

119. Alcohol and the breast, *Journal of the National Cancer Institute*, 1993;85:692, 722.

120. Yu, H., J. Berkel. Do insulin-like growth factors mediate the effect of alcohol on breast cancer risk? *Med Hypotheses*, 1999;Jun:52(6):491-96.

Nutritional Supplements for Breast Health

Exercises

Contents

*T*here are some health care practitioners who believe that we should get all our nutrients from food sources, while others believe that supplements are necessary for health preservation and for healing illness. My belief is that most of us suffer from at least some nutritional deficiencies due to depletion of nutrients from the soil and thus from our food. The mineral content of our foods is much less than it was 100 years ago. Our bodies need more nutrients to detoxify the pollutants in our air, water, and food; and our diets are often deficient in vital nutrients. The stress of living at this time, with its fast pace, uses up nutrient reserves; most of us don't absorb the nutrients we do take in because we are always on the go, interfering with the digestive process that needs us to relax for it to work properly. Supplementation of at least some nutrients is beneficial.

The following information is meant as a guide but not a prescription for some of the many supplements available to assist in the prevention of breast cancer. Get as many of them as you can through diet and find quality supplements from natural sources for the others. Work with a naturopath, nutritionist, or other professional in determining how to best use this information and what dosages to take.

Daily Therapeutic Amounts of Vitamins and Minerals Exercise

Review the nutrients and guidelines below with your health care provider and fill in the column with any supplements that are recommended for you, their dosages, and product name, if known. You will find combinations of these in many products, making a supplement schedule simpler. If you have an aversion to taking pills, write the food sources in the third column. Food sources or products that are derived from foods are better than synthetic vitamins.

Vitamins

Vitamin A

Though not nearly as effective as beta-carotene in preventing breast cancer, vitamin A, also known as retinol, is an important nutrient. It maintains the integrity of the body's skin — the outer skin as well as the mucous lining in the digestive and intestinal tract — leading to improved intestinal health, digestion and immunity. When this layer is healthy, it is less vulnerable to chemical carcinogens and parasitic or yeast infection. It prevents cancer from occurring on the inner lining of the stomach and lungs and on the skin. Vitamin A will help to improve the tissue tolerance for women undergoing chemotherapy or radiation so there is less damage to healthy cells. It helps cells repair themselves when they have been exposed to cancer-causing substances. It improves our body's ability to destroy tumors and increases the number of white blood cells. It causes phagocytes, a particular kind of white blood cell, to be more efficient at digesting toxins and potential carcinogens. Vitamin A prevents and reverses the effects of stress on the thymus gland by promoting its growth and reducing its shrinkage, which commonly occurs when we are stressed for long periods of time. The thymus coordinates the activity of our white blood cells, which are the warriors of our immune system. Vitamin A is more effective when taken with zinc and adequate vitamin E. Sufficient vitamin A has a sparing effect on vitamin C. Preformed vitamin A (animal derived) is fat soluble; it is stored in the liver and can be toxic when the liver's capacity to store it has been exceeded.

FOOD SOURCES: butter, cream, egg yolks, fish liver oil from cod, halibut, salmon, shark.
DOSAGE: 5,000–35,000 IU daily
CONTRAINDICATIONS: Chronic ingestion of over 100,000 IU of vitamin A daily in a susceptible person may result in toxicity. Only low doses should be used during pregnancy.

Beta-carotene, Other Carotenes, and Carotenoids

Derived from vegetables, Beta-carotene is converted to vitamin A in the body. Beta-carotene, which is more effective than vitamin A in breast cancer prevention, has been shown to reduce the risk of pre-menopausal breast cancer

• Daily Therapeutic Amounts of Vitamins and Minerals •

Nutrient	Dosage Range	Your Personal Dosage
Vitamin A	5,000–35,000 IU	
Beta-carotene or mixed carotenoids	10,000–100,000 IU	
B complex	50–100 mg	
Niacin (B3)	25–2000 mg (with medical supervision)	
B6	50–200 mg	
Folic acid	400–800 mcg	
B12	50 mcg	
Inositol	200–1800 mg	
IP6	800–7,000 mg	
Vitamin C	2,000–10,000 mg	
Bioflavonoids	100 mg per 500 mg of vitamin C	
Vitamin D	0–800 IU	
Vitamin E	400–800 IU	
Calcium	800–2,000 mg (less if cancer is present)	
Magnesium	300–800 mg	
Potassium	Food sources, 3000–6000 mg	
Iodine or Kelp	100–1000 mcg	
Molybdenum	100–500 mcg	
Chromium	200–600 mcg	
Selenium	100–300 mcg	
Zinc	20–100 mg	
Manganese	5 mg	
Coenzyme Q10	60–400 mg	
Alpha lipoic acid	50–600 mg	
Grape seed extract	60–300 mg.	
Modified citrus pectin	10–15 g	
Melatonin	3–20 mg	
NAC	500–1,500 mg	
Reduced glutathione	75–2,000 mg	
Digestive enzymes	1–2 capsules before &/or between meals	
Thymus extract	100–800 mg	
Flaxseed oil	2–8 tbps	
Probiotic + FOS	2 capsules	
Psyllium seed powder	1 tsp–1 tbsp	
Indole-3-carbinol	300 mg.	
Curcumin	1500–3000 mg	
Folliculinum 9CH	Dose on days 7, 21 and possibly 14	
Maitake D-fraction	1 mg per kg of body weight per day, which for a 150 lb woman is 34–68 drops daily	
Carnivora	1 capsule 3× daily before meals	
MGN-3	250–750 mg daily	

by up to 90%.[1] This is probably because beta-carotene acts as a far better antioxidant than does vitamin A. It is also possible that the other health benefits that are associated with eating many vegetables may contribute to breast cancer risk reduction associated with beta-carotene.

Beta-carotene is only one member of a large group of over 600 different carotenes, many of which are therapeutic. Each carotenoid has a slightly different effect, and may have a preferred site of action in our bodies. Some of the other carotenes are alpha-carotene, gamma-carotene, lycopene, cryptoxanthin, and lutein. Instead of just supplementing our diets with beta-carotene, we can consume a diet rich in vegetables which will contain other carotenes that collectively block the initiation and promotion of cancer by binding free radicals; increase the level of cytokines (interferon, interleukin, tumor necrosis factor) in the body, which help fight cancer; protect DNA from chemicals and radiation; help to produce anti-cancer enzymes in the digestive tract; increase the ratio of helper to suppressor T-cells, which improves the ability of the immune system to attack cancer cells; and increase the size, weight, and function of the thymus gland.

FOOD SOURCES: algae, seaweeds, dandelion greens, carrots, parsley, spinach, kale, broccoli, Brussels sprouts, sweet potatoes, winter squash, pumpkin, cantaloupe, asparagus, pink grapefruit, mango, papaya, peaches, and apricots. Beta carotene in produce is destroyed when exposed to light, oxygen, storage, and processing. Fresh and locally grown is best. Surprisingly, when foods high in carotenoids are cooked, they are up to five times more active in inhibiting cancer than when they are raw.[2]
DOSAGE: 25,000–100,000 IU daily. The upper limit of beta-carotene intake is unknown. Because it is stored in the skin, high doses will begin to affect skin pigmentation by producing an orange hue on the palms of the hands. This is not harmful because beta-carotene is water soluble and non-toxic. It is a sign that your body has enough of the vitamin. Find a supplement that contains a mixture of naturally occurring carotenes, rather than pure beta-carotene. The color of the supplement is important, and should be orange to red if it is still fresh.
CONTRAINDICATIONS: None known.

B Complex

The B complex vitamins are needed to convert carbohydrate into glucose, giving us energy. The B complex also helps strengthen cell membranes so they are less vulnerable to stress and is needed for the health of our nerves. Irritability, impatience, depression, and many

psychological disorders can often be helped with the B complex. A deficiency in the B complex will depress immunity and cause shrinkage of lymphatic tissue. The function of lymphatic tissue is to fight infections, cancer, and detoxify on the cellular level. These abilities are impaired with a B complex deficiency. An excess of estrogen, such as when women take the birth control pill, can deplete some of the B vitamins. If any single B vitamin is taken, the B complex should be taken along with it to prevent a deficiency of some of the other B vitamins. They work best when taken together, as they occur naturally in foods.

FOOD SOURCES: Brewer's yeast, wheat and rice bran, wheat germ, beans, nuts, seeds, eggs, bee pollen, liver, whole grain cereals, and leafy green vegetables. Some of them can be produced by our intestinal bacteria.
DOSAGE: 50 mg daily, with food. Do not use time-released B complex.
CONTRAINDICATIONS: None. Any excess is excreted and not stored. Be sure to take the B complex along with any single B vitamin.

Vitamin B3 (Niacin)

Niacin, niacinamide, and inositol hexaniacinate are all forms of vitamin B3 that are useful in the prevention and treatment of breast cancer. Niacin assists enzymes in the breakdown and use of proteins, fats, and carbohydrates. It is also utilized in blood sugar regulation and for detoxification in the liver. It improves circulation, delivering more nutrients to the cells and removing waste more efficiently. It reduces cholesterol levels in the blood and is necessary for the synthesis of adrenal and sex hormones. It keeps the skin healthy and is important for the health of the nervous system and digestive system. Niacin is stored in the liver, which requires this vitamin for the breakdown of estrogen. Consequently, a deficiency of niacin will lead to an excess of estrogen and an increased breast cancer risk.[3]

Some studies indicate that niacin is a common deficiency among cancer patients.[4] One of its effects is to promote the repair and proper replication of DNA, the genetic material of the cell, which is disturbed in the cancer process. Niacin is required to make the enzyme ADP ribose polymerase, used in DNA replication and repair.[5] ADP ribose polymerase is made from the cell's NAD, which contains nicotinamide, a form of niacin. When animals were fed a diet low in niacin, they showed a deficiency of both NAD and ADP ribose polymerase.[6] In humans, a deficiency of niacin can lead to 70% less NAD in the cell.[7]

Niacin is required to make coenzyme Q10 from the amino acid, tyrosine. Low niacin will cause decreased amounts of coenzyme Q10, which is a promising therapy in breast cancer prevention and treatment. When niacin is administered before radiation treatments, it increases its effectiveness.[8] Niacin has been found to prevent tumor growth. In one study, two groups of human cells were treated with carcinogens. The group given adequate niacin developed tumors at only one tenth of the rate as the group deficient in niacin.[9]

Dr Max Gerson used niacin as an important part of his therapy with cancer patients. He felt that it improved liver function, bringing glycogen into the liver and helped to remove cellular toxins. He used 50 mg six times daily with his patients for four to six months. To prevent the niacin flush, he advised dissolving the tablet on the tongue *after* a meal or glass of juice.[10] The niacin flush causes the capillaries to dilate, producing a short-lived red flushing and tingling of the body similar to a sunburn. It can be very alarming for some people, but harmless. It may last for about 15 minutes and can occur a few hours after taking niacin.

Niacin is also an important nutrient in sauna detoxification programs and is used in increasing amounts up to 4000 mg daily for approximately 20 days, with medical supervision.

FOOD SOURCES: lean meats, poultry, fish, eggs, peanuts, sunflower and sesame seeds, pine nuts, brown rice, brewer's yeast, wheat germ and bran, liver.
DOSAGE: 25–2000 mg daily. Higher dose to be used with supervision.
CONTRAINDICATIONS: It can cause liver damage at dosages higher than 2000 mg daily, so anything above this should be monitored with liver function tests. It is contraindicated in persons with gout, liver disease, peptic ulcers, and possibly diabetes. If the dose is too high, nausea will be experienced, sometimes followed by vomiting.

Vitamin B6 (Pyridoxine)

Vitamin B6 is important for fat and protein metabolism and overall immune function. It is needed in the metabolism of essential fatty acids and in the breakdown of estrogen. Supplementation with B6 results in lowered estrogen levels and higher progesterone, which both decrease breast cancer risk. A deficiency of B6 causes lowered immunity, with shrinkage of lymphatic tissue, and a decrease in numbers of white blood cells and activity of the thymus gland. Cancer patients often have low levels of B6.[11] B6 helps keep the balance of sodium and potassium, which regulates body fluid. It allows linoleic acid to function better in our bodies and is needed for the production of hydrochloric acid so that we digest our food better, with better absorption of protein and minerals. Alcohol, excess protein, and the use of the birth control pill can all trigger a deficiency of B6.

FOOD SOURCES: Brewer's yeast, sunflower seeds, wheat germ, tuna, beans, salmon, trout, brown rice, bananas, walnuts, hazelnuts, avocados, egg yolks, kale, bee pollen, liver, whole grain cereals.
DOSAGE: 50–200 mg daily.
CONTRAINDICATIONS: Use with caution if you have stomach ulcers.

Folic Acid

Deficiency of folic acid can trigger megaloblastic anemia and degeneration of the intestinal lining, leading to poor nutrient absorption. Folic acid helps block the division of rapidly dividing cells, such as occurs in cancer formation, and is specifically used to prevent cervical dysplasia. When folic acid is deficient, there will be shrinkage of lymphatic tissue and depressed immunity. Folic acid is needed for the production of DNA and for mental and emotional health. It stimulates hydrochloric acid production in the stomach, which helps to prevent intestinal parasites. It also assists liver function. It is destroyed by high temperatures, exposure to light, and when foods are left out at room temperature for long periods, as in salad bars. Consequently, it is a common nutritional deficiency.

FOOD SOURCES: green, leafy vegetables, liver, brewer's yeast, black-eyed peas, wheat germ and bran, beans, soy, lentils, asparagus, broccoli, Brussels sprouts, whole wheat, oatmeal, barley, almonds, split peas, and walnuts.
DOSAGE: 400 mcg daily in adults, 800 mcg during pregnancy and breast-feeding.
CONTRAINDICATIONS: None.

Vitamin B12

Vitamin B12 is important in protein, carbohydrate, and fat metabolism. It helps the conversion of beta-carotene to vitamin A and assists in the production of DNA and RNA, the genetic material in each cell. It assists the action of vitamin C and is essential for longevity. Vegetarians are sometimes deficient in B12, as it is uncommon in vegetarian diets. We should take a B complex that includes B12 on a regular basis if we are avoiding meat and dairy.

The absorption of B12 decreases with age and the use of laxatives will deplete B12 reserves. A B12 deficiency may take over five years to appear, after the body's stores have run out. A recent study found that if post-menopausal women had serum B12 levels below a certain threshold level, their breast cancer risk was increased.[12]

FOOD SOURCES: liver, kidney, meat, fish, egg yolks, poultry, yogurt, milk.
DOSAGE: 50 mcg daily.
CONTRAINDICATIONS: None.

Inositol and Inositol Hexaphosphate (IP6)

Inositol is part of the B complex found naturally occurring in high fiber foods, such as wheat bran, rice bran, and legumes. When bound to hexaphosphate, it forms IP6 or phytic acid. When properly combined with inositol, inositol hexaphosphate or IP6 forms two molecules of IP3 in the body. IP3 acts to prevent cancer by regulating cell division. When IP3 levels are low, cancer cells replicate out of control, whereas when there are high amounts of IP3 available, they cease to divide. In addition, IP6 promotes cell differentiation, a process whereby cancer cells become more normal. Animal studies have shown that the effects of IP6 occur within 24 hours of administration and persist for several days after a single dose.[13] Rats given 0.4% IP6 in drinking water, equivalent to a diet containing 20% bran, showed a 33.5% reduction in tumor incidence and 48.8% fewer tumors.[14] Evidence suggests that IP6 has a positive effect on tumor suppressor genes such as p53, which encourages genetically damaged cells to self-destruct.[15] The combination of inositol and IP6 is more effective than IP6 alone. It also enhances immune function and acts as an antioxidant. Studies have shown this combination to be effective against breast, prostate, lung, liver, skin and brain cancers, as well as leukemia and lymphomas. They can be used in conjunction with chemotherapy and radiation.

The maximum benefit is obtained from products that contain four parts IP6 to one part inositol. Zinc, iron, and calcium will be poorly absorbed if ingested with IP6, so take these supplements at a different time of day.

FOOD SOURCES: whole grains and beans.
DOSAGE: 800–1200 mg. IP6 and 200–300 mg. inositol as prevention; 4,800–7,200 mg. IP6 and 1,200–1,800 mg. inositol for individuals with cancer. It should be taken on an empty stomach.
CONTRAINDICATIONS: None.

Vitamin C

According to the lowest estimates, vitamin C can reduce the risk of breast cancer by 5–10% in menopausal and post-menopausal women. Higher estimates suggest that risk can be reduced for menopausal women by 16% and for post-menopausal women by 37%. Some studies concluded that the greater the amount of vitamin C that a woman routinely ingested from foods, the greater the reduction of breast cancer risk.[16] This vitamin acts as an antioxidant to prevent cellular and DNA damage from free radicals. Vitamin C helps to prevent tumor growth and the formation of metastases by building dense connective tissue and assists the activity of white blood cells, improving immunity. It is important in the production of interferon. Fruits and vegetables are the best dietary source of vitamin C. Chewable vitamin C tablets have a high sugar content and can lead to tooth decay.

FOOD SOURCES: citrus, strawberries, melon, tomatoes, green leafy vegetables, papaya, mangoes, cantaloupe, broccoli, potatoes, cabbage, green and red peppers, rose hips, and the Ayurvedic herb, amla.
DOSAGE: 2,000–10,000 mg daily in frequent small doses, preferably with food.
CONTRAINDICATIONS: Diarrhea may result at levels of 10,000 mg daily, at which point the dose should be reduced. Always increase or decrease vitamin C incrementally rather than starting at very high amounts or dropping the dosage suddenly.

Vitamin P (Bioflavonoids)

These are a very large group of over 4,000 antioxidants which prevent cancer-promoting substances from attaching themselves to cells and inhibit cancer cell growth and metastasis. They form the pigment in plants, as do the carotenes. Usually they concentrate in the peel, skin, or outer layer of the plant and are also present in tea and wine. Bioflavonoids include catechin, quercetin, rutin, and silymarin. They help to remove toxic copper from the body and prevent vitamin C from being destroyed. Bioflavonoids assist the body in using vitamin C to stimulate detoxification of chemicals, toxins, and drugs in the liver. A standard Western diet contains a daily dose of 500–1000 mg of bioflavonoids, while a vegetarian diet contains 5,000 mg, which protects us from cancer and inflammation. We need certain intestinal bacteria to activate bioflavonoids. The following chart summarizes some of the important bioflavonoids and their effects.

Bioflavonoid	What It Does	Found In
Quercetin	Toxic to cancer cells, indirectly improves immunity.	Ginger, echinacea, pau d'arco, St. John's wort
Rutin	Toxic to cancer cells, strengthens capillaries.	Buckwheat
Silymarin	Improves liver's ability to detoxify toxins.	Milk thistle
Aglycone, Kaempferol, Myricetin	Cancer fighting ability.	Green and black tea
Pycnogenol	Powerful antioxidant and cell protector, strengthens capillaries.	Pine bark, grape seed

FOOD SOURCES: citrus, berries, yams, soy, dark, leafy greens, milk thistle, broccoli, cabbage, squash and carrots, amla.

DOSAGE: 100 mg of bioflavonoids for every 500 mg of vitamin C; purchase vitamin C with bioflavonoids.

CONTRAINDICATIONS: None.

Vitamin D

Vitamin D is found mainly among dairy products such as milk and cheese. Because these foods have been linked with increased breast cancer risk, we should consume them infrequently. The easiest way to obtain vitamin D is by spending a little time in the sun. Studies show that the closer to the equator a population is, the less risk they have for breast cancer.[17] Sunshine causes the body to make its own vitamin D, which is then synthesized by the liver to become active vitamin D. The more receptors we have in our breasts for vitamin D, the greater the effect it has on tumor prevention as well as tumor treatment (vitamin D has been shown to reduce the size of malignant tumors in women with high amounts of vitamin D receptors).[18] To prevent skin cancer, we should be cautious about too much direct exposure to sunlight. Fifteen minutes towards the end of the day is probably sufficient.

Vitamin D is also a hormone that regulates the mineral balance of calcium and phosphorus. It stimulates their absorption from the intestine, works with parathyroid hormone to draw calcium out of bone tissue, and stimulates the reabsorption of calcium from the kidneys. Adequate vitamin D is crucial during and after menopause when the decline in estrogen and progesterone can lead to bone loss and osteoporosis.

FOOD SOURCES: dairy products, fortified soymilk, fish oils.

DOSAGE: For someone who avoids the sun and dairy products 800 IU of vitamin D daily is appropriate, while 400 IU would be adequate for those living in cloudy environments. No supplementation is necessary if you are regularly exposed to adequate sunlight. In its wisdom, the body will simply stop production when enough has been made from sun exposure. This safety mechanism is not present with supplementation.

CONTRAINDICATIONS: Overdoses of vitamin D are extremely toxic, resulting in deafness and blindness.

Vitamin E

Vitamin E refers to a group of eight fat-soluble compounds composed of four tocopherols (alpha, beta, delta, gamma) and four tocotrienols. It is stored in liver, muscle, and fat tissue. It is an antioxidant, working along with vitamin C to protect from cellular damage due to toxins, radiation, and aging. As an antioxidant, it protects the other fat-soluble vitamins and oils from oxidation, and we should take extra vitamin E when we consume higher amounts of unsaturated oils, such as flaxseed oil.

Vitamin E improves immune function and helps prevent shrinkage of lymphatic tissue. It protects the thymus gland and enhances the function of T-cells, our body's defense against cancer. Vitamin E works synergistically with selenium and will enhance its protective effect. One study found that vitamin E as alpha-tocopherol decreased risk of breast cancer in pre-menopausal women with a family history of the disease.[19] Recent studies suggest that vitamin E in the form of tocotrienols derived from palm oil inhibits both estrogen-positive and estrogen-negative breast cancer cells and is more effective than the alpha-tocopherol form of vitamin E.[20] When we use a vitamin E supplement for breast cancer prevention, we should purchase one that includes tocotrienols and mixed tocopherols.

FOOD SOURCES: cold-pressed vegetable oils, fresh wheat germ, raw seeds and nuts, egg yolk.

DOSAGE: 400–800 IU daily.

CONTRAINDICATIONS: It should not be taken with iron, but separated from it by eight or more hours. It may raise blood pressure in someone who has not used it; therefore, start at a low dosage and monitor blood pressure in anyone with hypertension. Use with caution in patients with chronic rheumatic heart disease.

Vitamin K

Vitamin K has demonstrated effectiveness in attacking the energy packets (ATP) of the cancer cells. It is usually manufactured in the intestines in the presence of healthy bacteria. (Hence a rationale for avoiding antibiotics and supplementing regularly with acidophilus and bifidus.) A synthesized form of vitamin K, vitamin K3, was developed to treat people who were incapable of producing their own vitamin K. This form of the vitamin reduces the risk of breast cancer more than the original form.[21] Vitamin K acts as a clotting agent, but when used with the anticoagulant warfarin its effectiveness in breast cancer treatment increased. Vitamin K and warfarin can be used in combination with conventional breast cancer drugs to reduce their toxic effect. This combination greatly increased life expectancy of cancer patients.

FOOD SOURCES: our own intestinal bacteria, cabbage, broccoli, turnip greens, lettuce, wheat bran, alfalfa sprouts, kelp, leafy green vegetables, cheese, egg yolks.
DOSAGE: 300–500 mcg daily.
CONTRAINDICATIONS: Excessive amounts of synthetic vitamin K may build up in the blood and cause toxic reactions.

Minerals

Calcium

Animal studies have shown that a low intake of calcium and vitamin D combined with a high fat diet can cause an increase in tumors of the breast from 37–75%, or approximately double. The tumors in the low calcium group also tended to be larger than those in animals fed a high fat diet with sufficient calcium.[22] High calcium intake is especially protective in preventing colon cancer.

Girls with low calcium levels during puberty may be at more risk for breast cancer later in life. In animal studies, reduced amounts of calcium and vitamin D during this critical growth period caused more breast cancer later in their lives than in animals that were fed sufficient amounts.[23]

A reasonable but difficult to achieve dietary level is 800–1500 mg daily depending upon age, pregnancy or lactation and sex, while the therapeutic dose range is between 1000–2000 mg. The majority of a calcium supplement is best taken at night because more calcium is lost at night and foods may interfere with absorption. However, if an individual has deficient stomach acid, it will not be absorbed on its own and would be better taken with a meal. Stomach acid levels tend to decrease as we age and should be checked yearly if there are digestive complaints or mineral deficiencies. A simple and inexpensive test called the Gastro-Test involves swallowing a capsule with a long thread in it, waiting 15 minutes, and then drawing the thread back up to measure the pH on the portion that entered the stomach.

Calcium should be taken with magnesium (in a 2:1 ratio) and vitamin D for proper absorption. Other minerals that enhance its absorption and utilization are boron and silica. High protein and high phosphorus intake (meats, soft drinks) promotes calcium loss. Cereal grains and fiber that are high in phytates decrease calcium absorption. Salt, sugar, and caffeine cause calcium loss. In summary, take your calcium before bed or with a meal that is low protein, low fiber, and without salt or sugar. Generally, avoid sugar, salt, caffeine, soft drinks, and high protein diets. In so doing, you will help to protect your breasts, colon, and bones.

Chelated minerals (aspartates, picolinates, amino acid chelates) are more bio-available than metallic minerals such as gluconates, lactates, sulphates, carbonates and oxides. Hydrochloric acid production can be stimulated with bitter herbs such as wormwood, gentian, goldenseal, and pippali. Lemon and apple cider vinegar before a meal also have a beneficial effect on hydrochloric acid production.

FOOD SOURCES: seaweeds (hijiki, arame, nori, kombu, dulse, kelp), sesame seeds, almonds, sunflower seeds, dairy, tofu and soy products, parsley, kale, broccoli, beet greens, shepherd's purse, kidney beans, lentils, nettle, horsetail, sage, barley, millet, quinoa, figs, and molasses.
DOSAGE: 800–2000 mg daily.
CONTRAINDICATIONS: Although calcium acts to protect against breast cancer, it may not be a good idea to take high amounts if you have cancer. Gerson found that calcium caused tumors to grow but was unclear why this would be so. The only minerals he advised taking if one had cancer were potassium and iodine.[24]

Magnesium

Magnesium reduced the incidence of malignant breast tumors by 50% in studies on rats. When used with vitamin C, selenium, and vitamin A the number of tumors declined even further. Cancer progression is partially due to nutrient deficiency, and magnesium is a common nutritional deficiency.[25] It is needed in the metabolism of glutathione, an important amino acid complex used by the liver and white blood cells.

Magnesium is the mineral that is responsible for chlorophyll's green color. Any green vegetable or seed will have some magnesium.

FOOD SOURCES: pumpkin seeds, nuts, brewer's yeast, soy, dried apricots, collards, seafood, whole grains, dark green vegetables, molasses.

DOSAGE: 300–800 mg daily.

CONTRAINDICATIONS: High amounts of magnesium can cause diarrhea in some individuals. If this happens to you, cut your dosage down and then gradually increase it to tolerance levels.

Potassium

Potassium is a mineral found in the body's intracellular fluid; only a small amount occurs in the extracellular fluid. Sodium and potassium help regulate water balance in the body, maintaining the fluids on either side of the cell wall. Potassium keeps the body fluids alkaline, which is important because cancer prefers an acid environment. It is necessary for normal growth, muscle contractions, and stimulates the kidneys to eliminate waste products. Thus, as a mineral, it is one of the body's detoxifiers. As part of a cancer prevention program, we want to keep a low sodium and high potassium balance to keep the body detoxifying and to prevent the accumulation of toxins in the cells. Normally, a potassium supplement is unnecessary unless we are retaining sodium. We can use foods high in potassium and low in sodium as a regular part of our diet (see pages 215 and 216).

FOOD SOURCES: navy beans, caraway seeds, dark cherries, dried apricots, lentils, walnuts, oranges, almonds, apple, avocado, peaches, banana, grapefruit, pineapple, potatoes, soybeans, squash, tomatoes, sage, and mint.

DOSAGE: 3000–6000 mg daily from foods.

Iodine

There is a link between iodine deficiency and fibrocystic breast disease, which sometimes increases a woman's susceptibility to breast cancer. Kelp, other sea vegetables, sodium iodide, or aqueous molecular iodine can be used as part of a treatment regime for fibrocystic breast disease. Women with breast cancer sometimes show iodine deficiency in a hair analysis. Iodine is needed as a raw material to synthesize thyroid hormones and there is a link between an unbalanced thyroid and breast cancer risk. Iodine is commonly deficient in our diets because it is deficient in the soil that is inland from the sea. Japanese women traditionally use kelp in their cooking, and it may be one of the nutrients (along with soy) that gives them roughly one quarter of the breast cancer rates present among women in the United States. In animal studies, kelp has been shown to prevent breast tumors.[26]

Dr Max Gerson used a form of iodine called Lugol's solution, half strength in a dosage of three drops, six times daily, as well as dessicated thyroid, in treating his cancer patients, believing that it restored the electrical potential of the cell and enhanced cellular activity. The thyroid gland absorbs 80 times more iodine than any other tissue but contains only 20% of the body's iodine content; the rest is found in the skeletal muscles, liver, central nervous system, pituitary gland, breasts, and ovaries. Gerson believed that the basal metabolic rate in cancer patients is often disturbed, being either very high or low, with a corresponding high or low iodine content of the blood. He was able to normalize these extremes with supplemental iodine. One of the functions of the thyroid gland is to improve oxygen levels in body tissues; cancer cells prefer low oxygen environments and do not thrive when the tissues are saturated with oxygen. This may be a rationale for assessing thyroid function in cancer patients.

Too much iodine can suppress the thyroid gland. Dosages need to be monitored by someone experienced with thyroid disorders and the use of iodine. Kelp is safer to use than liquid iodine.

FOOD SOURCES: sea salt, sea vegetables, fish, asparagus, garlic, lima beans, mushrooms, sesame seeds, soybeans, spinach, summer squash, and turnip greens.

DOSAGE: A reasonable dietary level is 150 mcg of iodine, while the therapeutic dose range is 100–1000 mcg daily. Start with a small dose of kelp and increase gradually.

CONTRAINDICATIONS: Side effects of too much iodine are weight loss, insomnia, anxiety, heart palpitations, acne, headaches, water retention, metallic taste in the mouth and skin sensitivities. Do not use iodine if you have a hyperactive thyroid or sensitivity to it.

Cesium and Rubidium

These are alkaline minerals found in tiny amounts throughout the earth's crust. Cesium may help protect against radiation toxicity. It has a high pH level and can change the acidic pH of the cancer cell to being alkaline. At a pH of 8 or so, cancer cells are non-viable. Mice fed cesium and rubidium showed a decrease in tumor sizes within two weeks. Cesium also helps decrease the pain commonly associated with malignancy. Cesium is considered moderately toxic and must be used with supervision.[27]

Molybdenum

This trace mineral aids in the mobilization of iron from the liver and helps with the oxidation of fats. It is a free radical scavenger and provides protection against chemical carcinogens. When molybdenum and vitamin C were added to the food supply in the Taihang Mountain range in northern China, the once prevalent esophageal cancer decreased its occurrence in that area. It also exerts a protective effect against stomach cancer. Animal studies have shown it to inhibit the formation of breast cancer.[28]

FOOD SOURCES: legumes, whole grain cereals, kidney, liver, milk, and dark green vegetables.
DOSAGE: 100–500 mcg daily.
CONTRAINDICATIONS: Toxicity can result in diarrhea, anemia, copper deficiency and low growth rate.

Chromium

Chromium is a common deficiency in North America because the soil does not contain an adequate supply and therefore neither does our food. A diet high in sweets and refined foods, North American staples, causes chromium to be used up quickly. Chromium deficiency will cause sweet cravings to increase, creating a vicious cycle of binging with further depletion of the mineral. Chromium is essential for the maintenance of proper blood sugar levels and for keeping blood levels of insulin low. When insulin levels are increased, the risk of breast cancer is increased threefold. The blood level of the related hormone, insulin-like growth factor-1, is also probably decreased by chromium, although I have not found this theory tested in any studies. The Harvard Nurse's Study found that when the levels of insulin-like growth factor-1 were higher in a woman's blood, her risk for breast cancer increased sevenfold. Therefore, if chromium can help keep the levels of insulin and insulin-like growth factors low, it may help to prevent breast cancer.

Chromium is an ingredient (along with niacin and amino acids) in a substance that the body makes called glucose tolerance factor, or GTF. Chromium stimulates the activity of enzymes involved in the metabolism of glucose for energy and the synthesis of fatty acids and cholesterol. It increases the sensitivity of cells throughout the body to insulin. Without chromium, insulin's activity at a cellular level is blocked, causing its levels to rise in the blood, and blood sugar levels to go up. It is a critical nutrient used in treating both hypoglycemia and diabetes.

One of the strategies involved in facilitating weight loss is to increase the sensitivity of cells to insulin, since high insulin levels in the blood lead to fat deposition and weight gain. Chromium supplementation has been found to increase lean body mass and decrease weight, and to lower cholesterol and triglyceride levels. Weight loss in itself will decrease breast cancer risk as there is less estrogen available when there is a decrease in body fat.

Several forms of chromium can be found on the market, including chromium polynicotinate, chromium enriched yeast, and chromium picolinate. The most effective one is chromium picolinate.[29]

FOOD SOURCES: brewer's yeast, liver, beef, whole wheat bread, beets, mushrooms.
DOSAGE: 200–600 mcg daily.
CONTRAINDICATIONS: None.

Selenium

Selenium is toxic at high doses but deficiencies are linked to a higher cancer incidence. Many geographic areas have soil deficient in this trace mineral. Its anti-cancer effects include the inhibition of the action of chemical substances, minerals, and viruses that cause cancer by repairing DNA damage; protection against UV light; reduction in tumor volume; and stimulation of the activity of natural killer cells to directly annihilate cancer cells. It protects the thymus gland from free radical damage. Selenium is essential for the conversion of the thyroid hormone T4 to the more active hormone, T3. The higher the selenium present in a person's tissues, the lower the breast cancer incidence, providing a toxic level has not been reached.[30] One study revealed that breast cancer patients had serum selenium levels of 41–51 ug/L, while healthy subjects had levels of between 73–89 ug/L.[31] Selenium also improves the synthesis and activity of glutathione, along with magnesium and zinc.

Selenium can be accurately measured through hair analysis. Selenium is more effective when there are high amounts of vitamin E in the blood and works with it to protect cell membranes.[32]

FOOD SOURCES: Brazil nuts, sunflower seeds, barley, brown rice, red Swiss chard, tuna, swordfish, lobster, oysters, herring, brewer's yeast, wheat germ and bran, whole grains, and sesame seeds.
DOSAGE: 100–300 mcg daily.
CONTRAINDICATIONS: Symptoms of selenium toxicity include hair, tooth and nail loss and dermatitis.

Zinc

Zinc is a common deficiency in our diets today because the soil has become deficient. Zinc is necessary for numerous enzyme systems in the body, including the detoxifying systems of the liver. It is essential for the metabolism of vitamin A, stabilizes cell membranes so they are less vulnerable to damage, and is needed for growth and repair. The pineal, pituitary, and thymus glands need sufficient zinc for proper function. Zinc increases thymus hormones and decreases shrinkage of the thymus due to stress or free radical damage. It increases the number of T-cells and improves phagocytosis, or the ability of certain white blood cells to digest toxins. It inhibits the growth of viruses. Zinc is important in the utilization of insulin, the hormone that regulates blood sugar. A zinc deficiency can manifest as an inability to taste with a subsequent loss of appetite. Zinc competes with copper for absorption in the small intestine, so if too much zinc is given, there will be a copper deficiency, and vice versa. Copper toxicity results in zinc deficiency.

One study found that zinc levels were decreased in women with breast cancer.[33] Another study found that women with breast cancer have higher serum copper and lower zinc levels that healthy controls.[34] Zinc levels can be monitored yearly through an oral zinc test or hair analysis. Supplementation of zinc should generally be taken away from meals, as eggs, milk, and cereal will decrease its bioavailability.

FOOD SOURCES: pumpkin seeds, sunflower seeds, almonds, walnuts, garlic, turnips, split peas, potatoes, lima beans, seafood, organ meats, mushrooms, brewer's yeast, soybeans, oysters, herring, eggs, and wheat germ.

DOSAGE: 20–100 mg daily.

CONTRAINDICATIONS: Excessive zinc may result in a copper deficiency, so consider supplementing a small amount of copper if zinc is used long term.

Manganese

As a trace mineral, manganese activates numerous enzymes, including those necessary for utilization of vitamin C. It helps in the synthesis of fatty acids and cholesterol. It nourishes the nerves and brain and is essential in the formation of thyroid hormone. The largest amounts of manganese are found in the pituitary gland, kidney, bones, liver, and pancreas. Manganese has been found to increase the activity of natural killer cells in mice through increased interferon production. Natural killer cells directly attack cancer cells.

FOOD SOURCES: whole grain cereals, egg yolks, nuts, seeds, green vegetables, pineapple.

DOSAGE: 5 mg daily.

CONTRAINDICATIONS: Toxicity results in weakness, irritability, psychological and motor disturbances, and impotence.

Other Nutrients

Coenzyme Q10

Coenzyme Q10 is a naturally occurring molecule similar to vitamin K and is necessary for the health of all human tissues and organs. Highest concentrations of it are found in the organs that need the most energy, such as the heart, liver, muscles, and cells of the immune system.[35] Its synthesis requires the presence of the amino acid, tyrosine, vitamins B2, B3, B5, B6, B12, folic acid, and vitamin C. Deficiencies of these nutrients (particularly B6) will lead to a deficit of coenzyme Q10. CoQ10 maintains the effectiveness of vitamin E and helps to prevent the breakdown of cell membranes. It works synergistically with the amino acid carnitine.[36] It is a component of the cellular respiration cycle from which metabolic energy is derived. It is used therapeutically in gum disease, cardiovascular disease, diabetes and immune disorders. It activates immune responsiveness and functions as an antioxidant. With aging, the body loses its ability to make CoQ10 from foods. In animals, it was able to prevent shrinking of the thymus gland and extended lifespan.[37] People with heart disease and cancer have a very low supply of CoQ10 in their tissues. As a supplement it strengthens the heart, normalizes blood pressure, improves energy and extends life. It improves the effectiveness of the immune system. CoQ10 is also helpful in preventing damage to the heart caused by chemotherapy drugs such as adriamycin.[38]

CoQ10 has been shown to be beneficial in treating breast cancer. In one study, 32 node-positive breast cancer patients were treated with conventional allopathic therapy as well as antioxidants (beta carotene, vitamin C, vitamin E, and selenium), essential fatty acids, and 90 mg of CoQ10 for 18 months. None of them died or showed evidence of metastases. Six showed partial tumor regression.[39] In one patient, the dosage of CoQ10 was increased to 390 mg; in one month, the tumor was no longer palpable, and in another month, mammography confirmed that it was gone. Another patient who had non-radical surgery with a proven residual tumor in the tumor bed was also treated with 300 mg of CoQ10. After three months, there was no residual tumor tissue. CoQ10 has been shown to cause tumor regression in five cases of breast cancer using a daily dose of 390 mg for a period of three to five years. One patient experienced disappearance of multiple liver metastases after 11 months on the therapy.[40] Another study of 200 women with breast tumors (80 malignant and 120 benign) found that CoQ10 concentrations in plasma were reduced both in patients with cancer and in women with benign lesions, compared to the control population of women with normal breast tissue. There were more severe reductions when the tumor volume was large, when the tumor grade suggested a bad prognosis, and when there were no hormone receptors in the breast tissue. On the other hand, plasma levels of vitamin E were the same in women with malignant or benign tumors as women in the control group. Breast cancer, therefore, is associated with a decreased level of plasma CoQ10.[41] CoQ10 is a promising therapy in breast cancer prevention and treatment.[42] These are very high doses as the usual therapeutic dosage is 20–60 mg. More research is necessary to see if similar results could be obtained at a lower dosage level.[43]

Q-Gel, a soluble form of coenzyme Q10, is more bio-available than other preparations of this nutrient, and lower doses may be sufficient to achieve the same effect, although research is lacking.[44] Because it is more soluble in fats, CoQ10 is best taken orally in soft gel form to maximize absorption.

FOOD SOURCES: highest in beef muscle and heart, lower in spinach, grains, beans, and some oils.
DOSAGE: For prevention, 60–300 mg daily. With breast cancer, 300–400 mg daily in divided doses.
CONTRAINDICATIONS: None, other than the high cost for high dosages.

Alpha Lipoic Acid

The amino acids cysteine and methionine help to synthesize alpha lipoic acid from linoleic acid. Alpha lipoic acid is produced in high amounts by the liver and in lower amounts by every cell. It has the extraordinary ability to prevent damage to the cell at the genetic level. It reduces the cancer-stimulating effect that environmental toxins have on breast cells. Because of our increasingly toxic environment, we need more of it these days than ever before in human history. Alpha lipoic acid inhibits the ability of cancer cells to become invasive or to metastasize.[45] It decreases our susceptibility to the damaging effects of ionizing radiation.[46] It is an excellent free radical scavenger and antioxidant, and enhances immune function by increasing the number of helper T-cells. Alpha lipoic acid increases the effectiveness and lifespan of other antioxidants, including vitamins C and E, quercetin, and

Coenzyme Q10.[47,48] It promotes the production of glutathione, a powerful antioxidant, immune stimulant, and detoxifier. It also decreases the toxic side effects of chemotherapy and regenerates the liver. It helps to reduce the formation of calcium oxalate crystals which interfere with liver function and can form gallstones. Alpha lipoic acid is one of the few substances that can chelate, or bind to, toxic metals such as lead, aluminum, mercury, copper, cadmium, and arsenic, and help to remove them from our bodies. This nutrient works synergistically with selenium, so we must ensure adequate amounts of selenium for optimal output.[49] By consuming foods high in the sulphur-bearing amino acids along with flaxseed oil, we maximize the amount of alpha lipoic acid that our bodies produce and protect ourselves from breast cancer and many other ailments.

FOOD SOURCES: red meat, liver, yeast, potatoes, leafy vegetables.[50,51]
DOSAGE: 50–100 mg daily for prevention; 300–600 mg daily with breast cancer.
CONTRAINDICATIONS: None; it is very safe with no adverse reactions reported.

Grape Seed Extract

Grape seed extract contains high amounts of bioflavonoids, including what are known as proanthocyanins and anthocyanins. These act as potent free radical scavengers, apparently 50 times more effective than vitamin E and 20 times stronger than vitamin C in neutralizing free radicals. They help to slow down the rate of DNA mutation when cells are exposed to carcinogens. Grape seed extract is particularly effective in preventing free radical damage to polyunsaturated oils, such as flaxseed oil. It maintains the integrity of the arterial walls and circulation, can improve eyesight, and helps to restore the elasticity, flexibility, and strength to the body's connective tissues. It will slow down the aging process in general.

FOOD SOURCES: None.
DOSAGE: 60–300 mg daily.
CONTRAINDICATIONS: None.

Modified Citrus Pectin

Modified citrus pectin is a special form of pectin that has been shortened through a laboratory process so that it can be absorbed through the intestinal wall. Otherwise, citrus pectin, obtained from the peel and pulp of citrus fruits, acts as a soluble fiber that is not broken down or absorbed.

Research has shown that certain cancer cell types have specific carbohydrate-binding protein molecules on their cell surfaces called galectins. The more advanced the cancer, the more galectins are produced. Higher galectin levels allow greater adhesion of cancer cells to each other so that they form colonies and facilitate the binding of cancer cells to distant sites, promoting metastases. Modified citrus pectin works by blocking the galectins on the surface of cancer cells so that they cannot adhere to other cells. It inhibits the clumping of cancer cells to each other and the adhesion of cancer cells to normal cells. The result is that cancer cells are less likely to thrive and are more easily destroyed by the immune system. Modified citrus pectin has an affinity for various cancer cell types, including breast, prostate, larynx, and melanoma. Modified citrus pectin is also able to bind to cholesterol in the bloodstream, helping to prevent arteriosclerosis. It is able to bind heavy metals, facilitating their excretion from the body.[52]

FOOD SOURCES: None — the citrus pectin from foods needs to be modified through a laboratory process.
DOSAGE: The recommended dosage is 15 g per day in three divided doses, although lower amounts are also beneficial.
CONTRAINDICATIONS: Well tolerated and safe, although there may be mild gastrointestinal complaints.

Melatonin

Melatonin is one of the body's first lines of defence in response to malignant breast cell growth, as we discovered in the chapter on Understanding the Hormone Puzzle. Increased melatonin keeps abnormal breast cancer cells under control, while a deficiency of melatonin allows breast tumors to form. Melatonin has been shown to prevent chemically caused breast tumors in studies on rats. It inhibits the replication of breast cancer cells in the laboratory by regulating cell division and multiplication.[53] It's as though it flips a breaker switch to turn off estradiol's activity on the breast cell. It may also actually lower estrogen levels.[54] Some scientists believe that melatonin competes with estrogen for the estrogen receptor sites, thus negating estrogen's activity. Women with late stage breast cancer achieved partial remission lasting an average of eight months when they were given high doses of melatonin in the evening (20 mg per day). Melatonin has been found to be highly effective at inhibiting estrogen-sensitive breast cancer cells but only minimally effective in inhibiting cancer cells that were not estrogen-sensitive. Melatonin increases the effectiveness of tamoxifen when used along with it and improves patient response to chemotherapy. Melatonin has an added benefit of decreasing anxiety.[55]

Melatonin can be taken to prevent breast cancer or used as part of a treatment for it, particularly if the cancer is estrogen receptor positive.[56] If melatonin is prescribed, all doses should be taken at bedtime, since morning administration has been found to stimulate cancer growth in animal studies, while evening dosing inhibits cancer.[57] It is illegal for over-the-counter sale in Canada, but is available at health food stores in the United States.

Interestingly, melatonin is a molecule that is present in many life forms, including plants. Melatonin is derived from its precursor, serotonin, which was identified in fruits and vegetables over 30 years ago, and many foods high in serotonin also contain melatonin. One study found that an average of 100 g of fruit or vegetable contained the following amounts of melatonin: banana, 47 ng; tomato, 25 ng; cucumber, 9 ng; beet root, 0.1 ng. The 'Sweet 100' variety of tomatoes contains about five times more melatonin than wild tomatoes.[58] Rice and corn contain melatonin. Herbs that contain melatonin include the Chinese herb *Scutellaria baicalensis*, St. John's wort flowers and feverfew. See also the discussion of ways of taking care of your pineal gland in the chapter on hormones in this book.

FOOD SOURCES: bananas, tomatoes, beet root, rice, corn, dessicated pineal gland, the Chinese herb *Scutellaria baicalensis*, St. John's wort flowers, and feverfew.
DOSAGE: For prevention, 3–9 mg nightly. With breast cancer, 5–20 mg nightly.
CONTRAINDICATIONS: Don't take it at any other time of day. Otherwise, appears to be very safe.

Natural Progesterone Cream

As we also learned in the hormone chapter, Dr John Lee maintains that breast disease and breast cancer are linked to 'estrogen dominance', or higher levels of estrogen without the opposing balance of progesterone. Estrogen causes excess multiplication of breast cells, while progesterone is responsible for the maturation of cells. The earlier the maturation is completed – that is, after a full-term pregnancy — the less prone we are to breast cancer. He considers premenstrual breast swelling and fibrocystic breast disease conditions of estrogen dominance that can be remedied by increasing natural progesterone levels. Women with low progesterone levels have 5.4 times more breast cancer than women with normal progesterone. Dr Lee recommends the cream for women with the following symptoms: water retention, fatigue, swollen or fibrocystic breasts, PMS, low libido, heavy or irregular periods, uterine fibroids, sweet cravings, weight gain, particularly on the hips and thighs, and symptoms of an underactive thyroid, such as cold hands and feet.

Natural progesterone cream is made from an extract of wild yam called diosgenin which is converted to progesterone in the laboratory. Diosgenin will not increase our progesterone levels; the lab conversion to progesterone is necessary. Many products are now available, although not easily in Canada, that contain natural progesterone. (You may need your medical doctor to prescribe it and a compounding pharmacist to make it for you). Depending on the concentration of progesterone, they will work differently. Dr Lee suggests a concentration of 400–500 mg progesterone per ounce at a dosage of ⅛ to ½ teaspoon of cream per day, for two to three weeks of the month. Normal progesterone production during a menstrual month is approximately 250 mg. The cream should be applied on various fatty areas of the body, rotating the areas of application.

Other more natural ways to help the body to make more progesterone rather than replacing it with the cream are to eat yams and soy, supplement with vitamin B6, vitamin E, boron, zinc, and selenium, and to use the herb chaste tree berry daily for up to a year.[59] The homeopathic remedy Folliculinum 9CH can be taken on days seven and 21 of your menstrual cycle as well. You can check your progesterone levels with a salivary hormone test available from Aeron Lab (San Leandro, California, tel. 800-631-7900 or fax. 510-729-0383) or from Diagnos Tech International Inc. (tel. 715-294-2149 or fax. 715-294-3921).

DOSAGE: Pre-menopausal women: ⅛ to ½ tsp daily between days 15 and 26 of your menstrual cycle. Menopausal women not on estrogen: same dosage over a two to three week period monthly. Menopausal women on estrogen: ¹⁄₁₆ to ¼ tsp daily over three weeks monthly.[60]

CONTRAINDICATIONS: Because it is a hormone, it should be used only when other natural therapies haven't worked. We are still not clear as to progesterone's role in breast cancer. Progesterone can become converted to metabolites that stimulate growth in breast cancer cells when cancer is present. For these reasons, it should be used with caution with women who have breast cancer, although at least one study has found it to be protective.[61] It will take more research until we know whether we should prescribe it or not for breast cancer patients. In the meantime, we can safely encourage the body to make its own progesterone

with the foods, vitamins, minerals, and herbs listed above. Use the cream with medical or naturopathic supervision and monitoring using saliva testing. Consult Dr. Lee's book for further information and best sources of the cream.

Liver Supplements

N-acetyl cysteine (NAC)

Cysteine is a sulfur-containing amino acid that helps our bodies make toxic chemicals and carcinogens harmless, as we learned in the chapter on Detoxifying Our Bodies. Because of this, it is important in the prevention and treatment of cancer. A thiol compound on the cysteine molecule helps to prevent the oxidation of sensitive tissues, which protects us from aging and cancer. In the liver, cysteine helps the small protein called glutathione detoxify carcinogens and chemicals, including some of the organochlorines. In the rest of the body it acts as a free radical scavenger. Cysteine works synergistically with vitamin C and is an essential element in many parts of the immune system.

Glutathione is made up of only three amino acids — cysteine, glutamic acid, and glycine. Glutathione is a powerful antioxidant and detoxifier, and the amount of cysteine present determines how much glutathione will be produced. N-acetyl cysteine is a modified form of cysteine that is converted back into cysteine in the body. It helps clear the cells of toxins, increases glutathione production and reduces the toxicity of chemicals. Glutathione is necessary for melatonin to work effectively. Women who take NAC experience fewer side effects from chemotherapy and radiation, but it may also make certain drugs less effective in targeting cancer cells. It is safe in doses of up to 3–4 g daily, even in pregnancy, but has a nauseating taste and smell. It is able to make less toxic many of the chemicals that cause breast cancer and assists our bodies in clearing them.

FOOD SOURCES: soy products (highest source), black beans, adzuki beans, chick peas, lentils, split peas, dried spirulina, nori, kelp, beef, avocados, almonds, sunflower seeds, butternuts, cottage cheese, fish, eggs, organic yogurt, wheat germ, oat flakes.

DOSAGE: 500 mg 1–3 times daily.

CONTRAINDICATIONS: Dosages higher than 7 g daily can be toxic.

Reduced Glutathione

Glutathione has five main functions in the body. Briefly, it protects the body against natural and man-made oxidants, which destroy cell membranes; helps the liver to detoxify poisonous chemicals and metals such as lead, cadmium, arsenic and mercury; is necessary for immune function, increasing the numbers and efficiency of various white blood cells; protects the integrity of the red blood cells; and acts as a brain neurotransmitter. The liver manufactures glutathione whenever extra cysteine is available. Magnesium and zinc deficiencies reduce glutathione levels. Selenium enhances glutathione synthesis and activity. Glutathione itself is poorly absorbed but reduced glutathione can be used as a supplement instead.

FOOD SOURCES: None. The body synthesizes it from three amino acids. Soy or pumpkin seeds are helpful.
DOSAGE: For prevention, 75–300 mg daily. With breast cancer, 1,600–2,000 mg daily.
CONTRAINDICATIONS: None. Best taken with antioxidant anthocyanidins, as from black currant and beet root.

What to Take During Surgery, Chemotherapy, and Radiation Treatments

How to Recover from Surgery Quickly

When I have patients scheduled for surgery, I usually recommend them to take several supplements before and after surgery. Vitamins A, C, and E can be taken after the surgery to keep the immune system strong and promote healing. (If vitamins C and E are taken before surgery, they may increase blood loss). Zinc taken before and after surgery will reduce the possibility of infection and assist in wound healing. To improve the ability of the liver to deal with the anesthetic, I recommend milk thistle tincture, NAC, and the homeopathic remedy, Phosphorus 6CH. The homeopathic remedy Arnica 30CH can be used two to three times daily to prevent excess bruising and bleeding. The remedy Calendula 30CH can be used after the surgery for a month or so to prevent infection and keloid formation along the scar. It encourages rapid healing of the skin, as do external applications of herbal oils from calendula, St. John's wort, and comfrey.

If you are pre-menopausal, schedule your breast surgery during the latter half of your menstrual cycle when progesterone levels are highest. A few, though not all, studies suggest that women who have their surgery between days 13–32 or on the first two days of their period have a better prognosis than women who have breast tumors removed during days 3–12 (where day one is the first day of your period).[62]

Chemotherapy, Radiation, and Antioxidants

Differing opinions exist in the naturopathic community about which supplements, particularly antioxidants, should be taken (or not taken) during chemotherapy and radiation treatments. The confusion arises because antioxidants may protect cells, including cancer cells, from the toxic effects of chemotherapy and radiation. Some practitioners, such as Dan Labriola, ND, believe that they may also prevent the destruction of some of the cancer cells remaining in the body. The patient who takes antioxidants will usually have fewer short and long-term side effects from chemotherapy and radiation, but the speculation is that years later a recurrence may be more likely to occur if a few cancer cells have survived because the antioxidant decreased the effectiveness of the drug or radiation treatment. At the present time, this is primarily a theoretical speculation that deserves consideration. In contrast, many studies have shown that various antioxidants augment the effectiveness of chemotherapy and radiation when taken singly or together. The chart on page 248 summarizes what is known so far about various antioxidants and their use with chemotherapy and radiation. More studies are needed to prove or disprove some of the beneficial or deleterious effects of taking antioxidants during chemotherapy and radiation treatments.

We do know that cysteine (or NAC) will reduce the anti-tumor effects of certain drugs that act as alkylating agents (cyclophosphamide, ifosfamide). On the other hand, it will protect the heart from damage induced by the drug, adriamycin.

In the July 1999 issue of the journal *Oncology*, Dan Labriola, ND, and Robert Livingston, MD, present guidelines for predicting interactions between chemotherapy drugs and antioxidants. Factors that should be considered before recommending supplements to women undergoing chemotherapy are the fraction of the drug effectiveness that depends upon its ability to generate free radicals; the nature of the free radicals generated by the drug; the dosage and concentration of the free radicals generated by the drug; the nature of the antioxidant; the concentration of the antioxidant; and the time that exists between the administration of the drug and the intake of antioxidants (before and after). These are difficult parameters to assess and will require the cooperation of an oncologist, pharmacist, and naturopathic doctor to

• Antioxidants and Their Use with Chemotherapy and Radiation •

ANTIOXIDANT	RADIATION	CHEMOTHERAPY
Vitamin A	• improves its effectiveness • decreases tumor size • increases survival time when administered with radiation in mice • improves response rate to radiation in humans	• does not interfere with methotrexate, cisplatin, etoposide, doxorubicin • does not reduce the effectiveness of chemo • increases the cytotoxic effect of chemo, reduces toxicity, increases survival time • protects the small intestine from damage due to methotrexate and improves intestinal absorption • use dosages between 15,000–50,000 IU/daily
Carotenoids	• improves its effectiveness	• beta carotene may interfere with the action of 5-fluorouracil • reduces the severity of mouth sores with high dose chemotherapy • more research needed
Vitamin C	• increases the effectiveness of radiotherapy in humans and in mice	• does not decrease the effectiveness of chemo • reduces the toxicity of Adriamycin • increases the effect of cyclophosphamide, vinblastine, doxorubicin, 5-fluorouracil, procarbazine, cisplatin, and paclitaxel • may increase the resistance to doxorubicin in resistant breast cancer cells but does not lead to resistance in cells that respond to doxorubicin • simultaneous administration of vitamin K can increase the activity of vitamin C
Flavonoids: Quercetin, Green tea, Genistein	• flavonoids increase the sensitivity of cancer cells to radiation *in vitro*	• green tea, quercetin and genistein increase the concentration of chemotherapy drugs in some resistant cell lines • quercetin increases the anti-tumor activity of cisplatin and busulfan in humans and does not interfere with the effectiveness of doxorubicin or etoposide • tamoxifen activity is decreased by tangeretin (from tangerines) in vivo and by genistein in vitro
Vitamin E	• increases the effectiveness of radiotherapy in mice when doses below 500 mg/kg are used (approximately 35,000 IU human dose) • more research needed	• no evidence that it reduces the effectiveness of chemo • increases the activity of 5-fluorouracil, doxorubicin, and cisplatin in humans
Selenium	• low selenium may reduce the lethal dose of radiation. Selenium may therefore decrease the effectiveness of radiotherapy • until more research is available limit selenium intake to less than 400 mcg/daily during radiotherapy	• decreases the toxic effect of cisplatin on the kidneys while improving its anti-tumor activity • increases white blood cell count when taken during chemo • may interfere with the effectiveness of the anti-tumor drug, bleomycin • no other evidence in humans suggests that selenium reduces the effectiveness of chemo

• Antioxidants and Their Use with Chemotherapy and Radiation •

ANTIOXIDANT	RADIATION	CHEMOTHERAPY
Coenzyme Q10	• may interfere with the effectiveness of radiotherapy if doses above 700 mg/day are used. • safe to use in doses of 100–400 mg/day	• reduces diarrhea and stomach irritation when used with doxorubicin • protects the heart from the toxic effects of doxorubicin • does not interfere with the effectiveness of doxorubicin • no evidence in humans suggests that CoQ10 reduces the effectiveness of chemo
N-acetylcysteine	• does not block the effectiveness of radiation	• does not interfere with the effectiveness of cyclophosphamide in humans • one out of two animal studies showed NAC to reduce the effectiveness of doxorubicin, but this was not confirmed in human trials; therefore, caution is required before using NAC with doxorubicin • NAC may inhibit the effectiveness of cisplatin; therefore, avoid NAC during use of cisplatin
Glutathione	• is not thought to interfere with radiotherapy	• decreases toxicity and increases the anti-tumor effect of cisplatin • more research is needed on the interaction between glutathione and chemotherapy
Melatonin	• increases the effectiveness of radiation and increases survival time when used with it • fewer side effects from radiotherapy when melatonin is used with it	• 20 mg/day of melatonin normalized platelet counts in breast cancer patients undergoing chemotherapy • increases survival time when used with tamoxifen, cisplatin, and etoposide • decreases weight loss during chemo • no evidence in humans suggests that it reduces the effectiveness of chemo

provide reasonable recommendations to a particular patient. If this is not possible, then Labriola and Livingston recommend that patients avoid alternative therapies during the time when chemotherapeutic drugs are most sensitive to interactions with antioxidants.[63] This time window will vary from one drug to the next.

The views of Labriola and Livingston met with criticism from two other authors, Davis W. Lamson, ND, and Matthew S. Brignall, ND. In the October 1999 issue of the journal *Alternative Medicine Review*, Lamson and Brignall present evidence to suggest that antioxidants do not reduce the effectiveness of chemotherapy or radiation when administered along with them but on the contrary may increase their effectiveness, as well as decrease adverse effects.[64] They surveyed the scientific literature and developed the guidelines presented in the chart on page 248. Combinations of antioxidants have been shown to act synergistically to reduce tumors in humans. When combined with chemotherapy and radiation they increase survival time and reduce toxicity.

Other supplements that one can safely take during chemotherapy and radiation are B3 (niacin), B6, inositol, IP6, kelp, chromium and modified citrus pectin. Niacin in particular is useful prior to and during radiation treatments. It is required to make the enzyme ADP ribose polymerase, used in DNA replication and repair.[65] When niacin is administered before radiation treatments, it increases its effectiveness, and will result in less damage to healthy cells.[66]

Herbs can be administered that protect the body's cells from the effects of chemotherapy without protecting the cancer cells. The main herbs used to restore the white blood cells and decrease the likelihood of infection are echinacea, goldenseal, astragalus, ligustrum, ganoderma (reishi mushroom), maitake and shitake mushrooms.

Essential oils can be used during radiation to protect from radiation burns. Niaouli oil and tea tree oil can be applied prior to treatment to accomplish this, while lavender with St. John's Wort oil can be used after radiation treatments are completed to stimulate rapid healing.

What to Take for Nausea During Chemotherapy Treatments

Ginger tea or ginger capsules can help relieve nausea but should be used cautiously in patients who have low platelets because ginger can inhibit blood clotting. Chemotherapy also has an anti-clotting effect, and the two used together may thin the blood to levels that are too low in patients whose platelets are reduced (60,000 or less), possibly causing hemorrhaging.[67] Nausea can also be counteracted with the Chinese medicinal mushroom called hoelen (fu ling) and the underground stem of pinellia. Collectively, these three herbs will reduce nausea, vomiting, and diarrhea. Catnip, peppermint, chamomile, and red raspberry can be used as alternatives to relieve nausea.

The acupuncture point P6, found three finger widths (about two inches) above the center of the wrist crease on the underside of the arm, relieves nausea when stimulated daily. Use acupressure or see an acupuncturist who can administer this treatment. You can also try taping a mung bean to this point and applying pressure several times daily, or purchase an anti-nausea wristband.

What to Take for a Low White Blood Cell Count During Chemotherapy and Radiation

Chemotherapy and radiation can suppress the white blood cells, the guardians of your immune system. Many natural substances can be used to protect them and to elevate them if they are low in number. The vitamins that are helpful are vitamins A, B6, B12, C, and E. Protective minerals include zinc, selenium and manganese. Herbs that sustain the white blood cells are astragalus, codonopsis, ligustrum, schizandra, millettia, white atractylodes, royal jelly, oldenlandria, pau d'arco, echinacea, goldenseal, and some of the herbal formulas, including the Immune Power Formula or the Immune Tonic Tea. Mushrooms that have a restorative effect include ganoderma (reishi mushroom), maitake, shitake, Zhu ling, Turkey Tail, and coriolus. Maitake D-Fraction and MGN-3 can also be considered.

What to Take for Anemia and Low Platelets During Chemotherapy Treatments

Chemotherapeutic agents often reduce red blood cell and platelet counts. To counter anemia, the herb yellow dock can be used in tincture form, at a dosage of 5–20 drops daily. Angelica is a Chinese herb that strengthens the spleen and increases the red blood cell count. The herb agrimony can increase platelets and stimulate blood clotting. Another Chinese herb used for restoring both the red and the white blood cell count is millettia. Deer antler is sometimes used for this purpose as well. Other blood builders include pumpkin seeds, oatmeal, dried apricots, beets, nettle, kale, and seaweeds.

How to Combat Fatigue During Chemotherapy and Radiation

Fatigue is a common symptom in women undergoing chemotherapy or radiation. To combat fatigue, consider using Siberian ginseng (30 drops, 3× daily), schisandra berry tincture (30 drops, 3× daily), astragalus in tea or tincture form, nettle tea, an ounce a day of fresh wheat grass juice, or the Immune Power Formula or Immune Tonic Tea described on pages 178 and 182.

Are Gelatin Capsules Harmful?

At the second World Conference on Breast Cancer, held in Ottawa in July 1999, Dr Samuel Epstein made women aware of the fact that gelatin capsules may contain estradiol. Normally cows are given estradiol to increase growth and milk production. It is administered through an implant positioned under the skin of their ears, where absorption is low. When cows are slaughtered, their ears are cut off and sold to rendering plants for the manufacturing of glycerol and gelatin. Gelatin is commonly used to make capsules for supplements. I have not been able to find any studies on this subject, but clearly it is a possible risk factor. Fortunately, some companies, such as Genestra, have switched to using veggie caps which will be free of estrogen contamination. Contact the suppliers of your capsules and request veggie caps. Try to find products that do not rely on gelatin capsules.

When to Take Supplements

The following guidelines are designed to take some of the confusion out of when the best times are to take your supplements.

Vitamins

Generally vitamins are taken with meals, with the exception of vitamin C which can be taken in divided doses throughout the day between or with meals.

Minerals

Minerals are usually taken with meals, with the exception of zinc, which is better taken between meals, and calcium, which can be taken with a meal or before bed, providing you have enough hydrochloric acid to absorb it on an empty stomach. Calcium and other minerals should not be taken with a high fiber meal. Iron and vitamin E should be taken eight hours apart.

Amino Acids

As protein molecules, amino acids are best taken with meals. These include NAC and reduced glutathione.

Herbs

Herbal formulas are best absorbed on an empty stomach, either ½ hour before or 2 hours after a meal. If herbs are used to improve digestion, they are taken 15–30 minutes before a meal.

Enzymes

If enzymes are used to digest food, they are taken immediately before or during your meal. If they are being used to control inflammation or digest toxins in the blood, they are taken between meals.

Probiotics (acidophilus and bifidus)

Depending on the type and the manufacturer, these can be taken either before or between meals.

Homeopathic Remedies

These are taken on an empty stomach, away from other supplements so that strong tastes or smells do not interfere with their subtle action, usually ½ hour or more before or after a meal.

Designing Your Supplement Schedule Exercise

Copy the chart on page 252. Fill in the times of day, amount of each supplement you need, and what it is doing for you. Tape it to your cupboard or refrigerator door until it becomes routine. Take a break every now and then from supplement taking when it feels like too much. Listen to your body's needs.

Summary

Our supplements will work better for us if we are mindful as we take them. Think of them as healers. We can potentiate their action with prayer and mental imagery. Follow this sequence as you take your supplements until it becomes automatic:

1) Thank the organisms or elements that have become your supplement.

2) Invoke a silent prayer or mantra that the supplement will add to your health and well being. Take a minute to formulate one that you can use over and over again – for example, *May I use the wellness you bring me to good end.*

3) Envision the cells of your body accepting what you put into it and using it for your maximum benefit. Picture the nutrients going to the parts of the body that need them or being directed by your body's innate intelligence to its target cells.

Though not easily quantifiable, the power of visualization and imagery in activating our immune system and assisting in healing is considerable, as we shall see in the next chapter.

Further Reading

Gerson, Max. *A Cancer Therapy: Results of Fifty Cases*. 3rd ed. Del Mar, CA: Totality Books, 1977.

Ontario Breast Cancer Information Exchange Project. *A Guide to Unconventional Cancer Therapies*. Toronto, ON: Ontario Breast Cancer Information Exchange Report, 1994.

Moss, R. *Cancer Therapy: The Independent Consumer's Guide to Non-Toxic Treatment and Prevention*. New York, NY: Equinox Press, 1992.

TIME OF DAY	SUPPLEMENT AND HOW MANY	WHAT IT'S DOING FOR YOU
On Arising:		
Before Breakfast:		
With Breakfast:		
Between Meals:		
Before Lunch:		
With Lunch:		
Between Meals:		
Before Dinner:		
With Dinner:		
Before Bed:		

References

1. Katsouyanni, K., et al. Diet and breast cancer: a case control study in Greece. *Int J Cancer*, 1986:38815-20.
2. Weed, Susun. *Breast Cancer/Breast Health!* Woodstock, NY: Ash Tree Publishing,1996:47.
3. Biskind, M.S., G.R. Biskind. Effect of vitamin B complex deficiency on inactivation of estrone in the liver. *Endocrinology*, 1942;31:109-14.
4. Inculet, R.I. et al. Water soluble vitamins in cancer patients on parenteral nutrition: a prospective study. *Journal of Parenteral Enteral Nutrition*, May-June 1987;11(3):243-49.
5. Jacobson, E.L. A biomarker for the assessment of niacin nutriture as a potential preventive factor in carcinogenesis. *Journal of Internal Medicine*, 1993;233:59-62.
6. Henning, S.M. et al. Male rats fed methyl - and folate – deficient diets with or without niacin develop hepatic carcinomas associated with decreased tissue NAD concentrations and altered poly (ADP-ribose) polymerase activity. *Journal of Nutrition*, Jan 1997;127(1):30-36.
7. Jacoson, E.L., et al. Niacin deficiency and cancer in women. *Journal of the American College of Nutrition*, 1993;12(4):412-16.
8. Kim, J. Use of vitamins as adjunct to conventional cancer therapy. 2nd *Denver Conference on Nutrition and Cancer*. Sept. 7-11, 1994.
9. Jacobson, M, E. Jacobsen. Niacin, nutrition, ADP-ribosylation and cancer. *The 8th International Symposium on ADP-ribosylation*, Texas College of Osteopathic Medicine, Fort Worth, TX, 1987.
10. Gerson, Max. *A Cancer Therapy: Results of Fifty Cases*. Del Mar, CA: Totality Books, 1958.
11. Folkers, K. Relevance of the biosynthesis of coenzyme Q10 and the four bases of DNA as a rationale for the molecular causes of cancer and a therapy. *Biochem Biophys Res Comm*, 1996;224:358-61.
12. Choi, S.W. Vitamin B12 deficiency: a new risk for breast cancer? *Nutr Rev*, 1999;Aug;57(8):250-53.
13. Shamsuddin, A.M., G.Y. Yang, I. Vucenik. Novel anti-cancer functions of IP6: growth inhibition and differentiation of human mammary cancer cell lines in vitro. *Anticancer Res*, 1996 Nov-Dec;16(6A):3287-92.
14. Vucenik, I., G.Y. Yang, A.M. Shamsuddin. Comparison of pure inositol hexaphosphate and high-bran diet in the prevention of DMBA-induced rat mammary carcinogenesis. *Nutr Cancer*, 1997;28(1):7-13.
15. Saied, I.T., A.M. Shamsuddin. Up-regulation of the tumor suppressor gene p53 and WAF1 gene expression by IP6 in HT-29 human colon carcinoma cell line. *Anticancer Res*, 1998 May-June;18(3A):1479-84.
16. Zhang, S. et al. Dietary carotenoids and vitamins A, C, and E and risk of breast cancer. *J Natl Cancer Inst*, 1999, Mar 17:91(6):547-56.
17. Ainsleigh, H.G. Beneficial effects of sun exposure on cancer mortality. *Prev Med*, 1993;22:132-40.
18. Colston, K.W., et al. Possible role for vitamin D in controlling breast cancer cell proliferation. *Lancet*, 1989;i:188-91.
19. Ambrosone, C.B. et al. Interaction of family history of breast cancer and dietary antioxidants with breast cancer risk. *Cancer Causes and Control*, Sept. 1995;6(5):407-15.
20. Guthrie, N. et al. Inhibition of proliferation of estrogen receptor-negative MDA-MB-435 and positive MCF-7 human breast cancer cells by palm oil tocotrienols and tamoxifen, alone and in combination. *American Society for Nutritional Sciences*, 1997.
21. Moss, R. *Cancer Therapy: The Independent Consumer's Guide to Non-Toxic Treatment and Prevention*. New York, NY: Equinox Press, 1992:78.
22. Jacobson E.A. et al. Effects of dietary fat, calcium, and vitamin D on growth and mammary tumorigeneis induced by 7,12-dimethylbenz(a)anthracene in female Sprague-Dawley rats. *Cancer Research*, 1989;49:6300-03.
23. Diet of teenage girls may increase their risk of breast cancer, *Primary Care and Cancer*, 1994;14(2):8.
24. Gerson, Max. *A Cancer Therapy: Results of Fifty Cases*. Del Mar, CA: Totality Books, 1958.
25. Ramesha A, et al. Chemoprevention of 7,12-dimethylbenz(a)anthracene-induced mammary carcinogenesis in rats by the combined actions of selenium, magnesium, ascorbic acid and retinyl acetate. *Jpn J Cancer Res*, 1990:1239-46.
26. Teas, J. et al. Dietary seaweed and mammary carcinogenesis in rats. *Cancer Research*, 1984;44:2758-61.
27. Moss, R. *Cancer Therapy: The Independent Consumer's Guide to Non-Toxic Treatment and Prevention*. New York, NY: Equinox Press, 1992:94.
28. Wei HJ, et al. Effect of molybdenum and tungsten on mammary carcinogenesis in Sprague-Dawley rats. *Chung Hua Chung Liu Tsa Chih*, 1987;9:204-07.
29. Astrup, A. et al. Pharmacology of thermogenic drugs. *Am J Clin Nutr*, 1992;55(1 Suppl):863-67.
30. Ladas, HD. The potential of selenium in the treatment of cancer. *Holistic Medicine*. 1989;4:145-56.
31. Ksrnjavi, H. and D. Beker. Selenium in serum as a possible parameter for assessment of breast disease. *Breast Cancer Research and Treatment*, 1990;16:57-61.
32. Moss, R. Cancer Therapy: *The Independent Consumer's Guide to Non-Toxic Treatment and Prevention*. New York, N.Y., Equinox Press, 1992:112.
33. Magalova, T., et al. Copper, zinc and superoxide dismutase in precancerous, benign diseases and gastric, colorectal and breast cancer. *Neoplasma*, 1999;46(2):100-04.
34. Magalova, T., et al. Zinc and copper in breast cancer. *Therapeutic Uses of Trace Elements*, 1996;65:373-75.

35. Haynes, J. Coenzyme Q10 and breast cancer. *Townsend Letter for Doctors and Patients.* Aug/Sept 1997:160-62.

36. Murray, M.T. *Coenzyme Q10.* Rocklin, CA: Prima Publishing, 1996:196-308.

37. Bagchi, D. A review of the clinical benefits of coenzyme Q10. *Journal of Advancement in Medicine,* 1997;10(2):139-48.

38. Takimoto, M. et al. Protective effects of CoQ10 administration on cardiac toxicity in FAC therapy. *Gan To Kogaku Rryoho,* 1982;9:1,116-21.

39. Lockwood, K., S. Moesgaard, T. Yamamoto, and K. Folkers. Progress on therapy of breast cancer with vitamin Q10 and the regression of metastases. *Biochemical and Biophysical Research Communications,* 1995;212:1,172-77.

40. Gaby, A.R. The role of coenzyme Q10 in clinical medicine: Part 1. *Alternative Medicine Review,* 1996;1:1,11-13.

41. Jolliet, P. et al. Plasma coenzyme Q10 concentrations in breast cancer: prognosis and therapeutic consequences. *International Journal of Clinical Pharmacology and Therapeutics,* 1998;36(9):506-09.

42. Ta, K., K. Mauro. Coenzyme Q10 and breast cancer. Toronto, ON: *Canadian College of Naturopathic Medicine,* April, 1999.

43. Lockwood et al. Partial and complete regression of breast cancer in patients in relation to dosage of coenzyme Q10. *Biochemical and Biophysical Research Communications,* 1993:1504-08; 1994, Mar 30.

44. Choopra, R. Relative bioavailability of coenzyme Q10 formulations in human subjects. *International Journal of Vitamin and Nutrition Research,* 1998;68:109-13.

45. Colacci, A., et al. Inhibition of chemically induced cell transformation by lipoic acid. *Proceedings of the Annual Meeting of the American Association of Cancer Research,* 1997;38:A2419.

46. Berkson, B.M. Alpha lipoic acid (thioctic acid): My experience with this outstanding therapeutic agent. *Journal of Orthomolecular Medicine,* 1998;13(1):44-47.

47. Challam, J. Alpha-lipoic acid: A new antioxidant backed up by solid scientific research. *The Nutrition Reporter,* 1996;7(7):1.

48. Berkson, B.M. Alpha lipoic acid (thioctic acid): My experience with this outstanding therapeutic agent. *Journal of Orthomolecular Medicine,* 1998;13(1):44-47.

49. Buckler, J., A.J. DeNault, V. Franc, T. Strukoff. Breast cancer treatment and prevention: limonene, lycopene and alpha-lipoic acid. Toronto, ON: *Canadian College of Naturopathic Medicine,* April, 1999.

50. Natureworks. *Alpha Lipoic Acid Fact Book.* New York, NY: Abkit, Inc., 1996:18-19.

51. Murray, M.T. *Encyclopedia of Nutritional Supplements.* Rocklin, CA. Prima Publishing, 1996:343-46.

52. Eliaz, I. The role of modified citrus pectin in the prevention of cancer metastasis. *Townsend Letter for Doctors and Patients,* 1999;July;192:64-65.

53. Blask, D., S. Wilson, F. Zalatan. Physiological melatonin inhibition of human breast cancer cell growth in vitro: Evidence for a glutathione-mediated pathway. *Cancer Res,* 1997;57:1909-14.

54. Tamarkin, L., C.J. Baird, O. Almeida. Melatonin: A coordinating signal for mammalian reproduction? *Science,* 1985;227:714-20.

55. Lissoni, P., S. Barni, S. Meregalli et al. Modulation of cancer endocrine therapy by melatonin: A phase II study of tamoxifen plus melatonin in metastatic breast cancer patients progression under tamoxifen alone. *Br. J. Cancer,* 1995;71:854-56.

56. Lissoni, P., S. Crispino, S. Barni et al. Pineal gland and tumor cell kinetics: serum labelling rate in breast cancer, *Oncology,* 1990;47:3:275-77.

57. Bartsch, H., C. Bartsch. Effect of melatonin on experimental tumors under different photoperiods and times of administration. *J. Neural. Transm,* 1981;52:269-79.

58. Dubbels, R. et al. Melatonin in edible plants identified by radioimmunoassay and by high performance liquid chromatography-mass spectrometry. *J. Pineal Research,* 1995;18:28-31.

59. Ledenac, M., S. Miranda, M. Pevac-Djukic. Breast cancer prevention research project: Role of progesterone. Toronto, ON: *Canadian College of Naturopathic Medicine,* April, 1999.

60. Lee, J. *What Your Doctor May Not Tell You About Menopause.* New York, NY: Warner Books, 1996: 275-78.

61. Jato, I. Neoadjuvant progesterone therapy for primary breast cancer: rationale for clinical trial. *Clinical Therapies,* 1997;19(1):56-61(discussion 2-3).

62. Cooper, L.S., et al. Survival of pre-menopausal breast carcinoma patients in relation to menstrual timing of surgery and estrogen receptor/progesterone receptor status of the primary tumor. *Cancer,* 1999,Nov.15;86(10):2053-58.

63. Labriola, D., Livingston, R. Possible interactions between dietary antioxidants and chemotherapy. *Oncology,* 1999, July:1003-07.

64. Lamson, D.W., M.S. Brignall. Antioxidants in cancer therapy; their actions and interactions with oncologic therapies. *Alter Med Rev,* 1999, Oct;4(5):304-29.

65. Jacobson, E.L. A biomarker for the assessment of niacin nutriture as a potential preventive factor in carcinogenesis. *Journal of Internal Medicine,* 1993;233:59-62.

66. Kim, J. Use of vitamins as adjunct to conventional cancer therapy. 2nd Denver Conference on Nutrition and Cancer. Sept. 7-11, 1994.

67. Jones, C. Allies in the breast cancer battle: herbs for prevention, treatment and healing. *Herbs for Health,* 1998,Jan/Feb:29-33.

Psychological Means of Preventing Breast Cancer

Exercises

Contents

Most, if not all, illness seems to have an emotional as well as a physical cause, including breast cancer. Tumors of all types may arise after a sudden shock, loss, or conflict. Women more prone to cancer of any kind are sometimes those who put the needs of others first and are perceived as 'good, kind, and nice'. They are often unable to express their anger or other negative emotions. As part of the healing journey, women can be encouraged to resolve old conflicts, identify their own needs, believe that they deserve to have those needs met, and identify and express anger constructively. We need outlets to express negative emotions (art therapy, bioenergetics) and exercises to improve self-esteem. We need to focus on resolving conflict, developing assertiveness, transforming limiting beliefs, understanding communication styles, and releasing anger, as well as using imagery and visualization. Our well-being is dependent upon our ability to heal ourselves psychologically as well as physically.

Resolving Conflict

Dr Hamer, a German medical doctor who developed a novel theory of the causes of cancer, believes that every cancer begins with a severe, acute conflict which occurs as a shock to the individual and registers an effect in the psyche, in the brain, and in a target tissue or organ. The conflict is followed by nervous system stress that may manifest as cold hands and feet, loss of appetite, weight loss, sleeplessness and anxiety, or a dwelling upon the conflict. It is the responsibility of the physician to explore with each cancer patient what incident may have occurred before the onset of the cancer which led to internal conflict. Dr Hamer feels that the type of cancer is determined by the characteristics of the initial traumatic occurrence, which registers in a particular part of the brain and in a specific location in the body. Hamer studied thousands of brain CT scans of cancer patients and was able to observe concentric rings around a target area of the brain which he called an HH or HAMERsche HERD. From

the brain location of the HH, a trained person such as Dr Hamer can accurately predict where in the body the cancer has occurred and what type of conflict preceded it. Dr Hamer has found this to be true for over 15,000 documented cases.

If, for example, the conflict has to do with a shock to the mother-child relationship, such as an unexpected accident in which the child is injured, this may manifest as a tumor in the left breast of a right-handed woman. If the conflict has to do with a partner, such as discovering that a husband has been unfaithful, it may manifest as a tumor in the right breast if the woman is right-handed. The woman's emotional reaction and thought processes at the time of the conflict determine which body part is affected. When the conflict is resolved, healing begins. The physical stress symptoms abate, the brain repairs itself, and the cancer growth stops.[1]

Part of the healing journey for cancer patients, therefore, is to identify and resolve the initial conflict that may have precipitated the illness. This may be facilitated through therapy, bodywork such as reiki, artmaking, or creative expression and dream analysis.

Becoming Assertive

Often difficulties with being assertive stem from mistaken beliefs about ourselves that devalue us in our own mind. We have learned these beliefs earlier in our lives, often from our parents, or have modeled our behavior on others with similar mistaken beliefs about themselves. We become passive or submissive, always putting the needs of others before our own, believing that what we want does not count. When we pass up opportunities for being assertive, we are often left with feelings of anger, resentment, defeat, or depression. Our needs are not being met, our feelings are not voiced. The accumulated frustration interferes with our physical well-being, causing stagnation in the liver in the Chinese medical model, decreased immune strength due to the effect on the hypothalamus, and a depletion in energy. When we are assertive, generally we feel empowered, have improved self-esteem, and more energy is freed up for living fully in the present. We aren't as likely to store our negative emotions in the tissues of the body if we express our needs and wants in a healthy assertive way. By first identifying our limiting beliefs we can begin the process of shifting towards establishing healthy rights for ourselves.

Exploring Your Beliefs Exercise

Read through the list of limiting beliefs on the left column of the chart on page 258 and see how many of them apply to you. Read out loud the parallel healthy belief and pause to notice how each statement makes you feel.

If you are in a group, pick a partner. Have one person read the limiting belief and comment to their partner on whether it is an accurate statement for them. Ask the partner to then read the healthy belief back to the first person using the word 'you' instead of 'I' and allow time for the first person to take in its effect. Whether you are alone or in a group, circle the healthy beliefs that have the most impact for you. Write these phrases on small recipe cards and keep them in the bathroom or another spot you visit frequently. Each day, repeat one or two of the healthy beliefs out loud as you look at yourself in the mirror. Continue to do this for 40 days or so. Notice how your responses change to people and events as your beliefs change. After 40 days move on to a different affirmation.

Communication Styles

Another step in learning to become assertive is to identify the three communication styles we use with one another. Here are three such styles.

Aggressive Style

Some examples of aggressive behavior are bullying, being pushy, fighting, threatening, blaming, and generally stepping on people without considering their feelings. The aggressive person believes that she has to be forceful to get what she wants. She has not experienced that her needs can be met through simply asking for what she wants or through dialogue and compromise. The advantage to this kind of behavior is that she usually doesn't get pushed around. The disadvantage is that people often will resent her pushiness and not want to be around her.

Passive Style

A person is acting passively when she lets others take control of her actions or thoughts. She will not stand up for herself; she will do what she's told. She disregards what she really feels and believes. She may be so cut off from or afraid of her feelings that she doesn't really know what she feels. The body can become a container for these repressed feelings and manifest them in physical symptoms. An underlying belief is that she does not deserve to have her needs met. She sees herself as being less important, less talented, than her family and friends. She often has an irrational fear of negative consequences that may happen if she expresses her needs honestly, and feels paralyzed. The advantage of being passive is that the person rarely experiences direct rejection. The disadvantage is that these women are taken advantage of, and store a backlog of resentment and anger, much of it unconscious. The anger will manifest in indirect ways, such as being chronically late or emotionally distant. Because she does not put herself first, she falls short of accomplishing or experiencing all that she can in her life. She may defer to a partner or her children, look to their successes for validation, and never really seek out avenues of fulfillment for herself. She may never discover who she really can be.

Assertive Style

A person who behaves assertively will stand up for herself, will not let others take advantage of her, and will express her feelings honestly. At the same time, she is considerate of others' feelings, and can acknowledge those feelings while holding her ground. The advantage of being assertive is that you usually get what you want without violating another's rights or causing anger or resentment. Assertiveness allows you to act in your own best interest and not feel guilty or wrong about it. Attack and blame, passivity and withdrawal are infrequent in a person who has mastered assertive behavior because they are recognized as poor communication styles causing confusion, misunderstanding, and ill will which usually do not fulfill our needs and wants. Before you can achieve assertive behavior, you must realize that your own life matters. Your needs, wants, goals, talents, and pleasures are important; you deserve to have them met. We can only be assertive when we place value in our own spiritual, physical, emotional, and mental well-being. We matter.

Most of us are able to act assertively in some situations but not in others. We may be assertive with our children but not with our partners or employers. We may be able to express ourselves honestly with a few friends but not with our parents or siblings. You can explore the areas where you lack assertiveness through the following exercises.

Limiting Beliefs	Healthy Beliefs
1 I should always try to be logical and consistent. Once I choose a direction, I should keep to it.	I am free to change my mind and decide on a different course of action.
2. I feel ashamed when I make a mistake. I should know the right answer in every situation.	It is okay for me to make a mistake. I don't have to be perfect. I can learn from my mistakes.
3. If someone gives me advice, I should follow it or take it seriously. They are most often right.	I can take advice and filter it through my mind, heart, and intuition before deciding to act on it. I trust myself.
4. I should respect other people's opinions, especially if they are in a position of authority. I should keep my differences of opinion to myself.	I have a right to express my opinion. My opinion matters.
5. I am being selfish if I put my needs before the needs of others, such as family members.	I have a right to put my own needs before the needs of others sometimes. I deserve to enjoy myself and experience fulfillment in my life today.
6. When I do something wonderful, I should not tell anyone. People would think that I am boasting and would dislike me. I feel embarrassed when someone compliments me.	I deserve to be recognized for what I do well. I appreciate well-earned compliments.
7. I should be flexible and adjust to other people's agendas, even when it is inconvenient for me.	I acknowledge my own desires and agenda before I adjust to those of another.
8. I always try to stay on people's good side. I don't want to make anyone angry.	I communicate my feelings honestly to people and am not responsible for their anger.
9. When someone else thinks that my feelings or responses are unreasonable, then I must be wrong.	I have a right to all my feelings and responses and I accept them as being valid for me.
10. I should keep my problems to myself. No one really wants to hear them or be there for me.	There are individuals who care about me and are willing to help me sort out difficulties.
11. When things are going poorly for me I shouldn't try to change them. It could be worse.	I deserve the best possible life for myself and can change my circumstances for the better.
12. If people ask me to do something for them, I respond to them right away. I often agree to something without thinking it through.	I can take whatever time I need before I fully commit to a favor or task.
13. If I am anti-social people will think that I don't like them. I am obliged to participate in social events even when I would rather be alone or doing something else.	I choose the social activities that appeal to me. I also choose to be alone at times to nurture myself.
14. I should always have a good reason for the way I feel and what I do.	It is all right for me not to know why I feel a certain way.
15. When someone is in trouble, I should help her.	I am not responsible for another person's problem or way of reacting. When I help, it is because I consciously choose to do so.
16. I should never interrupt people when they are speaking. If I ask questions, I appear stupid.	I have a right to interrupt in order to clarify a point or gather more information.
17. I should be sensitive to the needs and wishes of others, even if they are unable to express what they want.	I react to what is communicated to me directly.
18. I should always try to accommodate others. If I don't, they will dislike me and may not be there for me when I need them.	I have a right to say 'no' without feeling guilty.

Identifying Your Communication Styles Exercise

Please refer to the chart on page 260.

Passive

Identify situations in which you act passively or people with whom you are passive. For example, Sandra was at the hairdresser's and had brought in a photograph to the hair stylist of just how she wanted her hair cut. She was excited about the 'new look' and hoped it would create a more positive self-image for her. As the hairdresser began to cut her hair, he talked to her about the kind of cut that was 'in' and how it would suit her facial shape. He began cutting more of her hair than she had intended and soon had styled it to the cut he deemed appropriate for her. She was unable to speak throughout, but could only smile sweetly as she fumed inside. When finished, he raved about the cut to the other staff and clients in the salon as she sat miserably in her chair. She thanked him, paid the cashier, and burst into tears when she got to her car.

Aggressive

Identify situations in which you act aggressively, or people with whom you are aggressive. For example, Sheila works long hours at work to support her family. Her husband is an artist who earns less than she does. Although self-employed as a massage therapist, she does not schedule enough breaks for herself and consequently feels burnt out at the end of her week. When her four children awaken on Saturday morning, she is irritable, bothered by their noise, and frequently yells to break up their bickering. This causes further tension in the air, more tears, and intensifies the 'acting out' of her children.

Assertive

Identify situations in which you act assertively, or people with whom you are assertive. For example, Janet's older sister often came to visit in the evening several times a week around dinner-time. Janet was studying for a law degree, and though she enjoyed her sister's company, she needed time for her studies. She thought about the situation and then spoke to her sister, "I enjoy you coming over to be with us but my priority for the next two months is studying for my exams. Could you limit your visits to Wednesday evenings for now? That way I can plan to be with you and won't feel stressed about squandering my study time. We'll have a more enjoyable time together." Her sister responded positively, respected Janet's boundary concerning time, and Janet was able to do well on her exams.

Developing Assertive Behavior Exercise

A working model for becoming assertive contains the following components; see pages 261 and 262. By following this process you can develop successful assertive behavior.

If you follow this model step-by-step, then it will become automatic for you after practicing it several times.

The Healing Effects of Being Assertive

Remember that your body and particularly your immune system respond to what you believe about yourself and what you present to the world. Breast cancer and most illnesses bring us the opportunity to adopt a new persona that is different from the one we had when we became sick. We can change our negative beliefs about ourselves with repetition of positive beliefs, practice of healthy behavioral scripts, validation, and encouragement.

► **Action for Prevention:** In summary, assertiveness can be encapsulated in three steps:

1) Communicate your thoughts about a particular situation in a factual, non-blaming way.
2) Communicate your feelings about a particular situation using 'I statements'.
3) Communicate your wants clearly and specifically. ◄

More specifically, you can develop an assertive communication style in these ways:

1) Create a time and place to discuss your needs and feelings with the other person.
2) Refrain from judging or blaming the other person, but describe behavior objectively.
3) Describe your needs and circumstances clearly, using specific references to time, place, and frequency.
4) Express feelings calmly, rationally, and directly.
5) Stay with the particular problem or behavior that needs to be addressed without attacking the whole person.
6) Avoid putting down another person and calling it assertiveness.
7) Ask for specific, small, possible changes from the other person.
8) Ask for only one or two changes at a time.
9) Let the other person know what the benefit will be for them from the behavior change.

• Identifying Your Communication Styles •

Passive
Situations when I acted passively:
1)
2)
3)
4)
5)
Who are the people with whom I act passively (husband/partner, employer, children, sibling, particular friends, salespersons, etc.):
1)
2)
3)
What are the feelings in me during and after these interactions?
How would I like this to change?

Aggressive
Situations when I acted aggressively:
1)
2)
3)
4)
5)
Who are the people with whom I act aggressively?
1)
2)
3)
What are the feelings in me during and after these interactions?
How would I like this to change?

Assertive
Situations when I acted assertively:
1)
2)
3)
4)
5)
People with whom I act assertively:
1)
2)
3)
What are the feelings in me during and after these interactions?
How would I like this to change?

• Developing Assertive Behavior •

1 Examine and affirm your rights in each particular situation. Look at what you want out of it, what your needs are, and pay attention to your feelings. Release feelings of blame, the desire to hurt, and self-pity. Define your goal and keep it in mind as you negotiate for change. As you practice 'trying on' assertive behavior, write these things down for yourself before communicating to the other party so that you are clear and validate yourself.
Situation #1:
My rights:
What I want out of it:
My needs are:
My feelings around this are:
Situation #2:
My rights:
What I want out of it:
My needs are:
My feelings around this are:
Situation #3:
My rights:
What I want out of it:
My needs are:
My feelings around this are:
2. Arrange a time and place to discuss your concerns with the person involved that is convenient for both of you.
Situation #1:
Possible time and place:
Situation #2:
Possible time and place:
Situation #3:
Possible time and place:
3. Be specific as you define the problem. State matter-of-factly how you see the situation and share your opinion and beliefs in a calm and rational way. For example, you might say, " We have spent the last three weekends staying at home; it's time we did something adventurous together".
Situation #1:
Define the problem specifically:
Situation #2:
Define the problem specifically:
Situation #3:
Define the problem specifically:

• Developing Assertive Behavior •

4. Describe your feelings around the situation so that the other person has a better understanding of you and what the situation means to you. When communicating your feelings, own them by saying, "I feel _____ when_____." Do not blame the other person as you express your feelings, but instead let them know how their actions affect you. Refer to a specific action as you express your feelings rather than generalizing. For example, you could say, "When you arrive home late without calling, I feel discounted and unappreciated." Do not place labels on the other person such as 'inconsiderate' or 'passive-aggressive' but stick to the specific situation and the feelings it engendered in you.

Situation #1:

I feel:

When:

Situation #2:

I feel:

When:

Situation #3:

I feel:

When:

5. Express your wishes in a simple statement while being firm and specific. Clearly state your needs and what you want from the situation. For example, "I would really like the two of us to spend time alone together this evening."

Situation #1:

Simple statement expressing your request:

Situation #2:

Simple statement expressing your request:

Situation #3:

Simple statement expressing your request:

6. Reinforce the other person so that they will be more inclined to give you what you want. Tell them what the return will be for both of you. Describe the positive consequences of what will happen if your request is granted. For example, "If you put your pajamas on when I ask you to, then we will have time for a bedtime story." If these positive outcomes are not motivating for the other person or don't work, then describe negative consequences for failure to cooperate. For example, "If you do not put your pajamas on when I ask you to, then you'll have to go to bed without a story. I need time to myself tonight." Be sure that the negative consequence is something you can and will follow through with. You will lose your own and the other person's respect if you do not keep to your word. Think about the negative consequence before you say it and don't threaten the other person.

Situation #1:

Positive reinforcement:

Negative consequences:

Situation #2:

Positive reinforcement:

Negative consequences:

Situation #3:

Positive reinforcement:

Negative consequences:

10) Avoid threats or blame. Avoid negative consequences that you are not able to keep.

11) Keep your awareness on your rights and goals while being assertive.

Look at your scripts and see whether you are staying in line with these guidelines. Change what needs to be changed. Choose one of the scripts and role-play it with a partner, or by yourself using two chairs. Move from chair to chair as you role-play yourself and the other person. If you are with a partner, give each other feedback as to how it was received and how the person who delivered it felt before, during and after. Be vigilant with yourself over the next month and notice when you give up your assertiveness and act either passively or aggressively. Keep copies of these pages accessible so that you can remodel your behavior to become more assertive. Sit down and write out these steps and then address some of the situations that are causing you discomfort. Practice them with a friend or in front of a mirror first. Congratulate yourself after you have been assertive and incorporate it into a new-found sense of identity. Read your list of rights regularly to remind yourself who you are and what you deserve.

Negative Consequences of Internalizing Anger

Another possible emotional influence on our physical well-being is withheld anger. When we do not express our anger, we store it in our bodies where it can affect a particular area or cause generalized muscle tension. Typical sites for stored anger include the jaw, neck and shoulders, back, abdomen, liver, and reproductive organs. However, we can internalize it anywhere. This anger becomes energy held in, rather than energy expressed. Anger held in acts as a blockage to the free flow of energy in the body. This can have a paralyzing effect on us physically and emotionally, causing fatigue, lack of zest, flatness to our outward expression, and a thwarting of our impulses and intuition. We become stuck.

Repressed anger interferes with our relationships. When we are holding in anger, instead of expressing what we feel angry about, we can adopt a variety of tactics that express it indirectly. These can include avoidance; that is, we may avoid the person we are angry at or avoid the topic which triggers our anger. We may compensate for the underlying anger by appearing sweet and/or smiling. We may become passive-aggressive, acting out our anger unconsciously by undermining another person through our actions (for example, being chronically late for engagements). We may talk about surface things (weather, work, someone else) rather than the issue that is consuming or preoccupying us. This reinforces our emotional barriers and prevents intimacy and relationships of depth. We may become irritable or explosive. When we have a backlog of anger, it finds its own way to be released, either through generalized irritability or unwarranted explosiveness. We may even become self-destructive, developing addictions, destructive behavior patterns, and perhaps suicidal tendencies.

Acknowledging Your Anger Exercise

Think about a situation that easily angers you. Hold it in your mind. Walk around the room and notice where you feel the tension in your body, where the anger is seated. Find words to describe the feelings in that body part. Draw a picture of your body, focusing on the parts that hold the most tension, using particular images to express that tension. Write words beside the picture that further express the angry feelings in the body. If you are in a group, have each person talk about their picture. Recall previous situations where these same feelings have been triggered. Write them down. Is there a familiar pattern? List the times in your life that you have felt most angry.

Looking at the times in your life where you have felt most angry, identify the unmet need that lay beneath the anger. If relevant, identify the feelings of being hurt. Acknowledge them and their validity. Ask where these situations are asking you to grow. What leap are you required to make in your psyche to better deal with these situations and feel empowered rather than victimized? Draw another picture that represents what resource you would need to feel comfortable, protected or empowered so that anger is not internalized. Find an image that would help to heal the anger.

If you are in a group, work with a partner, communicating your feelings of anger, addressing your partner as though she is the person you are angry towards. If you are alone put a pillow on an empty chair and superimpose the person's face on the pillow. Address the pillow, communicating the feelings you have held inside. Alternatively, write a letter to the person who has stimulated your anger. You may or may not choose to mail it. Read the letter out loud, as though you are speaking to the person you wish to address. Notice how your body feels during and after these expressions that contain anger.

► **Action for Prevention:** The following 12 steps may assist you in transforming feelings of anger from a potentially destructive emotion into something with healing power.

1) Accept that anger is a valid emotion. It is okay to feel angry.

2) Acknowledge that you feel angry. Identify the part of the body that is holding the anger.

3) Identify whom you are angry with and/or what you are angry about.

4) Ask yourself if the anger is warranted or if it has been magnified by a previous situation not fully dealt with. Are you projecting your mother, father, or sibling onto the person you feel anger towards? Recognize it.

5) Identify what lies beneath the anger. Usually there is an unmet need or a feeling of being hurt.

6) Explore the unmet needs or feelings of being hurt within yourself first, and then with the other person. If possible, communicate your feelings by saying, "When you did such and such, I felt such and such." Communicate it without blame. Communicate your unmet need specifically; for example, "I need you to put down your newspaper and really listen to me when I speak to you." If you are unable to do this directly, then write a letter, choosing to mail it or not, or use a chair exercise and speak to the person as though they were sitting in the chair. Honor your unmet need and create a plan to meet it as soon as possible.

7) Check in again with the body part that was holding the anger. Ask it if it needs anything more from you. Consciously relax the area.

8) Discharge the anger physically. Use aerobic exercise, rebounding, running or swimming, martial arts, kundalini yoga, rowing, Dragon-boat racing, drumming, etc. to release the build up of muscle tension. Do this on a regular basis — two to three times weekly.

9) Channel any residual anger creatively. Do a drawing, painting, or sculpture which utilizes the energy of the anger and helps externalize it rather than turn it inward

10) Channel anger into a worthy cause or project. Help fight some of the injustices in the world and join forces with others who are helping to create global change for the better.

11) Recognize that by holding on to the anger you are hurting yourself. Choose to let go of it.

12) Give the outcome to the divine forces of the universe. Use prayer and meditation to help you access the state of forgiveness. Forgive the other person and pray for their well being. ◄

Sitali Breathing Exercise

Sitali breathing[2] is an ancient yoga practice to cool down anger and cleanse the body and mind.

1) Sit with a straight spine, eyes closed and focused up between the eyebrows. Open your mouth slightly, shaping the tongue into a 'U' shape and protruding it out slightly between your lips. If you are unable to curl the tongue, make the mouth into a beak shape with the tongue close to the lips.

2) Inhale through the curled tongue, as though sipping through a straw. Exhale through the nose. Slow the breath down so that you are breathing less than 4 breaths per minute. This may take practice.

3) Continue the same breathing pattern for 26 long deep breaths or for 11 minutes. Try it every morning and evening for 40 days.

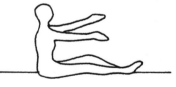

Kundalini Yoga Exercise for Releasing Anger

1) Sit with the legs stretched out in front of you, arms at your sides. Keeping the heels on the ground, bend the left knee and raise it. Then as you lower the left knee, raise the right knee so that you alternately move the knees up and down. 1–3 minutes.

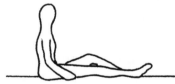

2) Continue the same leg motion as the first exercise. Stretch the arms straight out in front of you, palms facing down and alternately move the hands up and down coordinating them with the leg motion. Move fast and try to create a sweat.

3) Lie on your back with the arms at the sides. Raise and lower the pelvis so that the body from the shoulders to

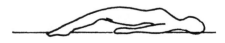

the ankles is lifted off the ground and then lowered back down. 3 minutes.

4) Same exercise as #3 but lie on your stomach instead of your back. 3 minutes.

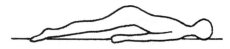

5) Cat stretch. Lie on your back with your arms stretched out to the sides. Inhale and bring the left knee into the chest and then cross it over the right leg to touch the left knee on the ground. Keep your arms fairly

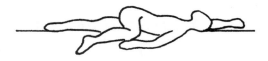

stationary. Exhale as you bring the leg back down to the original position. Then do the same to the opposite leg. Continue alternating legs. 3 minutes.

6) Relax on your back and breathe very slowly for 11 minutes.[3]

Give Your Anger to the Universe

Give the anger away. Recognize that the universe is a better container for injustices and negativity than your body. Practice letting it go, knowing that the law of cause and effect gives back to you what you put out and will do the same to others. It is not for us to judge another's actions. You can only do what is right and necessary for you to maintain your own truth and then leave the outcome to God or the universal energy field. You hurt yourself by holding on to the anger. Compose a letter of forgiveness and send thoughts of well being (as much as you are able to at this time) to the person you have the most anger towards. Create a space in you for this forgiveness to grow in time.

Mind-Body Connections in Health and Illness

Mind-body health is dependent upon our ability to acknowledge our feelings and to develop the means to express them. Quite often the emotional links are buried in the unconscious. Techniques to access these feelings are helpful as part of the healing process.

The researchers Nemiah, Freyberger, and Sifneos (1976) have suggested that people with psychosomatic illnesses have a defective pattern of associative connections between their cortex and their limbic system, in the pathway that links the higher brain to the emotional brain. Brain activity which is usually associated with emotions is not experienced in the higher cortical pathways of mind but is instead short-circuited through the hypothalamus and its linkage with the autonomic, endocrine, and immune systems. Psychosomatic symptoms become a form of body language that takes place of verbal (left hemisphere) and imagistic-emotional (right hemisphere language).[4] In other words, emotional states we cannot describe in words and pictures become bodily symptoms.[5]

A second theory explaining how emotional symptoms become expressed physically has been put forth by Erickson and Rossi (1979). In psychosomatic illness, there is a denial, suppression, and/or repression of right-hemisphere experience so the left hemisphere lacks the information needed to express the problem in words. The normal accessing and flow of information in the mind-body system is either blocked, short-circuited, or misguided so that the body is left to process information that would be better dealt with at the level of mind. Bodily symptoms are the result.[6]

Both of these theories are plausible. Any means by which we can recover buried emotions through touch, images, and words will be helpful in releasing symptoms from the body. These avenues include drawing, dreamwork, dialoguing with the ailing part, and bodywork. If we use these techniques regularly and actively listen to our emotions, we may avoid psychosomatic illness.

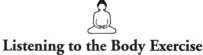

Listening to the Body Exercise

1) Draw an outline of your body on a large piece of paper, or if you are in a group, lay down on a large piece of bond paper and have another group member outline your body with marker or crayon.

2) Lie down beside your paper. Breathe slowly and deeply, allowing the abdomen to fill after each inhale and to fall gently after each exhale. As you breathe, allow relaxation to fill the body and mind. Continue long, deep breathing for a few minutes.

3) Survey the body piece by piece from the inside and notice any signals you are given from each part. Ask, "Do you have anything to tell me today?" as you let your awareness pass through each body part. Listen with your whole being to receive information from that part. It may come to you verbally, as in "I feel

Kali, be with us.

Violence, destruction, receive our homage.

Help us to bring darkness into the light,

To lift out the pain, the anger,

Where it can be seen for what it is —

The balance-wheel for our vulnerable, aching love.

Put the wild hunger where it belongs,

Within the act of creation,

Crude power that forges a balance

Between hate and love.

Help us to be the always hopeful

Gardeners of the spirit

Who know that without darkness

Nothing comes to birth

As without light

Nothing flowers.

Bear the roots in mind,

You, the dark one, Kali,

Awesome power.

— May Sarton

tired and unsupported" or as a feeling of tightness or pain, an image, or a memory of some sort. Listen to whatever information you are given and acknowledge that body part for having communicated with you. Write down the information you have been given or draw a picture of the feeling on the paper in the appropriate body part. Pay special attention to the areas where you have symptoms.

Start with your feet. Direct your awareness to your feet and listen for any signal from them. Move your awareness to the lower legs and knees and notice if there is anything they want to communicate with you. Keep your breathing slow and deep and be receptive to the feelings in your thighs and hips. Move your awareness up through your back. Continue listening to your body. Bring your awareness to the lower abdomen, listening to the reproductive organs, bladder, kidneys, large intestine, and small intestine. Maintain an attitude of receptivity. Breathe into the belly and chest fully and deeply. Listen for anything it may want to communicate to you. Be aware of the feelings you have associated with your breasts and what they are asking from you. Notice the sensations in your neck and shoulders, and down your arms. Is there anything that wants to be seen or heard at this moment? Now be aware of your face — the mouth, chin, cheeks, nose, eyes, and scalp. Allow stored feelings to come to the surface as you are ready to notice and recognize them. Let your awareness drift through the whole of the body as you allow it to communicate to you. As awareness of the feelings from each area come to you, write or draw them on the surrogate body beside you.

4) Tape your drawing on the wall and continue to interact with it daily — drawing or writing about your feelings as you experience them. Over time you will learn to honor your feelings and psychosomatic symptoms will be reduced.

Imagery and Visualization

Increasingly we are discovering the subtle and powerful linkages of mind and body through imagery. Jeanne Achterberg, author of *Imagery and Healing*, believes that the image can alter cellular mechanisms and the intelligence of the cell. Image can also shift the cellular machinery so that it performs unnatural functions. What we imagine in our minds has a direct correlation to how our body responds to life.

Achterberg has found that imagery is able to deeply affect the individual in the following ways. There is an unplanned, non-deliberate body-mind shift due to an event or to external environmental sensory stimulation; for example, the biggest effect on infertility is for a woman to call a fertility clinic to make an appointment, for women often become pregnant just knowing that they may receive help. On the other hand, walking into a typical doctor's office causes most people's white blood cell count to go down and blood pressure to go up.

Imagery can affect the body-mind if a woman adopts a new identity. She takes on a new persona, changes her previous life-script, and recreates herself as the character in the play. She 'imagines' and embodies this new identity with the inner commitment to helping herself. This is a deliberate effort of moving the mind-body in a healing way. *She becomes a different person from whom she was when she became sick.* The global shift or new persona pervades much of her life and can last for a long time (until there's another shift). For example, the cancer patient shifts from being a 'pleaser' or 'victim' and initiates life changes to do what she's always wanted to do for herself. She may appear selfish and different to those who have known her previously. Take a minute to think about this for yourself. What would your new life script look like if you could rewrite the character in the play? How would you be different? How would you act differently to those around you? Write a few lines on how your character would be different on a separate piece of paper. We do not have to have an illness to do this. Do it now. Life is short for all of us.

Imagery affects the body-mind through a conscious and deliberate attempt to connect directly to the workings of the cell. This may occur through hypnosis, biofeedback, or specific visualization of anatomical parts and physiological processes. There is a one-to-one relationship between the image and cellular function. For example, Achterberg has found that if we visualize that we have more T-helper cells and T-killer cells that improve our defense against cancer cells, we can actually increase their numbers.

Achterberg developed a drawing exercise to assess an individual's likely prognosis with an illness. Using 14 specific parameters, she was able to predict over 90% of the time who would die and who would go into remission from cancer. This is what she did. First, she ensured that the patient was in a comfortable position, preferably lying down. The patient listened to tape-recorded relaxation instructions and was given a brief education provided regarding the disease process, how treatment might be helping the patient, and how the immune system works.

The listener was advised to imagine these three factors in action. It was the listener's choice to imagine her cancer cells or white blood cells any way she chose: *"Describe how your cancer cells look in your mind's eye." "How do you imagine your white blood cells fight disease?" "How is your treatment working in your body?"* The patient was then asked to draw a picture of the body, the immune system, the cancerous process, and the treatment.

The interview protocol plus the drawings were scored according to the following 14 parameters:

1) vividness of cancer cell
2) activity of cancer cell
3) strength of cancer cell
4) vividness of white blood cells
5) activity of white blood cells
6) relative comparison of size of cancer and white blood cells
7) relative comparison of number of cancer and white blood cells
8) strength of white blood cells
9) vividness of medical treatment
10) effectiveness of medical treatment
11) choice of symbolism
12) integration of whole imagery process
13) regularity with which they imagined a positive outcome
14) ventured clinical opinion on the prognosis

These parameters were scored on a '1' to '5' scale (from negative to positive). Total scores were found to predict with 100% certainty who would have died or shown evidence of significant deterioration during the two-month period and, with 93% certainty, who would be in remission.[7] How many of us in the health profession are able to do this and then work towards reprogramming the body-mind towards healing?

Achterberg's work reinforces the fact that what we believe and imagine about our bodies has an incredible bearing on how we deal with an illness. Our minds create the most powerful drugs during the healing process. We can believe in our body's innate capacity to heal. We can familiarize ourselves with our immune system and visualize its components doing their jobs efficiently and perfectly.

So often the role of medical professionals is to create doubt in a patient's self-healing capacity, to place all hope in colored pills or radiation. We must reclaim our innate capacity to heal, and no matter what our choice of treatment is, believe in its power.

► **Action for Prevention:** Using Achterberg's findings, for people with cancer, we can develop imagery for healing by encouraging the following:

1) Portray the cancer cells as being few in number, small in size, weak in strength, and lacking vividness.

2) Portray the white blood cells as being vivid, very active, strong and powerful, large and abundant, and overwhelming the cancer cells. Believe more in the potency of your body's ability to heal than in the disease process, and understand that nothing is fixed — it is a process than can go either way.

3) Portray the naturopathic and medical treatments with vividness and effectiveness.

4) Choose strong, powerful, active imagery that is well integrated yet personal.

5) Practice the imagery frequently, at least twice daily. Keep drawing, over and over, until it's as powerful as it can be for a healing response. Draw so that you believe it.

6) Visualize that your body's healthy cells are easily able to repair any slight damage the treatment might cause; that the dead cancer cells are flushed from the body easily and completely; that at the end of the imagery, you are healthy and cancer-free.

7) See yourself accomplishing your goals and fulfilling your life's purpose — relate to your future rather than your past. Explore what your ideal future might be and shift your life in that direction so that your immune system responds with you. ◄

Activating Your Capacity to Heal Exercise

In addition to the methods of detoxifying our bodies and supporting its functions with a healthy diet and appropriate nutritional supplements, we can assist our immune systems through techniques of visualization and imagery. Consider drawing an outline of your body (full-size is best) showing the components of your immune system as you work through this exercise.

The Thymus Gland

Your thymus gland sits behind your upper sternum and is the commander-in-chief for many of your white blood cells, training them and telling them what to do. (Can you tell yourself what to do?) Tap the upper part of your sternum (which stimulates the thymus) as you repeat these phrases out loud, three times each.

"I am found behind your upper sternum, close to your heart. I am made stronger by your love."

"I call white blood cells from the bone marrow to me. I train them to co-operate and perform specific jobs. I send them out into the blood to patrol the body."

"I respond well to feelings of joy, hope, prayer and self-love. I need to feel supported."

"I need you to be relaxed for me to function well."

"I am strengthened by coordinated arm and leg movements on alternate sides (swimming, marching, yoga), tapping on the sternum, and brain hemisphere balancing."

"I am nourished by vitamins A, C, E, B complex, B6, folic acid, the carotenes, selenium, zinc, melatonin, thymus extract, coenzyme Q10, probiotics, digestive enzymes, burdock root, echinacea, goldenseal, European mistletoe, poke root, wild indigo root, amla, astragalus, and ganoderma."

The Spleen

Your spleen is located in the upper left part of the abdomen, beneath the diaphragm and behind your stomach. Tap the outer part of your body over your spleen as you repeat the following phrases out loud, three times each.

"I am found beneath your diaphragm and behind your stomach, and am the size of your fist."

"I am packed full of powerful, intelligent lymphocytes."

"The macrophages on duty in me identify and destroy all bacteria, viruses, and toxins as they circulate in the blood through me."

"I am an amazing filter for debris in the blood."

"I am nourished by burdock root, goldenseal, and echinacea."

The Liver

Place your hand over your liver on the right side of your body beneath the rib cage as you repeat the following phrases out loud, three times each.

"I am a magnificent factory for manufacturing lymphatic fluid."

"I am able to detoxify whatever comes my way."

White Blood Cells: Macrophage

Open and close your hands in front of you as though you are a macrophage engulfing and destroying foreign particles. Repeat the following phrases out loud, three times each as you continue the arm movement.

"I am able to attack, engulf, and digest invaders in the blood."

"I recognize what doesn't belong in this body; I will engulf, digest, and inactivate anything that is harmful to me."

"I like to hang out in the spleen, liver, lungs, lining of the

intestines, lymph nodes, nervous system, bone marrow, and connective tissue."

"I call on helper T-cells to come to the infection site."

"I am made more vigorous by shitake and maitake mushrooms, echinacea, burdock, zinc, European mistletoe, and goldenseal."

Helper T-cell

Move your arms as though you are beckoning helpers to come to your aid and repeat the following phrases out loud, three times each.

"I am well trained in the thymus gland."

"I respond quickly to the call of duty."

"I signal the other cells of the immune system to come and help when we need to defend this body."

"My numbers are increased by vitamin B6, zinc, and alpha lipoic acid."

Killer T-cell

Move your arms and hands as though you are shooting or targeting foreign organisms or cancer cells as you repeat the following phrases out loud, three times each.

"I recognize what needs to be destroyed and I destroy it."

"I protect the life of this body."

"Shitake and Turkey tail mushrooms make me a stronger warrior, as does MGN-3. So does the mistletoe preparation called Iscador and the mineral manganese."

B Cell

Punch out with alternate closed fists as though you are knocking down any enemies while you repeat the following phrases out loud, three times each.

"I can manufacture substances that make my enemies harmless."

"I recognize my enemies and can defend myself against them."

"I recognize what is harmful to me and can defend myself from it."

"I can quickly move to protect this body from what is harmful to me."

"My home is in the spleen and lymph nodes, but I travel wherever I'm needed."

"I have a helper who signals me to act."

Suppressor T-Cell

Use your hands to make the 'time out' hand gesture with the left hand flat, palm down, and the right fingers perpendicular touching it underneath to form the letter 'T'. Repeat the following phrases out loud, three times each.

"I know when to stop attacking."

"Things are safe now; I can be less aggressive at this time."

If you have cancer, you want to activate your Helper T-cells and decrease the activity of your suppressor T-cells.

Memory Cell

Make circles with the fingers of each hand and place them around your eyes, as though you are looking through binoculars. As you look around you, repeat the following phrases out loud, three times each.

"I recognize you from before and know how to deal with you."

"I will be around for a long time, watching for anything that is a threat to the life of this body."

"I will protect you for life."

▶ **Action for Prevention:** Choose one or more of these affirmations and repeat it out loud to yourself several times daily, particularly when you look in the mirror. Copy one out and tape it to your mirror to remind you.

I am a different person now from whom I was when I became sick.

I listen daily to the signals of my body and respond in ways that honor it.

I allow long held emotions to be released from my body in a healthy manner.

I believe in my body's capacity for self-healing. ◀

Script for Recovering from Breast Cancer Exercise

If you have breast cancer, you can follow this script as is or adjust it to better suit your particular needs and personality. Rehearse it one or more times daily as you are recovering.

1) Create a sacred space for yourself by changing your environment in such a way to set the stage for healing. This time is for you and your healing process. Ensure that you won't be disturbed. You might want to light a candle or incense, use a special blanket to cover yourself or arrange flowers in the room. *(Long Pause)*

2) Come sitting or lying down in a comfortable position. Support your neck and back with pillows if needed. Close your eyes. Give yourself permission to be still and to focus on relaxation and healing for at least twenty minutes. Open to a greater energy than yourself and invite it into your life. Imagine you can

feel a healing presence in the room with you. Visualize a powerful healing force assisting you now. Receive the presence of your higher self and spiritual guides and ask them to help you through this healing journey. Become aware of your breathing, … in and out through your nose, and notice the breath becoming slower and deeper. Experience your abdomen rising gently as you inhale and falling softly as you exhale. Feel your breathing for a few long, deep breaths. Inhale … Exhale … Inhale … Exhale … *(Medium Pause)* Listen to the sound of the breath as though you are listening to the sound of the ocean waves coming in … and going out. *(Medium Pause)* Inhale the smell of a pine forest and allow that scent to fill you with rejuvenating and healing energy. With each exhale notice more tension being released. Take a few very slow, long deep breaths to enjoy this fully. Each breath brings more relaxation than the one before it. *(Medium Pause)* Notice where you feel numbness, pain or discomfort in your body and breathe into those areas.

3) Feel more relaxed now, more relaxed with each breath. Give yourself permission to ignore all sounds in your environment and choose not to interact with thoughts that come to mind. As you breathe in, imagine a cleansing and peaceful warmth filling your body. Feel it spread from your head and neck down through the shoulders, chest and arms, to your back, abdomen, and pelvis, then down through your legs and feet as though you are a plant drinking in energy from the sun. Take your awareness to your feet and let any tightness and tension dissolve. Notice the muscles feeling loose and smooth and warm as though they have just been given a gentle massage. Relax your lower legs and let the muscles soften. Breathe relaxation into your knees and thighs. Notice them becoming warm and relaxed, as though being bathed by rays of light. Become aware of your hips, buttocks, and pelvic area. Allow the breath to circulate there like a gentle wind, bringing warmth and relaxation with it. Relax your hips and pelvis. Let go of any tension you experience there. Breathing slowly and deeply, be aware of the muscles in the abdomen and release any tightness or anxiety you find there. Watch it dissolve. Feel the muscles in your back, allowing them to relax and let go. Imagine you are lying on warm sand and release tension from your back into the earth. As you breathe fully and deeply, let go of any tightness or tension stored in your chest. *(Pause)*

4) Direct healing and relaxation to the area of your breasts. Pick a healing color and let this color completely fill and wash through the breast area. Feel it cleansing the area, bringing renewed vitality. Notice the feelings you have associated with your breasts. Watch and listen to those feelings, acknowledge them, and then release them. *(Pause)*

5) Imagine a nurturing female presence beside you. It may be someone in your life now, someone you have known in the past, or an energy that you invoke. *(Medium to Long Pause)* She brings grace into your life. She fills you with courage, acceptance and love. She brings healing to the area of your breasts. *(Pause)* She can respond at any time to your questions. The response may be in the form of words you hear internally, a feeling in your body, or an image. It may also come in a dream or an incident in your life. If you have a question for her, ask now — and be open to her response. *(Long Pause)* She reminds you of your own needs and when it is time for you to take care of yourself. She is available to you in your daily life. You have only to ask for her and listen to her response.

6) Now move your attention from the breast area, maintaining a long, deep breath, to your shoulders. Imagine healing hands massaging the shoulders as you allow tension to melt away. Let them become like soft wax. Allow relaxation to spread down your arms and to your hands. Let any stiffness or tightness be released. Open and close your fingers a few times and release constriction from your body and mind the way a butterfly releases itself from a cocoon. Open your mouth slightly and relax the muscles in your jaw. Relax your lips. Relax your cheeks, eyes, and eyebrows. Send the breath to your eyes as you feel them relax. Enable your eyes to see new choices available to you in your life. As you continue to breathe very slowly and deeply through your nose, become aware of your forehead and scalp. Allow them to relax and feel warm. Let any tension be released.

7) Now become aware of your whole body. If you notice pain, tension, or fear in any part of your body, send the breath there to soothe it. Inhale deeply … Exhale … Inhale … Exhale … With each breath, send your healing color through the entire body, washing it clean. Let that color permeate every cell, as though each cell receives pure air. Allow your mind to become very open, centered, and still. *(Long pause)*

8) Imagine a feeling of complete harmony, safety, and empowerment within yourself. Know that your body is a miracle and is in a state of constant change, responding to the myriad of messages it receives moment by moment. Your body is able to shift as your mind shifts. This body is your vehicle in this lifetime, and is meant to be used by you for a unique purpose, for your own life story. It has built-in mechanisms that protect it and heal it from illness, including cancer. You have millions of white blood cells, many of them targeted for healing cancer, active right now within your body. These cells are powerful allies. They help to protect your body from all diseases. As you imagine them, enliven them with an image that is fitting. It may be an archetypal religious figure or goddess, a historical person of power, an angel, an animal, or other image. Choose an image that has significance for you, that you can believe in, and that is vivid and powerful, as your white blood cells are. Feel and visualize that your white blood cells are fueled by the energy of this image. Internalize your image and let it feed the white blood cells. For example, you may imagine that the spirit of Joan of Arc is commanding your white blood cells into action, or that they are potent rocket ships set on a particular course and mission to destroy any loose cancer cells. You might use the image of a team of expert gardeners consciously and consistently weeding any unhealthy cells, or a pack of wolves ever on the alert for stray cancer cells. You might utilize the precision of an army of archers shooting arrows at cells that have become harmful to you. Take a moment to let an image become clear in your mind. Be sure that it is an image that you are comfortable with, and that fits your belief system. *(Pause)*

9) See your white blood cells as your helpers. There are millions of them to protect you, many more of them than there are cancer cells. The white blood cells are large, vivid, and clear in your mind. Give them energy. Imagine these being formed in the bone marrow, traveling to the thymus gland in the sternum where they are become potent, intelligent, determined, energized, and assigned specific tasks. Let them flow purposefully from there to the rest of the body. They are able to identify and attack any invaders in the body. They are controlled by a center in your brain. Feel their sense of direction and purpose in your mind, patrolling, engulfing, and attacking any stray cancer cells. Send the white blood cells into the breast area, keeping it healthy. Feel their courage and collaboration as they swiftly identify toxins, viruses, bacteria, and cancer cells, then execute a marvelous attack on whatever is harmful to you and your breasts. They are a fantastic clean up crew, protecting every millimeter of your breasts and body. They are determined to defend you to live your life to accomplish your soul's purpose. The more relaxed you are, the more powerful and capable they are of protecting you. *(Long Pause)*

10) Take some time to imagine whatever treatments you are taking working effectively in your body. If you are taking anything to strengthen your immune system, see and feel it activating and energizing your white blood cells with a spark of life, making them brighter and more alive. Picture and hear your white blood cells responding enthusiastically to the boost that you are giving them. Listen to their sound. Visualize any anti-cancer drugs or therapies going directly to the cancer cells and shrinking them hourly, until you are free of disease. See the medication affecting only the unhealthy cells, protecting what is healthy. See and feel the treatment interacting in a positive way with the rest of the body. Experience the treatment assisting your return to health and helping you to maintain perfect health. See, feel, and hear the body's debris being eliminated like a great river flushing through you. The liver effectively breaks down toxins, while the colon, kidneys, and skin are able to eliminate them.

11) As you finish, feel that your body is more relaxed, your defences against disease are stronger, and you are more able to participate in your medical treatment. You are resistant to cancer, immune to it. Visualize yourself as billions of molecules able to shift and move and connect to the web of life. Feel your connection to your surroundings, to an inner guiding force, to the living beings around you, and to your future. Stay with this feeling and know that you have skills and inner resources to cope with whatever comes your way. Imagine yourself in a state of perfect balance — mental, emotional, physical, and spiritual. Experience these working together. Congratulate yourself for having allowed time for healing and quiet reflection. As you begin to stretch, become more alert to your surroundings and at your own pace, go back to your daily living.

▶ **Action for Prevention:**

1) Learn to watch your thought processes. Identify with healing imagery and use it to replace self-destructive thoughts. Explore disturbing thoughts to understand their source, the need that lies beneath them, and ways to transform them. Remind yourself of the following:

    i) illness is not a form of punishment — you are not guilty;
    ii) others have recovered from the same illness;
    iii) your symptoms are a messenger and can be a catalyst for change;
    iv) you have an innate capacity to heal;
    v) the body is in a constant state of change — nothing is fixed — all is process.

2) Use meditation tools such as mantras, witnessing thoughts and feelings, attention to the breath, and eye focus to disengage from the temporary 'reality' created by your thoughts.

3) Use sensory stimuli to create healing responses. Through your waking day associate sensory experiences with healing processes (for example, when you turn on a water faucet, visualize any toxins, illness, or cancer cells being flushed out of your body; when you walk outside allow the wind to blow out any toxicity; when you hear music direct it to breaking up any tumors, etc.) so that many sensory experiences become a celebration of your body's self-healing ability. Make a list of all the ways you can use sensory stimuli to generate healing.

4) Use particular images that have power and significance for you. Find your totems — a rock, a tree, a piece of music, an animal — whatever contains healing power for you. Look for these in your dreams, honor them in your life. Place these images around you to remind you of healing. Believe in the power of nature to heal or in a spiritual force or deity. Identify with and pray to that higher power regularly, believing that it will heal you. Let a healing animal, person, or deity come to you in a state of relaxation and absorb the power of that animal or deity, letting it fight for you even as you sleep. Make a list of images that have power and significance for you.

5) Use imagery and visualization regularly, two to five times daily. Enter a relaxed state before using imagery. This usually takes a minimum of 11 minutes.

6) Remind yourself that the body-mind is in a constant state of change. If your mental state can change, so can the physical. ◀

Summary

During an illness, we often need help to generate a healing response. A health practitioner can assist by creating a safe and relaxed environment. You need an opportunity to feel deeply, and to get in touch with emotions which may have gone unnoticed far too long, resulting in disease. You can gently be coaxed into the future that is calling you and there realize the full meaning of your life. You can also utilize spiritual practises to attune to your innermost self and learn to walk with faith as your companion.

Further Reading

Achterberg, Jeanne. *Imagery in Healing: Shamanism and Modern Medicine.* Boston, MA: Shambhala, 1985.

Achterberg, Jeanne, Barbara Dossey, Leslie Kolkmeier. *Rituals in Healing.* Toronto, ON: Bantam Books, 1994.

Day, Charlene. *The Immune System Handbook.* North York, ON: Potentials Within, 1991.

Davis et al,. *The Relaxation and Stress Reduction Workbook.* 3rd ed. CITY: New Harbinger Publications, 1988.

References

1. Hamer, R.G. *The New Medicine: Questions and Answers,* handout.
2. Bhajan, Yogi. *Sadhana Guidelines for Kundalini Yoga Daily Practise.* Los Angeles, CA: Kundalini Research Institute, 1996:79.
3. Bhajan, Yogi. *Owner's Manual for the Human Body.* Los Angeles, CA: 3HO Foundation & Kundalini Research Institute. 1993:37.
4. Nemiah, J., H. Freygerger, P. Sifneos. Alexithymia: A view of the psychosomatic process. In D. Hill, ed. *Modern Trends in Psychosomatic Medicine. Vol. III.* London: Butterworth, 1976:430-39.
5. Rossi, E. *The Psychobiology of Mind-Body Healing.* New York, NY: W.W. Norton & Co. Inc., 1986:169.
6. Rossi, E. *The Psychobiology of Mind-Body Healing.* New York, NY: W.W. Norton & Co. Inc.,1986:170.
7. Achterberg, J. *Imagery in Healing.* Boston, MA: Shambhala, 1985:189.

Spiritual Practices for Preventing Breast Cancer

Exercises

Contents

We should not separate our spiritual health from the health of our body. Some of the spiritual links to breast cancer include the loss of a loved one, feelings of hopelessness and despair, an inability to be true to one's own nature, a life full of fear of what others may think, and loss of faith in God or the spiritual dimension.

A loss or grief from childhood that has never quite been healed or is reawakened by another loss in adulthood (such as the death of a loved one or loss of a relationship) can increase the likelihood of cancer.[1] Usually this second loss occurs one to five years before the diagnosis of cancer. Creating a safe environment to experience and express grief may be an important healing step. Seeking spiritual guidance, using prayer, and developing a relationship with God are important aspects in overcoming grief.

When a woman feels an underlying hopelessness and despair much of the time, this is filtered through the hypothalamus to affect the immune system and causes her to be more susceptible to cancer. The hopelessness may arise from perceiving that she is in an unhappy situation with no way out. Counseling is important to allow her to see positive choices available, and encourage movement towards one of those choices. Often we need to release guilt as we establish a new direction for ourselves.

There is a link between the level of stress in our lives and cancer. If we are not coping well with stress, then relaxation techniques, meditation, yoga or tai chi, time management training, and other coping techniques are important components of the therapeutic process.

Many of us live our lives in fear of what others may think. We suppress our own desires, intuition and direction. We follow a mental script of what we 'should' be doing rather than carving a niche in life that reflects our unique identity. We sacrifice ourselves to be 'good'. This killing of the spirit can contribute to cancer development as the life force is suppressed.[2]

Many people sense that their disease is a 'wake-up call'. What if we were to wake up to our spiritual needs and embark on a path of purification before a disease summoned us?

Living with Joy and Purpose

The feeling of joy and the sense of having a purpose in life are dependent upon our emotional and spiritual well-being, our prevailing attitudes, development of our potential, sustaining relationships, who we are in a state of 'being', and what we 'do' in life. A lasting sense of joy and purpose comes from inner direction rather than from outside expectations. It is the voice inside of us linked to our intuition and to the universal energy that guides us to living our destiny. Destiny is the path our life takes when we relate to our soul and listen to and obey our intuitive callings. Our soul is in the driver's seat. Fate is what happens to us when the soul is in the back seat and we let other people, parental expectations, societal norms, or 'shoulds' guide our lives. Disease sometimes manifests when we do the latter, as it can be the intelligence of the body-mind communicating to us that all is not well in the way we are living our lives. There may be some part of ourselves that we are not listening to or honoring, some aspect of unlived life. The psyche wants wholeness, integration of polarities and opposites, wants to embrace all parts of us.

Still, disease can also happen when we are living our lives fully. Why one woman should become ill and another may not is partially out of our control. We do not know what larger purpose is at work in the unfolding of our lives and in our dying. I believe that there is a time when each of us is slated to die and lessons we are meant to learn through our living and dying. The disease process can sometimes teach us those lessons more quickly. I also think that we have the capacity to change the time of our death by how we live our lives and how we respond to what is handed to us. Though the 'script' is there, we can rewrite it.

Breast cancer has many contributing causes. You did not cause your disease, nor are you responsible for curing it. If you have breast cancer, do not blame yourself. There are many causative factors that place all women at risk. However, if you orient your living to finding meaning, purpose, and joy, your immune system will respond positively to these cues and will help to protect you from breast cancer or to recover from it more quickly.

Your Unique Way of Being in the World

Lawrence LeShan, a psychologist who has worked with cancer patients for over 35 years, describes in his book *Cancer as a Turning Point* the spiritual methods he uses in treating cancer patients and claims that the cancer goes into remission roughly 50% of the time. When he had his clients review their past and try to address what was wrong with them using Freudian and psychoanalytic techniques, they did not get better;[3] but when he began to encourage patients to explore avenues for bringing meaning, fulfillment, and joy into their lives, they often became well. He noticed that in a large majority of his clients, there had been a loss of hope in ever achieving a meaningful and satisfying way of living previous to discovering first signs of the cancer. LeShan helped each client find her unique ways of being in the world and attempted to match these to a lifestyle and form of work which best suited her nature. When we recover our hope for living a satisfying and meaningful life, we strengthen our defences against cancer as our body and mind respond to our spiritual commitment to live. By finding our own unique and joyous way of being in the world, breast cancer will be less likely to find us.

Ethel's Story

LeShan tells the story about Ethel, a woman with metastatic breast cancer who had been told that there was nothing else that could be done medically for her. She consulted a psychiatrist and described herself, her experiences, and how for her whole life she had longed to travel aboard an ocean liner and see the world, but her life situation had prevented her from doing so. The best memories in her life were when she was newly married and working as a saleswoman in an exclusive clothing store in Chicago. She had children who were now grown and lived on the other side of the United States. The psychiatrist suggested to her that since her husband was dead and her children no longer needed her, there was nothing to hold her back now from taking a trip on an ocean liner. Her oncologists had told her that she had but two months to live. Ethel took all her money and invested it in a first-class cabin on the Queen Mary for a world cruise. Four months later she angrily stormed into her psychiatrist's office and complained that she had spent all her money and was still alive! The psychiatrist

was able to get her a job in a boutique on another ship. She loved the work and found it completely fulfilling. Over the years, the breast cancer shrank to half its original size with no further treatment. She kept in contact with her psychiatrist until he died eight years later.[4] What did Ethel do to generate self-healing? She rekindled and acted out a life-long dream. She let go of the mental obstacles that had previously thwarted the realization of that dream. She found a situation in life where she felt happy. She put everything on the line for herself. She made a commitment to her own happiness and her immune system responded.

▶ **Action for Prevention:** Strive to live a life in alignment with your true nature, where your passion and joy are kindled and you use your talents and gifts. ◀

But don't be satisfied with poems and stories of how things have gone with others.

Unfold your own myth, without complicated explanation, so everyone will understand the passage.[5]

— Rumi

Searching for Meaning and Purpose

Achievement is something we 'do' in the external world, while experience shapes who we 'are' internally. Meaning comes from both areas. In his book *Man's Search for Meaning*, Viktor Frankl writes about the ways in which we derive meaning from life. For our well-being, what we expect from life is not as important as how we respond to life's expectations of us, he suggests. Life is the teacher, continually presenting us with tests, choices, and opportunities. Daily and hourly we are being questioned by life and our answer can consist in right action and right conduct. Each of us is given tasks to fulfill, a piece to play on the world stage, and it is our responsibility to find our personal path that is in step with the grand scheme of things. This is the meaning of the word 'dharma' in Indian philosophy. Frankl called his method of responding to the world 'logotherapy' and wrote that we could discover the meaning in life in three different ways.

Meaning through Doing

The first way to find meaning is through creating a work or doing a deed. This includes meaningful work or a career, any artistic expression or something we make with our hands, as well as the day-to-day actions of our lives — greeting a friend, smiling at a stranger, writing a letter, making a charitable donation, doing volunteer work, buying organic food, etc. There are many deeds that can bring meaning to us, and for each of us they will be different. We can also bring meaning into the daily actions of our lives. Take cooking, for example. I can come home from work, throw a meal together, call my children and my husband to the table, dish out the food, and read while I eat. It isn't very meaningful. Another time, I can choose a meal plan with care, being attentive to color, nutrient value, delicious flavor, feeling gratitude for having so much good food available. I can chant or pray as I cook. I can decorate the table with flowers and candles, call the family in and have us pray or meditate together before we begin. I can bless the food by holding my hands over it. I can chew the food slowly and savor each bite. We can all talk about our day as we eat and meet together. I can deliver some of the extra food to a neighbor who is elderly. I have made the act meaningful. We can do the same for many of our daily tasks.

Meaning through Experience

The second way to gather meaning from life is by experiencing something or encountering someone. We may experience goodness, truth, beauty, nature, or culture. We can consciously deepen our experience of these by seeking out people or places with deep connections to us, by participating in events or occasions that are moving for us.

Goodness

To experience goodness, we can spend time with 'good' people and visit places where goodness is exemplified, such as in volunteer organizations, spiritual retreats, or healing centers. We can read books about people who exemplified goodness, such as Mother Theresa. If you were going to look for goodness, where would you go?

Truth

We can experience truth through studying the works of spiritual giants of whatever faith we find appealing. We can experience our own truth through meditation, contemplation, and emotional honesty in our interactions.

Beauty

We all recognize beauty in different areas. It may be in the human body, a rose garden, faces of children, a well-made machine, or a decorated home. When we surround ourselves with beauty, we feed ourselves meaning. It is also possible to 'see' beauty where we didn't see it before, and so add to our meaning 'bank'. When I was a young adult, I worked for several months as a nurse's aide in a ward with elderly patients who had senile dementia. My job involved dressing them, feeding them, and changing soiled diapers. I enjoyed the work, for I recognized beauty in most of the residents and appreciated who they were on a soul level, though their minds were fragmented. We can change the way we look at the world so that we see beauty more easily.

Nature

Nature is there for us to experience meaning. Running on the beach, walking in the woods, planting a garden, and travel to scenic places renews us spiritually. Where do you generally find meaning in nature? Is it by water, among trees, or in the mountains? Most of us have found our own sacred spots in nature where we felt rooted and joyous. How can you bring more of those experiences into your life?

Culture

Culture also provides a source of meaning for many. Music, dance, art, theater — each of these has the potential to deepen our connection to our spiritual natures.

Love

Of all interactions, it is loving encounters that bring us the most meaning. When we love another, we help them to actualize their potential, and when we are loved, we more easily realize more of our own potential. If we are feeling unloved, then we can make ourselves beacons of love and find people, plants, or animals that need our love. In giving it, we will receive it back. There are always organizations that need volunteers and plants and animals that need taking care of.

Moira was a patient in her seventies who noticed that the plants in my waiting area needed some care. She volunteered to come in weekly to water them, fertilize the soil as needed, transplant them into larger pots, and dust the leaves. She loved plants and would tell me at length what the needs of each of them were and how she would help them. She was grateful that I was taking care of her, and I was very grateful that she was tending to my plants. She continued to look after them for a year. After she died of a stroke, I could no longer walk by the plants without thinking of her, and often felt that she was still there invisibly caring for them.

Donna is another patient who is uncomfortable with people but loves cats. As a child she was sexually abused for many years. She shelters cats that are ailing and nurses them back to health. She is very sensitive to their psychological needs and describes their personalities to me, as a therapist might describe a client. It brings her great joy and meaning to care for them and is part of her own healing process.

In our culture we value achievement over experience.

Meaning through Our Attitude towards Suffering

The third way we can experience meaning, according to Frankl, is by "the attitude we take towards unavoidable suffering. When we suffer, we are challenged to change ourselves, and if the suffering is unavoidable, we can triumph in the way we bear it provided that we find meaning in it."[6] Suffering can be the hero's path, although it challenges us physically, emotionally, and spiritually. If suffering is avoidable, then we should remove its cause, whether it be physical, psychological, or political. If suffering is unavoidable, then, through our journey into the dark reaches of the soul, we can sometimes pass to the other side having gained in compassion, acceptance, tolerance, and wisdom. Illness is a great teacher. The illuminating qualities that illness can bring us might never have been gained if we were able to cure our sicknesses instantly. Many of us call suffering into our lives so that we can help others. Once we have felt pain, we sense others' pain. We are then more able to extend our hearts and minds in compassionate service.

▶ **Action for Prevention:** Strive to find meaning daily in what you do, what you experience, and through goodness, truth, beauty, nature, culture, and love. Build your 'meaning bank' by filling your life with experiences of depth. Find meaning in the attitude you take to suffering or to illness. Ask of every situation that's given to you what you can learn from it to help you grow. ◀

Finding Lasting Joy and Purpose Exercise

1) The first step in finding joy and purpose is *to acknowledge that you have a spiritual self.* People have called this the soul, inner guide, inner voice, Holy Spirit, higher self, etc. This aspect of us is divine, not bound by time or space, and is linked to a universal energy or universal mind. It is the God within linked to the God everywhere. It is not concerned with material possessions, success, or what others think. Even though you may not experience this aspect of yourself often, it is important to acknowledge its presence as a starting point. Close your eyes and take a minute now to link with your spiritual self.

2) The second step is to *create a relationship with your spiritual self.* As you create relationships with others through communication and time spent together, you can create a relationship between the mind and the soul. Most of us have been taught to relate to money, possessions, and outward pleasures rather than the soul. The mind must relate to the soul, be receptive to it. There are many forms that this can take, but essentially it is a daily spiritual practice. It is a regular setting aside of time to acknowledge and be with your spiritual self, a time of inner listening. It may be accomplished through one or more of the following practices: yoga and meditation; dreamwork; journal writing; creative activity such as drawing, painting, sculpture, music, poetry, dance; prayer and contemplation; service; and time spent in nature. As you acknowledge the soul's presence through a spiritual practice, you more easily recognize its voice and what it (or God) wants from you in the world. Take a moment to reflect upon what kind of spiritual practice best suits you and how you can establish it as a priority in your life. Make a commitment to explore alternatives or begin a regular spiritual practice.

3) The third step is to pay attention and *actively listen to the soul's calling.* This is often synonymous with listening to God's will. It is the voice of intuition that gently urges you to see situations clearly and to act in certain ways. It opens you up to a state of 'being' in the fullness of the moment, experiencing love within the transitory nature of life, and feeling the interconnectedness of everything. It asks you to act in the world, to do what you are most suited for, and to contribute to the improvement of the planet and the human condition. The calling of the soul usually requests that you express yourself uniquely, manifesting your talents and gifts in the world. It is the future pulling you to your potential. On some level, that potential is already manifest, only separated from you by time and space. You can answer the soul's calling, by asking yourself the following questions: Who am I? Why am I here? What did I come here to do? What is my passion? What is the potential in me that yearns for fruition? What did I come here to learn? What did I come here

to heal? Who did I come here to love? What did I come here to express? What did I come here to teach? What causes did I come here to serve? Who did I come here to be? What brings me the greatest joy? What can I do that reflects my beliefs and values? In the following exercises we will explore the answers to these questions.

4) The fourth step is to *agree to what is being asked of you.* This is often painful as the ego allows the soul to be in the driver's seat. Sacrifice is required. Taking risks and trusting the process of change is also often necessary. Like a snake shedding its skin, you are asked to release old belief systems that limit your growth and expanding identity. The old persona, the old clothes, don't fit anymore. Faith must also be your companion through this process — faith in yourself, faith in a higher power or God.

5) The fifth step is to *obey the guidance given to you from within,* to act on the stirrings of the soul, moment by moment, leap by leap. Illness sometimes pushes us more quickly to do this or gives us permission to pursue a direction we may not have taken otherwise. This path may not be easy, as it can demand constant surrender of the ego. It may be terrifying to obey the inner voice. You may feel that you are not worthy or up to the task and ask, 'Why me?' You need consistency, commitment and courage to carry it out. You often require a strong nervous system to act on your inner guidance. You may need support and validation from at least one other person.

6) The sixth step is to *realize what must die or be transformed in your life for the soul to be affirmed.* What do you need to say 'No' to in order to live a purposeful life that is in harmony with who you really are? If you are going to embrace a new way of living, then you must let go of parts of your old life that drain your energy, that reinforce negativity, or that no longer serve you. Sometimes you must let go of a relationship, shift careers, reassess friendships, give up comfort or wealth, and say 'no' to social engagements or responsibilities that you shouldered in the past. You can also change your life through attitudinal shifts. You can say 'no' to that part of you that reacts as a victim or is submissive, overly dependent, or concerned with what others think. You can transform your anger into love and forgiveness.

7) The last step is to *be fully present in your activity,* acknowledging the unseen hands that help you and the opportunities and soul responsibilities that come your

way at appropriate times. You can walk with an attitude of gratitude through life and welcome the joys and hardships of each day. You can actively accept what comes your way and meet it head on. As you are fully present, you become more aware of your relationship and interconnectedness to others. You can search for meaning in your present circumstances, in joy and in suffering. You can develop the ability to express gratitude for all that has been given to you, no matter how difficult. Every experience in life can be used as an opportunity to relate to the soul or spiritual self and to trust in something larger than yourself. You can release your resistance to the reality you've been handed and embrace the process of coming to terms with your life, or your death. You can release your need for control and acknowledge the mystery of living. You can act with commitment and integrity but surrender the outcome of your actions to a higher power or God.

Letting Go Exercise

Letting go is often part of a healing process. When you let go of the old, you create space for the new. When you release the past, you invite the future. Letting go frees up time and space so that you can dwell more fully in the present. You may need to let go of a past relationship and the expectations you had for it, or of your old identity and the restrictions and responsibilities you placed upon yourself. You may have to let go of an addiction that keeps you blunted emotionally — to work, television, overeating, alcohol, sugar, smoking, or drugs. It may be your time to let go of your 'busy-ness' to create time to feel joy in being. You may feel compelled to simplify your life, to let go of your compulsion to fill your emptiness with material things. The time may be right to let go of some of your possessions — clothes that you no longer wear, children's toys, a car you don't really need, books you have already read or will never read, or perhaps the really big ones — to let go of the house in order to travel or the job security that imprisons you in work you don't enjoy. Think about what life is asking you to let go of right now or what you could release to invite new energy into your life. Make a list below. Include past relationships, outdated ideas of who you are, material possessions, social obligations, old emotions of anger, guilt, or grief, addictions, and any excess physical or emotional baggage you carry around with you. If you are in a group, share three of the things you want to let go of with the other women.

Limiting beliefs to let go:	Guilt to let go:
Relationships to let go or transform:	Social obligations to let go:
Possessions to let go:	Expectations to let go:
Addictions to release:	Old emotions to let go:
What else to let go?	

Meditating for Inner Knowing Exercise

Often in life it is difficult to recognize the 'voice' above the chatter of the mind with its confusion, preconceptions, desires, and illusions. This inner knowing can be developed well through slowing down the breath to less than five breaths per minute and through specific breathing practices. The following technique co-ordinates both hemispheres of the brain to develop powerful insight and clear inner direction.

Sit with a straight spine, either cross-legged or in a chair. Have your upper arms against the rib cage with your elbows bent and your hands in front of the area between the breasts known as the heart center. Cross your hands, having both palms facing up, resting one palm in the other. Cross your thumbs. Have the fingers angled up comfortably.

Close your eyes and look at the point between the eyebrows. Then shift your gaze to look at the tip of the nose and keep it fixed there throughout the exercise. Follow this four-part breath sequence.

1) Inhale through the nose slowly, then exhale through the nose at the same pace.

2) Make your lips into a circle and inhale slowly through the mouth, then exhale through the mouth.

3) Inhale through the nose, exhale through the mouth.

4) Inhale through the mouth, exhale through the nose.

Continue for eleven minutes. Practice it daily for 40 days when you are confused or unsure where your direction lies.[7] Be receptive to an answer, letting it come in its own time.

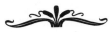

*A new moon teaches gradualness
and deliberation and how one gives birth
to oneself slowly. Patience with small details makes
perfect a large work, like the universe.*

*What nine months of attention does for an embryo
forty early mornings will do
for your gradually growing wholeness.[8]*

— Rumi

Confronting Your Death While Alive Exercise

The possibility of death brings into sharper focus our reasons for living. Whether you are well or not, imagine that it is time for you to die. Review your life in the following four areas: relationships; experiences you have had; actions and achievements; and qualities you have developed. Imagine that you are conversing with a spiritual mentor about the significance of your life. Have you done the things or lived the life you came here to live? Have you grown in the ways you needed to grow? Have you shared your talents and capabilities with the world? Write your impressions down.

1) Write a few sentences that summarize your satisfaction with your life. Write in the third person, as though you are an outside observer commenting on your life. Start the first sentence with, "In this life (your name) has …

(list what relationships you have developed, what you have experienced, talents you have developed, actions and achievements, and personal qualities you embody)".

Keep your phrasing positive. If you have had negative experiences, evaluate what the positive outcomes of those experiences were for you or what you have learned from them. For example, if you have lost a loved one, the positive outcome of that experience may be that you have become more compassionate to others as you empathize with their loneliness and pain.

2) On a separate piece of paper draw four things that you would like to complete, experience, accomplish, and nurture before you die. It is important to draw rather than write because we access more of the unconscious when we draw and it evokes more emotional content than the written word. In a group situation, it provides the participant with a picture to talk about which helps to remove inhibitions when talking about oneself.

The first image should reflect a relationship that you would either like to develop, heal from the past, or have in the future. It may be with someone you have not yet met. It may be with a family member with whom you have had conflict. It may be a special relationship with a child. It may be relationship with yourself, with nature, or with God.

The second image should be about an experience you would like to have before you die, something you have longed for. It could be a place you have wanted to visit, something you have wanted to do at least once, or a spiritual experience you have sought.

The third image should be about something you would like to achieve or accomplish. It could be about running a marathon, publishing a poem, obtaining a career promotion, devoting your energy to a mission, learning to ski or play an instrument etc.

The fourth image reflects the potential in you that you want to nurture and develop. This may be creative ability in drawing, painting, writing, cooking, music, or dance. It may be a talent you have in languages that prompts a desire to learn a new language. It may be a desire to learn something new that you would enjoy, such as astrology, Japanese literature, or bird-watching.

3) If you are in a group situation, share these exercises in the group by having each woman in turn read her life summary and talk about her images briefly. Listen to each woman's story, being present and respectful in silence. This will deepen the experience of the woman who is sharing her story and allow the group to actively empathize with her. Do not interrupt, give advice or console. By interrupting we potentially shut down a person's need to express freely and be fully heard.

▶ **Action for Prevention:** Live your life being aware of your death, so that you deepen relationships, experience life fully, achieve and accomplish your goals, and develop your talents and gifts. ◀

Expanding Your Joy Exercise

Joyful experiences and play help us to live our lives fully and renew our energy and creativity. When we connect to the miracle of each breath, we can bring joy into everyday moments. As women, we often sacrifice our personal joys for the needs of our families or career. It is valuable to put yourself first sometimes. Create balance between your inner life, family life, and career. This exercise will help you to access the states of 'being' and 'doing' that bring you the most joy and encourage you to bring more of these experiences into your life.

1) In the first column, make a list of the 'being' states that have brought you joy in the past or experiences that are possible for you in the near future. These will include your favorite forms of play and relaxation as well as the ways you connect to your inner self or soul. In the second column, recall the 'doing' states that have brought you joy and fulfillment or things you have always wanted to do but have put off. Think back to recall any aborted dreams or forgotten desires. These will also include the ways you express your unique talents and capabilities in the world. Joyful states are often ones where we lose track of time because of being absorbed in the moment. Aim for an equal number of entries in each column. For example, some 'being' states might include watching a sunset, having a bubble bath, or listening to a favorite piece of music. 'Doing' states could include horseback riding, teaching a skill, hosting a party, making pottery, traveling to the Galapagos, sky-diving, or swimming. Joy can also be an inner state that we bring to all our interactions. Because we feel joy, we can perform small acts of devotion or service, such as reading to a child, shoveling snow for a neighbor, or wishing someone a happy birthday.

2) If your list is short, then imagine what might bring you joy. What are the things you have watched others do that you have thought you would like to try? When you have exhausted your list, write beside each entry how often you would like this experience. Make it a

priority to manifest at least three of these experiences each month and set dates for activities that need some planning, such as a vacation. If you are in a group, share your list with other women.

Joyful 'Being' States (more passive)	Joyful 'Doing' States (more active)

Why Am I Here?

In order to answer the question "Why am I here?" we need to appreciate our unique qualities, gifts, talents, and capabilities. Think about what these are in you. What are the unique qualities that you perceive in yourself and the positive qualities that others have recognized? These might include qualities of optimism, insight, reliability, compassion, leadership, creativity, organizational ability, patience, assertiveness, sensitivity, grace, etc. Search for the hidden qualities that may lie buried in you that perhaps others don't see or you have not yet revealed to the world. Include those in your list, too. These may include such things as being forthright, adventurous, outrageous, wise, risk-taking, courageous. Add to your list the positive qualities you would like to embody in the future, the qualities you most admire in others. We all have unique gifts, talents, and capabilities. What were the gifts you came into the world with, have developed along the way or have wanted to develop? What are the talents you have not explored but which are calling you? What are the ways in which your creative energy expresses itself or has expressed itself in the past? Is it through writing, drawing, painting, acting, pottery, dance, cooking, dressmaking, athletic ability, music, weaving, gardening, carving — it is important to

find your avenues of self-expression and nurture them.

Rudolph Steiner believed that as we prepare to die, we should choose the seeds we want to develop for our next life. We may never master a particular skill or talent in this life, but the seeds we plant will make it easier for them to germinate the next time around. List your gifts, talents, and capabilities and ways in which you can develop them to increase your joy and to seed your future — whether it's the next 50 years or a future life.

Today, like every other day, we wake up empty and frightened. Don't open the door to the study and begin reading. Take down a musical instrument.

Let the beauty we love be what we do. There are hundreds of ways to kneel and kiss the ground.[9]

— Rumi

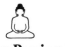

Finding Your Passion Exercise

The other aspect of understanding "Why am I here?" is recognizing where your passion lies. What do you feel very strongly about that you would love to give your energy to? Think about your past and about when life drew the most from you, when you felt as though what you were doing really mattered, either for yourself, for others or the planet. Whatever it is should be something you did gladly and looked forward to each day or something you recognized was your calling and your soul compelled you to do. Look for the things you love more than your own comfort or convenience, the things you could die for because you believe in them so strongly. Or what have you always wanted to do but have been unable to so far?

List those areas that you feel passionate about. It might be one of the arts, a particular sport, the environment, women's rights, health, education, mythology, folk music, preserving history, social justice, children, quiet study, or wildlife. Anything at all that excites your interest is fine. Include as many areas that you can think of. Circle the one that generates the most excitement.

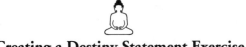

*Start a huge, foolish project,
like Noah.*

*It makes absolutely no
difference what people
think of you.*[10]

— Rumi

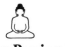

Creating a Destiny Statement Exercise

We have all been affected by what other people have said about us. If, as children, were we told we would 'never amount to anything', then we are more likely to have low self-esteem and lose sight of our potential. Our interests don't matter because we could never succeed at them anyway. If, on the other hand, we were told that we had

an exceptional ability in a particular area, or could do whatever we put our minds to, then the remembered phrase acts as a catalyst for our growth and success even many years later. Ingrained in the subconscious, it may steer us in a particular direction. Sometimes we are fortunate enough to have someone who recognizes us on a soul level bless us with a phrase that feeds our development. When I was in high school, one of my teachers was a priest; I felt 'seen' by him. During his travels one summer, he sent postcards to many of his students. I still remember his words to me, "To a delightful, beautiful, sensitive, feelingful person. Long may you bring happiness to all those

---

Construct the first part of your destiny statement by including three to six qualities, gifts, talents and capabilities. Begin the sentence with,

"I am a ....
.... person."

As the next part of your destiny statement, look over the list of things that bring you joy, both through 'being' and 'doing' and the list of things that excite your passion. Think about the direction that you would like your life to take from this point onward. Choose a few words from these lists that speak to you at this moment, generating excitement and fulfillment. Create a directional statement that is broad enough to be able to include these words and that will act as a compass to guide your actions. Phrase it in the present tense. Write the phrase below, beginning with the words,

"My destiny is ....
.... "

Combine both sentences together to create your destiny statement. Write it below.

" ....
....
.... "

Read your destiny statement out loud to yourself, looking in a mirror, three times daily for 40 days. As you go through your day, at different times do the following: Inhale and hold your breath. Mentally repeat your destiny statement three times. Exhale, mentally repeating it once on the exhale. Notice how your destiny statement changes you.

---

who come into your orbit." I repeated the phrase to myself for years afterwards, affirming the identity that he defined for me. It filled me with positive self-esteem and provided a foundation from which I evaluated and acted upon life choices.

In just this way, you can create a destiny statement for yourself that will remind you who you are and where your direction lies. You can repeat the statement regularly so that your thoughts and actions are congruent with this soul definition. In time, you will become 'who you really are'. The first part of the statement reflects the positive qualities you want to embody. The second part steers you in the direction your soul wants you to go. The whole sentence should be short enough that it is easy to remember, phrased in the present tense so that you are challenged to manifest it now, and inclusive enough to allow for unlimited becoming. Of course, if your direction changes, you can alter the destiny statement as needed.

Hey! Learn to hear my feeble voice

At the center of the hoop

You have said that I should make the tree to bloom.

With tears running,

O Great Spirit, my Grandfather

With running eyes I must say

The tree has never bloomed

Here I stand, and the tree is withered

Again, I recall the great vision you gave me.

*It may be that some little root of the
great tree still lives.*

Nourish it then

That it may leaf

And bloom

And fill with singing birds!

Hear me, that the people may once again

Find the good road

And the shielding tree.

— Black Elk

Creating a Meaning Mandala Exercise

Mandalas have been used in all cultures as symbols of the self, as meditation tools, and as expressions of healing and integration. They usually consist of a central point with symmetrical geometric radiations out from that point. Many forms in nature are expressions of a mandala — flowers such as daisies, peonies, and roses, microscopic diatoms that thrive in the oceans, and the growth rings of a tree are just a few such forms. In the human body, the iris of the eye and the shape of the breasts are examples of mandalas.

In this exercise you will make a 'meaning mandala'. It will help you to define where you derive meaning from your life and propel you to manifest that meaning. It will remind you of your soul's purpose here and how to live that purpose. It will help to integrate the divergent directions in your life and bring you stability when you lose your compass or your anchor. As you relate to your meaning mandala, you will mobilize your body's ability to heal. If you have lost one or both breasts, you can use a space on the meaning mandala to reclaim what they represent.

Using the diagram on the next page as a model, redraw it on a large piece of paper, at least 24 inches by 36 inches (the bigger the better). In the center of the inner circle write the words, 'I am Here'. This represents where you are presently situated in life. At the end of the spaces between two radiating lines at the outer edge of the largest circle, write words or phrases that answer the questions around the diagram. Between the radiating spokes list the progression of actions or experiences that would enhance or develop the meaning at the outer edge of the circle. These might include qualities to develop within yourself, tasks to do, other people to involve, phone calls to make, money to save, courses to enroll in, practice time, etc. Place this drawing on the wall where you can see it regularly to remind yourself of all you have to live for. Focus on the drawing as you do your rebounding exercises. Let it speak to you and remind you of the next step in manifesting your potential.

In time, as you begin to actualize the meaning and purpose of your life, use colored markers to fill in the spaces from the center outward. Use many colors and make the mandala vibrant with life. For every step you take to experience meaning, purpose, and joy, acknowledge it by filling in an area around the section associated with it. To make the mandala more powerful, draw

• Meaning Mandala •

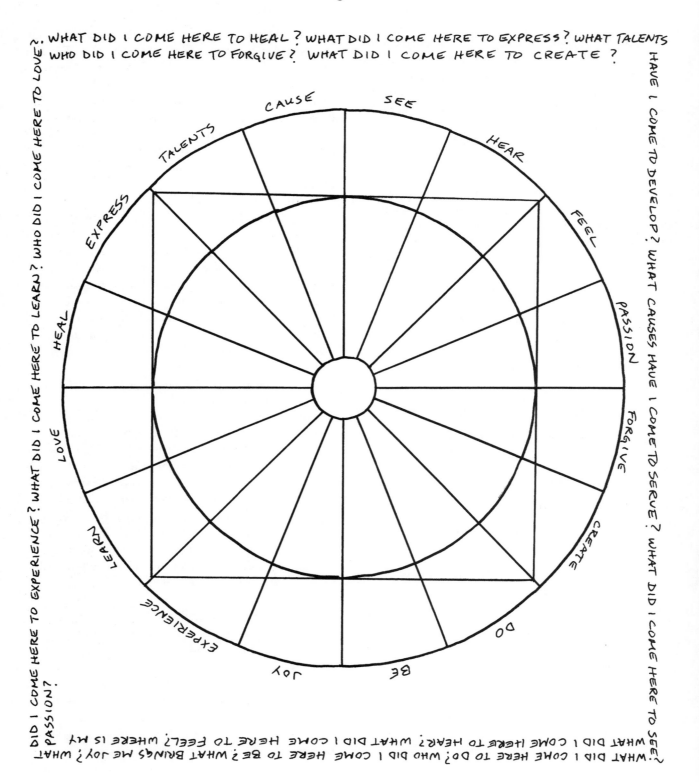

images around the outer circle that represent your goals or fulfilled self. You can also cut up magazines to make a collage with images that remind you of your purpose. Make the meaning mandala uniquely your own, as your life is. The meaning mandala will help you develop more of an active role in creating a satisfying, joyous life. Your body needs to know that you are serious about living for it to co-operate whole-heartedly with you in healing.

The Healing Dream

For over 1000 years, the Greeks believed that dreams were an integral component in healing. This healing tradition began with Asclepius, who was born in the thirteenth century B.C., who legend says died when he was struck by lightning sent by Zeus, and who became the Greek god of medicine. His symbol was the snake we still see used in many medical insignia. Not only did Asclepius cure the sick, but also on occasion he brought the dead back to life. He established over 300 temples in Greece, usually in a country setting near sacred springs and rocks with crevices into the earth, presided over by priests who were also physicians. Snakes were commonly present in the temples and were considered to be the incarnation of Asclepius. Healing was seen as a sacred tradition, and the physician-priests were required to take a sacred oath that evolved into what we now call the Hippocratic oath. Patients came to sleep in the temple to be treated with herbs, surgery, exercise, hydrotherapy, and the laying on of hands – and to receive a healing dream. The patient would do a cleansing fast and don white clothing. In the evening, she would make an offering at an altar, while the priest read a prayer on her behalf. She was told that she would be visited by Asclepius through the night in a dream and perhaps be healed. In the morning, the priest interpreted the patient's dream and told her what treatment should be carried out in response to the dream. If she was healed, she made another offering and went home. If not, she could stay longer.

Many patients inscribed their healing stories on stone tablets around the temple. Here is one story:

A man came to the temple with paralyzed fingers, skeptical of the cures he read on the inscriptions around him. He slept and dreamed that as he was playing dice under the temple, Asclepius came and stepped on his fingers, stretching them out. He then asked the man if he still disbelieved. When the man said 'No', Asclepius said that if he trusted in the future, he would be healed. When the man awoke his fingers were no longer paralyzed.[11]

In her book, *Life After Healing*, Sandra Ingerman describes how prayer and dreams can come together for healing. She herself had suffered terrible pain for years and prayed nightly for help to come to her in a dream.

Months later, she dreamt that suddenly as she was in her house a young, handsome Native American appeared from behind her couch and stated that he had always lived there, though she was unaware of it. He wore blue jeans and a blue work shirt and held a rattle made of extraordinary, translucent blue skin. He pointed to the location of her pain, told her she had a problem there, and shook his rattle over the area. She immediately felt the pain leaving her body and knew even in her sleep that she had been cured. When she awoke the pain was gone, and has not returned in ten years.[12]

In her practice as a psychologist Sandra Ingerman often uses prayer and dreams as part of the therapeutic process. She frequently prays that a healing dream be sent to her clients when they have given her permission to do so.

Lisa came to me for follow-up care after traditional breast cancer treatment several years earlier. A cat scan and X-rays suggested that the cancer had metastasized to one of her ribs, though the bone biopsy was negative. Her doctors told her that they believed it to be a metastasis, but because of the lack of confirmation from the biopsy, they would not treat it. It left her feeling afraid and in limbo, not sure whether she was going to live or die. She had the following dream:

I was standing in a large 3-story house on the edge of a cliff, something like the Scarborough Bluffs. The house was dilapidated and was crumbling even as I stood in it. It was about to fall into the ocean, as was I. Just then a hand appeared and pulled me out of the house as it tumbled over the cliff. I was safe.

I told her that I felt it to be a positive dream because she didn't fall over the cliff; an outstretched hand saved her. She could heal. Because of the inconclusive diagnosis, she had only her intuition to rely on and felt 'in her bones' that she was not going to die. Though the next few months were full of confusion, at different times she experienced distinct periods of elation when she felt connected to a source much greater than herself. During those months, I reminded her of her dream. Another CAT scan in three months showed that the lesion remained the same and there were no further metastases. In six months it had shrunk considerably.

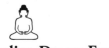

Invoking a Healing Dream Exercise

It is possible to invoke a healing dream using the Asclepian tradition as a model. Here are the steps you can use.

1) Decide to whom or what you will direct your prayer.

2) Be conscious through the day of creating an air of sanctity in your surroundings and in your self. You can do this by cleaning your living space, playing devotional or meditative music throughout the day, fasting or eating very pure foods, bathing with the intent to purify body and mind, and perhaps practicing yoga, meditation, or another purification practice. Through the whole day embody an attitude of quiet reverence in preparation for your healing dream. Let your home and your body become your temple or choose an outdoor location to receive the earth's healing energies.

3) Create a sacred spot inside or outside where you can establish an altar and make an offering. The location can be a place you revisit as needed. You can also visit or make a pilgrimage to an altar in an established place, such as a church, temple, synagogue, or healing shrine. The more frequently you visit the altar, the easier it will feel and the more it will work for you. We energize sacred spots with our devotion.

4) Place an offering at the altar, such as money, fruit, flowers, or time given in service to others.

5) Ask for a healing dream that will guide you in your journey to wellness or ask that you be healed. Often the less specific you are the better — leave it up to God or your unconscious to figure out how to heal you rather than trying to control the process.

6) Keep a paper and pencil beside your bed and tell your unconscious before you sleep that you are ready to receive a healing dream. If you receive a dream, write it down.

7) Reflect on your dream until you can discern its meaning or get help from someone skilled in dream interpretation, such as a Jungian analyst. A good book to help with dream analysis is *Inner Work* by Robert Johnson.[13]

8) Make another offering in the morning as thanks.

9) If you don't receive a dream, continue the process until you do. Be patient. You will eventually.

The Power of Prayer

As you discover your reasons for living, you can reinforce your belief that a new life is possible and that you deserve it. Prayer is one of the tools that can strengthen your belief or faith. Health practitioners, family, and friends will either add to your faith (consciously or unconsciously) or diminish it. Prayer is an innate faculty of humans, existing in all cultures in a variety of forms. It reminds us that we are spiritual beings first, living a human life.[14] Though our physical bodies are bound by time and space, our souls are not. Through prayer we connect to a higher source of power or energy. We don't have to do it all ourselves; we can draw on the unlimited power of the creator. We can gain access to a spiritual dimension to come to our aid. We are not alone. We call it God, the Infinite, or any name from the many world religions. At least some of the time prayer works to reverse diseases of all kinds. Spontaneous regression of cancer is possible but not predictable.

Prayer and visualization are inherently different. When we visualize, we consciously attempt to control an outcome in our body or in our life. It is accomplished through focused concentration, intention, and repetition. We attempt to fix ourselves or create the reality we want. When we pray we give up control. We surrender. We entreat a power greater than our own to help us. We admit that we need help; we can't fix the part of us that is broken. We are vulnerable. Though they are different, they are not mutually exclusive. Prayer and meditation are complementary practices that each have a place in a healing program. I once attended an imagery workshop in Toronto with Jeanne Achterberg and Frank Lawless. Jeanne said that she noticed that the Aids patients who did the best were the ones who were actively engaging the warrior archetype to be victorious over their disease but had given up trying to influence the outcome. In other words, do the best you can and leave the rest up to God. Visualization is 'doing'; prayer is 'leaving the rest up to God'. We need both. Whatever the outcome, we did the best we could. We are not responsible for the outcome. God is in charge.

While we pray we establish a conscious connection to the spiritual dimension within us and around us. That connection always exists but prayer is a vehicle that grounds us in the spiritual rather than the material. The spiritual dimension is much bigger and more powerful than the physical. Our attempts at attaining power or possessions in the material world often reflect our disconnection from our authentic spiritual selves. Eventually prayer can become a state of being, where we feel the connection to God or the Beloved all the time. Rumi was a Sufi poet who expressed this beautifully:

*You've read where it says that
Lovers pray constantly*

*Once a day, once a week, five times an hour,
is not enough. Fish like we are
need the ocean around us.*[15]

— Rumi

Illness as the Gateway to the Spirit

Prayer heals us spiritually. Often we turn to prayer in times of crisis or illness. It helps us psychologically through difficult times, though it may not outwardly change a particularly situation or reverse disease. If you are ill and prayer does not reverse your illness, even though you are doing the best you can through allopathic and complementary medicine and psychological change, you can consider the following.

Spiritual growth is not necessarily proportional to an improvement in physical health. Poor physical health, however, is often the gate through which we pass to explore our spirituality. Illness can be a path of purification for the mind, body, and spirit. Sickness is part of the natural order on earth. Plants and animals get sick and die, as we do. Perhaps the purpose of our lives is to link to the totality and divinity within ourselves and all around us. The length of your life is not as important as how fully you receive your soul and how well you live in accordance with your true nature and your values. If the soul is infinite, then an opportunity may exist for it somewhere else to express itself, perhaps through reincarnation or through another form. Who are we to know when or where that opportunity lies? Many things are beyond our control. That is as it should be. Reversing disease is not the ultimate goal. We are obliged to do all we can to live as fully as possible and to purify and heal as deeply as possible and then surrender the outcome of our efforts. Our soul never dies. Physical death can come sweetly as an exit point when we have finished our work here. It heralds a new beginning. For those of you who have

cancer, there is no formula that will result in spontaneous healing. You must create your own path, reclaim your authentic life. You may or may not be 'cured' but your living will be more vital.

People who are true to themselves and honor the experiences that come from the depths of their being are sometimes graced with a miraculous cure, however. They can but do not always have the following traits in common. They use surgery, medication, complementary medicine, and any other healing modalities that may be helpful. They do not desperately seek a miracle and are not determined to be healed of their disease. Rather, they believe that God's will is being done, no matter what the outcome. They live with gratitude for their lives despite their disease. They focus on 'being' and live fully in the present rather than getting caught up in 'doing'. They have a fighting spirit yet a capacity to surrender.

Types of Prayer

Several types of prayer are used in different religious traditions. They include *petition*, when we ask for something for ourselves; *intercession*, when we ask for something for others; *confession*, when we ask for forgiveness for a wrongdoing; *invocation*, when we call on the presence of God; *thanksgiving*, when we express gratitude for what we have received; and *submission*, when we accept God's will for us and surrender our personal will.

Patrons of Prayer

"Whom do I pray to?" you may ask. You can pray to the particular deities, saints, enlightened beings, or teachers associated with a spiritual tradition. You can pray to a divine spirit or energy that is all pervading, with no particular face. You can pray to the feminine creative power of the universe, known as Adi Shakti in India, or to the Virgin Mary in Christianity. You can pray to Jesus, Buddha, or Krishna. You can pray to one of the Greek goddesses, such as Athena. You can pray to the Greek healing God, Asclepius, or to Guru Ram Das, a healing divinity in the Sikh tradition. Saint Peregrine is the patron saint for spontaneous regression of cancer in the Christian tradition. While a young priest, he developed cancer in his leg and was scheduled for amputation. He prayed earnestly the night before surgery and dreamed he was cured. When he awoke, he was surprised to find that his dream had come true. In 1345 he died at the ripe age of 80 without any recurrence of cancer. He lived in service of those people afflicted with cancer, as many breast cancer survivors do today.[16]

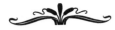

Go to the library and research world religions or talk to religious people if none of them seem right. We all have links to various teachers and saints. It's up to us to find out who they are, recognize and accept them. But for now, just pray. Make the connection in your heart to something larger and more powerful than yourself. Imagine you are plugging yourself in to a spiritual power, much as you plug in a light to receive electricity. The more you link with devotion to this higher power or being, the stronger your prayer will be. Over time, let there be intimacy between you and your spiritual source, and talk regularly to it as you would talk to a close friend who is a good listener. Remember the first law in physics, "for every action there is an equal and opposite reaction." There will be a response to your prayer, though it may not be what or when you expect it.

How to Pray Exercise

We all will find different ways to pray as we listen to the longing of our soul and follow its directives. If you feel a little inept entering the world of prayer, here are a few suggestions to get you started.

Create a Time and Space for Prayer
Create a time and space for prayer. As religious groups establish places of worship and set times for prayer, so too we can do this in our own homes. Find an area in your living space which you can designate as your place to pray. It may be in your bedroom, living room, a large closet or even outside. Claim your space with a blanket, pillow, or sheepskin that you can sit on for prayer. Over time you will associate this object with prayer and it will become easier to do — it may also be something to take with you when you travel. Create an altar if you like. Find some symbols that are meaningful to you and decorate the area with them. You might use religious pictures, natural objects such as flowers and shells, drawings or photographs. You want the images to be uplifting and transcendent so that they will help put you into a prayerful state. Change the symbols occasionally to create an ongoing relationship with your prayer space. Establish a regular time for prayer. Typically this is in the morning on awakening or in the evening before bed, but it can be any time. If you pray at the same time daily, you establish a habit in your psyche that makes it easier to sustain. Co-ordinate the times of prayer with your ultradian rhythms. Take your 10–20 minute breaks to unite body, mind, and spirit by listening to their signals. Then establish a routine.

Work. Keep digging your well.
Don't think about getting off from work.
Water is there somewhere.

Submit to a daily practice.
Your loyalty to that
is a ring on the door.

Keep knocking, and the joy inside
will eventually open a window
and look out to see who's there.[17]

— Rumi

Be consistent, even when it's difficult. Like any discipline, it requires practice. Think of it as exercising your spiritual muscle — spirit-building, rather than body-building.

Begin with a Gesture
Initiate your prayer time with a gesture. Whatever feels natural to you — you can touch your forehead to a sacred object, bow or genuflect, put your palms flat together at your heart center, or simply close your eyes — this gesture becomes a signal for your body and mind to enter into a prayerful state.

Decide on Type of Prayer
Decide which of the six types of prayer you will use at this time. Will it be a prayer for yourself, a prayer for another, a prayer of thanksgiving, a request for forgiveness, a call for God's presence, or a prayer for the ability to submit to divine will? Center yourself by focusing your attention on your breath rather than any distracting thoughts. Bring your awareness to the heart center, between the breasts, and adopt an attitude of reverence and devotion as though you are in the presence of a great spiritual being or power. Feel compassion, receptivity, and surrender to a higher will. Give up control.

Begin Your Prayer
Begin your prayer. Your prayer may be a feeling state without words that you maintain for a period of time. It may be a formal prayer that you recite one or more times until you feel finished. You might keep a little notebook in your prayer space and let your prayer come out as written thoughts or as letters or drawings to God. Find what works for you.

Finish with Thanks

Finish your prayer with a moment of gratitude for having had the opportunity to pray. Acknowledge yourself as a spiritual being living a human life.

Your Personal Prayer

Each of the spiritual traditions has a large body of prayers to choose from and to recite. If you have a religious heritage, you might begin to search for your personal prayer in some of these religious books or in the writings of the saintly persons associated with your tradition. Find a few prayers, read them out loud, and notice how they make you feel. Change the wording if necessary so that it has a greater effect upon you. Ideally a prayer will connect you to your spiritual identity on the inside and to an external spiritual source (they are really one and the same). It will increase your faith and generate a peaceful, relaxed state. It will augment your spiritual longing and stimulate your capacity to surrender to a higher will than your own.

With practice, prayer can replace worry and fear. You can use it when you feel overwhelmed with either of these emotions by putting your faith and trust in a force much greater than yourself. Once you have found or developed your own prayer, write it on a small card and carry it with you, perhaps in your wallet or written on a bookmark. Read it silently or out loud during your prayer time and recite it internally during the day, particularly when you feel a loss of faith or hope. Let it become a trusted companion. Here are some examples of prayers.

This prayer is a variation of a prayer by Saint Angela Merici of Brescia, who founded the Ursuline nuns. She experienced many mystical visions and was a woman of action, always ready to do God's work.[18]

O Divine Spirit, speak to me. Your servant is listening and is ready to obey You in all ways.

or

O my Soul, speak to me. I am listening and am ready to obey You in all ways.

This prayer was inspired by a prayer written by St. Richard of Chichester, who after severe misfortune was able to focus on gratitude rather than becoming bitter and angry.[19]

Thank you God, for all the blessings you have given me, and for the pain and suffering you carry for me. May I hold you more clearly, love you more dearly, and follow you more nearly each day.

This prayer was inspired by a prayer of Brother Charles

De Foucauld, who came to realize that self-discipline was necessary for saintliness, but that discipline is possible only with God's help.[20]

I give myself to You, to do what You will. Whatever You do with me, I thank You. I am ready for all, and I accept all. I offer You my soul with all the love in my heart.

This prayer is a variation of one by Saint Anthony Mary Claret, who founded the Claretian Order and was archbishop of Cuba.[21]

I believe, but let me believe more deeply.
I hope, but let me hope more surely.
I love, but let me love more completely.
I forgive, but may I forgive without limits.

The inspiration for this prayer comes from the Chandogya Upanishad, a sacred text in Hinduism.[22]

There is a Light that shines beyond all things on earth, and beyond the highest heavens. May this Light shine in my heart.

This prayer is taken from the Brihad-Aranyaka Upanishad.[23]

From ignorance lead me to truth
From darkness lead me to light
From death lead me to immortality.

This prayer was inspired by Buddhist teachings.[24]

Through impermanence, may I know what is eternal,
Beyond selfishness, may I know the Self
May my mind and heart know the peace of my soul

The Sikh poem, Sukhmani Sahib, is the inspiration behind this prayer.[25]

May I always remember You
In the void of emptiness, where I have no friends or relatives,
When I cross the wilderness, pursued by death,
When despair consumes me,
As I reflect on my wrongdoings.
May Your Name be my companion
And release me in a moment
Bringing peace and liberation.

▶ **Action for Prevention:** Design your own prayer or use a traditional prayer upon rising each morning and before bed. When you find yourself feeling a loss of hope, worry or fear, use a form of prayer as a centering device. ◀

Summary

My Prayer of Intercession for You

God bless you on your healing journey. My prayers are with you. May we all be blessed in our efforts to heal ourselves, each other, and the Earth.

Further Reading

Bolen, Jean Shinoda. *Close to the Bone: Life-Threatening Illness and the Search for Meaning*. New York, NY: Touchstone, Simon and Schuster Inc., 1996.

Canfield, Jack et al. *Chicken Soup for the Surviving Soul*. Deerfield Beach, FL: Health Communications, Inc., 1996.

Dossey, Larry. *Healing Words: The Power of Prayer and the Practice of Medicine*. New York, NY: Harper Collins, 1994.

Frankl, Viktor. *Man's Search for Meaning: An Introduction to Logotherapy*. Translated by Ilse Lasch. New York, NY: Pocket Books, 1963.

LeShan, Lawrence. *Cancer as a Turning Point: A Handbook for People with Cancer, Their Families, and Health Professionals*. Revised ed. New York, NY: Plume, Penguin Books, 1994.

Siegel, Bernie. *Love, Medicine and Miracles: Lessons Learned About Self-Healing from a Surgeon's Experience with Exceptional Patients*. New York, NY: Harper and Row, 1986.

Siegel, Bernie. *Peace, Love and Healing*. New York, NY: Harper and Row, 1989.

References

1. Psychosomatic Dimensions of Cancer Therapy. Dr. Bernard Greenwood. *Consumer Health Newsletter*, Jan./Feb. 1987; 8(1).
2. Excerpt from a tape made at the annual Cancer/Nutrition Convention of the Foundation for Alternative Cancer Therapies held at the Biltmore Hotel in New York City in May 1979. The speaker was Dr. Leo Roy.
3. LeShan, Lawrence. *Cancer as a Turning Point: A Handbook for People with Cancer, Their Families and Health Professionals*. New York: Penguin, 1994:21
4. LeShan, Lawrence. *Cancer as a Turning Point: A Handbook for People with Cancer, Their Families and Health Professionals*. New York: Penguin, 1994:72-73.
5. Barks, Coleman. *The Illuminated Rumi*. New York, NY: Broadway Books, 1997:11.
6. Frankl, Viktor. *Man's Search for Meaning: An Introduction to Logotherapy*. Translated by Ilse Lasch. New York, NY: Pocket Books, 1963:115.
7. Bhajan, Yogi. *Survival Kit: Meditations and Exercises for Stress and Pressure of the Times*. Compiled by S.S. Vikram Kaur Khalsa and Dharm Darshan K. Khalsa. San Diego, CA: K.R.I. Publications, 1980:27.
8. Barks, Coleman. *The Illuminated Rumi*. New York, NY: Broadway Books, 1997:49.
9. Barks, Coleman. *The Illuminated Rumi*. New York, NY: Broadway Books, 1997:31
10. Barks, Coleman. *The Illuminated Rumi*. New York, NY: Broadway Books, 1997:81.
11. Jayne, Walter Addison. *The Healing Gods of Ancient Civilizations*. New Hyde Park, NY: University Books Inc., 1962:240-303.
12. Ingerman, Sandra. *Welcome Home: Life After Healing*. San Francisco, CA: Harper-San Francisco, 1993.
13. Johnson, Robert. *Inner Work*. New York, NY: Harper and Row, 1986.
14. I heard this idea first in a lecture by Yogi Bhajan and have since read it in Jean Shinoda Bolen's book, *Close to the Bone*. New York, NY: Touchstone - Simon and Schuster, 1996:71.
15. Barks, Coleman. *The Illuminated Rumi*. New York, NY: Broadway Books, 1997:122.
16. Dossey, Larry. *Healing Words: The Power of Prayer and the Practice of Medicine*. New York, NY: HarperCollins, 1993:28.
17. Barks, Coleman. *The Illuminated Rumi*. New York, NY: Broadway Books, 1997:45.
18. Koenig-Bricker, Woodene. *Prayers of the Saints: An Inspired Collection of Holy Wisdom*. New York, NY: HarperCollins, 1996:59.
19. Koenig-Bricker, Woodene. *Prayers of the Saints: An Inspired Collection of Holy Wisdom*. New York, NY: HarperCollins, 1996:5.
20. Koenig-Bricker, Woodene. *Prayers of the Saints: An Inspired Collection of Holy Wisdom*. New York, NY: HarperCollins, 1996:47.
21. Koenig-Bricker, Woodene. *Prayers of the Saints: An Inspired Collection of Holy Wisdom*. New York, NY: HarperCollins, 1996:53.
22. Mascaro, Juan. *The Upanishads*. Toronto, ON: Penguin, 1965:113.
23. Mascaro, Juan. *The Upanishads*. Toronto, ON: Penguin, 1965:127.
24. Radhakrishan, Sarvepalli and Charles A. Moore. *A Sourcebook in Indian Philosophy*. Princeton: Princeton University Press, 1957:345.
25. Kaur, Sardarni Premka. *Peace Lagoon*. Pomona, CA: K.R.I. Publications, 1984:265.

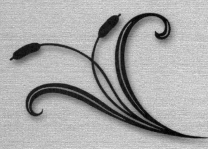

Summary of the Healthy Breast Program

Contents

The Daily Healthy Breast Program

On a daily basis, consider following this regime, consulting the Recipes for Breast Health section for creating variety in your meals.

Upon Rising

- skin brushing
- alternating hot and cold shower
- prayer
- powdered greens and water
- herbs
- 11 minute breathing exercise
- 15 minutes of yoga, Qiqong, tai chi, etc.
- 15–30 minutes of rebounding

Breakfast

- breakfast with vitamins and minerals

Snack

- vegetable juice

½ Hour Before Lunch

- powdered greens and water
- herbs

Lunch

- lunch with vitamins and minerals

Snack

- vegetable juice

½ Hour Before Dinner

- powdered greens and water
- herbs

Dinner

- dinner with vitamins and minerals

Before Bed

- Healthy Breast Drink
- prayer
- meditation or breathing exercises

The Annual Herbal Healthy Breast Program

Below is the basis for a herbal program in preventing and treating breast cancer, to be used in conjunction with other therapies which may include conventional breast cancer treatments. It may be modified depending upon your risk factors and the type and staging of the cancer. Please work with a naturopathic doctor or herbalist before embarking on this program.

For Prevention

Healthy Breast Formula (or Hoxsey Formula):
(p. 175, 173)
20 drops twice daily, for 4 weeks on, 1 week off, or
30 drops three times daily for three months, twice yearly

Liver Loving Formula (or other liver formula):
(p. 130, 131)
20 drops twice daily, for 6 weeks on, 2 weeks off
Use in a stronger dosage 1–2 times yearly for a liver cleanse.

Immune Power Formula: (p. 178)
30 drops twice daily, before dinner and before bed, for 3 months in the winter

For Breast Cancer Recovery

Healthy Breast Formula (or Hoxsey Formula):
(p. 175, 173)
40–100 drops three times daily, for 4 weeks on, 1 week off
Continue for 5 years after diagnosis and then take it for 3 months twice yearly

Liver Loving Formula (or other liver formula):
(p. 130, 131)
40 drops three times daily, for 6 weeks on, 1 week off.
Continue for 5 years, then take 30 drops twice daily, continuously

Goldenseal/Echinacea Tincture:
30 drops twice daily, for 3 weeks on, 2 weeks off
Repeat this pattern for 5 years, then as needed for infection

Immune Power Formula: (p. 178)
(or other immune enhancing formula):
30–100 drops three times daily
Continue 6 weeks on, 1 week off for 5 years
Then take 30 drops three times daily for 3 months, twice yearly.

The Breast Health Data Sheet for Patient Monitoring

Complete the questionnaire on pages 294, 295 and 296 yourself, bringing it up-to-date at least once each year, and provide copies to your health practitioners so that they can have clear records of what you have been doing and how you are responding

If you wish, please send a copy of your finished questionnaire every six months to me, Sat Dharam Kaur ND, so that I can keep track of your progress and judge the success of The Healthy Breast Program. It will also allow me to modify the program each year.

You can access new information about The Healthy Breast Program and order many of the herbal formulas and supplements in this book through my web site: www.healthybreastprogram.on.ca, by telephone (519-372-9212 or 519-372-2755), or by mail (Sat Dharam Kaur, ND, 534 8ᵗʰ St. A East, Owen Sound, ON, N4K 1M9, Canada). Thank you for your participation. God bless you.

Responsibilities of Patients in *The Healthy Breast Program*

1) To complete *The Breast Health Balance Sheet* and provide this to your medical and naturopathic doctor.

2) To practice breast self-exam and breast mapping once monthly and to notify your naturopathic doctor and your medical doctor of your findings.

3) To have your doctor perform a clinical breast exam with you every 6 months and to follow-up with any recommended testing procedures as your finances allow.

4) To complete a one-week *Diet Diary* at least once monthly and provide a copy to your health care professional.

5) To comply with your health care practitioner's recommendations regarding the taking of supplements and to inform him/her of any side effects or financial difficulties that require you to alter your regimen

6) To maintain regular visits with your health care practitioner (every 1–3 months).

Guidelines for Health Care Professionals

The following guidelines have been written for health care professionals using *The Healthy Breast Program*. They provide a convenient, practical review of the program for both practitioners and patients and suggest how you, the patient, can cooperate with your health care professional to make *The Healthy Breast Program* work for you. When both you and your health care professional understand the approach, prevention and treatment of breast cancer is optimized.

If you are a health care professional using *The Healthy Breast Program*, show this guideline to your patient, while introducing her to the book. Ask her if there is anything she would rather not work on with you. Ask her which areas she would like to address first, after the material in the initial four visits is covered. Be flexible in your approach, responding to your patient's needs and taking time to be fully present. You needn't follow this sequence in order, but I would recommend that you attempt to address the following areas within the first year of the initial visit. Some of these 'visits' will require more than one appointment, depending on the patient. When the patient has established the components of the program in her everyday life, or at least is familiar with them, consider scheduling visits every three months rather than once monthly. The visits in these guidelines correspond to the structure of the book.

Visit 1 (1½ hours): Assessing Risk Factors

❑ Have patient fill out a standard intake form and *The Breast Health Data Sheet* from this book before the visit. At the end of the visit, ask her to complete *The Breast Health Balance Sheet, Life Map, Diet Diary*, and *BBT* chart at home before the next visit. Make copies of these forms before hand or mark them in the patient's copy of the book.

❑ Take patient history, including family history. Listen to the whole story. Record specifics about any breast tumors and past breast history. Keep homeopathic remedies in mind and repertorize for subsequent visit. Ask for a copy of the pathology report.

❑ Ask about emotional links to their breast health: what happened before the appearance of the tumor; was there an unresolved conflict that preceded it?.

❑ Ask about any medications or supplements they have been taking so far; list dosages.

The Breast Health Data Sheet For Patient Monitoring — Page 1 of 3

Name:		Address:		
Tel:	Fax:		E-mail:	
Age:	Birthdate: (M/D/Y)		Breast Exam Date: (M/D/Y)	

Personal History

1.	Age when periods began		Age when periods stopped	
2.	Length in days between menstrual cycles			
3.	Number of live births			
4.	Age at birth of first child			
5.	Total number of months spent breast-feeding			
6.	Number of bowel movements	per day		per week
7.	History of fibrocystic breast disease? ☐yes ☐no		Other breast disease?	When?
8.	Dates of previous mammograms		Frequency	
9.	Family history of breast cancer? ☐yes ☐no		Who, and at what age were they diagnosed?	
10.	Family history of ovarian, endometrial or prostate cancer?		Who, and at what age?	
11.	Personal history of breast cancer? ☐yes ☐no		If yes, complete the following:	
12.	Location of tumor L R		Size of tumor	
13.	Grade of tumor cells	Cancer stage 0 I II IIB III IV	Estrogen or Progesterone receptor + or − (circle which)	
14.	How many lymph nodes removed		Spread to the lymph? ☐yes ☐no	
15.	Bone metastases? ☐yes ☐no	If yes, where?	When?	
	Other metastases? ☐yes ☐no	If yes, where?	When diagnosed?	
16.	Current weight	Previous normal weight	Height	
17.	Any recurrence of breast cancer? ☐yes ☐no		If yes, when and where?	

Hormone Profile and Predictive Tests

1.	Saliva estrogen quotient $\text{Estrogen quotient} = \dfrac{\text{Estriol}}{\text{Estrone} + \text{Estradiol}}$		and date of test
2.	Ratio of C2 to C16 estrogen		and date of test
3.	Saliva progesterone (days 20–23)		and date of test
4.	TSH _____free T_4 _____free T_3 _____rT_3 antimicrosomal ab_____ antithyroglobulin ab_____	basal body temp. ☐normal ☐high ☐low	date tested:
5.	Melatonin level at 3:00 a.m.		
6.	IGF-1 in serum	IGF-2 in serum	date of test

7.	AMAS test.			When?	
8.	urinary equol	urinary daidzen	urinary enterolactone		urinary enterodiol
9.	Stool or blood glucuronidation rate				
10.	Tumor markers				
11.	pH of urine (note a.m or over 24 hrs)			pH of saliva	
12.	Monthly breast self exams? ☐yes ☐no			Breast mapping? ☐yes ☐no	
	Attach copy of breast map.				
13.	Other tests				

Previous Medical Treatments for Breast Cancer

1.	Surgery? ☐yes ☐no	If yes, date(s)	lumpectomy mastectomy (circle one)
2.	Tamoxifen? ☐yes ☐no	If yes, dates of use	
3.	Raloxifene? ☐yes ☐no	If yes, dates of use	
4.	Chemotherapy? ☐yes ☐no	If yes, names of medication and dates of treatment	
5.	Radiation? ☐yes ☐no	If yes, when and number of treatments	
6.	Other?	Dates	

Past and Present Risk Factors

1.	History of birth control pill use?	☐yes ☐no	Age with use and for how long?
2.	History of estrogen replacement therapy?	☐yes ☐no	Age began and for how long?
	Type of ERT		
3.	History of fertility drug use?	☐yes ☐no	How often?

Attach a copy of your completed Breast Health Balance Sheet.

Naturopathic Treatments and Therapies for Breast Health

1.	Evening meditation practice?	☐yes ☐no	When did you begin?
	Type of practice and duration		
2.	Rebounding	☐yes ☐no	When did you begin and for how many minutes daily?
	How many days per week?		

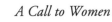

3.	Hours of aerobic exercise weekly			
4.	Contrast showers?	☐yes ☐no	Skin brushing?	☐yes ☐no
5.	Have you done a cleanse for yeast and parasites?	☐yes ☐no	When?	
	What did you use, dosage and for how long			
6.	Have you done a liver cleanse?	☐yes ☐no	When?	
	What did you use, dosage and for how long?			
7.	Have you done a sauna detoxification program?	☐yes ☐no		
	If yes, how many minutes in the sauna each time and what was the frequency?		How much B3?	

Attach copy of Dietary Tips for Breast Health.

Attach copy of a two-week diet diary.

Attach copy of Daily Therapeutic Amounts of Vitamins and Minerals.

Herbal Formulas

1.	Are you taking a lymphatic cleansing formula? ☐yes ☐no Circle which, if any of the following: Hoxsey Formula Healthy Breast Formula Essiac Floressence		
	When did you begin?	How many drops?	How many times daily?
2.	Are you taking a liver cleansing formula? ☐yes ☐no Circle which of the following? Liver Loving Formula Milk thistle / Dandelion Other (list herbs)_____		
	When did you begin?	How many drops?	How many times daily
3.	Are you taking an immune enhancing formula? ☐yes ☐no Circle which of the following: Immune Power Formula Astragalus Combo (St. Francis Herbs) Other (list herbs)_____		
	When did you begin?	How many drops?	How many times daily
4.	List other therapies you may be doing or taking for breast health: (Attach another sheet if necessary)		
5.	Please comment on which therapies you feel are most beneficial to you and how you are feeling overall.		
6.	Is there anything else you think should be included in The Healthy Breast Program?		

❑ Physical exam; reserve breast exam and breast mapping for second visit if time is a factor.

❑ Review the structure of *The Healthy Breast Program* with the patient and ask her to tell you in the next visit if she is willing to commit to it or if she is uncomfortable/has questions about any piece.

❑ Educate patient about any other Healthy Breast Components available in your area. For example, The Canadian College of Naturopathic Medicine offers a Healthy Breast Nutrition support group (once weekly for 8 weeks); Yoga & Rebounding for Breast Health (once weekly for 1½ hrs); Breast Self-Exam Drop-In Clinic (bimonthly for 3 hours at a time); Mind-Body Relaxation Course (2½ hours once weekly for 8 weeks).

Prescribe:

❑ **Diet Changes:** Give the patient a copy of the *Healthy Breast Diet* and ask her to begin to implement dietary changes. Specifically, prescribe kelp or seaweeds, flax-seed oil and freshly ground flaxseeds (2 tbsp minimum of each). Consider psyllium seed powder or other bowel cleansing formula, Greens + or other green powdered supplement containing spirulina.

Cautions:

❑ **Hypothyroid and Brassicas:** If hypothyroid, monitor the effect of soy and the raw brassicas on TSH and thyroid function (TSH sometimes goes up after consistent intake of soy and raw brassicas). That's why it's a good idea to test TSH beforehand. Make sure they are including sea vegetables and/or kelp tablets with these foods to counteract their goitrogenic effect.

❑ **Soy Allergy:** If allergic to soy, increase other phytoestrogens, decrease soy. Miso and tempeh may be easier for some individuals to digest as long as there is not a Candida problem.

❑ **Wheat Allergy:** If allergic to wheat bran, increase psyllium.

Homework for the Patient:

❑ Fill out *Breast Health Data Sheet* and *Breast Health Balance Sheet* found in this book.

❑ Complete a *BBT* chart for at least two weeks to screen thyroid function; if low, continue to monitor progress.

❑ Complete a *Life Map*, showing environmental links to breast cancer in places you have lived.

❑ Complete a *Diet Diary* for at least one week

❑ Read *The Healthy Breast Diet*.

Homework for the Practitioner:

❑ Review the patient's present supplement protocol and ensure that the following nutrients are provided; CoQ10 (100–400 mg), antioxidant formula (containing vitamin C plus bioflavonoids, vitamin E, zinc, selenium, grapeseed), chromium, niacin, folic acid, B complex, NAC or reduced glutathione. Consider what is known about pros and cons of antioxidants during chemo and radiation and evaluate dosages.

❑ Fill out the chart, *Daily Therapeutic Amounts of Vitamins and Minerals* for the patient with what you are recommending at this time, listing dosages and brand names if known. Prepare to explain to her what each supplement is used for.

❑ **Herbal Medicine:** Lymphatic formula (Floressence, Hoxsey or Healthy Breast Formula), liver formula (Milk Thistle Combo or Liver Loving Formula), immune tonic (Astragalus Combo or Immune Power Formula). (If breast cancer is present, all three should be done simultaneously. If needing prevention, do a lymphatic formula with a liver formula consistently and use an immune formula only if there seems to be an immune weakness from the history. See the *Annual Herbal Healthy Breast Program* on page 292 as a guide for dosages).

❑ **Consider:** Alpha lipoic acid, potassium, inositol and inositol hexaphosphate (IP6), melatonin if estrogen receptor positive tumor or if on Tamoxifen (may have to refer or use St. John's wort or evening meditation), thymus extract or thymuline 9CH, modified citrus pectin, digestive enzymes, indole-3-carbinol, curcumin, goldenseal, echinacea, bloodroot, juniper, Maitake D-fraction, MGN-3, carnivora.

❑ **Homeopathic Differential Diagnosis:** Come up with one.

Visit 2: Hormones

❑ Review *Breast Health Balance Sheet* and counsel as to ways to decrease breast cancer risk. Start with a few changes and set target dates for the implementation of those changes (for example, sleep in a dark room, decrease exposure to electromagnetic fields in specific ways, begin exercising more, wear a less restrictive bra, assess dental fillings, eliminate use of plastic packaging on foods, use water filter, etc.) Keep coming back to this chart in repeat visits until all the possible changes have been made.

❏ Review *Diet Diary* and suggest a few simple changes. Be sensitive to the patient's capacity for change. Instruct that you will do a more thorough diet review in the next visit.

❏ Review BBT and thyroid function. Check if BBT is consistently below 97.8 F. Ask about previous thyroid tests and physicals associated with low thyroid (easy weight gain, hair loss, cold, constipated, depression, heavy prolonged menses, insomnia or needing to sleep a lot, infertility, dry skin, eczema, headaches, high cholesterol). If temperature is low or high, complete thyroid tests which include TSH, free T3, free T4, reverse T3, antithyroglobulin, and antimicrosomal antibodies. All of these need to be done to see where the problem lies in the thyroid system. They can be done through DiagnosTech International Inc. Also check adrenal function through the Koenigsburg test or salivary cortisol. Check salivary progesterone too. A low temperature could be related to one or all of these (thyroid, adrenals, progesterone).

❏ Perform clinical breast exam along with breast mapping for the patient; instruct in how to perform a Brest Self Exam (BSE) and request she does it monthly. Draw your findings on the map and suggest the patient refer to the map monthly and record any changes. Set up clinical breast exam for patient every 6 months, recording the next date for both of you. Request that she bring in her breast map from her own BSE practice every 6 months when you perform a clinical breast exam. Refer for further testing if anything unusual.

❏ Talk about the importance of long, deep breathing in correcting and maintaining balanced rhythms in the bodymind. Explain the significance of ultradian rhythms and their relationship to melatonin production and cell division. One nostril should be dominant for 90–120 minutes, then both open for 20 minutes, then the other nostril dominant for 90–120 minutes. This cycle helps to regulate hormone balance and cell division, among other things. It is shortened during periods of stress. The slower the breath, the more balanced the glands. Watch the patient breathe, timing the number of breaths per minute and the number of seconds for the inhale and the exhale. Teach her the alternate nostril series and have her practice it in the

evening before bed. Encourage her to slow the breath down to less than five breaths per minute while doing so and to become more aware of her breathing patterns in her daily life. Each inhale should be equal in length to the exhale. If possible, ask her to complete the *Ultradian Rhythm Cycle Chart* on page 83 for one day.

❏ Review Life Map and assess potential risk and necessity for sauna detoxification in future if chronically exposed to environmental estrogens or carcinogens.

❏ Ask any questions for the homeopathic differential diagnosis.

Prescribe:

❏ Lifestyle changes to improve the score on the *Breast Health Balance Sheet*.

❏ Daily breathing exercises; complete the *Ultradian Rhythm Cycle Chart* for one day.

❏ Complete *Daily Therapeutic Amounts of Vitamins and Minerals* form.

❏ Continue with BBT and *Diet Diary*.

❏ If low thyroid function is apparent, then consider DiagnosTech blood test for TSH, T4, T3, reverse T3 and antimicrosomal antibodies. Prescribe Thyroidinum 9CH once daily and/or other thyroid balancers (Unda 21 and 1000, Bladderwrack Combo, BMR Factors, iodine, selenium, zinc, tyrosine – what you prescribe depends on what parameters are off). If, over time, patient is unresponsive to these therapies, suggest desiccated thyroid from her medical doctor. Restore adrenal function if it is low as determined by the Koenigsburg test or physical exam findings. Balance progesterone with chaste tree berry, zinc, selenium, boron, B6, E and/or progesterone cream if it is low. Use Phonix detoxification remedies C-26, C-23, and C-6 to remove environmental chemicals that may be disrupting thyroid function.

❏ If fibrocystic breast disease, recommend supplements to help. Vitamin E, mixed tocopherols — 600 IU daily. Kelp tablets and/or iodine in one of the following forms: aqueous molecular diatomic iodine, 0.07 to 0.09 mg per kg of body weight daily for 6 months (preferred type of iodine but only available by prescription from a medical doctor); or Lugol's Solution (sodium iodide), 5 to 10 drops daily, depending on body weight. Evening primrose oil combined with twice as much flaxseed oil, 2–3 g daily. Vitamin B6, 50 mg, 3× daily with meals and a B complex. Coenzyme Q10, 60–200 mg daily. Chaste tree berry, 30 drops t.i.d. or progesterone cream, if indicated by low amounts of progesterone in saliva, 2 oz per month or 15–20 mg per day. Xiao Yao Wan, 8 pills, 3× daily and/or milk thistle and dandelion tincture, 25 drops, 3× daily for liver support. Dietary use of turmeric, soy, and rosemary.

❏ Assess necessity to do saliva tests for hormone levels and recommend the following if patient can afford it (all are recommended): estradiol, estrone and estriol and estrogen quotient; progesterone (particularly if PMS symptoms or history of fibrocystic breast disease); melatonin (particularly if depression or insomnia); C2 and C16 estrogens (available from DiagnosTech); IGF-1 (particularly if obesity, family history of diabetes or high carbohydrate/sugar diet); urinary phytoestrogens (not available yet).

Visit 3 (1 hour, 1–3 weeks later): Diet and Digestion

❏ Review how the patient is doing physically and emotionally and if she is having any difficulties with the program so far.

❏ Assess the *Ultradian Rhythm Chart* of the patient; if it is not normal, recommend breathing exercises or meditation at least twice daily. Help her to choose times that will work for her, with one of them being before bed.

❏ Go over the details of the *Healthy Breast Diet* and assess what is possible and helpful to this particular patient. Come up with compromises if they are unable to do pieces of it. Avoid being rigid but be firm.

❏ Assess whether there may be a deficiency of HCl (trouble digesting beans, bloating, undigested food in stool, low mineral absorption, constipation, weak nails, pH of urine >7.2). Test HCl using the gastrotest, available from HDC Corporation (tel. 408-954-1909 or fax. 408-954-0340) or HCl challenge as needed. Do oral zinc test.

❏ Explain how estrogen metabolism can be manipulated in a positive way through diet, exercise, and supplements, using the diagram How to Manage Your Estrogen in Appendix 1.

❏ Provide recipes or cookbook suggestions to patient.

❏ Assess bowel function. Keep track of number of bowel movements daily or weekly and adjust diet, supplements, or exercise to ensure at least two per day. Three is ideal.

❏ Assess pH balance through daily testing of a.m. urine and saliva or 24 hour urine for several weeks. Correct through acid/alkaline food chart. Recommend more potassium foods in particular if acid.

❏ Assess fiber intake and figure out what she needs to do to get 30 g per day.

❏ Assess fat intake and counsel regarding the protective fats (olive, flaxseed and pure fish oils) and how cooking practices and diet can be changed to utilize these. Restrict saturated and other unhealthy fats to less that 15% of calories or eliminate them altogether. Achieve a ratio of 2:1 Omega 3: Omega 6 oils. Include minimum of 2 tbsp of unheated flaxseed oil in diet daily. Assess the amount of Omega 6 oils she consumes through nuts, and seeds, vegetable oils or evening primrose oil and reduce these if necessary.

❏ Talk about water intake and water filters and recommend an affordable filter; for example, reverse osmosis or carbon block filter. Ensure that she drinks at least 1½ liters of water daily, up to 3 liters during chemotherapy and radiation.

❏ Assess mineral content of foods and suggest a hair analysis to reflect mineral status. Pay attention to toxic minerals and deficiencies of zinc, selenium, iodine, boron, magnesium, chromium, molybdenum, manganese. When hair analysis comes back, recommend ways to balance mineral status or remove toxic minerals.

Prescribe:

❏ Suggest homeopathic remedy based on constitution and location and quality of the tumor.

❏ Refer to a breast cancer support group or individual therapist. This will increase life expectancy and quality of life according to studies.

❏ If low HCl, supplement with a few drops of wormwood tincture or bitter foods before meals or mindfulness to increase HCl. Relax before eating and chew well. Consider enzymes.

Homework for the Patient:

❏ Continue making changes to incorporate *The Healthy Breast Diet*. Keep a *Diet Diary* for one week each month and bring this to your naturopathic doctor.

❏ Fill out the chart, *Dietary Tips for Breast Health* for two weeks and bring it to the next visit. Attempt to do more of it over time; don't expect to do it all at once.

❏ Keep monitoring thyroid function through the BBT chart.

Visit 4 (1 hour; 1–4 weeks later): Detoxification

❏ Review how patient is doing physically and emotionally, and question if she is having any difficulties with the program. Praise her for everything she has managed to do; acknowledge how difficult it is.

❏ Educate the patient in the body's methods of detoxification. Show pictures of liver, bowel, and kidneys.

❏ Review what she has been doing so far to detoxify: liver formula, increased fiber, blood cleansing herbs, water.

❏ Review the protocol for sauna detoxification and talk about what would be realistic for the patient. Create a plan for sauna detoxification aiming for 100 hours of sauna time. Consider measuring DDE and PCB levels in blood or fat before and after sauna detoxification.

❏ Educate patient about homeopathic detoxification and recommend a 45–180-day detox program using Phonix C-23 (liver), C-26 (kidney), and C-3 (lymph). These were found to decrease PCPs about 78% in 2 months. For the first 3 days, use Phonix C-23, 3 times per day, 20–60 drops after a meal, then stop. For the next 3 days, use Phonix C-26, 3 times per day 20–60 drops after a meal, then stop. For the next 3 days, use Phonix C-3, 3 times per day, 20 drops after a meal. Continue cycling them like this for 45–180 days. Use the longer time with cancer patients.

❏ Review the need for and use of enemas and judge whether in your opinion this patient would benefit from coffee enemas or other enemas and decide upon a frequency schedule; if not using enemas, ensure that she is having at least two bowel movements daily and is taking a herbal fiber supplement which may include bentonite.

❏ Assess whether yeast and parasites may be a problem for this patient, and if so, suggest a cleanse for a limited amount of time, following strategies in the book to do so if necessary. Consider recommending a yeast and parasite cleanse once or twice a year for three months as a matter of course, using your clinical judgement. Consider a comprehensive digestive stool analysis and parasitology with Great Smokies Diagnostic Laboratory if digestive symptoms are present.

❏ Review the patient's supplements; any questions or concerns.

Prescribe:

❏ Possible supplementation with probiotics and FOS, the use of the gemmotherapies Juniperus and Rosmarinus for improved liver drainage and repair, antiparasitic and antifungal formulas.

❏ Implement a sauna detoxification program and/or enemas if they were recommended.

❏ Implement a homeopathic detoxification program

❏ Implement a yeast/parasite cleanse if it was recommended.

❏ Keep a diet diary for one week and bring it to the next visit.

Visit 5 (1 hour, 2 to 4 weeks later): Lymphatics

❏ Review diet diary and suggest changes.

❏ Review patient's ability to practice the breathing exercises or meditation. Suggest a class if she is having difficulty. Recommend her to a relaxation/visualization/meditation program.

❏ Ask about how the patient is feeling physically and emotionally

❏ Monitor progress during the sauna detox, homeopathic detox, and the intestinal cleansing.

❏ Educate patient about the function of the lymphatic system and the importance of regular exercise and deep breathing.

❏ Assess how much aerobic exercise the patient does weekly, outside of normal activity. Impress upon her that what is needed is 4 hours of exercise weekly or 35 minutes a day. This will decrease breast cancer risk 30–60% and improve estrogen metabolism. Help the patient set up an aerobic exercise program that will be enjoyable and which she can maintain for life. It may be walking, rebounding, cycling, a fitness class, dancing, jogging, etc. Consider asking patient to fill out a 2-week exercise log.

❏ Talk about the value of rebounding for improved lymphatic circulation and breast health. If possible, demonstrate the rebounding exercises from the *Ultimate Rebounding Workout* or suggest she practice with the video. Recommend a rebounding and yoga program.

❏ Discuss the importance of wearing a bra that it is not too restrictive. After removing one's bra, there should be no red marks from increased pressure. This will impede lymphatic circulation.

❏ Review with the patient the methodology of skin brushing and contrast showers and encourage her to practice them daily. Demonstrate how to use a skin brush.

❏ Recommend use of Healthy Breast Oil 3 or more times weekly.

Homework for the Patient:

❏ Begin a daily exercise program that can be maintained for life, exercising at least 4 hours weekly. Keep a two week exercise log and bring it to the next visit.

❏ Begin rebounding daily for whatever length of time you can sustain, increasing it to at least 15 minutes daily over time.

❏ Purchase a bra that is not restrictive.

❏ Integrate skin brushing and contrast showers into your daily routine.

❏ Keep a diet diary for one week.

❏ Begin using Healthy Breast Oil or essential oils of lavender, juniper, rosemary, frankincense, lemon.

Visit 6 (1 hour, 2 to 4 weeks later): Immune System and Traditional Chinese Medicine

❏ Assess diet, breathing practice, exercise, sauna detoxification, review supplements.

❏ Ask patient to draw a large outline of her body. Review the components of the immune system one at a time and ask her to draw them on the picture (thymus gland, spleen, bone marrow, hypothalamus, pituitary, macrophages, T-helper cells, T-killer cells, T-suppressor cells, Kupffer cells, etc.) Read the statements in the book about each of these and do the arm movements or make up arm movements for them while repeating the phrase. Then draw each one in the picture. The various types of white blood cells can be drawn along the side. Explore with the patient how she can use imagery to make these immune system components work better. The imagery should involve as many senses as possible and use cues from her everyday environment. Help the patient find a metaphor for her T-helper cells and her T-killer cells that is personal yet powerful. Include in the drawing symbols for the

supplements she is taking that energize her immune system. Work out guidelines for a script for the patient to use in a regular visualization. Include references to the supplements she is using in the script. For homework, ask the patient to write out her script and make her own visualization tape, using the one in the book as a reference. Listen to the tape daily.

❏ Assess pulse, tongue and history and evaluate patterns of disharmony according to TCM. Recommend any additional herbal formulas or acupuncture to correct patterns of disharmony. If on chemo or radiation, recommend tonics — e.g., royal jelly and ganoderma, caulis millettia tablets, astragalus/oldenlandria tea. Create a plan for acupuncture treatments or refer to a TCM practitioner for a series of treatments. You may also recommend regular classes in Qiqong or yoga.

Homework for the Patient:

❏ Write out a visualization script and make a visualization tape and bring them to the next visit.

❏ Begin treatments in acupuncture, Qiqong and/or yoga, if recommended.

Visit 7 (1 hour, 2 to 4 weeks later; may take several visits): Emotional Issues

❏ Review the visualization script and suggest any changes that might improve it. Ask what her response has been to listening to the tape. Ask her what cues she can place in her environment to remind her of her own innate capacity to heal and of the strength of her immune system. This may include pictures on the wall, affirmations, plants, photographs, places she visits, healing foods, token objects to touch, massage oil, music or specific sounds, smells, essential oils.

❏ Explore issues around family, nurturing, abandonment, guilt, loss, sexuality, separation, intimacy to uncover any buried emotions that may be connected to the appearance of the tumor or to her breasts in general. Explore ways to heal any of these, perhaps referring to a therapist or bodyworker.

❏ Assess whether the patient feels trapped in an unhappy situation with no way out. Suggest counseling sessions so that she can seek resolution, discover unrecognized options, and be supported through psychological change. Women in either group or individual therapy have a longer life expectancy and better quality of life than control groups.

❏ Review the chart *Limiting Beliefs / Healthy Beliefs* and examine which of the limiting beliefs feel true to the patient. Have her read the healthy belief to replace it. Read the healthy belief back to the patient, using the word "you" and ask her how it feels to receive that statement. Ask her for examples of how in her life she displays the limiting belief and how her thoughts and actions would be different if she lived the healthy beliefs. Have her write out the healthy beliefs she needs as affirmations and repeat them 3× daily, out loud, in front of a mirror for 40 days. Suggest that she take risks to act out the healthy beliefs.

❏ Examine issues of buried anger with the patient and help her to bring these out and allow safe expression of them. Encourage a process (it may take several months) of moving from anger to forgiveness. This may require referral to a therapist.

❏ Assess whether this patient is able to act assertively or not. If not, review the assertive model and encourage her to use this model at least three times before the next visit.

❏ Consider homeopathic remedies or flower essences to help the patient on the emotional level.

Homework for the Patient:

❏ Redo visualization tape if necessary, listen to it one or more times daily. Place cues in your environment to remind you of your innate capacity to heal.

❏ Create a plan to improve your emotional well-being, working with the above issues with your naturopathic doctor, therapist or bodyworker.

❏ Read your healthy beliefs out loud while looking in the mirror, at least three times daily for forty days. Begin to take risks to act on the healthy beliefs.

❏ Acknowledge anger, express it, identify steps to resolve it and move to forgiveness with assistance from someone skilled in helping with this process.

❏ Act assertively at least three times before your next visit.

Visit 8 (1 hour, 2 to 4 weeks later; may take several visits): Meaning Mandala

❏ Review with patient how she is changing emotionally. Discuss her attempts to act assertively and the outcome of these attempts. Role-play with her, allowing her to act assertively with you in a particular situation that is difficult for her.

❏ Review the healthy beliefs, and how much closer she feels she has moved to accepting them.

❏ Ask her to write out a list of the things that bring her the most joy, through both 'being' and 'doing' states.

❏ Ask her to write out another list of her gifts, talents, and capabilities.

❏ Ask her to write out a third list of the things about which she feels the most passionate, that contribute to the meaning in her life and give her a sense of purpose and fulfillment. This will include both 'things to do' and 'ways of being'. (These may be given as homework the previous visit)

❏ From looking at these three lists, guide her in writing out a *Destiny Statement*. The first part of the statement will describe her most important qualities, the second part will describe her direction. Have her write the destiny statement out on a card and read it to herself daily. Read it back to her and ask her how it feels to receive it.

❏ Ask the patient to make yet another list of the things that need 'letting go' in her life. Included in this list are specific limiting beliefs, relationships, addictions, guilt, social obligations, expectations, negative emotions and anything else she can think of. Over time, check in to see what progress is being made with this list. Ask her to focus on one at a time for several weeks.

❏ Give the patient a large piece of paper with markers and other colored materials and have magazines and scissors and glue available to cut out and paste pictures. Show her the diagram for the meaning mandala and have her begin to make her own, first with words, then with drawings or cut out pictures. Have her finish it at home or in the next visit. Suggest that she put the meaning mandala up on a wall where she can see it while she does her rebounding. Ask her to bring the mandala back in the future (at least every 3 months) and keep encouraging her to act in the areas her energy wants to move.

❏ Review the types of prayer and explore whether this patient might find a practice of prayer acceptable or beneficial. If so, encourage her to find or to create prayers that resonate with her belief system.

Homework for the Patient:

❏ Complete a *Meaning Mandala* and hang it where you can see it regularly. Seek to actualize more of the meaning mandala each month, with organized action steps.

❏ Find a form of prayer that works for you and integrate it into your life.

❏ Read your destiny statement to yourself daily.

Guidelines for Follow-Up Visits:

❏ Ask that your patient complete a *Diet Diary* for one week each month and review it at least once every three months.

❏ Perform a clinical breast exam on your patient twice yearly and request that she bring in her *Breast Map* to these visits.

❏ Perform a hair analysis annually.

❏ Check saliva and thyroid hormone levels annually for a few years, then less often if they are stable.

❏ Keep coming back to the *Meaning Mandala* in follow-up visits

❏ After the first year, if the patient is stable in the program, schedule visits every 3 months or so.

❏ Assess whether a yeast and parasite cleanse may be beneficial for three months once or twice yearly.

❏ After the initial sauna detoxification is complete, recommend a weekly sauna and do the homeopathic detox annually for 45 days or longer.

❏ Let your patient know about Rachel Carson Day and about ways in which she can contribute to environmental reform.

❏ Link up to other women following *The Healthy Breast Program* through the support group directory listed on the web site: www.healthybreastprogram.on.ca and help set up new support groups.

❏ Continue following the program, adjusting the supplements annually.

Actions for Prevention Summary

Chapter 1 — *What Are Your Risk Factors for Developing Breast Cancer?*

Mother or Sister with Breast Cancer

Avoiding the other risk factors wherever possible, actively participating in environmental reform, strengthening immunity, and adopting a health-promoting lifestyle can prevent breast cancer, even when the genetic predisposition exists.

Female Relatives with Ovarian or Endometrial Cancer

Follow The Healthy Breast Program when you are at higher risk because of relatives with ovarian, endometrial, or prostate cancer.

Waist-to-Hip Ratio

Follow the dietary guidelines of The Healthy Breast Program.

Having Children Early

Have children before age 30 and closer to age 20 if possible. It will decrease your breast cancer risk and be healthier for your children. The younger you are when you conceive, the less vulnerable your breasts will be and the lighter will be the toxic load you pass on to your children through breast milk.

Breast-Feeding

Adopt a chemical free lifestyle (including avoiding animal fat) as early as possible in life and cleanse the body before conceiving. Detoxify weekly and annually with saunas, homeopathic preparations, and liver and bowel cleansers. Breast-feed your children for at least six months.

Age

Take antioxidants regularly or get them from your food to slow down the aging process and to protect your DNA from damage.

Exercise

Regular exercise (four hours weekly) is part of a prevention program. We can encourage our daughters to develop a regular exercise program before puberty (age 10 onward) that they can maintain for life.

Prescription Drugs

Find a practitioner who uses natural substances such as herbal, nutritional, and homeopathic formulas and alter your diet and lifestyle to deal with health ailments. Use pharmaceutical drugs only if your symptoms cannot be controlled through natural means. Educate yourself on the side effects of prescription drugs and herbal remedies before you take them.

Dental Problems

Take care of your teeth, brushing and flossing regularly. Visit a dentist who does not use mercury amalgam fillings and who can test for low grade infections that may not show up on an x-ray. Try to avoid root canals.

Immune Deficiency and Allergies

If your immune system is weakened, follow an immune-strengthening program using herbs, diet, and nutrients.

Constipation

Drink 8–10 glasses of water daily, use wheat bran, flaxseeds, and 6–9 servings of fruits and vegetables daily to up your fiber content and encourage more regular bowel movements. Exercise four hours weekly and practice rebounding daily

Monthly Breast Self-Exams

Perform monthly breast self-exams, map your breast topography and keep a written record of your findings to stay in touch with your breasts. Teach your daughters to do the same.

Cigarette Smoking

Stop smoking and avoid second-hand smoke. Consult an acupuncturist, naturopathic doctor, or self-help group to help you stop smoking.

Hair Dyes

Avoid hair dyes containing carcinogenic substances. Use henna or natural dyes instead.

Breast Implants

Avoid breast implants and consider surgical removal if you already have them.

Wearing a Bra

Don't wear a bra unless you have to; take it off as soon as you are able to; use a cotton stretchy bra without under-wires if you can.

Chapter 2 — *Getting to Know Your Breasts*

Breast Self-Examination (BSE) Exercise

Become an expert at performing monthly breast self-exams. Take time to explore and befriend your breasts at least once weekly.

Fibrocystic Breast Disease

1) Decrease your exposure to environmental estrogens.
2) Reduce unhealthy dietary fats to less than 15% of total calories, but do use flaxseed oil and olive oil.
3) Increase consumption of fresh fruits and vegetables, fiber, and phytoestrogens; decrease or eliminate meat.
4) Eliminate methylxanthines found in coffee, black tea, and chocolate.
5) Drink 8 or more glasses of water daily to promote bowel movements and elimination.
6) Assist liver function with herbs and nutritional supplements.
7) Correct thyroid function and iodine deficiency.
8) Normalize estrogen to progesterone ratios; and estrone to estriol levels.
9) Achieve appropriate weight and reduce body fat to 20–22%; maintain a regular exercise program.
10) Correct essential fatty acid deficiency with a 2:1 Omega 3: Omega 6 ratio.
11) Correct deficiencies of vitamin E, B6 and coenzyme Q10.

The AMAS Blood Test (Antimalignin Antibody in Serum)

Consider having the AMAS or the Immunicon test done annually if you are under 50. If you are over 50, also consider the AMAS test annually, as it can pick up the presence of any cancer when it is only 1 mm large, which is more sensitive than a mammogram. If a positive result comes back, then have a mammogram to determine where the cancer might be.

Thermography

If you are under 50, have annual thermography screening with the AMAS test. If you are over 50, consider a yearly mammogram along with the above two tests.

Mammography

If you are under 50, have a mammogram only as needed for diagnosis of a suspected lump. Use the AMAS or Immunicon test annually. If you are over 50, have an annual mammogram, or as another option, use the AMAS or Immunicon test and thermography on alternate years instead of a mammogram.

Ultrasound

Use an ultrasound to confirm the presence of a cyst, and if a cyst is not present, choose one or more of the other tests to rule out breast cancer.

Fine Needle Aspiration

Use fine needle aspiration when appropriate as a diagnostic tool for breast cysts that may have a cancerous component.

Biopsy

Use a core or open surgical biopsy to confirm or rule out breast cancer if other tests are inconclusive.

Other Predictive Tests

Consider carrying out some of the above tests annually to detect your susceptibility to breast cancer. Make appropriate changes in your diet, lifestyle or supplement schedule to move towards more favorable values, thus protecting you from a breast cancer diagnosis.

Homeopathic Remedies

Use appropriate homeopathic remedies for breast ailments, while keeping the whole person in mind.

Chapter 3 — *Understanding the Hormone Puzzle*

Estrogen's Impostors

We can look at this piece of the hormone puzzle and help protect ourselves from breast cancer by:

1) Decreasing our exposure to the xenoestrogens and carcinogens in general. We must become active in fighting the production and use of these chemicals, and remove them from our homes and environments.

2) Increasing the phytoestrogens and other protective foods in our diets.

3) Strengthening immunity using vitamins, minerals, herbs, and nutritional substances as well as through psychological and spiritual growth.

4) Increasing our own melatonin levels through a meditation or visualization practice.

5) Enhancing the body's detoxification ability through improving liver function.

6) Improving elimination through the colon and skin (saunas) to decrease our load of "in house" estrogens, environmental estrogens, and toxins.

Breakdown of Estrogen

When we examine this piece of the estrogen puzzle, we see that we can increase our protection from breast cancer by consuming raw foods from the brassica family, along with sea vegetables, avoiding xenoestrogens, and assisting the liver to detoxify.

Elimination of Estrogen

Looking at this piece of the estrogen puzzle we are able to decrease our risk of breast cancer by avoiding meat and saturated fat, consuming a high fiber vegetarian diet with the addition of wheat bran, psyllium, legumes, and flaxseeds, and ensuring that we have two or more bowel movements daily. From an understanding of estrogen metabolism (see Appendix 1: How to Manage Your Estrogen) we can recognize that there is much we can do to prevent breast cancer. We can become proactive in protecting our breasts.

Estrogen Quotient

Check your ratio of C2 estrogen to C16 estrogen and your sex hormone profile yearly through a saliva or urine test to evaluate your balance of estrogens and risk of breast cancer. This can be used as a routine annual test to assess women at risk for breast cancer, followed by work at prevention with diet changes and nutrient supplementation.

Early Onset of Menstruation, Late Menopause

Do not consume animal products while pregnant or breast-feeding. Do what you can to stall puberty in your daughters by keeping lights out at night, eating organic food, eliminating or drastically reducing animal products in their diets, giving them flaxseed oil regularly while limiting other fats, and protecting them from environmental exposure to estrogen-mimicking chemicals. Become aware of and fight the use of these chemicals. This is the call to arms, the call to women. We must protect the fertility of ourselves, other species, and the earth.

Shorter Menstrual Cycles

Consult a practitioner of Traditional Chinese Medicine, a naturopath, herbalist, or homeopath to help you regulate your periods. Decrease your breasts' ability to absorb estradiol by eating plants rich in phytoestrogens, which bind to breast cell receptors and prevent estradiol, estrogen replacement therapy and organochlorine estrogen-mimickers from entering the breast cell where they could promote cancer. These plants include tofu and soy products, flaxseeds, lentils, dried beans and their sprouts, pumpkin seeds, and herbs such as red clover, licorice root, turmeric, and fenugreek.

Birth Control Pills

Do not use the birth control pill for longer than five years or before the age of 20; preferably, avoid it altogether. Investigate other methods of birth control such as the Justisse method, and the use of condoms and the diaphragm.

Hormone Replacement Therapy

Maintain your calcium status from age 35 onward, ensuring 800–2000 mg daily depending on age, pregnancy and breast-feeding. Consult Dr Gaby's book, *Preventing and Reversing Osteoporosis*, and Dr John Lee's book, *What Your Doctor May Not Tell You About Menopause*, for alternatives to estrogen replacement therapy in reversing osteoporosis. If you are at high risk for heart disease, adopt the dietary guidelines in this book and supplement with vitamin E, magnesium, coenzyme Q10, and grapeseed. Consult a naturopathic doctor for a full program in reducing risk for heart disease and in dealing with menopausal symptoms. Consider the use of Chinese or Western herbal formulas and natural progesterone cream for menopausal symptoms. Avoid hormone replacement therapy except as a last resort and continue it for less than five years. Make sure your hormone replacement therapy contains estriol to offset the tumor enhancing effects of estradiol and estrone, as outlined in Dr Gaby's book, as well as natural progesterone cream, as described by Dr Lee. Increase your estriol levels naturally with the inclusion of sea vegetables (for iodine), flaxseeds, soy products, and other phytoestrogens.

Fertility Drugs

Before you intend to conceive, detoxify your liver, colon, and whole body using the methods outlined in the Healthy Breast Program or other detoxification regimes. Avoid all stimulants, including coffee, and follow an organic vegetarian diet for three months. Before you resort to fertility drugs to become pregnant, consult with a practitioner of Traditional Chinese Medicine or a naturopathic doctor. There are many natural ways to increase fertility without putting yourself at risk.

Pregnancy

If you are pregnant, take stock of your environment. Learn whether there are industries, farms, toxic waste sites, plastic recycling plants, or sewage treatment plants around you that are releasing organochlorines, dioxin, furans, pesticides, formaldehyde etc., or if these are in your water supply. If possible, for the first four months of your pregnancy, move to a less polluted area. Filter your water using a reverse osmosis or charcoal filter. Avoid animal products and fish. Don't overdo it on the phytoestrogens during pregnancy, which the diet in this book recommends to prevent breast cancer; instead, eat more beans and nuts and less tofu. Use more almond milk and less soy milk during pregnancy and breast-feeding.

High Estrogen Levels During Pregnancy

Avoid using, ingesting, or inhaling all chemicals while pregnant. Eat organic food and avoid animal protein while pregnant, including milk. If you are not breast-feeding your child, or are supplementing breast milk, be cautious about only using soy-based formulas because of their possible hormonal action. Use almond milk and organic goat milk as alternatives. Drink filtered water and attach a filter to your shower.

Reducing Estrogen Production to Protect Our Breasts

1) Rid our bodies of environmental chemicals before we conceive through the intensive use of saunas, homeopathic formulas, and a liver and bowel detoxification program so that we do not pass on our accumulated load of environmental estrogens to our children.

2) Stall puberty in girls by encouraging athletic activity, utilizing diets high in phytoestrogens such as soy and flaxseeds (in Japan, girls reach puberty at age 14–17), limiting their consumption of meat and fat to minimize estrogen intake and re-absorption from the intestines, decreasing exposure to environmental estrogens or "xenoestrogens", increasing elimination of xenoestrogens through improving liver function and the regular use of saunas. Decrease exposure to light and electromagnetic fields at night to increase melatonin production. Prevent obesity in our daughters, since puberty is partially triggered when a certain level of fat is present in a young girl's body.

3) Encourage higher circulating amounts of estriol and lower amounts of estradiol through vegetarian diets high in phytoestrogens, fiber, and the brassica family (cabbage, broccoli, Brussels sprouts, cauliflower, kale, sea vegetables, etc.) and through normalizing or improving thyroid and liver function.

4) Decrease dietary fats with the exception of flaxseed oil, extra virgin olive oil and uncontaminated cold water fish oils and encourage women to watch their weight, particularly after menopause.

Low Progesterone

When you are pregnant for the first time, realize that you will decrease your breast cancer risk by having the child rather than terminating the pregnancy. If you have premenstrual breast tenderness, fibrocystic breast disease, or breast cancer, have your progesterone levels checked through a salivary hormone test. If it is low, take vitamins B6 and E and increase your foods or supplements containing zinc, boron, and selenium. Evaluate mineral status yearly using hair analysis. Increase soy foods. Consider using one or more of the progesterone-enhancing herbs and work with a practitioner familiar with their use. Use the natural progesterone cream only if the other therapies are unsuccessful at raising progesterone, as the cream is not curative – it only supplies you with progesterone for its duration of use.

High Prolactin

Screening for prolactin levels may show susceptibility to breast cancer. Normalize thyroid function to lower prolactin. Avoid dairy.

Increased Growth Hormone

Ban the use of growth hormone in agricultural practice and keep your children away from dairy products.

Thyroid Function

Check your thyroid function annually with a temperature test, If it is low, follow-up with a blood test that measures TSH, T4, T3, reverse T3, and thyroid autoantibodies. If it is underactive, consume sea vegetables, use kelp and dulse powder as seasonings on your food, and regularly use bladderwrack, bee pollen, spirulina or chlorella algae, wheatgrass, oats, watercress, saw palmetto berries, damiana, guggul, and/or globe artichoke. Ensure adequate intake of iodine, selenium, zinc, and flaxseed oil. Make sure your progesterone and adrenal hormone levels are normal. Massage coconut oil into the soles of your feet nightly. Detoxify annually following the guidelines in this book or using other methods to remove hormone-disrupting chemicals. Work with a naturopathic doctor and a medical doctor to normalize any thyroid dysfunction. Establish routine sauna use. Actively participate in reducing environmental damage due to chemicals through the choices you make as a consumer and through activism. This is a critical time. We are all needed to work together in restoring the earth.

High Insulin Levels

Keep your insulin levels low by avoiding sweets, alcohol, refined carbohydrates, and saturated fats. Exercise regularly. Decrease insulin resistance with the use of chromium, alpha lipoic acid, and flaxseed oil. Eat foods with a low glycemic index.

High Insulin-like Growth Factors-1 and 2 (IGF-1 and IGF-2) Levels

Have your saliva or serum levels of IGF-1 and 2 checked annually and adopt a diet using carbohydrates with a lower glycemic index. These include most beans, barley, the Brassica family, green beans, tomatoes, sea vegetables, powdered greens, cherries, plums, grapefruit, peaches, apples, and pears. Include flaxseed oil and chromium in your diet or supplement schedule. Avoid sweets. Eliminate or drastically reduce saturated fat. Aim for a 2:1 ratio of Omega 3 to Omega 6 fatty acids.

Decreased Melatonin

There are ways to take care of the pineal gland and melatonin production through lifestyle practices, diet, and herbal and nutritional supplementation. The way many of us live is geared to upset pineal function and we should attempt to balance our lifestyle before resorting to any "quick fix". Here are guidelines for taking care of your pineal gland:

1) Avoid shift work. It confuses your body's rhythms and will interfere with melatonin production.

2) Spend at least 20 minutes outside in natural light (without sunglasses) in the early part of the day. This may help melatonin levels to be higher at night.[139]

3) Sleep in a dark room, with no light shining in from the street. Melatonin production is lower when we are exposed to light at night. Low intensity light (50 lux) is acceptable but levels of 500 lux or higher suppress melatonin release. If need be, wear a mask over your eyes as you sleep.

4) Keep regular hours, preferably going to bed early and getting up early.

5) Avoid excessive exposure to electromagnetic radiation, which interferes with melatonin production. Do not sleep within three feet of an electrical outlet or device.

6) Exercise regularly. One hour daily on a stationary bicycle can double or triple melatonin levels.[140]

7) Ensure adequate consumption of foods high in tryptophan or melatonin, along with vitamins B3, B6, calcium, magnesium, zinc, and NAC or foods containing cystine (see chapter seven). Consider supplementation with 5-HTP or St. John's wort.

8) Avoid the other factors which interfere with pineal function — alcohol, caffeine, recreational drugs, nicotine, intense electromagnetic fields, bright lights and medications such as beta-blockers, diazepam, haloperidol, chlorpromazine, and ibuprofen.

9) Practice a meditative or breathing exercise one or more times daily, particularly before bed.

10) If you have breast cancer, especially if it is estrogen receptor positive, consider supplementing with 5–20 mg of melatonin one half hour before bedtime (8:00–10:00 p.m.) with medical supervision. If you are at high risk for breast cancer, use 3–9 mg of melatonin nightly as prevention.

11) Monitor melatonin levels annually through saliva testing. (DiagnosTech International Inc. or Aeron Labs).

Kundalini Yoga Exercises for Balancing the Pineal Gland

Practice the Alternate Nostril Series or Kundalini Exercises for activating melatonin at least once daily, one hour before bedtime. If you are able to, practice it at another time in the day as well, perhaps upon rising. If you have breast cancer, practice this or other breathing or meditative exercises up to five times daily at two-hour intervals to increase melatonin levels and normalize cell division. Combine these breathing breaks with the practice of visualization and prayer.

Chapter 4 — *Environmental Impact on Breast Health*

X-rays and Mammograms

We can insist that government and industry develop safe, renewable energy sources such as wind and solar power. We can reduce our energy consumption by building more energy-conserving homes and using fewer electrical devices. We can install our own wind and solar powered units wherever possible or buy power from those people who have done it for us. We can join a movement to ban all nuclear power and weapons testing, such as the Campaign for Nuclear Phaseout in Ottawa (tel. 613-789-3634). We can write to our politicians and object to the burning of plutonium fuel bundles at electrical generation sites such as the Bruce nuclear station on the shores of Lake Huron in southern Ontario.

Generally, pre-menopausal women should avoid mammograms unless a lump is present and breast cancer is suspected. A woman over age 50 with high risk factors should consider having a mammogram every one to two years but also listen to her intuition and her body's signals. Thermography, the AMAS or Immunicon blood test, and the other diagnostic procedures described in Chapter 2 are useful alternatives to detect early cancers and pose no risk. We can protect ourselves somewhat from radiation by including the following foods in our diets: broccoli, cabbage, miso, vegetables high in carotenes (squash, carrots, yams, cantaloupe), burdock root, Reishi mushrooms, seaweed, lentils and other dried beans, and the trace mineral selenium (found in nettles, astragalus, kelp, burdock, and milk thistle seeds).[20]

Electricity and Electromagnetic Fields

We can protect ourselves and our children by removing sources of extra low voltage electromagnetic fields from the bedroom, by moving our beds at least 2 1/2 feet away from electrical outlets, and by minimizing our proximity to them during the day. We and our children can stay the required distance from computer video display terminals (2 feet from the front; 4 feet from the sides), and minimize their use while pregnant (less than 20 hours per week). We can use less electricity and fewer of the modern electrical conveniences to conserve energy globally, decreasing our participation in the nuclear industry. (What can you live without? The dishwasher, the dryer, or the TV?) Turn off all electrical appliances when not in use. Buy a wind-up watch rather than one with a quartz crystal or battery — they too emit electromagnetic energy. Buy or rent a gauss meter and measure the electro-magnetic field emissions around your home. Keep work areas away from the place where electricity enters your home. Limit your use of cordless and cell phones to emergencies and brief conversations.

Petrochemicals, Chlorinated Chemicals, and Formaldehyde

We can become aware of the products that contain form-aldehyde and get them out of our homes as well as refrain from putting them on our bodies. Limit your exposure to petrochemicals, and insist that chlorine not be added to your fuel. Use your car less often, relying on public transportation, your bicycle, or your legs more often. Move your residence closer to your workplace or move more of your work into your home office.

Pesticides

Buy organic food and/or grow your own food if possible. Find a way to establish a community garden or green-house with like-minded people. Connect with local organic growers. Plant fruit and nut trees on your property. Peel your fruits and vegetables, especially if they have been waxed, or wash them with a vegetable wash or diluted vinegar to remove surface pesticide residues.

If you can't buy all organic food, the foods that contain the most pesticide residues in decreasing order among Canadian grown varieties, for example, are celery, carrots, apples, head lettuce, sweet peppers, fresh beans, leaf lettuce, strawberries, and blueberries. Imported foods highest in pesticide residues are red, bell, and green peppers, oranges, strawberries, spinach, green beans, grapes, head lettuce, pears, apples, tomatoes, cherries, peaches, Mexican cantaloupes, celery, apricots, and cucumbers. You can try to buy these organically grown, grow them yourself, or avoid them. To find out more about what pesticides and herbicides are in your foods and which foods are safest, view the web site: www.food-news.org. To help you to grow organic food, visit the web site: www.organic-growers.com.

Talk or write to your local, provincial and municipal governments about banning pesticide use in public parks, playgrounds, and golf courses. Call your airline and request that they not spray the airplane with pesticides before takeoff, which most of them do. About 20 towns and villages, all in Quebec, have passed bylaws restricting pesticide spraying on private and public green spaces. The town of Hudson, Quebec, (population 5,000) takes 10–12 companies to court each year for illegal spraying. Its bylaw against pesticides was passed eight years ago.[54] We can learn from this small town and push for a moratorium on pesticide use in our own cities. It is much easier to win the battle against pesticides on the municipal level rather than the federal level, so start there. We can accomplish what Hudson has in our own communities.

Educate people about the hazards to children from pesticide use. If you are a medical doctor, call the Environmental Health Committee of the Ontario College of Family Physicians at (416) 867-9646 and request a copy of Pesticides and Human Health. Pass it on to your patients. Contact the World Wildlife Fund Canada (tel. 416-489-8800 or 800-26-PANDA, or fax. 416-489-3611) and ask for a number of free copies of "Reducing Your Risk from Pesticides" and circulate these among friends, neighbors, grocery stores, farmers, businesses, schools, hospitals, etc. For more information on pesticides and alternatives to pesticides, contact the Northwest Coalition for Alternatives to Pesticides in Eugene, OR (tel. 541-344-5044, fax. 541-344-6923, E-mail: info@pesticide.org, and web site: www.efn.org/~ncap/). They publish the quarterly Journal of Pesticide Reform and supply fact sheets on pesticides and their alternatives.

Alternatives to PVC

Avoid using PVC and plastics in general. PVC can be identified by a number 3 in the recycling symbol. If you are a retailer, you can choose not to stock PVC plastics and label your store PVC free — have a fact sheet available to consumers so they too can make healthy choices. As a consumer, encourage your retailers to phase out PVC; IKEA and The Body Shop have stopped selling products containing PVC. Make appointments with store managers and educate them about PVC. Discard your PVC blinds and any other sources you can change. Design and build a PVC free house. Talk to builders and carpenters about the health and environmental hazards of PVC. Do not buy plastic children's toys and call your credit card company to ask them to make the cards out of something other than PVC.

Bio-based polymers are made of natural raw materials, such as wood, cotton, horn or hardened protein, and raw rubber. One example is Biopol, made from chemicals produced by bacteria that have been fed sugar. These products degrade easily and can be composted. We need to investigate and develop their large-scale use.

Ask your supplement manufacturers to package your vitamins and herbs in glass rather than plastic bottles. Choose manufacturers that use glass. PVC is not part of a sustainable future for life on earth.

Dioxins

If there is a hospital near you, inquire as to whether its incinerator burns PVC plastic. Start or join a campaign to ban the production and incineration of PVC and chlorine based chemicals. Buy unbleached, chlorine-free paper products and ask your stores and photocopy shops to stock them for you. If there is a PVC manufacturer in your area, find out how much dioxin is released annually, and protest to local, provincial, state, and federal officials. Although the number 3 in the recycling symbol can often identify PVC, not all plastics are labeled, making it difficult to know which ones contain PVC. Companies consider their formulas trade secrets and are not required to disclose whether they contain PVC or not. We can insist to government, retailers, and the plastic companies that they label their products "PVC free" or "Contains PVC" so that we can exercise our right to choose. Until then, refrain from buying plastics. Eliminate or limit your consumption of meat, fish, and dairy to reduce dioxin exposure.

Phthalates

For the sake of your children and future generations, avoid phthalates, which are added to PVC toys and are linked to cancer, kidney damage, and may interfere with your children's ability to reproduce. Urge your retailers not to sell PVC toys and pressure your municipal, provincial, state, and federal governments to ban the use of PVC plastic. Urge your daycares and schools to eliminate PVC and plastic toys in general. Tell your friends and relatives not to buy plastic toys for your children. Put pressure on toy manufacturing companies like Mattel, Hasbro, Playskool, Safety 1st, Gerber, and Disney to stop using PVC in their products. Explain to your children the hazards in their plastic toys in a way they can understand, and then discard them, replacing them with wood, cloth, or other natural fibers.

Buy oils or fatty foods in glass rather than plastic containers. Use waxed paper or butcher paper to wrap sandwiches and other foods in, and especially do not microwave food in plastic containers or plastic wrap. Use ceramic or glass containers instead.

Bisphenol-A

If you consume canned foods, call the manufacturer to ask whether bisphenol-A is used to line the can. If yes, express your concern about its capacity as a hormone disruptor and its impact on breast cancer. Stop using the cans. Buy food in glass jars or cans without the liners. Call the toll free numbers on the food packaging you buy and ask whether there are PVC, phthalates, nonylphenol ethoxylates, or bisphenol-A in any of it.

If your dentist suggests a new plastic coating for your children's teeth, ask her if she can guarantee in writing that it contains no bisphenol-A or other hormone disrupting chemical. Whenever possible, ask your dentist to use ceramic fillings on your teeth, and pressure the dental industry to test all their filling materials for estrogenic or carcinogenic activity before experimenting with them on children and the general public. Insist on mandatory release of names of ingredients used in dental fillings before you allow them into your mouth.

Contact the World Wildlife Fund (tel. 416-489-8800 or 800-26-PANDA or fax. 416-489-3611) and ask for a number of free copies of "Reducing Your Risk: A Guide to Avoiding Hormone-Disrupting Chemicals" and circulate these among friends, neighbors, businesses, schools, hospitals, etc.

Nonylphenol Ethoxylates

Use glass, ceramic, or stainless steel in containers for foods and beverages. Take cotton or hemp bags or cardboard boxes to the supermarket to load your groceries. Choose not to buy plastic packaging or containers. Call the companies whose products you buy and ask them to switch to non-toxic containers. Avoid industrial or super-strength cleansers. Use environmentally friendly soaps such as those made by Nature Clean or create your own cleansers. You can also often buy ecological cleansers in bulk at health food stores, recycling a glass or cardboard container.

PCBs (Polychlorinated Biphenyls)

Avoid animal products, particularly if you hope to have children who are breast-fed. Detoxify regularly with saunas to eliminate PCBs through your sweat. Follow the sauna detoxification outlined in this book before conceiving. Take your children into the sauna with you once a week.

Perchloroethylene (PERC)

Talk to your dry cleaner about switching to 'Green Clean' methods and find out from Environment Canada or the USEPA if there is an outlet available in your city. Take the time to wash selected clothing by hand or buy clothes that don't need dry cleaning.

2,4- dichlorophenoxyacetic acid (2,4 -D)

Notice the number of residents in your area who use pesticides on their lawns and gracefully educate them about risks to their health. Minimize your use of carpeting in the home, using hardwood floors and natural fiber throw rugs instead. If you do have carpets, steam clean once or twice yearly with non-chlorinated cleansers. Insist on shoe removal in your home. Do not allow outdoor pets onto carpeted areas.

Trichloroethylene (TCE)

Minimize your use of processed foods and stock your kitchen with what you need to cook from scratch. Filter your drinking water using a reverse osmosis or carbon filter.

Disinfecting of Sewage, Drinking Water and Chlorinated Pools

We can consider opting out of the toxic soup most cities call water by filtering stored rainwater, spring water, or groundwater from a drilled well. If this is not possible, then install a reverse osmosis or charcoal filter to your water supply and shower head. We can install composting toilets that recycle human waste and contribute nothing to global pollution. They also avoid the water wasting of flush toilets and the many chemicals used to clean up sewage. For information on composting toilets contact one of the following manufacturers: Sun-Mar Composting Toilets, Burlington, ON (tel. 905-332-1314); Storburn Pollution Free Toilet, Brantford, ON (tel. 800-876-2286); BioLet (tel. 800-6BIOLET); Envirolet Composting Toilet Systems, Scarborough, ON (tel. 800-387-5245); or Clivus Multrum (tel. 800-4CLIVUS).[89] We can insist upon safe, non-chlorine purification methods in our drinking water and swimming pools, such as ozonation and the use of grapefruit seed extract.

The Pulp and Paper Industry

Buy totally chlorine free paper products (toilet paper, diapers, sanitary products, tampons, and paper packaging) or recycled paper that is chlorine free. Talk to your supermarket managers to have them stock these items, or buy them from ecological or health food stores. Use TCF paper for printing and photocopying. Recycle the paper products that you do use.

Create a Safer Environment

If you live in a high polluting province or state, or close to an industry that releases any amount of organochlorines, put pressure on your municipal, provincial, state, or federal elected leaders to enforce regulations banning the production and release of organochlorines and other toxic chemicals. Put pressure on the industries themselves to stop production. Find out what quantities of environmental hormone disruptors are in your air and water supply and where they are coming from. In the United States, you can easily find out who is polluting in your area through visiting the web site: www.scorecard.org/. A similar site is planned for Canada by the end of 2000 and can be accessed through www.net/cela/. Unite with other activist groups and use the many resources available, as listed in the resource directory at the back of this book.

There are three excellent films on the environmental links to breast cancer that you can show in your communities. One is called Exposure: Environmental Links to Breast Cancer and comes with an excellent resource guide and handbook to accompany the film. You can order it from Women's Network on Health and the Environment (517 College St., Ste 233, Toronto, ON, M6G 4A2, tel. 416-928-0880). Another is called Hormone Copy-Cats and can be ordered from the World Wildlife Fund Canada (90 Eglington Ave E, Ste 504, Toronto, ON, M4P 2Z7, tel. 416-489-8800 or 800-26-PANDA or fax. 416-489-3611). The third film is called Rachel's Daughters, a reference to Rachel Carson, founder of the environmental movement, which also comes with an excellent Community Action and Resource Guide, available from Light-Saraf Films (264 Arbor St, San Fransisco, CA 94131, tel. 415-469-0139).

Chapter 5 — *Detoxifying Our Bodies*

Overall Detoxification

To enhance detoxification generally, we should do the following daily: ensure 3 or 4 bowel movements through the use of fiber and enemas, drink at least two liters of water to flush the kidneys, take herbs or nutritional substances to cleanse the liver and kidneys, sweat through exercising and the use of saunas, use a skin brush to stimulate the lymphatic system and the skin, and practice breathing exercises to detoxify the lungs.

The Liver's Detoxification Pathways

We can improve Phase 1 detoxification with the following nutrients:[1]

1) Niacin, riboflavin, copper, zinc, vitamin E, vitamin A, calcium, and magnesium are needed as cofactors in making Phase 1 enzymes.

2) Indole-3-carbinol from the raw brassicas, such as cabbage, broccoli, bok choy, and cauliflower, which promotes the conversion of estrone to the C2 estrogen, rather than the harmful C16 estrogen.

3) Isoflavones found in soy and limonene (present in oranges and tangerines).

4) Amino acids from protein, essential fatty acids, and complex carbohydrates in our diets.

5) The herbs *Schizandra chinensis, Curcuma longa,* milk thistle *(silybum marianum), Rosmarinus officinalis, Capsicum frutescens, Calendula officianalis, Solidago vigaurea* and *Sassafras albidum.*

We can improve Phase 2 detoxification with the following nutrients:

1) Cysteine (or NAC), methionine, choline, vitamins B6, B12, B5, and C, molybdenum, folic acid.

2) Foods from the brassica family, limonene, Omega 3 fatty acids (flaxseed oil and fish oils).

3) The herbs *Rosmarinus officinalis, Curcuma longa,* or turmeric.

The Liver Flush

Schedule a time to do a 10-day liver flush. If you can, do it within the next month. Prepare yourself physically and psychologically with relaxation and breathing exercises daily, a vegetarian diet, and consciously releasing negative thought patterns, old resentments, and anger.

Look at a calendar for the next year. Block in future 10-day periods when you will do the liver flush, up to four times per year. Block in the 6–8 week periods when you will take a liver loving herbal formula, overlapping it with the liver flush. You may choose to do it one to four times yearly, or continuously if you are recovering from breast cancer.

Taking Care of Your Liver

1) Food combining enhances digestion. Proteins and starches should be eaten at different meals. Avoid combining sweets and proteins. Regularly eat foods that assist the liver — beets, garlic, dandelion, cabbage and the other brassicas, turmeric, rosemary, seeds, lemon, grapefruit, apple cider vinegar. Use fresh organic vegetable juices regularly, such as a mixture of beet, carrot, celery and cabbage.

2) Reduce fat in your diet, eliminating saturated fats of animal origin. Have 2–6 tsp of unsaturated fat (such as flaxseed oil) daily. Reduce sugar in your diet. When eaten in refined form, sugar lowers the effectiveness of liver enzymes, decreases immunity. and favors the growth of yeast and parasites.

3) A weekly 'resting' of the digestive system will benefit the liver. Eat only when hungry, and not too close to bedtime, ideally before 6:00 p.m. Massage the liver daily.

4) Exercise daily, and use saunas regularly, as some toxins are only eliminated through perspiration.

5) Increase fiber and water intake to ensure at least two bowel movements daily.

6) Use the 'Lemon Aid' cleanse as described below or other cleansing diet as needed (early spring and fall are prime times).

7) Anger, anxiety, and other negative emotions can impede liver function. Be aware of your feelings and appropriately release emotions — exercise or find a good listener.

8) Vitamins C and E, beta-carotene, selenium, and zinc are antioxidants, protecting the liver. Take them regularly or obtain them through diet.

9) Recommended teas are dandelion, licorice, and ginger. Milk thistle rebuilds a damaged liver.

10) At least two times a year, take a herbal liver formula and go on a liver and bowel-cleansing program for 6–8 weeks. If you have breast cancer, do it continuously,

with short breaks every 3 months. In this way, you will decrease the chemical load in the body and eliminate excess estrogen. Once or twice a year do the liver flush. Consider using castor oil packs to detoxify your liver as well.

11) Cleanse the body of yeast and parasites twice yearly for at least 6 weeks at a time.

Ensure Parasite Protection

It is much easier and cheaper to prevent parasites in the first place than it is to eliminate them. Our first method of contact with them is usually through the skin and mouth. The following guidelines will help to protect you and your children.

1) Always wash your hands before eating.

2) Wash your hands with soap and water after going to the bathroom, changing diapers, or handling pets.

3) Keep your fingernails short and use a nailbrush to scrub beneath them.

4) Wipe off the toilet seat before sitting on it or squat above the toilet. Wear rubber gloves while cleaning the bathroom. Clean bathrooms daily or at least twice weekly. Pinworm eggs and trichomonas can be found under toilet seats. Trichomonas can also be spread through mud and water baths and sauna benches.

5) Use sterilized lens preparations to clean contact lenses and remove them before swimming.

6) Don't walk barefoot in areas frequented by dogs, cats, raccoons, etc.

7) If you travel frequently, eat out regularly, have pets, or visit mountainous regions, have a complete parasite exam twice a year. Use a purged stool and rectal mucous exam to check for infection. Be aware that parasites don't always show up in a stool sample even when they are present.

8) Breast-feed your children as long as you can. Human milk has antibodies that protect against amoeba and giardia.

9) Keep young children away from puppies and kittens that have not been regularly dewormed. Prevent them from kissing house pets or being licked by them. Empty kitty litter boxes daily while wearing gloves. Disinfect litter boxes frequently with boiling water and grapefruit seed extract. If you are pregnant, wear disposable gloves and a mask while changing the litter box or have someone else do this task to avoid risk of toxoplasmosis. Keep children away from snails or

have them wear gloves while playing with them. Be sure they wash thoroughly after contact with these and other animals. Freshwater snails are the intermediate host of schistosomiasis, a blood fluke. Keep pets and their bowls out of the kitchen.

10) Do not allow children to eat dirt or play in areas where there are animal droppings. Encourage children to keep their fingers out of their mouths and not to bite their fingernails.

11) Damp mop or vacuum bedrooms and bathrooms weekly (don't sweep) to eliminate eggs that may be in dust. Keep bedrooms well aired.

12) Bathe or shower daily.

13) If pinworms are present, launder bedding and personal clothing daily, wear close-fitting underwear to bed, and don't share a bed with other family members.

14) Keep toothbrushes in closed containers to avoid exposure to bathroom dust.

15) Drink filtered water. Use reverse osmosis or carbon block filters. Always boil or filter water from rivers or streams to eliminate giardia.

16) If you eat fish, use varieties that are commercially blast-frozen. Cook until it is flaky and white. Bake at 400°F, eight to ten minutes per inch of thickness. Avoid sushi.

17) If you are a meat eater, cook at 325°F or higher and use a meat thermometer to check that the internal temperature is 170°F.

18) Avoid oral-anal sex to prevent transmission of trichomonas, pinworms, ascaris, giardia, strongyloides, and Entamoeba histolytica. Use condoms when engaging in sexual intercourse unless you know that your partner is free of parasites.

19) Wash your fruits and vegetables before eating them.

20) Avoid the use of antibiotics unless absolutely necessary. These disturb the ecology of organisms in the intestines and can cause an overgrowth of *Candida albicans* in the body which can damage the cells in the stomach that produce hydrochloric acid. Hydrochloric acid, when present in sufficient amounts, will kill most parasites when they enter the stomach so they cause no further damage. The gastric analysis test (available from HDC Corporation, 408-954-1909) can determine if enough stomach acid is present. Antibiotics also eliminate the bacteria that convert phytoestrogens into a usable weak estrogen.

Use Natural Anti-Parasitic Substances

Because parasites are a prevalent health problem but are difficult to diagnose, it behooves each of us to do a routine parasite cleanse twice a year, during the time of the full moon, for a minimum of six weeks each time. A combination of wormwood, black walnut, cloves, male fern, goldenseal, grapefruit seed extract, and Unda #39, or Cina would tackle most varieties. We may have particular sensitivities to different products, so starting with a low dosage or testing energetically for compatibility is advised.

Normalize Stomach Acid

Once a year, check your stomach acid through use of the Gastro test (available from HDC Corporation, 408-954-1909). Correct it with one of the available methods if it is low.

Eliminate Candidiasis

Once or twice yearly, do a Candida cleanse along with the parasite cleanse. Work with a practitioner to decide which supplements to use. Use the anti-yeast supplements for at least two months. Do it at the same time as you do the parasite cleanse.

Take Fiber Supplements

Cleanse your intestines with a fiber formula at least twice yearly for six weeks at a time, or use a fiber formula continuously, particularly if you have cancer. Use wheat bran and psyllium regularly, unless you are allergic or sensitive to them. Maintain a high fiber content in your diet, at least 30 g daily. Be sure to drink sufficient water, about two liters daily, while taking a fiber supplement.

Use Enemas

Choose a time period in which you will cleanse the colon and decide which method you will use — either a fiber supplement or a series of enemas or colonics. Work with your health practitioner. Consider a six week period, twice yearly for the fiber supplement, or enemas three times a week, for several weeks at a time, one to three times per year. If you have cancer, more frequent enemas may be necessary. Mark these times in your yearly calendar and start as soon as possible. Do it under supervision of a health care practitioner familiar with detoxification regimens.

Squat

Squat on the toilet at home or use a small 10-inch stool that to place your feet on while having a bowel movement.

Reintroduce Good Bacteria

Supplement your diet with probiotic organisms including Lactobacillus acidophilus and Lactobacillus bifidus as well as the growth medium FOS. Include asparagus, onions, Jerusalem artichoke, and/or burdock root as a regular part of your diet.

Conserve Enzymes

1) Include sprouts as a regular part of your diet because they are high in enzymes. For breast cancer prevention, some of the best sprouts to use are clover, broccoli, pea, green lentil, chickpea, mung bean, and sunflower. If you eat these at the beginning of a meal with salad, the increased enzymes will help to digest the rest of the meal.

2) Include fresh raw juices as part of your daily diet.

3) Consume at least 50%–80% of your food raw.

4) Cook food on low heat or for shorter periods. Soak beans and grains overnight to increase their enzyme content and decrease their cooking time. Use a slow cooker for bean and grain dishes and stir fry for short periods.

5) Use supplemental enzymes before meals to help digest your food and between meals to detoxify the blood and to break down the fibrin coat of cancer cells. If you have breast cancer, consider using proteolytic enzymes several times daily between meals. Supplement your diet with probiotic organisms including *Lactobacillus acidophilus* and *Lactobacillus bifidus* as well as the growth medium FOS.

Bottled Water

Drink 2–3 liters of filtered water daily, using a reverse osmosis or carbon block filter. Other choices for kidney cleansing are to add lemon juice to your water in the morning, use dandelion regularly (it's in the liver formula), drink green juices (including some parsley and watercress), and use beets regularly, which cleanse the kidneys and liver.

Chart Your pH

Monitor your urinary and salivary pH for several weeks and attempt to normalize. This will improve your absorption of minerals and relieve many symptoms related to pH imbalance. In general, your diet should consist of 80% alkaline-forming foods (sea vegetables, fruits, vegetables, millet, kidney beans, adzuki beans, tofu) and 20% acid-forming foods (grains, seeds and nuts, flaxseed and olive oil, asparagus, cranberry, plums, prunes, lentils, animal protein).

The Sauna Detoxification Program

1) Encourage the building of saunas in our communities, or build our own.

2) Undergo a medically supervised three-week sauna detoxification program every one to five years, the frequency depending upon our toxin exposure, age, and general health. This would be a wonderful ritual for women to do together in their efforts to prevent breast cancer, connect with each other, and to feel better generally.

3) Develop the ritual of the family sauna, having a weekly sauna with our partners and children. In this way we will release toxins regularly, not giving them time to build up to high levels. If we don't have a family, then we can find a group of sauna-lovers to sweat with regularly.

4) Before getting married, spend at least a few days sweating it out and considers doing the full sauna detoxification program together, especially if the couple intends to have children in the future.

5) At least three months before you conceive, do the full sauna detoxification program. Toxins continue to be released for several months after the therapy is completed, so do the cleansing well in advance of conception.

A Cleansing Diet

Consider a cleansing diet or fast one or more times a year for several days if you do not have cancer. Consider the Mung Beans and Rice Diet if you have cancer.

Chapter 6 — *Activating the Lymphatic and Immune Systems*

Spleen

You can support the activity of your spleen through lifestyle, diet, and herbs.

1) Like the rest of the lymphatic and immune systems, the function of the spleen and its white blood cells is compromised by stress, and periods of relaxation are essential.

2) In Traditional Chinese Medicine, sugar and excessive sweets are recognized as harming the spleen; therefore, you should limit your sweet intake to occasional use.

3) You can use the herbs burdock root, goldenseal, echinacea, astragalus, and codonopsis to nourish the spleen when necessary.

Thymus Gland

You can support the work of your thymus gland with nutritional supplements, herbs, and exercises.

1) You can use the antioxidant nutrients alpha lipoic acid, vitamins A, C, E, zinc, selenium, melatonin to protect the thymus from shrinking when you are under stress as well as vitamins B6 and B12.

2) Since the thymus secretes its hormones under para-sympathetic stimulation when you are relaxed, you can develop a meditation practice and find ways to take 20-minute relaxation breaks regularly.

3) Bovine thymus extract and homeopathic thymuline 9CH have a modulating and strengthening effect on the gland and can be taken as directed by a naturopath or holistic doctor.

4) The following herbs can be used to improve thymic function: echinacea, licorice, European mistletoe, astragalus, maitake and shitake mushrooms, and reishi.

5) Exercises that involve coordinated arm and leg movements on alternate sides strengthen the thymus — you can swing your arms as you walk and avoid carrying heavy bags on one side, and can march, swim, and do yoga.

Dry Brush Massage

1) Buy a long handled, natural bristle brush, with a brush pad about the size of your own hand. If you can't find a natural bristle brush, you can substitute a natural plant fiber vegetable brush, a bath glove made of twisted hog's hair, or a loofah mitt

2) Start with the soles of your feet. Brush in a circular motion as you move up your body, feet to legs, hands to arms, back to abdomen, and chest to neck. The face and inner thighs are sensitive areas and can be avoided. Brush with as much pressure as is comfortably possible until your skin feels pleasantly warm (this is usually about five to 10 minutes). The massage is best performed when you rise in the morning and before you go to bed at night.

3) You can increase the cleansing qualities of a dry brush massage if you follow it with an alternating hot-cold shower (hot for three minutes, cold for 30 seconds), repeating the hot-cold pattern three times.

4) Make sure that you wash your brush every two weeks with soap and water to remove the debris that may have moved from your skin to your brush, and then dry it in a warm place. Use a separate brush for each family member. The scalp is not ignored, as increased blood flow to it will help keep your hair healthy and growing. Irritated portions of your skin are avoided so as not to damage them. Increased blood flow to the surrounding areas will assist in its healing.

Hydrotherapy and Contrast Showers

Have a contrasting shower at least once daily, preferably in the morning as you begin your day. If you are recovering from any illness, consider having an additional one before bed.

Rebounding Exercise

Rebound 5–30 minutes once or twice daily while listening to your favorite music.

Going Braless

Choose a bra that is cotton, has no underwires, allows the breasts to move a little, and wear it less than 12 hours daily, or go braless. Don't wear your bra to bed.

The Lymph Flush

Use the lymph flush when you feel sensitivity or swelling in your lymph nodes or with lymphedema.

The Hoxsey Formula

As part of a breast cancer prevention program, consider taking the Hoxsey formula for three months once or twice a year, the frequency and dosage being dependent upon your risk factors. Take it continuously with short breaks every six weeks if you are recovering from breast cancer.

Essiac

As part of a breast cancer prevention program, consider alternating the Essiac formula with the Hoxsey formula or use The Healthy Breast Formula. Take Essiac or FlorEssence for three months when you are not taking the Hoxsey formula, once or twice a year. If you are recovering from breast cancer, use both of them simultaneously.

Immune Activating Formula or Tea

As prevention, consider using an immune activating formula or tea for 1–3 months per year, particularly during the winter, or whenever you are most prone to infections. If you are recovering from breast cancer, use one of the formulas or a similar formula continuously with short breaks every six weeks. Drink Pau d'arco tea and decaffeinated green tea regularly, and use Chyavan Prash. Use antioxidants, meditation, thymus extract, echinacea, licorice root, European mistletoe, astragalus, maitake, shitake, and reishi mushrooms and co-ordinated exercise to strengthen your thymus gland.

Chapter 7 — *The Healthy Breast Diet*

Organic Food

Call the makers of your favorite brands of foods and tell them you would like them to use organically grown crops in their products. Insist on an organic section in your local supermarket. Transform your lawn by growing your own vegetables in a front or backyard garden or push your city government into establishing community gardens. Many communities offer direct weekly deliveries from farms or organic food depots to your home. If you are so inclined, grow your own broccoli, red clover, alfalfa, and sunflower seed sprouts in your kitchen or grow lettuce in indoor window boxes. Investigate the principles of permaculture to transform our cities into green oases.[1]

Vegetarianism

Consume six to nine servings of vegetables and fruits daily. Follow a primarily vegetarian diet.

Raw Foods

Be sure that at least 50% of your vegetables are raw. Consume two salads daily at the beginning of your meals. If you cannot digest raw food, cook it lightly and use supplemental digestive enzymes. Use red clover, mung bean, and broccoli sprouts regularly.

Beneficial Brassicas

Consume at least one half cup or about 14 oz of members of the brassica family daily.[11] Have coleslaw several times a week, add cabbage to salads, consume raw broccoli and cauliflower with hummus or other bean dips, and add broccoli sprouts to your main dishes and salads. Use fresh juices including cabbage, kale, bok choy, garden sorrel, watercress, or collards daily. Lightly steam kale, Brussels sprouts, and the other brassicas and have them as a side dish or mix them in a tofu stir-fry. Use the brassicas with seaweeds or dulse powder whenever possible.

Benefits of Broccoli Sprouts

Buy or grow your own mung bean, red clover, broccoli, sunflower, and alfalfa sprouts and consume them daily or several times weekly. Use them in salads, on top of bean dishes, added to stir fries, or mixed with vegetable juices. Aim for at least six cups weekly. Consume them at the beginning of the meal so that their enzyme power will assist in digesting your food. See the recipe section for details on growing various sprouts. For a great book on sprouts and sprouting, read *The Hippocrates Diet and Health Program* by Ann Wigmore. Consume 2 tsp twice daily of a cereal grass supplement, mixed in water or juice, such as Greens+ or Barley Green.

Garlic, Onions, and Leeks

Eat a raw onion and one to three cloves of garlic daily. Make potato leek soup when leeks are in season and freeze for year round use.

Sea Vegetables

A simple way to incorporate sea vegetables into your diet is by sprinkling dulse or kelp powder on your food and adding it to soups, juices, salad dressings, and bean dishes. Use it to replace salt. A side portion of soaked and drained hiziki or arame can become a regular part of your meals. Most children like to munch on nori sheets or dried dulse as snacks or have them with rice during mealtimes. Have two tablespoons of sea vegetables daily.

Dandelion Root and Leaves

Eat dandelion greens and root in season.

Fresh Vegetable Juices

Consume freshly pressed vegetable juice two to five times daily, using carrot, beet, and cabbage as the base and adding other vegetables and sprouts for variety.

Lycopene: Tomatoes, Grapefruit, Watermelon, Guava

Consume tomatoes or tomato products regularly, at least twice weekly unless contraindicated by joint pain or allergy.

Flavonoids and Limonene: Citrus Juices and Peel

Include freshly squeezed organic citrus juices in your diet regularly, or simply eat citrus several times a week, if not daily. Save the peels and as long as they are organic, grate a little over your salad or consume them in a tea daily. If you have a known allergy to citrus, avoid it. Drink mint tea regularly and make dill a familiar kitchen herb.

Include organic cherries and cherry juice in your diet and use lavender oil on your skin.

Fats to Avoid

Avoid all products that say "hydrogenated" or "partially hydrogenated" on their labels.[30]

Decrease saturated fat content to not more than 5 % of your caloric intake, or less than 7–10 g daily.

Omega 6 Fatty Acids

Consume small amounts of Omega 6 oils in the form of raw unsalted nuts and seeds. These can include sunflower, sesame, pumpkin seeds, and almonds. Two tablespoons daily is a reasonable amount. Balance it with a higher amount of flaxseed oil. If you have cancer, do not use these seeds – take only flaxseeds and flaxseed oil until the cancer is gone.

Fats to Use

If you are in good health, consume 1–2 tbsp of flaxseed oil daily, along with 2 tbsp of ground flaxseeds. If you have a degenerative condition, like arthritis, diabetes or cancer, take 3 to 5 tbsp of the oil daily with 2–4 tbsp of seeds. Individuals with cancer metastases can take 6 to 7 tbsp daily along with 6 to 7 tbsp of ground seeds daily. Six tablespoons of ground flaxseeds contain 2 tablespoons of oil.

Use a small amount of extra virgin olive oil daily.

Types of Fiber

Consume equal amounts of wheat bran (if tolerated) and psyllium daily, approximately one tablespoon of each. Eat 30 g of fiber daily, using beans, raw fruits and vegetables, and whole grains to do so.

Beans

Consume 1–2 cups of beans daily, particularly soybeans, fava beans, yellow peas, pinto beans, green lentils, garbanzo beans, black turtle beans, mung beans, adzuki beans, bush beans, navy beans, baby lima beans, black-eyed peas, lentils, and kidney beans.

Evaluating Fiber Content

Consume 30 g of fiber daily. This is equivalent to one serving of high fiber cereal, one cup of cooked beans, two pieces of whole grain bread, one serving of cooked whole grains such as brown rice, quinoa or millet and six servings of fruit or vegetables. Minimize flour products such as bread, baked goods, and pasta. Focus on whole grains instead.

Soy: Genistein and Daidzen

Each day you should eat either ½ cup of firm tofu or tempeh, 1½ cups soy milk, ¼ cup soy nuts, or some combination of these, aiming for 35–60 g of soy protein daily.

Include miso in your diet several times a week, perhaps as miso soup. You may also supplement with quality soy protein powder, mixed with fruit to make a shake. Find soy products that are organic and non-genetically modified, since the common pesticides used on soy are ones that can promote breast cancer. Be sure your soy milk has no added oil or sugar.

Balance the high salt content of miso with high potassium foods eaten in the same day. If you have high blood pressure or kidney disease, have miso only once or twice per week. If you have a problem with candidiasis, avoid miso and minimize tofu until you clear the excess yeast from your body. The isoflavones in miso are more easily absorbed from the small intestine than those from other tofu products and lead to a higher urinary output of equol, meaning that miso exerts more activity as a weak estrogen than other soy products. This is because genistein and daidzen exist in miso in an unconjugated form, whereas they are conjugated and less bio-available in tofu, soy milk, and soybeans.

Protection for Infants and Daughters before Puberty

Be cautious about consuming high amounts of soy while pregnant or when trying to conceive. Give your children moderate amounts of soy early in life and higher amounts before and through puberty.

Bacteria, Antibiotics, and Phytoestrogens

Use herbal medicines first before resorting to antibiotics when you need to fight an infection. Try to avoid antibiotics. If you must take them, use probiotics or 'good bacteria' while taking antibiotics and for a month afterward. Consider using immune enhancers such as astragalus, goldenseal and echinacea intermittently instead of antibiotics to protect from secondary infections. Generally avoid antibiotics unless absolutely necessary.

Flaxseeds and Other High Lignan Foods

Eat flaxseeds any way you can. Buy a small electric coffee grinder and add them ground to pancakes, muffins, cookies, breads, cereals, or even sprinkled in salad. Grind them daily so that the oil does not become rancid with storage. Freshly ground flaxseeds should be consumed within 15 minutes of grinding. Aim for two to four tablespoons (25–50 g) daily. If you have more than 2 tbsp. daily, you may need extra vitamin B6. They can also be mixed with juice.

Mung Bean Sprouts and Coumestrol

Eat mung bean sprouts several times a week aiming for 3 cups weekly. Add them to salads, on top of bean dishes, mixed in juices, or munch them on their own.

Not Too Much Protein

Consume approximately 30–60 g of vegetarian protein daily.

Sulphur-Bearing Protein in Combination with Flaxseed Oil

We should aim for 500 mg twice daily of sulphur-containing protein in combination with at least 2 tbsp of flaxseed oil daily. To prevent breast cancer, vegetarian sources are best, which include soy nuts, pumpkin seeds, sunflower seeds, oatmeal, beans, tofu and all soy products, broccoli, kale, kelp, and spirulina. Spirulina is an especially high source and is one of the main ingredients in Greens+.

Low Sodium / High Potassium Foods

Eat 3000–6000 mg of high potassium fruits and vegetables daily to help with cellular detoxification.

Shitake and Maitake Mushrooms

Eat shitake mushrooms daily (or at least twice weekly) for a month followed by a seven-day break. Buy them fresh, dried, or as a tea. Use them in stir-fries, sandwich spreads, casseroles, and soups.

Rosemary, Sage, Thyme, and Turmeric

Have one teaspoon of turmeric powder daily, or supplement with curcumin. Sauté onions, ginger, and garlic in water and olive oil and add turmeric before adding other ingredients for a stir-fry. Use a little in a tofu sandwich spread and add it to soup and bean dishes or boil it with basmati rice.

Ginger

To improve digestion, maintain the health of the intestines and protect from parasites, use rosemary, sage, thyme and ginger regularly to season your foods.

Rotate Your Foods

To follow a five-day rotation diet, prepare a diet plan where you attempt to eat a particular food only once every five days, with the exception of the 'fabulous five' phytoestrogens, the brassicas, flaxseed oil, and garlic. Eat these daily unless you have reason to believe that you are reacting negatively to them. Rotate your grains and beans. Tofu and soy products can also provoke sensitivities in some people. If you experience symptoms after ingesting frequent amounts of soy products, then decrease soy consumption to every four days rather than having it daily. Use some of the other foods and herbs containing phytoestrogens instead of relying on soy. Avoid known food sensitivities.

Foods with a Low Glycemic Index

Let most of your diet consist of foods with a low glycemic index. If you do consume foods from the high category, combine them with fiber, healthy oils such as flaxseed and olive oil, or protein.

Fish

Avoid fish, unless you know it is not contaminated with chemicals, and then have it seldom. Eat fish no more than once weekly and only if you crave it. Try to find fish from clean waters. Use flaxseed oil to obtain Omega 3 fatty acids. If you have breast cancer, do not eat fish.

Dairy

Avoid or limit milk products and products that contain casein, such as soy cheese.

Sweets

We should limit our sweets to a treat perhaps once weekly and otherwise use fruit to satisfy a sweet craving. Discourage a desire for sweets in your children by restricting their intake of processed sweets from infancy onward. If children are not given sweets, they often will not crave them as adults.

White Flour Products

Avoid white flour products. Use instead whole grains and a limited amount of whole grain baked goods.

Processed Food

Avoid processed food and food packaged in plastic.

Alcohol

Drink less than two to three alcoholic beverages weekly, preferably drink none.

Salt

Avoid salt.

Coffee

Avoid coffee.

Chapter 8 — Nutritional Supplements for Breast Health

Use nutritional supplements as prescribed by your health practitioners.

Chapter 9 — Psychological Means of Preventing Breast Cancer

The Healing Effects of Being Assertive

Assertiveness can be encapsulated in three steps:

1) Communicate your thoughts about a particular situation in a factual, non-blaming way.
2) Communicate your feelings about a particular situation using 'I statements'.
3) Communicate your wants clearly and specifically.

Acknowledging Your Anger Exercise

The following 12 steps may assist you in transforming feelings of anger from a potentially destructive emotion into something with healing power.

1) Accept that anger is a valid emotion. It is okay to feel angry.
2) Acknowledge that you feel angry. Identify the part of the body that is holding the anger.
3) Identify whom you are angry with and/or what you are angry about.
4) Ask yourself if the anger is warranted or if it has been magnified by a previous situation not fully dealt with. Are you projecting your mother, father, or sibling onto the person you feel anger towards? Recognize it.
5) Identify what lies beneath the anger. Usually there is an unmet need or a feeling of being hurt.
6) Explore the unmet needs or feelings of being hurt within yourself first, and then with the other person. If possible, communicate your feelings by saying, "When you did such and such, I felt such and such." Communicate it without blame. Communicate your unmet need specifically; for example, "I need you to put down your newspaper and really listen to me when I speak to you." If you are unable to do this directly, then write a letter, choosing to mail it or not, or use a chair exercise and speak to the person as though they were sitting in the chair. Honor your unmet need and create a plan to meet it as soon as possible.

7) Check in again with the body part that was holding the anger. Ask it if it needs anything more from you. Consciously relax the area.
8) Discharge the anger physically. Use aerobic exercise, rebounding, running or swimming, martial arts, kundalini yoga, rowing, Dragon-boat racing, drumming, etc. to release the build up of muscle tension. Do this on a regular basis — two to three times weekly.
9) Channel any residual anger creatively. Do a drawing, painting, or sculpture which utilizes the energy of the anger and helps externalize it rather than turn it inward
10) Channel anger into a worthy cause or project. Help fight some of the injustices in the world and join forces with others who are helping to create global change for the better.
11) Recognize that by holding on to the anger you are hurting yourself. Choose to let go of it.
12) Give the outcome to the divine forces of the universe. Use prayer and meditation to help you access the state of forgiveness. Forgive the other person and pray for their well being.

Imagery and Visualization

Using Achterberg's findings, for people with cancer, we can develop imagery for healing by encouraging the following:

1) Portray the cancer cells as being few in number, small in size, weak in strength, and lacking vividness.

2) Portray the white blood cells as being vivid, very active, strong and powerful, large and abundant, and overwhelming the cancer cells. Believe more in the potency of your body's ability to heal than in the disease process, and understand that nothing is fixed — it is a process than can go either way.

3) Portray the naturopathic and medical treatments with vividness and effectiveness.

4) Choose strong, powerful, active imagery that is well integrated yet personal.

5) Practice the imagery frequently, at least twice daily. Keep drawing, over and over, until it's as powerful as it can be for a healing response. Draw so that you believe it.

6) Visualize that your body's healthy cells are easily able to repair any slight damage the treatment might cause; that the dead cancer cells are flushed from the body easily and completely; that at the end of the imagery, you are healthy and cancer-free.

7) See yourself accomplishing your goals and fulfilling your life's purpose — relate to your future rather than your past. Explore what your ideal future might be and shift your life in that direction so that your immune system responds with you.

Activating Your Capacity to Heal Exercise

Choose one or more of these affirmations and repeat it out loud to yourself several times daily, particularly when you look in the mirror. Copy one out and tape it to your mirror to remind you.

I am a different person now from whom I was when I became sick.
I listen daily to the signals of my body and respond in ways that honor it.
I allow long held emotions to be released from my body in a healthy manner.
I believe in my body's capacity for self-healing. ◀

Script for Recovering from Breast Cancer Exercise

1) Learn to watch your thought processes. Identify with healing imagery and use it to replace self-destructive thoughts. Explore disturbing thoughts to understand their source, the need that lies beneath them, and ways to transform them. Remind yourself of the following:

   i) illness is not a form of punishment — you are not guilty;
   ii) others have recovered from the same illness;
   iii) your symptoms are a messenger and can be a catalyst for change;
   iv) you have an innate capacity to heal;
   v) the body is in a constant state of change — nothing is fixed — all is process.

2) Use meditation tools such as mantras, witnessing thoughts and feelings, attention to the breath, and eye focus to disengage from the temporary 'reality' created by your thoughts.

3) Use sensory stimuli to create healing responses. Through your waking day associate sensory experiences with healing processes (for example, when you turn on a water faucet, visualize any toxins, illness, or cancer cells being flushed out of your body; when you walk outside allow the wind to blow out any toxicity; when you hear music direct it to breaking up any tumors, etc.) so that many sensory experiences become a celebration of your body's self-healing ability. Make a list of all the ways you can use sensory stimuli to generate healing.

4) Use particular images that have power and significance for you. Find your totems — a rock, a tree, a piece of music, an animal — whatever contains healing power for you. Look for these in your dreams, honor them in your life. Place these images around you to remind you of healing. Believe in the power of nature to heal or in a spiritual force or deity. Identify with and pray to that higher power regularly, believing that it will heal you. Let a healing animal, person, or deity come to you in a state of relaxation and absorb the power of that animal or deity, letting it fight for you even as you sleep. Make a list of images that have power and significance for you.

5) Use imagery and visualization regularly, two to five times daily. Enter a relaxed state before using imagery. This usually takes a minimum of 11 minutes.

6) Remind yourself that the body-mind is in a constant state of change. If your mental state can change, so can the physical.

Chapter 10 — *Spiritual Practices for Preventing Breast Cancer*

Your Unique Way of Being in the World

Strive to live a life in alignment with your true nature, where your passion and joy are kindled and you use your talents and gifts.

Meaning through Our Attitude towards Suffering

Strive to find meaning daily in what you do, what you experience, and through goodness, truth, beauty, nature, culture, and love. Build your 'meaning bank' by filling your life with experiences of depth. Find meaning in the attitude you take to suffering or to illness. Ask of every situation that's given to you what you can learn from it to help you grow.

Confronting Your Death While Alive Exercise

Live your life being aware of your death, so that you deepen relationships, experience life fully, achieve and accomplish your goals, and develop your talents and gifts.

Your Personal Prayer

Design your own prayer or use a traditional prayer upon rising each morning and before bed. When you find yourself feeling a loss of hope, worry or fear, use a form of prayer as a centering device.

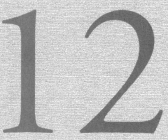

Recipes for Breast Health

The food which we are about to eat

Is Earth, Water, and Sun, combined through the alchemy of many plants.

Therefore Earth, Water, and Sun will become part of us.

This food is also the fruit of the labor of many beings and creatures.

We are grateful for it.

May it give us strength, health, joy.

And may it increase our love.

— Unitarian Prayer

Contents

Breakfast Dishes

Buckwheat

Place the water and dulse powder in a large saucepan and bring to a boil. Add the buckwheat gradually to prevent the water from bubbling over the pot. Reduce the heat to low, cover and allow to simmer until water is absorbed (15–20 minutes). Remove from heat and allow to cool for 5–10 minutes. Using a damp wooden spoon, gently mix the grain from top to bottom while still in the pot.

Cover again and allow to stand for 5–10 minutes. Grind the flaxseeds in a small coffee grinder. Serve sprinkled over the cereal with the wheat bran and top with soy milk.

Yields 3 servings.

Ingredients:

2 cups	water
1 cup	buckwheat
¼ tsp	dulse powder
2 tbsp	flaxseeds
1 tsp	wheat bran

Quinoa

Rinse quinoa, either by using a strainer or by running fresh water over the quinoa in a pot. Drain excess water. Place quinoa and water in a 1½ quart saucepan and bring to a boil. Reduce to a simmer, cover, and cook until all of the water is absorbed (10–15 minutes). The quinoa is done when all the grains have turned transparent. Grind flaxseeds in a small coffee grinder and sprinkle over cereal. Serve with soy milk.

Yields 2 servings.

Ingredients:

1 cup	water
1 cup	quinoa
2 tbsp	organic flaxseeds

Buckwheat, Flax, and Quinoa

Place the water in a 1½ quart saucepan and bring to a boil. Add buckwheat and quinoa and simmer for 15 minutes. Grind the flax seeds in a small coffee grinder. Serve the grains topped with ground flaxseeds and soy milk.

Yields 4 servings.

Ingredients:

4 cups	water
1 cup	buckwheat
1 cup	quinoa
2 tbsp	flaxseeds

Millet Cereal

Grind millet in a grinder or food processor. Combine ground cereal and water in a small pan. Stir constantly and bring to a boil. Turn heat to low and simmer 10–15 minutes, stirring continually to prevent sticking. Sprinkle on 2 tbsp of freshly ground flaxseeds and 1 tbsp wheat bran for each serving. Serve with soy milk and a small amount of honey, stevia, or maple syrup.

Yields 4 servings.

Ingredients:

1 cup	millet
2½ cups	water
2 tsp	flaxseeds
1 tsp	wheat bran

Mixed Grain and Seed Cereal

Mix the first four ingredients and store in a large glass jar. Grind cereal mix in a small electric grinder or food processor. Combine ground cereal and water in a small pan. Stir constantly as you bring to a boil. Turn heat to low, cover, and let simmer 10–15 minutes. Stir frequently to prevent sticking. Add 1 tbsp wheat bran and 2 tbsp freshly ground seed combination to each serving. Serve with soy milk.

Yields 4½ cup dry mix; 1 cup dry mix makes 4 servings cooked cereal.

Ingredients:

1 cup	hulled barley
1 cup	millet
1 cup	whole oats
1 cup	amaranth
1 tsp	wheat bran
2 tsp	sesame seeds
2 tsp	pumpkin seeds
2 tsp	flaxseeds
	To cook cereal:
1 cup	cereal mix
3 cups	water

Breakfast Kasha

Heat ghee in a 2-quart pan or 10-inch skillet. Add onion, garlic, and dulse. Sauté until onion is soft. Add kasha to onion mixture and stir well. Add boiling water, reduce heat to low, cover, and allow to set for 15 minutes. Remove lid, add parsley and tomato, and fluff before serving. Top each serving with a small amount of Bragg's if desired.

Yields 4–6 servings.

Ingredients:

2 tsp	ghee
1	small onion, chopped
1	clove garlic, minced
1 cup	kasha
2 cups	boiling water
¼ cup	chopped parsley
½	tomato, chopped
½ tsp	dulse or kelp powder Bragg's liquid aminos

Kasha with Sunflower Seeds

Grind the kasha in a blender, a coffee mill, or handmill. In a 2-quart saucepan, blend the kasha with 1 cup water until smooth, then add the remaining water and dulse powder. Bring to a simmer, stirring constantly until it thickens. Cover and simmer for 15 minutes, stirring occasionally and adding water as needed. When the kasha has finished cooking, add the sunflower seeds and serve. Allow each person to season individual portions with tamari or Bragg's to taste.

Yields 4 servings.

Ingredients:

1 cup	kasha (buckwheat groats)
4 cups	water (or more for thinner consistency)
½ tsp	dulse powder
½ cup	raw sunflower seeds
	Tamari or Bragg's liquid aminos to taste

Oatmeal with Blueberries

Mix the apple cider and water together in a small pot and bring to a simmer. Add the oats and rice cereal and cook slowly for 15 minutes or until the rice cereal is done. Stir in flaxseeds and blueberries.

Yields 4 servings.

Ingredients:

1 cup	rolled oats
½ cup	rice cereal or ground short grain rice
3 tbsp	flaxseeds, freshly ground
2 cups	apple cider
1 cup	water
½ cup	organic blueberries

Apple Porridge

Place the apple in a blender and blend until smooth. Bring water to a boil in a medium saucepan and add apple blend, oats and cinnamon. Cook 5–10 minutes until creamy. Remove from heat and stir in ground flaxseeds. Serve as is or with soy milk.

Yields 1–2 servings.

Ingredients:

1	apple, peeled and chopped
⅓ cup	rolled oats
⅓ cup	water
¼ tsp	cinnamon
1 tbsp	freshly ground flaxseeds

Whole-Grain Pancake Mix

Combine all ingredients and store in an airtight container.

Use whisk to mix ingredients well. Lightly oil griddle with ghee or olive oil and cook, flipping with a spatula until both sides are done.

Yields 6 cups dry mix; 2 cups dry mix yields 10 pancakes.

Ingredients:

1½ cups	buckwheat flour
1½ cups	barley flour
1½ cups	spelt flour
¼ cup	soy flour
¼ cup	cornmeal
½ cup	dry powdered soy milk
2 tbsp	(+ 1 tsp) baking powder

To make pancakes or waffles:

2 cups	pancake mix
1 tbsp	freshly ground flaxseeds
2 tsp	freshly ground sesame seeds
2½ cups	water
½	banana, mashed or
2 tbsp	apple sauce (optional)
	ghee or olive oil

Tofu Miso Soup

Add the mushrooms and tofu to the water in a pot. Bring to a boil, then simmer for 10 minutes. Reduce the heat to very low, and add snow peas and pureed miso. Simmer for 2 more minutes. Place in serving bowls. Garnish each bowl with a few nori strips and scallions.

Ingredients:

6 cups	water or soup stock
6	large shitake mushrooms, soaked and sliced
½	cake tofu, cubed
1	dozen snow peas, with stems removed
4 tsp	miso, pureed in a little water
	toasted nori strips
	scallions

Baked Goods

Oat Crackers

Mix all ingredients together except water. Then mix in enough water to make a firm dough. Cool slightly. Spoon onto a greased cookie sheet, gently pressing them flat. Bake at 400°F for 15 minutes or until brown.

Ingredients:

2 cups	quick cooking rolled oats
½ tsp	baking powder or
½ tsp	baking soda
1 tsp	cinnamon
1 tbsp	tahini
⅓ cup	organic raisins
1	banana, mashed
½ cup	boiling water
	extra oats

Flaxseed and Apple Sauce Muffins

Using a food processor or coffee grinder, mill the flaxseed until it looks like cornmeal. In a large mixing bowl, whisk together flaxseed, spelt flour and the baking powder. Mix thoroughly together the molasses, apple sauce, soy milk, ghee and egg replacer.

Lightly grease muffin tins with ghee. Spoon the batter equally and bake in a 350°F oven for 18 minutes or until done.

Yields 12 muffins.

Ingredients:

2 cups	flaxseeds
1¼ cups	spelt flour
1 tbsp	baking powder
½ cup	black strap molasses
⅓ cup	unsweetened apple sauce
¼ cup	plain soy milk
¼ cup	ghee
½ cup	egg replacer

Appetizers

Hummus

Soak the garbanzos over night in 3 cup of water. Drain. Using new water, cook until tender (2–4 hours). Drain and save the liquid. Mash the garbanzos with a fork (or in a blender). Add the remaining ingredients, plus enough of the liquid to make it spreadable. Top with parsley. Chill for a few hours.

Ingredients:

1½ cup	garbanzo beans (chick peas)
¾ cup	liquid from chick peas or water
¼ cup	lemon juice
¼ cup	tahini
1 tsp	dulse powder
4	garlic cloves, crushed
¼ cup	flaxseed oil
1 tsp	Bragg's liquid aminos
4	shitake mushrooms, boiled (optional)
½ tsp	fresh rosemary (optional)
	sprig of parsley

Guacamole Dip

Peel the avocados and mash with a fork. Add lemon juice and other ingredients to taste. Serve on crackers or use as a vegetable dip. Go easy on it as it is high in calories.

Ingredients:

1 or 2	ripe avocados
	lemon juice, to taste
1	clove chopped garlic
	finely chopped onion or scallion
½ tsp	coriander (optional)

Herb Oil

With food processor running, drop onion and garlic in and process until minced. Add herbs and dulse powder and process until chopped (20 seconds). Add rest of ingredients and process until well mixed. Use as is, or transfer to a dark glass jar and freeze until ready to use. Fill the glass jar only ¾ full to prevent breakage.

Yields 1 cup.

Ingredients:

1	green onion or ½ of small onion
2	cloves garlic, chopped
¼ cup	packed tarragon, basil, mint parsley or cilantro leaves
¼ tsp	dulse powder
1 tsp	lemon juice
	Dash cayenne
¼ cup	extra virgin olive oil
¼ cup	flaxseed oil

Tomato Spread

With food processor running, drop onion and/or garlic in and process until minced. Add tomatoes and dulse powder and process until chopped (20 seconds). Add rest of ingredients and process until well mixed. Use as is, or transfer to a dark glass jar and freeze until ready to use. Fill the glass jar only ¾ full to prevent breakage. Use on toast, pasta, baked potatoes, or baked tofu.

Yields ½ cup.

Ingredients:

1	green onion or ½ small onion
2	cloves garlic
½ tbsp	fresh tomatoes
1 tsp	dulse powder
1 tsp	lemon juice
	dash cayenne
¼ cup	extra virgin olive oil
¼ cup	flaxseed oil

Soups

Cream of Asparagus Soup with Dill

Sauté onion in a little water plus olive oil until soft. Cut asparagus into small pieces. Add to onion and sauté a few more minutes. Add stock, oats, and dulse powder; bring to a boil. Simmer 15 minutes. Transfer to a blender and puree. Reheat if necessary. Add lemon juice to taste and serve garnished with dill.

Yields 6 servings.

Ingredients:

2 tsp	extra-virgin olive oil
1	onion, chopped
1	bunch asparagus, washed and trimmed
5 cups	vegetable stock or water
½ cup	rolled oats
½ tsp	dulse powder
	freshly squeezed lemon juice

Garnish: Fresh dill

Squash-Ginger Soup

Sauté onion, garlic and ginger in a little water plus oil until transparent, about four minutes. Add squash and potatoes and cook, stirring occasionally, for five minutes. Stir in arrowroot flour, until dissolved. Add vegetable stock or water, 1 cup at a time. Stir in mustard, cinnamon and vinegar. Simmer uncovered, stirring occasionally, over medium-low heat for 30–45 minutes, or until sauce is thick and vegetables are tender. Season to taste with fresh basil, cayenne, and dulse powder.

Yields 4 servings.

Ingredients:

1	onion, diced
3	cloves garlic, minced or crushed
1 tsp	grated ginger
2 tbsp	extra virgin olive oil
1	large butternut squash, peeled, seeded and chopped
2	potatoes, peeled and chopped
2 tbsp	arrowroot flour dissolved in
2 tbsp	of cold water
3 cups	vegetable stock or water
2 tbsp	prepared mustard
¾ tsp	cinnamon
2 tbsp	apple cider vinegar
⅛ tsp	cayenne pepper
1 tsp	dulse powder
½ tbsp	fresh basil

Miso Soup with Ginger

Place wakame in small bowl of water and soak for 5 minutes. Put 6 cups of water in a 3-quart pot and bring to a simmer. Remove wakame from water and chop into small pieces, removing the spine. Add chopped wakame and shitake mushrooms to soup. Simmer for 10 minutes, adding ginger, parsley, and tofu cubes in the last minute or 2 of cooking time. Pour a bit of broth into each serving bowl and dissolve 1 tbsp miso into each bowl. Fill bowl with soup and stir gently. Garnish each bowl with scallions.

Yields 4 servings.

Ingredients:

4"	piece of wakame
6 cups	water
6	shitake mushrooms, sliced
1 tbsp	grated ginger root
¼ lb	firm tofu, cut into cubes
4 tbsp	miso
¼ cup	chopped parsley

Garnish:

2	scallions, thinly sliced

Carrot-Ginger Soup

Boil water or vegetable stock. Chop the onion, celery and carrots and add to water. Add the dulse powder, Bragg's, basil, garlic and ginger. Reduce heat and simmer, covered, for 10–15 minutes until the carrots are tender. Remove 1½ cup of the sliced carrots from the soup and set them aside. Strain the remaining soup reserving the broth, and puree the vegetables in a blender. Recombine the carrots, puree, and the broth. Stir well and bring the soup to a gentle boil. Season with dill to taste.

Yields 4 servings.

Ingredients:

1	onion
2	celery stalks
5 cups	carrots, cut in ⅛" rounds
4 cups	water or vegetable stock
½ tsp	dulse powder
½ tsp	Bragg's liquid aminos
½ tsp	basil
3	cloves garlic, chopped
2 tsp	ginger, chopped or grated
	fresh dill to taste

Carrot-Squash Soup

Bring water and vegetables to a boil in pot, add spices and reduce to simmer. Skim off any foam from the top. Simmer until vegetables are tender, then drain vegetables, reserving the broth. Remove bay leaves. Process the cooked vegetables in small batches in a blender or food processor, adding the cooking broth, as necessary.

Add almond butter and ginger to the last batch. When soup is all blended, thin with water if necessary. Add the fresh herbs to the soup and reheat gently, stirring often.

Ingredients:

1	butternut squash, peeled and cubed
3 cups	carrots, sliced
4–5 cups	water or vegetable stock
1 cup	chopped onion
2	cloves garlic, crushed
1 cup	celery, sliced
½ tsp	ground cinnamon
1 tsp	coriander
½ tsp	nutmeg
2	bay leaves
½ tsp	dulse powder
1 tbsp	almond butter
	2" piece of fresh ginger, peeled and grated
1	bunch fresh cilantro, dill or parsley, finely chopped

Barley and Kidney Bean Soup

Wash the barley and beans. Layer the ingredients in the pot in the following order: first the onion, then mushrooms, barley and kidney beans. Add tomato sauce and water. Bring to a boil, reduce the flame and simmer until the beans are almost done, about 2 hours. Add celery and parsley and cook for another 10 minutes. Season with Bragg's. Garnish with broccoli sprouts.

Ingredients:

½ cup	barley
¼ cup	kidney beans
1	onion, chopped
1	stalk celery, finely chopped
½ cup	chopped parsley
4	shitake mushrooms
3 cups	stewed tomatoes or tomato sauce
3 cups	water Bragg's liquid aminos
	broccoli sprouts

Vegetable Soup with Millet

Place the millet, vegetables, turmeric and water in a 2-quart soup pot; bring to a boil, reduce heat, cover, and simmer for 10 minutes. Add garlic and Bragg's and simmer for 5 minutes more. Stir. Chop the parsley into fine pieces and place a teaspoonful on top of each serving of soup.

Yields 4 servings.

Ingredients:

1–1½ cups	cooked millet
2 cups	baked squash or turnips
	cooked turnip greens
5 cups	water
1 tsp	turmeric powder
1	clove garlic, chopped
2 tbsp	Bragg's liquid aminos
1	handful parsley

Salads and Dressings

Cucumber Mint Salad

Combine vegetables and toss with lemon and oil mixture.

Ingredients:

1	English cucumber, sliced
3	carrots, grated
2	bunches of radishes, sliced
¼ cup	onions, thinly sliced
3	tomatoes, sliced
¼ tsp	garlic
1 tbsp	fresh mint, chopped
2 tbsp	lemon juice mixed with
2 tsp	flaxseed oil

Watercress Salad

Wash watercress, lettuce and cabbage by placing leaves in a sink full of cold water. Drain and repeat. Spin or pat dry. Tear greens into bite-size pieces and place in a large salad bowl. Add cucumber and set aside. Place all ingredients for dressing in a small jar, cover, and shake well. Pour half of the dressing on the salad and toss. The remainder of the dressing will keep in the refrigerator for at least a week.

Yields 6 servings and ⅔ cup vinaigrette.

Ingredients:

Salad:

1	bunch watercress, tough stems removed
½	head red leaf lettuce
½ cup	red cabbage, finely sliced and chopped
1	cucumber, thinly sliced

Dressing:

⅓ cup	flaxseed oil
¼ cup	apple cider vinegar
1 tsp	tamari or Bragg's liquid aminos
1 tsp	chopped fresh oregano (or ¼ tsp dried)
½ tsp	chopped fresh rosemary

Green Salad

Wash the lettuce, pat dry, and cut into thin slices. Wash the watercress and cut the thick stems into small pieces. Wash the celery, and cut into thin slices on the diagonal. Peel and thinly slice the cucumber. Combine the vegetables together in a salad bowl. Toss lightly. Place in individual bowls and top with Tofu-Ginger Dressing.

Yields 4 servings.

Ingredients:

½	head leaf lettuce
1	bunch watercress
2	stalks celery
½	cucumber, peeled and sliced finely
½ cup	broccoli or red clover sprouts

Mustard Green Salad with Tofu-Dill Dressing

Wash mustard greens and lettuce by placing leaves in a sink full of cold water. Drain and repeat. Spin or pat dry. Tear greens into bite-size pieces and place in a large salad bowl with radishes and sprouts on top. Set aside.

Place all ingredients for dressing in a blender and blend until smooth and creamy. Dress salad with about ¾ cup of the dressing before serving and toss well. The leftover dressing will keep in the refrigerator for about a week.

Yields 6 servings and 1½ cups dressing.

Ingredients:

Salad:
½ bunch mustard greens
½ head green leaf lettuce
½ bunch red radishes, sliced
handful mung bean sprouts

Dressing:
½ lb silken tofu
2 tbsp apple cider vinegar or lemon juice
1 tbsp fresh dill (or 1 tsp dried)
½ cup water

Tabouli

Place bulgur in a mixing bowl. Pour boiling water over bulgur; cover and let stand 15 minutes. Fluff grain with fork. While grain is cooling to room temperature, chop vegetables. Add parsley, scallions, cucumber, tomato, and mint to cooked bulgur; toss together.

Blend lemon juice, oil, and tamari with a fork. Pour over bulgur and vegetables; toss again. Serve immediately or store in refrigerator in covered glass container.

Yields 4 servings.

Ingredients:

Salad:
1 cup whole-wheat bulgur
1 cup boiling water
⅓ cup finely chopped parsley
2 scallions, finely chopped
½ cup cucumber, chopped into small pieces
½ cup tomato, chopped into small bites
¼ cup chopped mint

Dressing:
¼ cup freshly squeezed lemon juice
3 tbsp extra-virgin olive oil
1 tbsp tamari or Bragg's liquid aminos

Cole Slaw with Sprouts

Combine cabbage, scallions, carrot and sprouts in a large mixing bowl. Mix dressing ingredients together. Toss salad.

Yields 6 servings.

Ingredients:

Salad:
3 cups shredded green cabbage
3 scallions, finely sliced
½ cup grated carrot
1 cup broccoli or red clover sprouts

Dressing:
2 tbsp flaxseed oil
2 tbsp extra-virgin olive oil
3 tbsp balsamic vinegar
¼ tsp dulse powder

Four Colour Salad

Mix the beets, carrots, cabbage and seeds together in a bowl, tossing with the dressing. Arrange the parsley around the edges of the bowl and serve.

Yields 4 servings.

Ingredients:

Salad:

2	medium beets, peeled and shredded
3	medium carrots, peeled and shredded
½ cup	cabbage, shredded
	few sprigs parsley
1 tbsp	pumpkin seeds
1 tbsp	sunflower seeds

Dressing:

1 tbsp	flaxseed oil
1 tbsp	lemon juice
¼ tsp	dulse powder
	squirt of Bragg's liquid aminos

Purple and Green Salad

Wash and tear the spinach into small pieces and mix with the other ingredients. Toss with the dressing.

Yields 6 servings.

Ingredients:

Salad:

2 cups	shredded purple cabbage
2 dozen	cherry tomatoes
1 cup	chopped parsley
2 cups	raw spinach
⅓ cup	raw pumpkin seeds

Dressing:

1 tbsp	flaxseed oil
1 tbsp	apple cider vinegar
½ tsp	dulse powder
	squirt of Bragg's liquid aminos

Potato Salad with Dill

Add potatoes to a large pot of boiling water. Cook 15–20 minutes until just tender. Drain and cool in a mixing bowl. Add peppers, green onions and cucumbers.

In a separate bowl, mix the dill, lemon juice or vinegar, mustard and honey. Add the oil slowly and stir vigorously, until the dressing is smooth and thick. Pour it over the potatoes, stirring it in well. Store any excess dressing in a dark glass bottle in the fridge.

Ingredients:

Salad:

4 cups	new red potatoes, scrubbed and cubed
6 cups	water
1 cup	red peppers, sliced
½ cup	green onions, diced
1 cup	English cucumber, cubed

Dressing:

⅓ cup	fresh dill, chopped finely
¼ cup	lemon juice or apple cider vinegar
1½ tbsp	Dijon mustard
½ tsp	honey
½ cup	flaxseed oil

Quinoa Salad

Optional garnishes: Tomatoes cut in wedges or broccoli, alfalfa or red clover sprouts

Rinse quinoa with warm water and drain through a fine strainer. Place quinoa in a 3-quart pan with water; bring to a boil. Turn heat to low, cover, and simmer for 15 minutes. Add drained hiziki or arame and let mixture sit on very low heat, uncovered, for an extra 5 minutes so it dries out. This makes the grain fluffier for salads. Toss quinoa with fork and let cool.

Add carrots, parsley, cucumber, red pepper, seeds, and garlic to quinoa; mix thoroughly. Combine lemon juice, oil, and Bragg's. Pour over quinoa and toss well. Garnish with tomatoes and sprouts if desired.

Ingredients:

Salad:

1⅔ cup	dry quinoa
3⅓ cups	water
1 cup	chopped carrots
¾ cup	chopped parsley
½ cup	cucumber, finely chopped
½ cup	red pepper, finely chopped
⅓ cup	sunflower seeds
4	cloves garlic, minced
½ cup	soaked hiziki or arame

Dressing:

⅓ cup	freshly squeezed lemon juice
2 tbsp	flaxseed oil
1 tbsp	extra-virgin olive oil
1 tbsp	Bragg's liquid aminos

Bean and Cabbage Salad

Mix the drained beans, vegetables and sunflower seeds in a bowl. Make the dressing in a separate bowl and stir. Pour the dressing over the salad and toss gently. Chill for at least 2 hours before serving.

Yields 7 cups.

Ingredients:

Salad:

2 cups	green beans, gently steamed and sliced
1 cup	red cabbage, shredded and cut into 1" pieces
1 cup	black beans, cooked and drained
¼ cup	chopped onion
2	cloves garlic, chopped finely
½ cup	celery, diced
½ cup	carrot, finely chopped
½ cup	red pepper, diced
½ cup	parsley, chopped
¼ cup	raw sunflower seeds

Dressing:

⅓ cup	freshly squeezed lemon juice
1 tbsp	extra-virgin olive oil
3 tbsp	flaxseed oil
2 tsp	tamari or Bragg's liquid aminos
½ tsp	dulse powder

Marinated Beet Salad

Combine vinegar, dulse powder, sweetener and dill. Pour over beets and chill for several hours. Before serving add the onions and cucumbers. Top with sprouts.

Yields 5 servings.

Ingredients:

5	cooked beets, sliced ¼" thick
1	medium onion, sliced thinly and separated into rings
1	medium English cucumber, sliced
1 tsp	dried or fresh dill
½ cup	apple cider vinegar
½ tsp	dulse powder
½ tsp	honey or maple syrup
1 cup	sprouts

Sesame Salad Dressing

Blend all ingredients together in a blender until nearly smooth. Refrigerate in a dark closed glass container.

Ingredients:

¼ cup	extra virgin olive oil
¼ cup	flaxseed oil
¼ cup	sesame seeds or tahini
2 tbsp	fresh lemon juice
½ tsp	dulse powder
1 cup	chopped parsley (optional)

Avocado Dressing

Mash avocado with fork. Shake all ingredients together in a jar, or put everything into a blender or food processor and blend until quite smooth. Keep in a closed dark glass bottle in the refrigerator and use within 3 days. Yields 1 cup.

Ingredients:

2 tbsp	flaxseed oil
1	large ripe avocado
3 tbsp	lemon juice
¼ tsp	dulse powder
½ tsp	rosemary
	dash cayenne
	dash garlic powder

Tofu-Ginger Dressing

Grate the fresh ginger very finely. Combine the ingredients in a blender and puree until creamy.

Yields 4 servings.

Ingredients:

½ tsp	fresh ginger, grated
1	8-oz cake soft tofu
¼ cup	water
2 tbsp	flaxseed oil
2 tbsp	lemon juice
¼ tsp	dulse powder
½ tsp	rosemary
½ tsp	Bragg's liquid aminos

Lemon Tahini Dressing

In a small bowl, combine lemon juice and tahini and blend for 2–3 minutes. Add the remaining ingredients, one at a time, mixing well after each addition until the dressing is light and creamy. Store in a capped dark glass bottle in the refrigerator and use within 2 weeks. Avoid exposure to oxygen by keeping the lid on the bottle when not in use.

Ingredients:

4 tbsp	lemon juice
2 tbsp	tahini
2 tbsp	flaxseed oil
½ tsp	dulse powder
3 tbsp	barley miso
2 tsp	prepared mustard
4 tbsp	water

Grain Dishes

Wild Rice and Quinoa

Keeping grains separate, rinse under cold water before cooking. Bring water to a boil. Add wild rice. Simmer 45 minutes. Add quinoa and simmer 10 more minutes, covered. Add hiziki and cook 5 more minutes. Remove from heat and allow it to steam, covered for five minutes. Fluff with a fork.

Serve on a bed of red cabbage with broccoli and red clover sprouts.

Yields 2–4 servings.

Ingredients:

½ cup	wild rice
½ cup	quinoa
1½ cups	water
¼ cup	hiziki

Quick Veggie Rice

Sauté chopped onions in water with a little oil. When transparent, add cinnamon, bay leaf, cumin, turmeric, rice and vegetables. Sauté two minutes and add 3 cups of water. Bring to a boil, add dulse powder and coconut milk and simmer, covered, over low heat. Cook for 20 minutes (35–40 minutes for brown rice).

Garnish with coriander leaves or sprouts and serve with a bean dish.

Yields 2 servings.

Ingredients:

1	small onion, chopped
1 tsp	olive oil
1	small stick of cinnamon
1	bay leaf
1 tsp	turmeric powder
1 tsp	ground cumin
1 cup	basmati rice
½ cup	wild rice
1 cup	mixed chopped vegetables (potato, carrots, peas, beans)
4 cups	water
	dulse powder to taste
⅓ cup	coconut milk

Garnish:
coriander leaves, red clover or broccoli sprouts

Healing Lemon Rice

Bring water to a boil. Add rice and turmeric powder and simmer, covered until done (20–30 minutes).

Gently heat water with a little oil in frying pan and sauté garlic, red or green pepper and mushrooms until tender. Stir this into the cooked rice. Squeeze lemon over the rice. Mix well, but try not to mash the rice.

Yields 4 servings.

Ingredients:

2 cups	white basmati rice
4 cups	water
1½ tsp	turmeric powder
1 tbsp	extra virgin olive oil
1	red or green pepper, chopped
2	cloves garlic, chopped
4	shitake mushrooms, sliced (optional)
1	lemon, to be squeezed

Couscous

Measure out the couscous and set aside. Boil an equivalent amount of water in a medium sized pot. Add couscous, cover and remove from heat. Let stand 5–10 minutes. Place couscous in a bowl and fluff with a fork before serving.

Ingredients:

½–⅓ cup	dry couscous per person
	Equivalent amount of water

Millet Casserole

Wash and drain the millet and chop the onion. Sauté the onion in a little water plus oil in a 3-quart saucepan over medium heat. Chop the red pepper and the celery and add to the onion, stirring well before each addition. Now add the turmeric, millet, water, and dulse and bring to a boil. Reduce heat, cover, and simmer for 40 minutes or until millet is done.

Yields 4 servings.

Ingredients:

3 cups	millet
1	medium onion
1 tbsp	extra virgin olive oil
½	red bell pepper
3	stalks celery
5 cups	water
2 tsp	turmeric powder
1 tsp	dulse powder

Vegetable Kasha

Place a small amount of water in a pot and begin to sauté onions, garlic and mushrooms. Add ghee and continue to sauté until onions are transparent. Add carrot and sauté 3 more minutes. Add chopped parsley and buckwheat and sauté another 4 minutes, stirring occasionally. Add boiling water and dulse powder. Cover and simmer for 25 minutes or until all the water is absorbed. Garnish with sprouts.

Ingredients:

1 cup	buckwheat groats, roasted
2 cups	boiling water
½ tsp	ghee
1	onion, finely chopped
2	cloves garlic, finely chopped
3	shitake mushrooms, sliced
1	carrot, chopped
¼ cup	chopped parsley
½ tsp	dulse powder
	broccoli, sunflower, mung bean or red clover sprouts

Shitake Brown Rice

Soak the mushrooms in ½ cup water for 15 minutes. Remove the hard stem with a knife. Slice the mushrooms and then cut into small pieces. Wash rice and place all ingredients in a pot. Bring to a boil. Reduce heat and simmer, covered, for 1 hour or until rice is done. Season with Bragg's. Add a small amount of flaxseed oil once served.

Ingredients:

1 cup	brown rice
2	shitake mushrooms
2 cups	water
1 tsp	dulse powder
	Bragg's liquid aminos
	flaxseed oil

Bean Dishes

Red Lentils and Butternut Squash Puree

Wash and drain lentils. Put lentils, squash, and water in a small pan. Bring to a boil. Reduce heat and simmer, covered for 25–30 minutes. Puree in a blender with parsley. Sauté onions and garlic in a little water plus olive oil, adding turmeric, dulse and curry powder. Stir into the lentil mixture. Garnish with broccoli or red clover sprouts.

Yields 1½ cups.

Ingredients:

¼ cup	dried red lentils
½ cup	butternut squash, peeled and cut into small chunks
1½ cups	water
1 tbsp	chopped parsley
	extra virgin olive oil
2	cloves garlic, minced
2	medium sized onions, chopped
½ tsp	turmeric powder
½ tsp	dulse or kelp powder
	Curry powder, to taste
	broccoli or red clover sprouts

Navy Bean Soup

Wash and soak navy beans 2–8 hours. Drain. Bring them to a boil in 4 cups water, with sea vegetables and bay leaves for one hour, covered, or pressure cook 40 minutes. Beans should be very soft. Slice leeks in half lengthwise and wash very well to remove all dirt; slice finely. Dice onion. Sauté leeks and onion in a little oil. When the beans are soft, add the sautéed leeks to them. Add 2–3 cups of water if needed for a creamy consistency. Add chopped carrots, broccoli and red pepper. Simmer 20–30 minutes over low heat. Puree part of the beans to make a smoother soup. Chop fresh herbs and add them to the soup with the miso. Garnish with broccoli or red clover sprouts.

Ingredients:

1 cup	navy beans
1–2	strips kombu or wakame
2–3	large leeks
1	onion
1	clove garlic, finely chopped
2–3	bay leaves (optional)
1 tsp	olive oil
3	carrots, finely chopped
4	broccoli florets, finely chopped
1	red pepper, finely chopped
	White or light miso to taste
	Fresh or dried basil or dill

Mung Beans and Rice

Rinse beans and rice. Bring water to a boil, add rice and beans and let boil over a medium flame. Prepare vegetables. Add vegetables to cooking rice and beans. Heat a little water with olive oil, or use ghee to sauté onions, garlic and ginger over a medium-high heat. Add spices (not herbs). When nicely done, combine onions with cooking mung beans and rice. You will need to stir the dish often to prevent scorching. Add herbs. Continue to cook until completely well done over a medium-low heat, stirring often. The consistency should be rich, thick and soup-like, with ingredients barely discernible. Garnish with red clover or broccoli sprouts.

Yields 4–6 servings.

Ingredients:

1 cup	mung beans
1 cup	basmati rice
9 cups	water
4–6 cups	chopped assorted vegetables (carrots, celery, zucchini, broccoli, etc.)
2 tbsp	olive oil or ghee
2	onions, chopped
⅓ cup	minced ginger root
4	cloves garlic, minced
2 tsp	turmeric powder
½ tsp	pepper
1 tsp	(heaping) garam masala
1 tbsp	sweet basil
2	bay leaves
	seeds of 5 cardamom pods
	Bragg's liquid aminos or soy sauce to taste

Black Bean Soup

In a small bowl, cover the sun-dried tomatoes with boiling water and set aside. In a soup pot, sauté the onions, garlic, and cayenne in little water with the oil for about 5 minutes, stirring frequently, until the onions are translucent. Add the cumin, dulse powder, ⅓ cup water, and the juice from the tomatoes. Break up the tomatoes by squeezing them into the soup pot, or chop them coarsely right in the can and add them to the pot. Cover and bring to a boil. Lower the heat and simmer, covered, for 5 minutes. Add the black beans and their liquid, and continue to simmer, stirring occasionally to prevent sticking. Drain and chop the softened sun-dried tomatoes. Add them to the soup and cook for 5–10 minutes longer, until the onions are tender. Stir in the cilantro and remove the soup from the heat. Puree half of the soup in a blender or food processor and return it to the pot. If the soup is too thick, add some water or tomato juice. Reheat gently.

Yields 4–6 servings.

Ingredients:

10	sun-dried tomatoes (not packed in oil)
1 cup	boiling water
1½ cups	finely chopped onions
3	garlic cloves, minced or pressed
2 tbsp	olive oil
1 tsp	ground cumin
1 tsp	dulse powder
¼ tsp	cayenne pepper
⅓ cup	water
3 cups	undrained canned tomatoes (28 oz can)
4 cups	undrained cooked black beans (two 16 oz cans or 2 cups dry beans)
¼ cup	chopped fresh cilantro
	additional water or tomato juice

Lentil Soup

Wash lentils and combine with celery, carrots, red pepper, onion, garlic, dulse powder, pepper and water in a large saucepan. Bring to a boil. Reduce heat and simmer 35 minutes or until vegetables are tender. Remove from heat and add Bragg's, lemon juice and parsley.

Yields 4 servings.

Ingredients:

1 cup	dried split red lentils
3	stalks celery, coarsely chopped
2	medium carrots, finely chopped
1	red pepper, chopped
1	onion, chopped
2	cloves garlic, finely chopped
6 cups	water
1 tsp	dulse powder
¼ tsp	freshly ground pepper
1 tsp	Bragg's liquid aminos
½ cup	parsley, finely chopped
2 tsp	lemon juice

Lentil Burgers

Preheat oven to 350. Gently sauté the garlic, onion, celery and carrots in water and olive oil in a large pot until they soften slightly. Add the lentils, water, and dulse powder and simmer for about an hour until the lentils are soft and the liquid is absorbed.

Add 2 tbsp of the flour, and the spices and mix well, cooking for 2 more minutes. Let the mixture cool until it is not too hot to handle. Form patties of the mixture, about ½" thick. Coat each patty with some of the remaining flour. It will make about 18 patties. Oil a baking tray and place the patties on the tray. Grill for 15 minutes on one side, then flip them and grill for 10 more minutes. Serve with Lemon-Tahini Dressing and broccoli or red clover sprouts.

Ingredients:

2 tbsp	extra virgin olive oil
2	cloves garlic, finely chopped
1	onion, chopped
1	celery stalk, chopped
1 tsp	dulse powder
2	carrots, finely chopped
1 cup	green lentils
2 cups	water
4 tbsp	spelt flour
½ tsp	ground ginger
½ tsp	cumin
½ tsp	turmeric powder

Gingered Lentil Sandwich Spread

Gently saute the mushrooms in a little water and olive oil. Add to cooked lentils and put all ingredients in a food processor or blender; blend until smooth. If using a blender, blend ¼ of the mixture, then add the rest a little at a time. Will keep in the refrigerator for several days.

Yields 2 cups.

Ingredients:

2 cups	cooked lentils
2 tsp	extra-virgin olive oil
1 tbsp	grated gingerroot
1 tbsp	whole-grain mustard
1 tbsp	flaxseed oil
3	shitake mushrooms, sliced
2	scallions, sliced
1 tsp	dulse powder
1 tsp	fresh rosemary
¼ cup	water
	Bragg's liquid aminos to taste

Bean Salad

Steam the green and yellow beans until just tender. Mix all ingredients together and serve with avocado dressing.

Ingredients:

1 cup	cooked kidney beans
½ cup	cooked chickpeas
2 cups	steamed green beans, cut into 1½ " pieces
1 cup	steamed yellow wax beans, cut into 1½ " pieces
1	red pepper, finely chopped
½ cup	parsley, chopped
1	onion, finely chopped

Curried Chickpeas

Prepare chickpeas. Heat water with the oil in a cooking pot and add cumin seeds. When the seeds turn brown, add the chopped onions. Allow them to cook for one minute on medium heat and then add the garlic. Cook until onions are light brown, then add the ginger. Cook for 1–2 minutes. Add paprika, turmeric, cayenne and coriander powder. Stir and cook for another minute. Then add chopped tomatoes or tomato paste to the mixture. Stir and sauté for a few minutes more. Add the chickpeas to the above mixture along with 2 cups of water (use the water from cooking the chickpeas). Let the mixture simmer for a few minutes. Add garam masala. Serve with rice. Sprinkle with chopped coriander leaf or broccoli, sunflower, red clover or alfalfa sprouts.

Yields 4–6 servings.

Ingredients:

5 cups	cooked chickpeas (two 19 oz cans or 2½ cups dry)
4 tbsp	extra virgin olive oil
1½ tsp	cumin seeds
1	large onion, peeled and chopped
2 tsp	garlic, minced or crushed
3–4 tsp	grated fresh ginger
½ tsp	turmeric powder
3 tsp	coriander powder
1 tsp	paprika powder
¼ tsp	cayenne powder
1	large tomato, chopped
¼ tsp	garam masala (optional)
2 cups	water
	fresh coriander leaf, chopped or sprouts (broccoli, red clover, sunflower)

Lentil Rice Casserole

In a pot, sauté onions in a little water plus olive oil until translucent — approximately three minutes. Add spices and cook two minutes, stirring. Add lentils, rice and water and bring to a boil. Reduce heat to simmer and cook for 15 minutes. Stir in the cubed tofu. Preheat oven to 400°F. Oil casserole or loaf pan and dust with cornmeal.

Remove lentil-rice mixture from heat and pour into prepared baking dish. Cover tightly and bake for 30 minutes at 400°F, then reduce temperature to 350°F, and bake uncovered for another 35 minutes. Remove from oven and allow to stand for 20 minutes. Serve with spicy onions.

Spiced onions: Place a skillet over medium heat and add water with the olive oil. Add onions and turn heat to low. Add spices and cook slowly until the onions are limp (approximately 10 minutes). Add lemon juice and stir mixture constantly for two minutes. Top each serving of casserole with 1 tbsp of onion mixture. Serve with greens.

Yields 4 servings.

Ingredients:

1 tbsp	extra virgin olive oil
2 cups	onions, diced
1½ tsp	dulse powder
¼ tsp	cardamon powder
¼ tsp	turmeric
½ tsp	ground cumin
¾ cup	red lentils, rinsed and drained
¾ cup	brown rice, rinsed and drained
1 cup	tofu, cubed
3⅓ cups	water or stock
	olive oil and cornmeal for pan

Spicy Onions:

1 tbsp	olive oil
1½ cups	onions, slivered
¼ tsp	cardamon powder
½ tsp	turmeric powder
¼ tsp	ground cumin
2 tbsp	lemon juice

Chickpea Shitake Supreme

In a large pan or pot, sauté the chopped onion and mushrooms in a little water plus the oil until browned.

In a blender, blend the cashews, sesame seeds, flour and dulse powder with the water. Add the cooked onion-mushroom mixture and continue to blend. Return this sauce to the pan and add the peas and chickpeas. Bring to a boil, then simmer covered for approximately 15–20 minutes, until it thickens. Serve topped with sprouts.

Yields 4–6 servings.

Ingredients:

1	onion, chopped
2	shitake mushrooms, chopped
1 tbsp	extra virgin olive oil
½ cup	cashew pieces, raw, unsalted
4 tsp	sesame seeds
¼ cup	spelt flour
½ tsp	dulse powder
2 cups	of water
1½ cups	green peas
2 cups	cooked chickpeas
	(one 19 oz can or 1 cup dry)
	broccoli, sunflower, mung bean or clover sprouts

Potato Lentil Casserole

Set oven to 375°F.

In a frying pan, gently sauté the onions, garlic, pepper, celery or zucchini and mushrooms in a little water plus oil until tender. Layer the sautéed vegetables and uncooked lentils in a casserole dish, starting and finishing with a vegetable layer and sprinkling each layer with parsley and thyme.

Slice the potatoes thinly and lay them on top of the casserole. Warm the water and dissolve the miso in it. Pour over the casserole (it should completely cover the lentils and vegetables). Cover and bake for one hour at 375°F, removing the lid for the last 15 minutes to brown potatoes. Serve with a little extra stock and fresh rosemary.

Yields 6 servings.

Ingredients:

2	onions, chopped
2	cloves garlic, minced or crushed
1	red pepper, sliced
2	stalks celery, or 1 zucchini, chopped
1 tbsp	extra virgin olive oil
1 cup	shitake or maitake mushrooms, sliced
1 cup	red lentils, rinsed thoroughly
3 tbsp	fresh chopped parsley
2½ tsp	thyme
2	large potatoes, scrubbed but not peeled
1½ cups	water or stock
2 tsp	miso
	rosemary, to taste

Chickpea Spinach Loaf

In a large bowl, combine all ingredients except onions, mushrooms and spices and mix well.

Using a skillet, sauté onion, mushrooms and spices in water with a little oil until soft, then add to the bowl. Moisten with water, stock or tomato juice if too stiff. Press into loaf tin and bake at 350°F for about one hour or until loaf comes away from sides of tin. Delicious hot, or cold in sandwiches. Freezes well baked or unbaked.

Yields 4 servings.

Ingredients:

2 cups	cooked chickpeas, mashed (one 19 oz can or 1 cup dry)
1 cup	cooked brown rice (½ cup dry)
1 tbsp	extra virgin olive oil
	small bunch spinach, cooked and chopped
4	shitake mushrooms, sliced
3	carrots, grated
2 tbsp	chopped parsley
3	small tomatoes, chopped
1 tbsp	tahini
1	onion, chopped
1 tsp	ground cumin
1 tsp	coriander
1 tsp	turmeric
1 tsp	dulse powder
½ tsp	cardamom
½ tsp	chili powder

Vegetable Dishes

Potato Pockets

Thaw frozen corn and peas. Scrub potatoes. Bake in oven at 400°F for 45–55 minutes until done.

Cut potatoes in half. Scoop out centers, place in bowl, and add corn, peas, dulse powder, ghee and parsley. Mix ingredients together, adding a little water if the mixture is dry.

Put mixture back inside potato skins. Place under oven broiler for 5–10 minutes until browned. Serve immediately, topped with sprouts.

Yields 4 servings.

Ingredients:

4	large potatoes
1 cup	sweet corn (fresh or frozen)
1 tbsp	ghee
¼ cup	peas
¼ tsp	dulse powder
	several sprigs of fresh parsley or dill (or 1 tsp dry)
	broccoli or red clover sprouts

French Carrots

Scrub and cut the carrots diagonally into thin slices. Pour ½ inch water into a 2-quart pot. Add the carrots. Cover and steam over low heat for 8–10 minutes or until just soft.

Uncover the carrots and drain off excess water. Add flax oil and stir to coat the carrots. Chop the parsley. Add the parsley, toss gently, and serve at once.

Yields 4 servings.

Ingredients:

2 lb	carrots
2 tbsp	flax oil
1	small handful parsley

Stuffed Baked Squash

Prepare rice. Cut tops off squash, slice in half lengthwise and scoop out seeds and pulp.

In a pan, sauté celery, mushrooms and herbs in a little water plus oil. Combine this mixture with rice, nuts and Bragg's. Fill cavities of squash with rice mixture, and bake covered at 350°F for one hour, or until squash is tender.

Yields 4 servings.

Ingredients:

3 cups	cooked wild rice (1½ cup dry)
2	butternut squash
1 tbsp	extra virgin olive oil
2	stalks celery, chopped
½ cup	shitake mushrooms, chopped
½ tsp	thyme
½ tsp	sage
½ tsp	rosemary
½ cup	chopped nuts
1 tbsp	Bragg's liquid aminos

Baked Squash

Preheat oven to 350°F. Cut the squash in half and scoop out the seeds. Place the pieces face down on an oiled baking pan and bake for 1 hour until soft. Remove squash from oven and serve immediately. Drizzle flaxseed oil over each serving, if desired.

Yields 4 servings.

Ingredients:

1	medium acorn squash
	olive oil
	flaxseed oil

Vegetable Bean Patties

Bring stock to boil. Add lentils and turn off heat. After 30 minutes of soaking, turn on heat and simmer until lentils have softened (about 45 minutes).

Meanwhile, heat water and add mushrooms, onion, celery, red pepper and carrot. Steam until softened (10 minutes). Add spices and garlic. Stir together cooked lentils, vegetables and remaining ingredients. Add more liquid if mixture is dry and crumbly or more flour if mixture is wet and runny. Shape into patties. Cook both sides on a lightly oiled baking sheet under a broiler.

The mixture can be kept in the refrigerator for up to a week or made into patties, individually frozen on a cookie sheet and stored in freezer bags. Can be cooked without thawing. Serve with broccoli, red clover or sunflower sprouts.

Yields 6 patties.

Ingredients:

5 cups	vegetable stock, tomato juice, or water
2 cups	brown lentils, cleaned
2 tbsp	water
2 cups	onion, diced
½ cup	shitake mushrooms, chopped
½ cup	celery, finely diced
½ cup	red peppers, finely diced
½ cup	carrots, finely chopped
3	cloves garlic, minced or crushed
2 tsp	ground cumin
1 tsp	sage
	Pinch of cayenne
	Extra virgin olive oil
½ cup	quick cooking oats
½ cup	spelt flour
¼ cup	tahini
2 tsp	prepared mustard
½ tsp	dulse powder

Split Pea Puree in Nori

Wash peas and scrub carrot. Put peas, carrot, dulse powder, garlic and water in a small pan. Bring to a boil. Reduce heat and simmer, covered for 20–30 minutes. Puree in a blender with ¼ of a nori sheet. Serve rolled in a nori sheet.

Yields 3 servings.

Ingredients:

¼ cup	dried green split peas
½	carrot, sliced
1¼ cups	water
½ tsp	dulse powder
2	cloves garlic
	chopped nori sheets

Peppers with Basil

In a frying pan, gently heat the oil in a little water, then stir-fry the onion and garlic until the onion turns limp. Stir in the pepper pieces, oregano, dulse and pepper, then sauté over medium heat for about 15 minutes or until the pepper pieces soften, stirring occasionally.

Stir in the basil, rosemary and lemon juice. Serve immediately.

Yields 4 servings.

Ingredients:

2 tbsp	extra virgin olive oil
1	medium-sized onion, chopped
2	cloves garlic, crushed
4	large red peppers, seeded and chopped
1 tsp	oregano
½ tsp	dulse powder
¼ tsp	pepper
4	tbsp finely chopped fresh basil (or dried)
½ tsp	fresh rosemary
2 tbsp	lemon juice

Brassica Dishes

Scrumptious Red Cabbage and Carrots

Bring 1½ cups of water to a boil in a pot. Meanwhile, scrub carrots, slice on a diagonal and add to the pot. Add the chopped red cabbage, apple cider vinegar and maple syrup. Cover pot with a lid and let simmer 10–15 minutes.

Add the lemon juice and the water to the arrowroot. Stir well and then add to the vegetables. Allow to simmer gently and thicken for 5–10 minutes, stirring occasionally.

Yields 6–8 servings.

Ingredients:

1½ cups	water
4	large carrots
1	medium sized red cabbage (4 cups), chopped
¼ cup	apple cider vinegar
¼ cup	maple syrup
3 tbsp	lemon juice
1 tbsp	water
2 tbsp	arrowroot as thickener

Steamed Broccoli with Pumpkin and Flaxseeds

Separate the broccoli flowerets from the stems and trim ¼ inch from the stem bottoms. Peel off the thickest part of the skin and slice the stems crosswise in thin pieces. Place the broccoli stems and water in a 2 quart pot with a steamer. Steam 3 minutes. Place the pumpkin seeds and flowerets on top, cover, and steam for 3 minutes more or until bright green. Sprinkle on ground flaxseeds when serving.

Yields 4 servings.

Ingredients:

1	bunch broccoli
½ cup	water
½ cup	pumpkin seeds
¼ cup	freshly ground flaxseeds

Vegetarian Cabbage Rolls

Bring the water to a boil. Add the brown rice and simmer, covered, for 45 minutes or until done. Set aside.

Sauté the onions, garlic and mushrooms in a little water and olive oil for 5 minutes. Add the carrots and red pepper and steam gently with the onion mixture, adding a little more water if needed.

Mix the rice and sautéed vegetables together in a bowl with the ginger and dulse powder.

Preheat oven to 325°F.

In a large pot of boiling water, blanch the cabbage leaves for 30 seconds. Drain, and immerse the leaves in a bowl of cold water until cooled. Remove and pat dry. Slice a layer off the thickened stem of each leaf to make rolling easier. Spread out the leaves flat on a large working surface. Fill each leaf with an equal amount of stuffing and roll them from the stem end forward, tucking in the sides as you complete the roll. Place the rolls, seam side down, in a layer in a baking dish and pour the tomato sauce over top. Bake for 30 minutes or until the leaves are tender. The recipe can be doubled and layered in the baking dish with tomato sauce between the layers. They freeze well.

Yields 4 servings.

Ingredients:

1 cup	brown rice
2 cups	water
1 cup	chopped onion
2	cloves garlic, chopped finely
1 tsp	extra virgin olive oil
1 tbsp	water
¼ cup	dry hiziki or arame, soaked in 1 cup water
3	medium carrots, chopped finely
1	red pepper, chopped finely
6	shitake mushrooms, sliced
1 tbsp	grated, peeled ginger
1 tsp	dulse powder
10	large green cabbage leaves
½ cup	tomato sauce

Sea Vegetables

Hiziki with Sweet Potatoes

Rinse the hiziki with cold water. Soak in 4 cups warm water for 30 minutes. Drain hiziki and discard soaking water.

Peel the sweet potato and cut into French fry type slices ¼" thick. In a heavy pot or wok heat the water and steam the sweet potatoes for five minutes, stirring steadily. Add the oil and cook another two minutes. Add the hiziki, and stir-fry for 30 seconds. Add the broth, maple syrup and tamari or Bragg's. Bring to a simmer. Cover, reduce heat and simmer for four minutes.

Uncover, turn up the heat and boil away most of the liquid, stirring gently (this should take only a few seconds). Sprinkle the sesame seeds on top.

Yields 2 servings.

Ingredients:

¼ cup	dried hiziki
1	large sweet potato
1 tbsp	water
1 tsp	extra virgin olive oil
3 tbsp	water or vegetable broth
1 tsp	maple syrup
1 tbsp	tamari or Bragg's liquid aminos
1 tbsp	sesame seeds (toasted in a dry frying pan)

Dulse Salad with Lemon-Tahini Dressing

Soak the dulse in cold water. Meanwhile, cut the other vegetables for the salad. Clean the soaked dulse well, removing any pebbles. Pat dulse dry. Combine dulse, cabbage, red onion, red pepper, carrots and celery with vinegar; refrigerate for an hour or so. Combine all ingredients for dressing in a blender and blend until smooth. Serve the salad on a lettuce leaf with 1 tbsp dressing on top. Leftover dressing will keep in the refrigerator for a week.

Yields 4 servings.

Ingredients:

Salad:

1 cup	dried dulse
½ cup	shredded cabbage
1	red onion, sliced into thin rounds
1–2	stalks celery, cut into bite-size pieces
1	red pepper, chopped finely
1	carrot, chopped
1 tbsp	apple cider vinegar
4	red leaf lettuce leaves

Dressing:

¼ cup	tahini
1	clove garlic
2–3 tbsp	freshly squeezed lemon juice
½ tsp	tamari or Bragg's liquid aminos
½ cup	water

Vegetarian Sushi

Rinse rice in a sieve, then combine with water in covered pot and simmer for 40 minutes. In a small pot over low heat mix vinegar and maple syrup. Mix sauce into cooked rice and let cool. Lay nori, shiny side down, on bamboo sushi mat or cutting board. Using a quarter of the rice, cover the nori with an even layer of rice, leaving a one inch strip uncovered at the top. Place thinly sliced fillings such as red, green or yellow peppers, cucumber, carrot, avocado, etc. across width of the nori approximately a third of the way up the sheet. Roll up slowly and firmly using the mat, or keeping it tight with your fingers. Slice the roll into one inch slices with a wet knife. Serve with pickled ginger, Bragg's for dipping and wasabe, a spicy Japanese condiment similar to horseradish.

Yields 4 servings.

Ingredients:

1 cup	short-grain brown rice
2 cups	water
2–4 tbsp	rice vinegar
2 tsp	maple syrup
4	sheets nori
	Thin slices of vegetables: carrot, peppers, cucumber, avocado, etc.

Millet and Nori Rolls

Cook the millet with the water, turmeric, carrots, onions and garlic over low heat until the millet is soft, about 40 minutes. Add the ginger, dulse powder, cayenne, Bragg's, lemon and flaxseed oil. Cut tofu into ¼" slices, about 1½" wide, and steam. Spread the mixture over the bottom third of each nori sheet to ¼" deep. Layer tofu slices on top. Sprinkle on the red pepper pieces and top with a layer of sprouts. Roll the nori sheet from the bottom up, and seal the roll by moistening the top edge of the nori sheet with a little water.

Yields 2 servings.

Ingredients:

1 cup	millet, soaked overnight in 3 cups water
2	medium sized carrots, finely chopped
1 tsp	turmeric powder
1	red pepper, finely chopped
2	medium onions, diced
1	clove garlic, finely chopped
1 tsp	freshly grated ginger
2 tsp	lemon juice
1 tbsp	flaxseed oil
1	block firm tofu, cut ¼" and steamed
1 tsp	dulse powder
¼ tsp	cayenne pepper
1–2 tsp	Bragg's liquid aminos
	nori sheets
	broccoli, red clover, sunflower or alfalfa sprouts

Hiziki Salad

Wash the hiziki and soak it in warm water for 5 minutes. Place it in a saucepan and boil it for 15–20 minutes in enough water to cover it. Remove from heat, drain and let cool. Slice the hiziki into 2-inch pieces. Break the lettuce leaves into bite-sized pieces. Arrange the vegetables in a bowl and place the hiziki on top. Serve with tofu salad dressing.

Ingredients:

½	head romaine lettuce
½	cucumber, finely sliced
½ cup	broccoli, red clover or alfalfa sprouts
½ cup	parsley, chopped
1	red pepper, chopped
1	yellow pepper, chopped
½	medium onion, sliced into thin rings
1 cup	cooked hiziki

Wakame Salad

Wash the dry wakame and soak it in water for 10 minutes. Boil it with enough water to cover it for 2–3 minutes. Rinse under cold water, drain and slice it into 1-inch pieces. Break the lettuce into small bite-sized pieces. Mix the wakame, lettuce, sprouts, tomatoes and sliced cucumbers together in a bowl. Serve with a lemon-tahini salad dressing.

Ingredients:

1 cup	cooked wakame
1	head romaine lettuce
1	cucumber, finely sliced
½ cup	broccoli, red clover or alfalfa sprouts
2	tomatoes, quartered and sliced

Sprouts

The Benefits of Growing and Eating Sprouts

1) Sprouts are a quick, enjoyable, easy and inexpensive way to have a regular supply of organic greens throughout the year. They will grow indoors in any climate and require very little space.

2) Sprouts are good sources of vitamins A, B complex, C, D, E, G, K and U. They contain the minerals calcium, magnesium, phosphorus, potassium, sodium and silicon in a form that the body is easily able to utilize. The nutrients in grains, seeds and legumes increase when they are sprouted.

3) Sprouted grains and legumes provide all eight essential amino acids, which are easily absorbed when sprouts are eaten.

4) Sprouts are very high sources of enzymes which are catalysts that initiate and control the body's chemical reactions. Cancer is often thought of as a disease of enzyme deficiency.

5) Because they have a high level of simple sugars, sprouts are a good source of quick energy.

How to Make Sprouts

What You Will Need:

- 10 glass jars, either mason jars or larger ones with a wider mouth

- screen mesh or cotton unbleached cheesecloth to cover the mouths of the jars

- 10 wide rubber bands to secure the mesh or cheese-cloth

- dish drainer to angle the jars in upside down to drain between rinses

- filtered water

- organic untreated seeds — broccoli, red clover, alfalfa, mung bean etc.

The Sprouting Process:

The sprouting process consists of the following 4 stages:

1. The Dry Stage:
Store the seeds in sealed glass container in a cool, dry place, such as the refrigerator, freezer or root cellar. This lengthens their shelf life. Only raw seeds will sprout.

2. The Soaking Stage:
Nuts, seeds, grains, beans and legumes should be soaked before sprouting and ideally before use. This step removes enzyme inhibitors from the seeds and is the incubation period before sprouting. If seeds are soaked longer than 12 hours, the water should be changed. See the sprouting chart below for guidelines as to how long particular seeds need to be soaked. Measure out the correct amount of seed and place it a glass jar. Add at least twice the amount of water as seed. Soak for the prescribed length of time.

3. The Sprouting Stage:
When the seeds have soaked for the correct length of time, pour off the cloudy water or feed it to your house plants. Rinse the seeds again. Place the jar so that the seeds stay well-drained yet moist. They need adequate air circulation, and are best kept warm and in a dark or semi-dark location during the germination and initial sprouting stages. Rinse and drain the growing sprouts at least every 12 hours. In summer heat, rinse in cool water every 6 hours. Broccoli and cabbage sprouts tend to mold easily and should be rinsed every 4 hours. A few drops of food grade hydrogen peroxide can be added to the rinse water to deter mold.

4. The Greening Stage:
When the sprouts have developed their first 2 leaves, place them in strong indirect sunlight for 1–2 days to green them up. Broccoli sprouts have the highest amount of sulforaphane at 3 days, so would ideally be eaten at this time.

Sprouting Chart

Listed on the opposite page are some of the more common seeds to sprout. The asterisk* denotes the most popular choices.

• Sprouting Chart •

Seed Type	Dry Measure	Soak For	Sprout For	Yields	Length at Harvest	Tips
Pumpkin	1 cup	4 hrs	24 hrs.	2 cups	1/8"	
Sunflower*	1 cup	4 hrs	24 hrs.	2½ cups	¼"–½"	
Adzuki bean*	½ cup	8 hrs	3 days	4 cups	1"	pressure NB
Mung*	⅓ cup	8 hrs	4 days	4 cups	2"	pressure NB
Chick peas*	1 cup	12 hrs	3 days	4 cups	1"	good protein
Lentils*	¾ cup	8 hrs	3 days	4 cups	1"	whole bean
Green peas	1½ cup	8 hrs	3 days	4 cups	1"	
Pinto beans	1 cup	12 hrs	3 days	4 cups	1"	
Alfalfa*	3 tbsp	5 hrs	5 days	4 cups	2"	delicious
Broccoli*	3 tbsp	5 hrs	3 days	3 cups	1½"	spicy
Cabbage	3 tbsp	5 hrs	5 days	4 cups	1½"	
Fenugreek	¼ cup	6 hrs	5 days	4 cups	2"	rids mucous
Mustard	3 tbsp	5 hrs	5 days	4 cups	1½"	spicy
Onion	¼ cup	5 hrs	5 days	3 cups	1½"	
Radish	3 tbsp	6 hrs	5 days	4 cups	2"	spicy
Turnip	3 tbsp	6 hrs	4 days	4 cups	1½"	
Red clover*	3 tbsp	5 hrs	5 days	4 cups	2"	good taste

Beans and legumes should be soaked in very warm water to convert starches to complex sugars.
Small vegetables should be soaked in cool water.
Broccoli and cabbage sprouts should be rinsed 3 times daily to prevent mold.

Growing Baby Greens in Soil

Some seeds are better grown in a thin layer of soil. These include wheatgrass, sunflower baby greens and buckwheat greens. Wheatgrass must be juiced because its fiber is indigestible. It acts as a powerful stomach, liver, pancreas, and circulatory cleanser. It is a rich source of minerals and is abundant in vitamin B17, more commonly known as laetrile, which has proven anti-cancer activity. It is composed of 70% chlorophyll after the water is extracted. Ideally, wheat grass juice should be used within 30 minutes after being pressed. Because it is so cleansing, wheat grass juice may cause nausea after drinking as little as one oz. One should start with a small amount daily and then increase to 2–4 ozs daily. Sunflower greens contain all the essential amino acids and are considered a complete food. They have a high amount of vitamin D which helps to prevent breast cancer and are rich in chlorophyll. They act as an excellent cleanser and rebuilder and have a delicious nutty taste. They make a lively addition to salads, sandwiches, and soups.

Mung and Cabbage Crunch

Mix vegetables together. Toss with dressing.

Yields 5 servings.

Ingredients:

2 cups	mung bean sprouts
1 cup	shredded purple cabbage
15	cherry tomatoes
½ cup	chopped parsley
1 tbsp	raw sunflower seeds
1 tbsp	raw pumpkin seeds

Dressing:

1 tbsp	flaxseed oil
1 tbsp	apple cider vinegar
¼ tsp	dulse powder

Mixed Sprout Salad

Place the mung bean sprouts and half of all the other sprouts into a large bowl and mix together. Add the chopped red pepper to the sprouts along with the sesame salad dressing. Decorate the top with the rest of the sprouts and serve.

Yields 6 servings.

Ingredients:

2 cups	mung bean sprouts
1 cup	sunflower seed sprouts
½ cup	alfalfa sprouts
½ cup	broccoli sprouts
½ cup	clover sprouts
2	red peppers, chopped

Mung Bean and Broccoli Delight

Blend the sauce ingredients together until creamy. Place the vegetables in a bowl and pour the sauce over the vegetables. Toss gently and let sit for 30 minutes before serving.

Yields 6 servings.

Ingredients:

2 cups	of broccoli florets
2 cups	mung bean sprouts
1 cup	broccoli sprouts
1 cup	red peppers, chopped

Sauce:

2 tbsp	flaxseed oil
2 tbsp	Bragg's liquid aminos
1 tbsp	coriander
¼ tsp	cayenne
¼ cup	sesame seeds, soaked for 2–3 hours, or tahini

Tofu and Soy Dishes

Baked Tofu-Eggplant Pasta Spread

Lightly oil a cookie sheet with olive oil. Mix together the tofu, eggplant, tomato slices, onion and green onion slices, and garlic. Sprinkle the mixture with a little olive oil — stir gently. Sprinkle with the dried herbs and freshly ground black pepper. In a bag, shake together the dry yeast and bread crumbs. Spread it over the tofu. Shake sesame seeds over all. Bake at 375°F until it sizzles and eggplant is tender, 25 or more minutes. Meanwhile, boil the pasta as directed. Keep warm. Spoon the tofu/eggplant mixture over the individual pasta servings.

Yields 4–6 servings.

Ingredients:

1½ cups	silken tofu, cubed to one inch
1	eggplant, peeled, cut into one inch cubes and sprinkled with lemon juice
1 tbsp	extra virgin olive oil
3	medium tomatoes, thickly sliced
½ cup	thinly sliced onions
3	green onions, chopped
2	cloves garlic, finely chopped
½ tsp	oregano
½ tsp	thyme
¼ tsp	cayenne
½ tsp	dulse powder
	Good tasting nutritional yeast
	Black pepper
	Whole-wheat bread crumbs
	Sesame seeds
1 lb	whole-wheat, rice, spelt or spinach pasta (linguini or spaghetti)

Tofu and Red Pepper Sauce

Marinate tofu with Bragg's, tomato sauce, garlic and chili powder, for 1–3 hours. Then bake until browned on an oven tray at 350°F. In a large pan heat water with the oil and gently sauté onions and bell pepper for about two minutes or until tender. Add corn. Mix water with arrowroot flour; add to sautéed peppers. Transfer baked tofu to serving dish, pour pepper mixture over baked tofu, sprinkle with fresh parsley, and serve with rice.

Yields 4 servings.

Ingredients:

2	blocks tofu (500g/16 oz), diced
3 tbsp	Bragg's liquid aminos
¼ cup	tomato sauce
2	cloves garlic, chopped
½ tsp	chili powder
2 tbsp	extra virgin olive oil
1	large onion, thinly sliced
1	small red thinly sliced bell pepper
1 cup	fresh corn
½ cup	water
1 tbsp	arrowroot flour
¼ cup	fresh chopped parsley

Tofu Teriyaki

Cut tofu into large bite-sized squares and place in bowl. Blend remaining ingredients. Pour over the tofu. As time allows, marinate for one hour or longer.

Remove tofu from marinade and place in a small casserole dish along with ½ cup marinade. Bake uncovered in preheated 375°F oven for one hour, gently stirring and basting with marinade every 20 minutes.

Garnish and serve with rice and salad.

Yields 4 servings.

Ingredients:

2	blocks firm tofu (500 g/16 oz)
¼ cup	tamari or Bragg's liquid aminos
3 tbsp	lemon juice
3 tbsp	maple syrup
½ cup	orange juice
1 tsp	grated fresh ginger
3	cloves garlic, minced or crushed
¼ tsp	dry mustard
2 tsp	grated orange peel

Garnish:

chopped parsley or fresh coriander

Scrambled Tofu and Vegetables

Heat a little water plus oil in a frying pan. Add the celery and carrots and cook. Then add the shitake mushrooms, green onions, red pepper and turmeric and sauté for 1–2 minutes.

Crumble tofu with a fork and mix it into the sautéed vegetables. Cover and cook for 3–5 minutes. Season with lemon juice to taste. Garnish with onions, red clover or broccoli sprouts and serve.

Yields 2–3 servings.

Ingredients:

2–3 tbsp	olive oil
1	celery stalk, sliced
2	carrots, sliced
4	shitake mushrooms
1	red pepper, chopped
3	green onions, finely chopped
½ tsp	turmeric
2	blocks firm tofu (500 g/16 oz)
	lemon juice, to taste

Garnish:

2	green onions, sliced or red clover or broccoli sprouts

Baked Tofu

Preheat oven to 350°F. Lightly oil a baking sheet. Dip tofu slices into a bowl of nutritional yeast, coating both sides, and place them on the baking pan. Bake at 350°F for 15 minutes on one side, then turn over. Sprinkle a little more yeast on the tofu. Bake 10 more minutes until lightly browned. Squirt each piece with a little Bragg's. Serve with vegetables, rice or pasta.

Ingredients:

1–2	cakes firm tofu, cut into ¼" slices
	good tasting nutritional yeast
	olive oil
	Bragg's liquid aminos

Baked Shitake Tempeh

Slice tempeh in half and cut into 2 inch strips. Sauté mushrooms in a little water plus oil. Mix garlic, sesame seeds and water in a bowl and add tempeh and mushrooms. As time allows, marinate for one hour or longer. Turn mixture into a baking pan and bake in 350°F oven until browned (about 45 minutes to an hour) turning 2–3 times while baking.

Sauce: Sauté tomatoes, ginger, garlic and sesame seeds in a little oil or water. Add water or broth and Bragg's or tamari and simmer for 10 minutes. Sprinkle in arrowroot and stir mixture until it thickens.

Serve with baked tempeh.

Yields 3 servings.

Ingredients:

1	(340 g/12 oz) package tempeh
2	cloves garlic, minced or crushed
2 tbsp	sesame seeds
4	shitake mushrooms, sliced (optional)
1 tbsp	extra virgin olive oil
2 tbsp	water

Sauce:

3–4	tomatoes, chopped
2 tsp	grated fresh ginger
2	cloves garlic, minced or crushed
2 tbsp	sesame seeds
1 tbsp	water
	extra virgin olive oil
1 cup	water or vegetable broth
¼ cup	Bragg's liquid aminos or tamari
1 tbsp	arrowroot or cornstarch

Tofu Spinach Pasta

In a small pot of simmering water, poach tofu three minutes. Drain and set aside. In a pan, heat a little water and oil over medium heat. Add onions, garlic, spinach or kale, bay leaf, dulse, basil, oregano, and thyme. Cook, stirring occasionally, about 10 minutes or until onions are translucent, reducing heat to low after 3–4 minutes. Discard bay leaf. In food processor, puree the onion mixture with tofu and miso until smooth and creamy.

Meanwhile, in a large pot of boiling water, cook pasta until tender but firm and drain. Immediately toss with tofu mixture. Season with pepper and fresh rosemary.

Yields 4 servings.

Ingredients:

2	blocks soft tofu (500 g/16 oz)
2 tbsp	olive oil
2	onions, diced
2 cups	kale or spinach, chopped
1	bay leaf
2	cloves garlic, finely chopped
½ tsp	dulse powder
½ tsp	dried basil
½ tsp	oregano
½ tsp	thyme
¼ cup	light miso
500 g	(1 lb) fettucine, linguine, or other long noodles
	pepper and rosemary to taste

Deluxe Tofu Vegetable Scramble

Place water and oil in a 10-inch skillet on medium heat. Add onion, garlic, and scallion; sauté for several minutes, stirring in turmeric powder, cumin and coriander. Add red pepper and cabbage. Continue to sauté until vegetables are soft.

Crumble tofu into skillet with vegetables and stir. Add tomato sauce, tamari or Bragg's and parsley. Stir until everything is well mixed.

Yields 4 servings.

Ingredients:
2–3 tsp	extra virgin olive oil
½	medium onion, chopped
2	cloves garlic, minced
1	scallion, finely chopped
½	red pepper, chopped
½ cup	finely chopped red cabbage
1 tsp	cumin
½ tsp	coriander
1 lb	firm tofu
2 tsp	turmeric
½ cup	tomato sauce
1 tbsp	tamari or Bragg's liquid aminos
2 tbsp	chopped parsley

Tofu Cabbage with Ginger

Press and drain the tofu, then cut it into chunks. Cut the cabbage into shreds. Press the garlic, grate the ginger, and mix these two with the olive oil.

Cook the tofu in a little water and extra virgin olive oil to brown it. Add the ginger-garlic paste and continue cooking another minute or so. Remove from the pan.

Cook the cabbage lightly over moderate heat, using the same pan with water and olive oil. Add the tofu back in.

Season with tamari or Bragg's, adding more ginger or garlic to taste. Serve when everything is hot.

Yields 4 servings.

Ingredients:
1	block of tofu
	small head of cabbage (green, red, or Chinese)
2	large or 3 smaller cloves of garlic
1½	piece of fresh ginger root
1 tbsp	extra virgin olive oil
	tamari or Bragg's liquid aminos

Cheesy Tofu Sauce

Sauté onion and garlic in a little water and oil until slightly brown. Add other vegetables and cook for a few minutes longer. Steam tofu for 3 minutes. Blend steamed tofu and all other ingredients until smooth. Use thick in casseroles, or thin with water and serve hot over pasta dishes.

Ingredients:
2–3	green onions
2–3	cloves garlic
1 tbsp	olive oil
1 pkg.	tofu, drained and steamed
1 tbsp	miso
½ tsp	dulse powder
	Fresh rosemary, basil or dill
Optional:	carrots, red bell pepper, extra onion

Tofu Mayonnaise

While food processor is running, drop in garlic and fresh herbs to mince. Add rest of ingredients and blend smooth. May be used as a dip for vegetables, as well as a substitute for mayonnaise.

Ingredients:
1 pkg.	silken tofu
1–2	cloves garlic, minced
	Fresh dill, minced or dried dill
1 tbsp	miso or Bragg's liquid aminos
1 tbsp	fresh lemon juice
½ tsp	flaxseed oil

Veggie Tofu

Cut tofu into bite-sized pieces and sauté in water and oil. Add diced onion, grated ginger and Bragg's. Sauté until onions are soft, then remove from heat and set aside.

Place ½ inch of water in a covered frying pan or large pot and steam celery and carrots. Add other vegetables such as green pepper, frozen peas, whole kernel corn or green beans. After veggies are cooked, drain off excess water and add the tofu-onion mixture. Serve with rice or other grain.

Yields 6 servings.

Ingredients:

2	blocks firm tofu
2 tbsp	olive oil
1 cup	onion, diced
½"	of ginger, peeled and grated
2 tbsp	Bragg's
2	stalks of celery, sliced
2	small carrots, sliced
2 cups	of other chopped vegetables

Baked Tofu with Lemony Miso Sauce

Arrange tofu slices in a baking dish so that they are like dominoes, leaning upright against each other. Sprinkle the grated ginger over the tofu. Blend the miso and lemon juice together with a fork and add cold water, mixing to make a creamy sauce of medium thickness. Spoon the sauce over the tofu. Bake at 350 for 20 minutes. Garnish with scallions.

Yields 4 servings.

Ingredients:

2	cakes firm tofu, cut into ¼" slices
1 tbsp	miso
2–3 tsp	lemon juice
½"	piece of ginger, grated or finely chopped
	water
	scallions

Baked Tofu Jazz

Layer the tofu to cover the bottom of a baking dish. Marinate in lemon juice for at least one hour. Sprinkle the minced ginger and garlic evenly over the tofu. Sauté the mushrooms in a little olive oil in water. When they are cooked, layer them over the tofu. Mix together in a food processor the cooked yam (without the skin) and the tomato sauce. Add a squirt of Bragg's to taste. Spoon it over the tofu and mushrooms, spreading it evenly on top. Bake at 350°F for 25 minutes.

Ingredients:

2	cakes firm tofu, cut into ¼" slices juice of
3	lemons (juice)
2 tbsp	finely grated ginger
5	cloves garlic, minced
1½ cups	sliced shitake mushrooms
2	medium sized yams, baked or steamed
⅓ cup	tomato sauce
	Bragg's liquid aminos to taste

Tofu Sandwich Spread

Gently sauté the mushrooms, garlic and turmeric in a little water and olive oil. In a bowl, mash the tofu with the tahini using a fork or potato masher. Add lemon juice and tamari or Bragg's. Mix the mushroom mixture, carrot and red pepper in with the tofu. Chop the rosemary and stir it in. Use in sandwich making, on crackers, or stuff in cooked manicotti pasta. Serve with broccoli or red clover sprouts. Keeps refrigerated for 1 week.

Yields 3 servings.

Ingredients:

½ lb	tofu
2 tsp	tahini
	sliced green onions, to taste
½ cup	grated carrot (optional)
½	of a red pepper, chopped finely (optional)
3	shitake mushrooms, sliced (optional)
½ tsp	turmeric powder water
1 tsp	extra virgin olive oil
2	cloves garlic (optional)
½ tsp	tamari or Bragg's liquid aminos
1 tsp	fresh lemon juice
1 tsp	fresh rosemary

Tofu Casserole

Add a small amount of water to the miso and mix it with a fork or in a blender until it is creamy. Place all ingredients in a glass baking dish. Stir with a spoon, basting the ingredients with the liquid mixture. Bake at 350°F for 45 minutes or until potatoes are done, stirring and mixing the ingredients every 15 minutes.

Yields 4 servings.

Ingredients:

2	blocks firm tofu, cubed
2 tsp	turmeric
1½ tbsp	miso
¾ cup	water
3	red potatoes, cut into bite sized pieces
3	onions, cut into bite sized sections
1 cup	of broccoli florets
3	carrots, cut into ¼ inch rounds
5	whole cloves garlic
2 tsp	grated ginger
2 tsp	dulse powder

Liver Lovers

Beet Borscht

Bring the water or vegetable stock to a simmer. Add beets and onions and simmer 15 minutes. Add lemon juice and honey and simmer 10 more minutes. Add cabbage, simmer 15 more minutes. Add the dill and parsley just before serving.

Yields 8 servings.

Ingredients:

7 cups	water or vegetable stock
4 cups	beets, chopped or shredded
1 cup	green cabbage, shredded
½ cup	onion, finely chopped
1 tbsp	lemon juice
2	cloves garlic, chopped
2	bay leaves
1 tsp	dulse powder
1 tsp	honey
⅓ cup	fresh dill, finely chopped
½ cup	fresh parsley, finely chopped

Beet and Sprout Winter Salad

Using an electric blender, blend the water and the tofu until the mixture is creamy. Refrigerate.

Meanwhile, cover the beets with cold water, bring to a rolling boil and cook, covered, just until the skins easily come away from the beets (1 hour or more).

Remove the beets and hold them under running water for the skins to slip off under your finger tips.

Slice the beets into ¼ inch strips.

Transfer to a bowl. Mix in the tofu mixture and refrigerate until cold. Garnish with sprouts.

Yields 6–8 servings.

Ingredients:

3	large beets, well scrubbed
	a little water
2	blocks silken (soft) tofu
	broccoli, red clover, alfalfa, or sunflower seed sprouts

Apple-Beet Salad

In a large pot, steam beets until tender. Let cool. Whisk together dressing ingredients. Toss with apples and beets.

Yields 3 servings.

Ingredients:

6	beets, cooked and diced
2	apples, diced

Dressing:

⅓ cup	flaxseed oil
2 tbsp	cider vinegar
1 tbsp	Dijon mustard
1	clove garlic, minced
½ tsp	maple syrup

Lemony Beets and Rice

Sauté the onions and garlic in a little water at first, then the oil. Add the spices and cook until the onions are translucent. Add the beet and dulse powder, and then mix it well with the cooked rice or millet. Add lemon juice and serve while still hot. Top with broccoli sprouts.

Yields 3 servings.

Ingredients:

2	onions, chopped
2	cloves garlic, finely chopped
1 tbsp	water
1 tbsp	extra virgin olive oil
1 tsp	mustard seeds
1 tsp	freshly ground black pepper
½ tsp	cumin
½ tsp	turmeric powder
1	large beet, cooked, peeled and diced
½ tsp	dulse powder
3 cups	cooked brown rice, wild rice or millet
	juice of 1 lemon
	broccoli sprouts

Dandelion Potato Salad

Wash and scrub the roots clean and chop into slices. If you don't like the natural bitterness of dandelion leaves, soak in salty water for 30 minutes then rinse, drain and chop.

Steam or boil chopped roots with potatoes until tender. Meanwhile, sauté onion and garlic for five minutes in water with a small amount of olive oil. Add dandelion leaves, cover and cook over a low heat for two minutes. Drain roots and potatoes, and put in a serving bowl along with the leaves and onions.

Mix oil and vinegarwith dulse into a dressing and toss salad, seasoning to taste.

Yields 4 servings.

Ingredients:

2 cups	sliced dandelion roots
2 cups	dandelion leaves
4 cups	cubed potatoes
1 tsp	olive oil
2	large onions, diced
2	cloves garlic, minced or crushed
2 tbsp	flaxseed oil
2 tbsp	cider vinegar
½ tsp	dulse powder

Desserts

Jam-Filled Mochi

Preheat oven to 400°F. Break mochi into squares. The block is usually scored so that it can be broken easily into 2-by-2-inch squares.

Place squares on cookie sheet and put in oven. Bake until mochi puffs up (10–12 minutes). Remove from oven. Open each square and put a tsp or 2 of jam inside. Serve immediately.

Yields 6 mochi squares.

Ingredients:

1	block mochi
	all-fruit jam

Banana Ice Cream

Place 2 frozen bananas at a time with a proportional amount of the other ingredients in a food processor and blend until creamy. Serve immediately. Cannot be refrozen. This makes a delicious summer treat.

Ingredients:

6	ripe bananas, peeled and frozen
½ cup	soy milk
1 tbsp	carob powder
½ cup	fresh walnuts

Peach Crisp

Combine the peaches, arrowroot and water. Place them in a baking dish, spreading them out evenly. Mix the oats and maple syrup together. Spread evenly over the peach mixture. Cover the dish and bake at 375°F for 20 minutes or until peaches are cooked. Remove the cover and brown the topping for the last 7 minutes.

To make a blueberry crisp, use 1 quart of blueberries and bake for a shorter time. For apple crisp, bake for 20–30 minutes.

Ingredients:

10–12	peaches, peeled and sliced
2 tbsp	arrowroot flour
¼ cup	water
1 cup	rolled oats
2 tbsp	maple syrup or barley malt

Squash Pudding

Preheat oven to 400°F. Wash yam and cut in half. Place yam face down on an oiled cookie sheet and put in oven. Cut squash in half and scoop out seeds. After 20 minutes, put the squash face down on the cookie sheet with the yam halves and bake both for 40 minutes more or until tender.

Let the vegetables cool until you can comfortably handle them. Scoop out the insides of the yam and the squash. Blend the insides with soy milk and cinnamon in a food processor, with a hand mixer, or by hand using a potato masher. Put mixture in a baking dish, cover, and keep warm in a low-temperature oven until served.

Yields 6 servings.

Ingredients:

1	yam
1 or 2	butternut squashes
¼ cup	soy milk
½ tsp	cinnamon

Tofu Pudding

Mix all three ingredients together in a blender and serve fresh.

Yields 4 servings.

Ingredients:

1	package silken firm tofu
2	bananas
2 tsp	carob powder

Carob Tofu Berry Delight

Place the tofu, berries, jam, lemon juice, and carob powder in a food processor. Process until smooth. Spoon into glass bowls and serve.

Ingredients:

1	package (10½ ozs) firm or extra-firm low-fat tofu
1 cup	raspberries, blueberries, strawberries or blackberries, frozen and unsweetened
½ cup	fruit sweetened jam
1 tsp	fresh lemon juice
1 tsp	carob powder

Creamy Carob Fudge

Mix dry ingredients together in a small bowl. Add soymilk and blend thoroughly. Stir in flaxseed oil. Eat immediately.

Ingredients:

2 tsp	carob powder
2 tsp	soyprotein powder
5 tsp	soymilk
1 tsp	flaxseed oil

Soyberry Smoothie

Mix all ingredients together in a blender. Blend until smooth, adding more soymilk if necessary.

Ingredients:

2	bananas
¾ cup	frozen berries
1 tbsp	soyprotein powder
¼ cup	soymilk
1 tsp	flaxseed oil
1 tbsp	ground flaxseeds (optional)

Juices

Add spirulina, dulse powder and/or ground flaxseeds to your juices whenever possible.

Carrot, Cabbage and Beet Juice

Scrub or peel, if not organic, ¾ lb of carrots, ½ beet and a 3 inch wedge of red or green cabbage. Juice and drink slowly.

Carrot and Apple Juice

Prepare ¾ lb of cleaned carrots and one apple, peeled if it is not organic. Juice and drink slowly.

Carrot, Beet and Celery Juice

Prepare ¾ lb of carrots, ½ beet and 2 stalks of celery. Juice and drink slowly

Carrot, Spinach and Apple Juice

Carefully wash spinach, removing all dirt. Peel one apple and ¾ lb carrot if they are not organic. Juice and enjoy.

Carrot, Cabbage and Apple Juice

Prepare ¾ lb carrots, a 3 inch wedge of cabbage and a peeled apple. Add ¼ tsp dulse powder to the final juice.

Carrot, Celery, Parsley and Garlic Juice

Combine ¾ lb carrot, 2 celery stalks, a handful of parsley and a garlic clove. Juice and sip slowly, chewing before you swallow.

Carrot, Cucumber, Beet and Cabbage Juice

Use ¾ lb carrots, ½ beet, ½ cucumber and a 2 inch wedge of cabbage. Add ¼ tsp dulse powder. Juice and sip slowly.

Carrot, Apple, Cabbage, Broccoli Sprouts and Red Clover Sprouts

Combine ¾ lb carrot, 1 apple, a 2 inch wedge of cabbage, ½ cup of broccoli sprouts and ½ cup of red clover sprouts. Juice and chew before you swallow.

Carrot, Beet, Cabbage, Broccoli and Red Clover Sprouts, Garlic

Combine ¾ lb carrot, a 2 inch wedge of cabbage, 1 cup of sprouts and 2 garlic cloves. Add ½ tsp dulse powder. Juice and enjoy.

Carrot, Beet, Cabbage and Flaxseeds

Combine ¾ lb carrot, 1 beet, a 2 inch wedge of cabbage and juice them. Add 1 tbsp freshly ground flaxseeds and stir. Chew before you swallow.

Healing Beverages

Red Ginger Punch

Drop the dried herbs in a litre of boiling water. Cover and allow the tea to steep on simmer for fifteen minutes. Meanwhile, peel and slice the ginger root. Add to the small saucepan of boiling water. Reduce the heat to low and gently simmer for ten minutes.

Pour the frozen peach juice into a large jug. Into the same jug, strain the herb tea and the ginger root liquid. Stir well. Refrigerate until very cold.

Yields 8–10 servings.

Ingredients:

1 litre	water, boiling in large saucepan
4 tsp	dried red raspberry (or 4 teabags)
4 tsp	dried red clover (or 4 teabags)
6	slices of ginger root, ¼" thick
2 cups	water, boiling in small saucepan
1 can	frozen peach juice

Yogi Tea (©Yogi Bhajan*)

Make at least four cups at one time. The measurements may be adjusted to your taste, but only slightly. Do not vary too far on the cloves or cinnamon. Bring the water to a boil. Add the cloves, cardamom, peppercorn and cinnamon.

Boil for at least 30 minutes, then turn off heat, add the black tea and let steep for five minutes. Stir in the soy milk and briefly bring to a boil. When it reaches a boil, immediately turn off the heat source. Strain and serve with honey or maple syrup.

Instead of adding the milk immediately, the spice liquid may be stored in the refrigerator until you are ready to drink it. Then, heat up the tea and add the soy milk. (The original recipe used whole cow's milk but this is unsuitable for *The Healthy Breast Program*)[1]

Ingredients:
For each serving:

10 oz	water
3	whole cloves
4	whole green cardamon pods, cracked open
½	cinnamon stick
4	whole black peppercorns
½ cup	of soy milk
2	slices of fresh ginger root
¼ tsp	black tea, such as Jasmine

The Healthy Breast Drink

Simmer the turmeric powder in the water in a ladle over the stove for 3 minutes. Warm the soy milk in a small pot on low heat, to just below boiling. Turn off heat. Add the turmeric powder, sweetener, and banana to the soy milk and blend. Drink once daily.

Hint: You can make a turmeric paste by mixing 3 tbsp turmeric with ½ cup water and cook gently for 1–2 minutes. Store this in a covered glass jar in the fridge and use 1 tsp of this mixture per cup of soy milk.

Ingredients:

½ tsp	turmeric powder
2 tbsp	water
1 cup	soy milk
½ tsp	honey or maple syrup or ½ banana

---

*Bhajan, Yogi. Foods for Health and Healing. Berkeley/Pomona, CA: Spiritual Community/KRI Publications, 1983:128

Almond Milk

Pour boiling water over the almonds. Let soak for 5 minutes. Remove the skins. In the blender, place ½ cup blanched almonds, 3¾ cups water, 4¾ tbsp honey or maple syrup. Blend until smooth. Strain to remove pulp and store liquid in a sterilized glass jar. Repeat process with remaining ingredients.

Ingredients:

1 cup	raw almonds
7¼ cups	water
9½ tbsp	honey or maple syrup

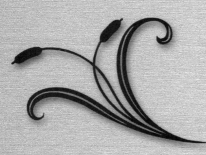

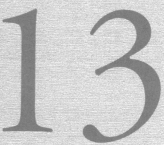

Other Resources

Contents

Resource Directory

Organizations for Further Information and Activism

Canada

Alliance of Breast Cancer Survivors, 20 Eglinton Ave, W, Suite 1106, Toronto, ON M4K 1K8. Tel: (416) 487-0584. Newsletter often contains articles on breast cancer and the environment.

Breast Cancer Action Montreal, 5890 Monkland Ave, Montreal, QC, H4A 1G2. Tel: (514) 483-1846

Breast Cancer Action Ottawa, Billings Bridge Plaza, PO Box 39041, Ottawa, ON K1H 1A1. Tel: (613) 736-5921. Campaigns against pesticide use.

Breast Cancer Prevention Coalition, 1102 Kitchen Sideroad, RR1, Coldwater, ON L0K 1E0. Tel. (701) 686-7457.

Breast Cancer Research and Education Fund, 266 St Paul St, St. Catharines, ON L2R 5N2. Tel. (905) 687-3333. Focuses on environmental links to breast cancer.

Campaign for Nuclear Phaseout, 1 Nicholas St, Suite 412, Ottawa, ON K1N 7B7. Tel: (613) 789-3634 or Fax: (613) 241-2292. Web site: www.cnp.ca. Has publications on safe alternatives to nuclear issues.

Canadian Breast Cancer Network, 207 Bank St, Suite 102, Ottawa, ON K2P 2N2. Tel: (613) 788-3311, Fax: (613) 233 1056.

Canadian College of Naturopathic Medicine, 1255 Sheppard Ave E, North York, ON M2K1E2. Tel: (416) 486-8585. Web site: www.ccnm.edu. Teaching and Support for The Healthy Breast Program.

Canadian Coalition for Nuclear Responsibility, Web site: www.ccnr.org

Canadian Environmental Law Association, 517 College St, Suite 401, Toronto, ON, M6G 4A2. Tel: (416) 960-9392 or Fax: (416) 960-9392, E-mail: cela@web.net, Web site: www.net/cela/

Canadian Naturopathic Association, 4174 Dundas St W, Toronto, ON. Tel: (416) 233-1043.

Canadian Women's Health Network, c/o Women's Health Clinic, 2nd Floor, 419 Graham Ave, Winnipeg, MB R63 0M3. Tel: (204) 947-2422 ext. 134, Fax: (204) 943-3844, E-mail: cwhn@web.net.

Commission for Environmental Cooperation, 393 rue St.-Jacques O, bureau 200, Montreal, QC H2Y 1N9. Tel: (514) 350-4300, Fax: (514) 350-4314, Web site: http://www.cec.org. Publishes *Taking Stock: North American Pollutant Releases and Transfers*.

David Suzuki Foundation, 2211 West 4th Ave, Suite 219, Vancouver, BC V6K 4S2. Tel: (604) 732-4228, Fax: (604) 732-0752. E-mail: solutions@davidsuzuki.org, Web site: www.davidsuzuki.org

Environmental Health Committee of the Ontario College of Family Physicians, 357 Bay St, Toronto, ON, Tel: (416) 867-9646. Has a four page publication called *Pesticides and Human Health* that is an excellent resource.

Greenpeace Canada, 185 Spadina Ave, Toronto, ON M5T 2C6. Tel: (416) 345-8408. http:// www.greenpeacecanada.org. Many excellent publications on environmental effects of chemicals are available from them.

International Institute of Concern for Public Health, Dr. Rosalie Bertell, President. 710-264 Queen's Quay West, Toronto, ON M5J 1B5. Tel: (416) 260-0575, Fax: (416) 260-3403. Focuses on the effects of nuclear power and radiation.

LiceBusters, Karen Tilley, founder. Toronto, ON. (416) 537-8639. Sells LiceMeister comb for removing nits, an essential oil mixture for deterring lice and a handbook on how to beat the bugs. Offers a nitpicking service to distressed parents.

National Pollutant Release Inventory (NPRI), Environment Canada, Hull, QC. Tel: (819) 953-1656, Fax: (819) 994-3266, E-mail: npri@ec.gc.ca, Web site: http:// www.doe.ca/pdb/npri.html. Access to data on which industries are polluting; what and where.

Ontario Breast Cancer Information Exchange Project (OBCIEP), 2075 Bayview Ave, Toronto, ON M4N 3M5, Tel: (416) 480-5899, Fax: (416) 480-6002. Encourages co-operative activity among organizations which have a role in breast cancer.

Ontario Naturopathic Association, 4174 Dundas St, W, Toronto, ON. Tel: (416) 233-2001.

Pollution Probe, 12 Madison Ave., Toronto, ON M5R 2S1. Tel: (416) 926-1601, E-mail: pprobe@web.net.

Teldon of Canada, 1-800-663-2212. Sells Green Power and Green Life juicers.

Voice of Women for Peace, 736 Bathurst St, ON M5R 2R4. Tel: (416) 537-9343, Fax: (416) 531-6214.

Wellspring, 81 Wellesley St, East, Toronto, ON M4Y 1H6. Tel: (416) 961-1928, Fax: (416) 961-3721. Relaxation and visualization approaches to cancer.

Willow, Ontario Breast Cancer Support and Resource Center. 785 Queen St East, Toronto, ON, M4M 1H5. Tel: (416) 778-5000, Fax: (416) 778-8070. Great resources available.

Women's Network on Health & the Environment (WNH&E), 517 College St, Suite 233, Toronto, ON, M6G 4A2. Education and activism on environmental links to breast cancer and women's health issues. Sells the video, *Exposure: Environmental Links to Breast Cancer* and Publishes *Connections.* Subscription $20.00/year (Cdn.) Tel: (416) 928-0880, Fax: (416) 531-6214, E-mail: weed@web.net, Web site: www.web.net/~weed/.

World Conference on Breast Cancer, 841 Princess St, Kingston, ON K7L 1G7. Tel: (613) 549-1118. Fax: (613) 549-1146. E-mail: brcancer@kos.net. Have developed a Global Action Plan for Breast Cancer Prevention based on input from delegates at the conference in Kingston in July 1997. International conference scheduled every 2 years.

World Wildlife Fund Canada, 90 Eglinton Ave E, Suite 504, Toronto, ON, M4P 2Z7. Tel: (416) 489-8800, Toll-free 1 800 26 PANDA, Fax: (416) 489-3611. Web site: www.wwfcanada.org/hormone-disruptors/index.html. Excellent brochures on pesticides and hormone disrupting chemicals free to the public, *Hormone Copy Cat* video available for loan or purchase.

Wylie Mycologicals. R R #1 Wiarton, ON NOH 2TO. Tel: (519) 534-1570, Fax: (519) 534-9045, E-mail: wylie@interlog.com. Supplies fresh shitake and maitake mushrooms, fresh and dry, and home growing kits.

The United States of America

Aeron Life Cycles Clinical Laboratory, 1933 Davis St., Ste. 310, San Leandro, CA 94577. Tel: (510) 729-0375, 1-800-631-7900, Fax: (510) 729-0383. Web site: http://www.aeron@aeron.com. Measures hormone levels in saliva as requested by a medical or naturopathic doctor.

Breast Cancer Action, 55 New Montgomery St, Suite 624, San Francisco, CA 94105. Tel: (415) 243-9301, Fax: (415) 243-3996. Web site: www.med.Stanford.EDU/bca/index.html

Breast Cancer Fund, 282 Second St, San Francisco, CA. Tel: (415) 543-2979, Fax: (415) 543-2975. Web site: www.breastcancerfund.com.

Cancer Prevention Coalition, 520 N Michigan Ave, Suite 410, Chicago, IL 60611. Tel: (312) 467-0600, Fax: (312) 467-0599.

DiagnosTech International, Inc., 375 280th St., Osceola, WI 54020. Tel: 888-342-7272 or (715) 294-2144, Fax: (715) 294-3921. Saliva hormone testing and blood testing for thyroid function.

Food and Water, RR1 Walden, VT 05873. Tel: (802) 563-3300, Fax: (802) 563-3311. Resources on food irradiation and toxins.

Greenpeace USA, 847 West Jackson Blvd., Chicago, IL 60607. Tel: (312) 563-0600.

Immunicon Corporation, 1310 Masons Mill II, Huntingdon Valley, PA 19006-3525. Tel: (215) 938-0100, Fax: (215) 938-0437. E-mail: Immunicon@Immunicon.com. Website: www.immunicon.com. Cancer blood test.

Immuno Laboratories, 1620 W. Oakland Park Boulevard, Fort Lauderdale, Florida 33311. Tel: 1-800-231-9197. Fax: 954-739-6563, Web site: http://www.immunolabs.com. For accurate ELIZA testing for food sensitivities and Candidiasis.

Journal of Pesticide Reform published by the Northwest Coalition for Alternatives to Pesticides (see below).

Meridian Valley Clinical Laboratory, Kent, WA. Tel: (253) 859-8700.

National Action Plan on Breast Cancer. Web site: www.napbc.org

National Alliance of Breast Cancer Organizations (NABCO), 1180 Ave of the Americas, 2nd Floor, New York, NY 10036. Tel: (204) 719-0154, Fax: (212) 689-1213.

New Action Products (NAP). 147 Ontario St, Buffalo, NY 14207. Tel: (716) 873-3738, Fax: (716) 873-6621, Web site: http://napherbs.com. Has the herbs for making Essiac if you are unable to get them at a local supplier.

Northwest Coalition for Alternatives to Pesticides, P.O. Box 1393, Eugene, OR. Tel: (541) 344-5044, Fax: (541) 344-6923, E-mail: info@pesticide.org, and Web site: http://www.efn.org/~ncap/. They publish the quarterly *Journal of Pesticide Reform* and supply factsheets on pesticides and their alternatives. Membership of $25/year includes quarterly.

Nuclear Information and Resource Service (NIRS), Washington, DC. Web site: www.nirs.org

Oncolab Inc., 36 The Fenway, Boston, MA 02215. Tel: (617) 536-0805 or 1-800-9-CATest, Fax: (617) 536-0657. For ordering the AMAS test.

Pesticide Action Network North America. Web site: igc.apc.org/panna

Rachel's Environment and Health Weekly. Web site: www.monitor.net/rachel. A great resource on connections between environmental connections and human health. You can subscribe free by E-mailing to Rachel at rachel-weekly-request@world.std.com with the single word "subscribe" in the message.

Rainbow Serpent: The Plutonium Free Future Women's Network, PO Box 2589, Berkeley, CA 94702. Tel: (510) 540-5917, Fax: 540-6159, E-mail: pff@1gc.apc.org.

3HO International Kundalini Yoga Teachers Association (IKYTA), Route 2, Box 4, Shady Lane, Espanola, NM 87532. Tel: (505) 753-0423, Fax: (505) 753-5982, Web site: www.yogibhajan.com/ikyta.html. Contact them to find a certified kundalini yoga teacher in your area.

Toxic Release Inventory (TRI), US Environmental Protection Agency, Washington, DC. Tel: 1-800-535-0202 within the United States or for on-line data access call (202) 234-8494. Web site: www.rtk.net

Women's Community Cancer Project (WCCP), 46 Pleasant St, Cambridge, MA 02139. Tel: (617) 354-9888, Fax: (617) 497-6787. Offers materials for action-for-prevention.

Women's Environment and Development Organization (WEDO), 355 Lexington Ave, 3rd Floor, New York, NY 10017-6603. Tel: (212) 973-0325, Fax: (212) 973-0335, E-mail: wedo@igc.apc.org, Web site: www.igc.apc.org/wedo/frmain.html. Publishes action for prevention materials and newsletter. Global organization based in New York.

World Resources Institute. Web site: www.wri.org

ZRT Laboratory, 12505 NW Cornell Rd, Portland, OR, 97229. Tel: (503) 469-0741, Fax: (503)469-1305, E-mail: dtzava@aol.com, Web site: salivatest.com. Saliva hormone testing.

Glossary

adaptogen: a substance that helps us adapt to stressors of all kinds.

adrenal gland: a gland that sits on top of the kidneys and secretes various hormones, some of which help us adapt to stress.

angiogenesis: the process of blood vessels growing, sometimes to feed cancer cells.

antibacterial: inhibits or kills bacteria.

antibiotic: a substance used to kill bacteria.

anti-cancer: prevents or stops the initiation, promotion or progression of cancer.

antifungal: prevents or stops fungal growth.

anti-inflammatory: prevents or stops inflammation.

antioxidant: substances that protect the body from free radical (oxidative) damage. These include vitamins A, C, E, the carotenes, selenium, co-enzyme Q10, grape seed, milk thistle, gingko biloba, amla and many others.

antiviral: prevents or stops viral infections.

areola: area of pigment around the nipple.

atypical cells: cells that are slightly abnormal and could progress to cancer.

axilla: armpit.

benign: not cancerous

Biomedical Center: the Mexican clinic that uses the Hoxsey Formula as a standard treatment for cancer.

biopsy: removal of tissue from the body for diagnostic purposes, usually through aspiration or surgery.

bone marrow: the soft, inner core of the bones where blood cells are made.

bone scan: a test using radiation to look for metastases in the bones.

Brassicas: the vegetable family that includes broccoli, cauliflower, Brussels sprouts, kale, Swiss chard.

BRCA1: gene linked to high risk of breast cancer.

breath of fire: a breathing exercise commonly used in kundalini yoga as taught by Yogi Bhajan.

C-2 metabolite (2-hydroxyestrone): a breakdown product of estrogen metabolism that is inactive and harmless. Also known as "good estrogen".

C-16 metabolite (16-hydroxyestrone): a breakdown product of estrogen metabolism that is recycled, active and potentially harmful. Women with breast cancer have nearly five times more of the C16 metabolite than women without. Also known as "bad estrogen".

calcifications: small calcium deposits visible in a mammogram that are occasionally indicative of breast cancer.

carcinogen: substance that can cause cancer.

cell: basic unit of biological growth in an organism.

chemotherapy: use of drugs to kill cancer cells in the body.

chromosomes: found in the cell nucleus and contain the genes made of DNA.

clinical study: a review of the records of people with a particular disease.

complementary medicine: a group of substances and practises that are natural, have a long use and can be used alongside drug treatments.

contraindicated: not to be used.

cortisol: hormone produced by the adrenal gland.

coumestrol: phytoestrogen found in high quantities in mung bean sprouts.

cyst: a fluid-filled sac or growth.

daidzen: phytoestrogen found in soy and other foods.

DDT: an organochlorine pesticide now banned in the United States but still used in Mexico and third world countries.

DES: diethylstilbestrol, a synthetic form of estrogen previously given to pregnant women to lower the risk of miscarriages. Now linked to increased reproductive organ and breast cancers.

DNA: deoxyribonucleic acid, which contains genetic information in a double spiral configuration and is found in the nucleus of each cell.

doubling time: how long it takes a group of cells to double in number.

duct: a narrow tube through which fluid passes.

carcinoma in situ: a group of atypical cells with a clear boundary, which is reversible without invasive treatment but may at some point progress to cancer.

edema: swelling caused by fluid build up between the cells.

eczema: skin ailment characterized by itching, redness, soreness.

endometrium: the tissue lining the uterus which fills with blood during the menstrual cycle, to be released during the menstrual period.

estrogens: hormones made by the ovaries, adrenals, fat cells and placenta which tend to promote breast cancer. Certain environmental chemicals and plant chemicals can also act as estrogens.

estrogen metabolism: bodily processes which make, use and eliminate estrogen.

estrogen receptor: special site in a cell to which estrogen attaches, allowing it to be active within the cell.

fibroadenoma: fibrous tumor of the breast.

fibrocystic breast disease: benign lumps in the breasts that fluctuate with the menstrual cycle.

free radicals: oxygen molecules with unpaired electrons which interfere with normal cellular functions. They are produced in the body from radiation, cigarette smoke, cooked and rancid oils, smog, chemicals and pollutants, and normal bodily processes. Antioxidants help to eliminate them.

FSH: hormone from the pituitary gland that stimulates the ovary to produce estrogen.

genes: cellular material composed of DNA that control physical and biochemical traits in all living things.

genistein: a phytoestrogen found in high amounts in soy, clover sprouts and the herb baptisia, among others.

Gerson therapy: an alternative cancer therapy utilizing vegetable juices, extra potassium and iodine, coffee enemas and a vegetarian diet.

glucuronic acid: a substance to which estrogen binds in the liver.

glucuronidation: the process of estrogen binding to glucuronic acid.

glucuronide conjugate or complex: the substance formed when estrogen binds to glucuronic acid.

homeopathy: a system of healing based on the principle of "like cures like" and utilizes very diluted amounts of herbs, minerals and other substances as remedies.

hyper: too much, overactive.

hypothalamus: area in the brain that controls hormonal functions and stimulates the pituitary gland.

hypo: too little, underactive.

immune system: network of organs, glands and specialized cells and proteins that defend the body from bacteria, viruses, fungi, parasites and cancer.

immunoglobulins: IgA, IgD, IgE, IgG, and IgM are antibodies active throughout the body.

indole-3-carbinol: a plant chemical found in the Brassica family that is able to decrease the amount of the C-16 metabolite from estrogen

initiation: the process of beginning something, such as damage to the DNA that turns on oncogenes, and starts cancer.

interferon: a protein produced by the immune system that inhibits viruses and activates T-cells.

intraductal: within the duct.

intraductal carcinoma: cancerous tumor within the breast duct.

invasive breast cancer: cancer growing beyond the original site into the surrounding tissue.

isoflavones: plant estrogens found in flaxseeds and other foods.

isothiocyanates: a group of plant chemicals found in the Brassica family that have anti-cancer activity.

kidneys: organs which filter waste from the blood.

kundalini yoga: a system of teachings which include physical postures, breathing exercises and mantras that is thousands of years old. It was brought to North America in 1969 by Yogi Bhajan.

liver: the body's main organ of detoxification and hormone breakdown.

lignan: a type of plant fiber that decreases breast cancer risk, found in flaxseeds.

lobules: milk-producing breast tissue.

lumpectomy: breast surgery to remove a lump.

lymphatic fluid: clear fluid that circulates among the cells and through the lymphatic vessels.

lymph nodes: cleansing stations packed with white blood cells that filter lymph; the major ones are found in the armpits, groin, neck and abdomen. Metastatic cancer cells can sometimes be found in the lymph nodes.

lymphatic system: a complex array of capillaries, vessels, ducts, cells, nodes and organs that maintain the fluid environment and cleanse cellular debris.

lymphatic vessels: small tubular structures that carry lymph to and from lymph nodes.

lymphedema: swelling caused by the build up of lymphatic fluid usually caused by damage to or removal of lymph nodes.

lymphocytes: specialized white blood cells that target viruses and cancer cells.

macrobiotic diet: an eating plan which focuses on brown rice, soy products, vegetables, occasional fish and excludes meat, dairy products and eggs.

macrophage: a large cell that can surround and digest foreign substances in the body. Found in the liver, spleen and elsewhere.

malignant: cancerous

mastitis: breast infection.

mammogram: picture of the breasts taken with an X-ray.

mass: a group of cells.

mastectomy: surgical removal of a breast.

melatonin: a hormone produced by the pineal gland that has an anti-cancer effect. It is produced in the dark and proximity to electromagnetic radiation decreases production.

menopause: when the menstrual periods stop permanently.

metabolism: natural biochemical processes that occur in the body, liberating nutrients and energy.

metastasis: cancer of the same type as the original cancer but which is located in a distant part of the body. Typical sites for breast cancer metastases include the liver, lungs, bone and brain.

methylxanthine: chemical found in coffee, tea, chocolate that causes cystic changes in the breasts.

naturopathy: a medical system based on helping the body to heal itself through detoxification, strengthening areas of weakness and the use of natural substances and non-invasive therapies.

oncogene: a normal gene that initiates cancer when it is damaged or activated. We know of about 100 of them at present.

oncologist: a medical doctor who specializes in treating cancer.

osteoporosis: loss of bone density that is common in postmenopausal women.

pectoralis major: muscle beneath the breasts.

phagocytes: cells that surround, eat and digest cell waste, toxins and small organisms.

phyto-: from a plant

phytochemical: natural chemical made by a plant. Many phyochemicals protect us from cancer.

phytoestrogen: plant substance that mimics estrogen but is generally protective from breast cancer.

pituitary gland: a gland in the brain behind the eyes that secretes hormones to regulate the other glands.

platelets: components of the blood that stop bleeding and repair blood vessels.

progesterone: hormone produced by the ovaries that acts in partnership with estrogen.

prognosis: a medical doctor's prediction of the probable outcome of a disease.

protocol: a particular program used in treating a specific disease.

recurrence: return of a cancer after it had disappeared.

remission: shrinkage of a tumor or disappearance of cancer.

side effect: undesirable result of using a substance for healing.

soy products: include tofu, tempeh, soy milk, soy sauce, tamari, Bragg's liquid aminos.

species: different genetic variations of the same organism.

spleen: an organ that is part of the immune system and houses red and white blood cells.

synergistic: a group of 2 or more substances working together in a way that is greater than the sum of each of the individual substances.

T-cells: specialized white blood cells that protect the body from viruses and cancer and are activated by the thymus gland.

tamoxifen: a hormonal drug which blocks the uptake of estrogen, used in breast cancer treatment.

tissue: group of cells of the same type that make up a particular body part.

tonify: strengthen, improve the function of a particular organ or body system.

tumor: a benign or malignant mass of abnormal cells.

virus: a very small organism that can only survive in the cells of another species and can cause disease.

white blood cells: lymphocytes, basophils, eosinophils, monocytes and neutrophils that destroy bacteria, parasites, viruses, toxins and damaged or abnormal cells.

xenoestrogen: non-natural substances that mimic estrogen, which include many environmental chemicals.

Bibliography

Achterberg, Jeanne. *Imagery in Healing: Shamanism and Modern Medicine*. Boston, MA: Shambhala, 1985.

Achterberg, Jeanne, Barbara Dossey, Leslie Kolkmeier. *Rituals in Healing*. Toronto, ON: Bantam Books, 1994.

Arnot, Bob. *The Breast Cancer Prevention Diet*. New York, NY: Little, Brown and Co., 1998.

Austin, S. and Cathy Hitchcock. *Breast Cancer: What You Should Know (But May Not Be Told) About Prevention, Diagnosis and Treatment*. Rocklin, CA: Prima Publishing, 1994.

Barks, Coleman. *The Illuminated Rumi*. New York, NY: Broadway Books, 1997.

Bhajan, Yogi. *Kundalini Yoga for Youth and Joy*. Eugene, OR: 3HO Transcripts, 1983.

Bhajan, Yogi. *Healing through Kundalini: Specific Applications*. Compiled by Vikram K. Khalsa and Alice Clagett. Eugene, OR: 3HO Transcripts, 1987.

Bhajan, Yogi. *Owner's Manual for the Human Body*. Los Angeles, CA: 3HO Foundation and Kundalini Research Institute, 1993.

Bhajan, Yogi. *Sadhana Guidelines for Kundalini Yoga Daily Practise*. Los Angeles, CA: Kundalini Research Institute, 1996.

Bhajan, Yogi. *Survival Kit: Meditations and Exercises for Stress and Pressure of the Times*. Compiled by S.S. Vikram K. Khalsa and Dharm Darshan K. Khalsa. San Diego, CA: Kundalini Research Institute, 1980.

Bhajan, Yogi. *The Kundalini Yoga Manual*. Claremont, CA: KRI Publications, 1976

Bensky, D. & A. Gamble. *Chinese Herbal Medicine Materia Medica*. Seattle, WA: Eastland Press, 1986.

Boericke, W. *Homeopathic Materia Medica and Repertory*. Delhi, India: B. Jain Publishers Pvt. Ltd., 1996.

Bolen, Jean Shinoda. *Close to the Bone*. New York, NY: Touchstone - Simon and Schuster, 1996.

Boyle, W. & A. Saine. *Lectures in Naturopathic Hydrotherapy*. East Palestine, OH: Buckeye Naturopathic Press, 1988.

Braverman, Eric. *The Healing Nutrients Within*. New Canaan, CT: Keats Publishing, 1987.

Brinker, F. *An Introduction to the Toxicology of Common Botanical Substances*. Portland, OR: National College of Naturopathic Medicine, 1983.

Clark, Hulga. *The Cure for All Diseases*. San Diego, CA: ProMotion Publishing, 1995.

Clorfene-Casten, Liane. *Breast Cancer: Poisons, Profits and Prevention*. Monroe, ME: Common Courage Press, 1996.

Colborn, Theo, D. Dumanoski, J. Peterson Myers. *Our Stolen Future*. New York, NY: Penguin, 1996.

Commission for Environmental Cooperation. *Taking Stock: North American Pollutant Releases and Transfers 1995*. Montreal, QC: CEC, 1998.

Davis et al. *The Relaxation and Stress Reduction Workbook*. 3rd ed. New York: New Harbinger Publications, 1988.

Dharmananda, Subhuti. *A Bag of Pearls*. Portland, OR: Institute for Traditional Medicine and Preventive Health Care, 1990.

Dharmananda, Subhuti. *Chinese Herbology*. Portland, OR: Institute for Traditional Medicine and Preventive Health Care, 1989.

Dossey, Larry. *Healing Words: The Power of Prayer and the Practice of Medicine*. New York, NY: HarperCollins, 1993.

Epstein, S. and D. Steinman. *The Breast Cancer Prevention Program*. New York, NY: Macmillan, 1997.

Erasmus, Udo. *Fats that Heal, Fats that Kill*. Burnaby, BC: Alive Books, 1993.

Falcone, Ron. *Natural Medicine for Breast Cancer*. New York, NY: Dell Publishing, 1996.

Frankl, Viktor. *Man's Search for Meaning: An Introduction to Logotherapy*. Translated by Ilse Lasch. New York, NY: Pocket Books, 1963.

Gerson, Max. *A Cancer Therapy: Results of Fifty Cases*. Erd ed. Del Mar, CA: Totality Books, 1977.

Guernsey, H. *The Application of the Principles and Practice of Homoeopathy to Obstetrics.* New Delhi, India: B. Jain Publishers Pvt. Ltd., 1988.

Gittleman, Ann Louise. *Guess What Came for Dinner?* Garden City Park, NY: Avery, 1993.

Gofman, John. *Preventing Breast Cancer: The Story of a Major, Proven, Preventable Cause of This Disease.* 2nd. ed. San Francisco, CA: Committee for Nuclear Responsibility, 1996.

Gupta, D., R. Attanasio & R. Reiter. (Eds.) *The Pineal Gland and Cancer.* Tubingen, Germany: Muller and Bass, 1988.

Hobbs, C. *Foundations of Health: Healing with Herbs and Foods.* Capitola, CA: Botanica Press, 1992.

Hole, J. *Human Anatomy and Physiology.* Dubuque, IA: Wm. C. Brown Publishers, 1984.

Holmes, P. *The Energetics of Western Herbs.* Vol. I and II. 2nd ed. Berkeley, CA: NatTrop Publishing, 1993.

Hubbard, L. R. *Clear Body, Clear Mind.* Copenhagen, Denmark: New Era Publications Int., 1990.

Ingerman, Sandra. *Welcome Home: Life After Healing.* San Francisco, CA: Harper-San Francisco, 1993.

Jayne, Walter Addison. *The Healing Gods of Ancient Civilizations.* New Hyde Park, NY: University Books, Inc., 1962.

Johnson, Robert. *Inner Work.* New York, NY: Harper and Row, 1986.

Joseph, Barbara. *My Healing from Breast Cancer.* New Canaan, CT: Keats Publishing, Inc., 1996.

Kaur, Sardarni Premka. *Peace Lagoon.* Pomona, CA: K.R.I. Publications, 1984.

Kent, James Tyler. *Lectures on Homeopathic Materia Medica.* New Delhi, India: Jain Publishing Co., 1983.

Keuneke, Robin. *Total Breast Health.* New York, NY: Kensington Books, 1998.

Khalsa, Gururattan K. *Transitions to a Heart-Centered World through the Kundalini Yoga and Meditations of Yogi Bhajan.* San Diego, CA: Yoga Technology Press, 1988.

Koenig-Bricker, Woodene. *Prayers of the Saints: An Inspired Collection of Holy Wisdom.* New York, NY: HarperCollins, 1996.

Kroeger, Hanna. Parasites: *The Enemy Within.* Boulder, CO: Hannah Kroeger Publications, 1991.

Krohn, Jacqueline, Frances Taylor, MA, and Jinger Prosser, LMT. *Natural Detoxification: The Complete Guide to Clearing Your Body of Toxins.* Point Roberts, WA: Hartley and Marks Publishers Inc., 1996.

Kushi, Michio. *The Cancer Prevention Diet.* New York, NY: St Martin's Press, 1993.

Lad, V. & D. Frawley. *The Yoga of Herbs.* Santa Fe, NM: Lotus Press, 1986.

Lawless, Gary. *First Sight of Land.* Nobleton, ME: Blackberry Books, 1990.

Lee, John R. *What Your Doctor May Not Tell You About Menopause.* New York, NY: Warner Books Inc., 1996.

LeShan, Lawrence. *Cancer as a Turning Point: A Handbook for People with Cancer, their Families and Health Professionals.* New York, NY: Penguin, 1994.

Lilienthal, S. *Homeopathic Therapeutics.* New Delhi, India: Indian Books and Periodicals Syndicate, 1890.

Love, S. *Dr. Susan Love's Breast Book.* New York, NY: Addison-Wesley Publishing Co., 1995.

Mascaro, Juan. *The Upanishads.* Toronto, ON: Penguin, 1965.

Michnovicz, J. *How to Reduce Your Risk of Breast Cancer.* New York, NY: Warner Books, 1994.

Mollison, B. *Introduction to Permaculture.* Tyalgum, NSW, Australia: Tagari Publications, 1991.

Moss, R. *Cancer Therapy: The Independent Consumer's Guide to Non-Toxic Treatment and Prevention.* New York, NY: Equinox Press, 1992.

Murphy, Robin. *Homeopathic Medical Repertory.* Pagosa Springs, CO: Hahnemann Academy of North America, 1993.

Ontario Breast Cancer Information Exchange Project. *A Guide to Unconventional Cancer Therapies.* Toronto, ON 1994.

Papp, Leslie. "Cancer - The Enemy Within." *The Toronto Star,* Saturday, November 21, 1998, A28.

Pizzorno, J. & M. Murray. *A Textbook of Natural Medicine.* Seattle, WA: John Bastyr College Publications, 1985.

Radhakrishan, Sarvepalli and Charles A. Moore. *A Sourcebook in Indian Philosophy.* Princeton, NJ:: Princeton University Press, 1957.

Rogers, S. *Wellness Against All Odds.* Syracuse, NY: Prestige Publishing, 1994.

Rossi, Ernest. *The Psychobiology of Mind-Body Healing.* New York, NY: W.W. Norton, 1986.

Rossi, Ernest. *The 20 Minute Break.* Los Angeles, CA: Jeremy P. Tarcher Inc., 1991.

Roy, Rob. *The Sauna.* White River Junction, VT: Chelsea Green Publishing Company, 1996.

Santillo, Humbart. *Food Enzymes: the Missing Link to Radiant Health.* Prescott, AZ: Hohm Press, 1993.

Santillo, Humbart. *Intuitive Eating.* Prescott, AZ: Hohm Press, 1993.

Siegel, Bernie. *Love, Medicine and Miracles: Lessons Learned About Self-Healing from a Surgeon's Experience with Exceptional Patients.* New York, NY: Harper and Row, 1986.

Siegel, Bernie. *Peace, Love and Healing.* New York: Harper and Row, 1989.

Simonton, O. C., S. Simonton, and J. Creighton. *Getting Well Again.* Los Angeles, CA: Tarcher, 1978.

Singer, S. & S. Grismaijer. Dressed to Kill: *The Link Between Breast Cancer and Bras.* Garden City Park, NY: Avery Publishing Group, 1995.

Singh, R. *Self-Healing: Powerful Techniques.* London, ON: Health Psychology Associates, 1997.

Steinman, D. *Diet for a Poisoned Planet.* New York, NY: Crown Publishing, 1990.

Steingraber, Sandra. *Living Downstream: An Ecologist Looks at Cancer and the Environment.* Reading, MA: Addison-Wesley Publishing Co. Ltd., 1997.

Tierra, M. *Planetary Herbology.* Santa Fe, NM, Lotus Press. 1988.

Weed, S. *Breast Cancer? Breast Health!.* Woodstock, NY: Ash Tree Publishing, 1996.

Wigmore, A. *The Hippocrates Diet and Health Program.* Wayne, NJ. Avery Publishing Group. 1984.

Wigmore, A. *The Sprouting Bible.* Wayne, NJ. Avery Publishing Group. 1986.

Wigmore, Ann. *The Hippocrates Diet and Health Program,* Garden City Park, NY: Avery, 1983.

Appendix 1: How to Manage Your Estrogen: The Estrogen Pathway

Points of Influence and Interference

1) Cholesterol levels will be increased by a diet high in fat. When cholesterol is high, there is often increased weight gain and estrogen levels will rise, causing a greater risk of breast cancer.

2) Progesterone will help to prevent breast cancer, but it is not certain if it inhibits or stimulates breast cancer when cancer cells are already present. Many women have a progesterone deficiency, as measured by saliva tests, which will increase breast cancer risk. Progesterone levels can be normalized with vitamins B6 and E, and the minerals boron, zinc, selenium, and possibly iodine. The herb chaste tree berry will normalize progesterone after six months of use, as may the herb stoneseed. The use of soy products increases progesterone levels. Environmental chemicals can interfere with progesterone, particularly hexachlorobenzene.

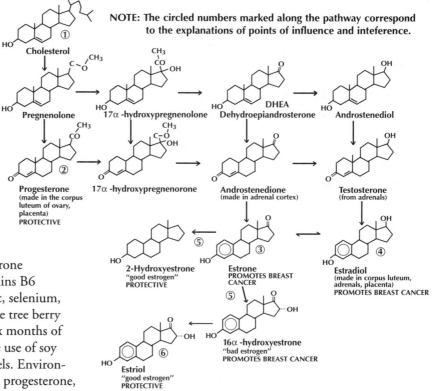

NOTE: The circled numbers marked along the pathway correspond to the explanations of points of influence and inteference.

3) Estrone, a strong estrogen that can promote breast cancer, is made in fat cells from the adrenal hormone, androstenedione. Generally, the more body fat we have, the higher our levels of estrone. Therefore, decrease body fat to lower estrone levels and protect from breast cancer.

4) Estradiol, the strongest estrogen, can promote breast cancer. Estradiol levels are increased by a diet high in meat and fat, which encourage the growth of a particular intestinal bacteria that is able to cause estradiol to be reabsorbed through the gut wall. Thus to decrease estradiol levels, maintain a diet low in meat and fat.

5) Estrone can be converted in the liver to either 2-hydroxyestrone, which protects from breast cancer, or 16α-hydroxyestrone, which strongly promotes breast cancer. This conversion happens during the liver's phase one detoxification process. Supplements that assist this process are vitamins A, B2, B3, E and the minerals copper, zinc, calcium, and magnesium. Soy foods, turmeric, flaxseed oil, fresh rosemary, limonene (from citrus peel), cayenne, calendula, schizandra, solidago, and sassafras also assist this process. The

family of foods known as the brassicas, which include broccoli and cabbage, contain a substance called indole-3-carbinol, when eaten raw. Indole-3-carbinol strongly pushes estrone to form the protective estrogen metabolite, 2-hydroxyestrone. Substances that interfere with this process and will cause more of the estrone to be pushed towards the harmful 16α-hydroxyestrone include alcohol, cigarettes, bad fats, car exhaust, barbituates, valium, antihistamines, dioxin, pesticides, paint fumes, and caffeine.

6) Estriol is a weak estrogen that generally acts to protect us from breast cancer, except when its levels are exceedingly high. Estriol levels are elevated in pregnancy and for several years after childbirth, helping to balance the effects of estradiol and estrone as strong and potentially harmful estrogens. The substances listed above that assist the liver in phase one detoxification will increase the levels of estriol, as may dietary iodine. The ratio between the three estrogens should be 1 part estradiol, 1 part estrone, and 8 parts estriol, except during pregnancy when estriol levels are higher.

7) Phase two liver detoxification prepares estrogen for elimination through the colon. Estradiol and estrone are joined to glucuronide to form a glucuronide conjugate that is ready for excretion. This process is favored by cysteine (NAC), methionine, choline, vitamins B3, B6, B12, C, folic acid and the mineral molybdenum. Foods that help include limonene (citrus peels), flaxseed oil, rosemary, turmeric, soy, oatmeal, the brassicas, beans, and spirulina. Substances which interfere with phase two detoxification include tartrazine dyes, NSAIDS, the birth control pill, cigarettes, phenobarbitol, and a protein deficiency.

8) Certain bacteria in the gut are able to split the glucuronide conjugate meant for excretion so that estrogen is reabsorbed. These bacteria are assisted by a diet high in meat and fat. Therefore a diet low in meat and fat means less circulating estrogen.

9) Elimination of estrogen through the colon is enhanced by a high fiber diet which includes wheat bran and psyllium.

10) Estrogen is prevented from binding to its receptor sites in the presence of both phytoestrogens (from foods) and xenoestrogens (from chemicals). Phytoestrogens are weak estrogens (similar to estriol) that are easily broken down by the body and are considered protective. They are found in flaxseeds, soy, clover and mung bean sprouts, legumes, and pumpkin seeds. Xenoestrogens are not easily broken down, can persist in our fat cells over our life times, and can have a synergistic effect that promotes breast cancer.

Index

Please note: this index sorts numbers before letters.

parts of, 162–163
lymph nodes, 162–163
lymphedema, 168

M

macrophage, 163, 164, 169, 170, 182, 216, 268
magnesium, 40, 42, 79, 240
maitake, 182, 214
mammary glands, 36
mammograms, 49, 93
mandrake, 175
massage, dry brush, 164–165
mastitis, 45
meaning, *see also under* purpose, 275–285
meat, 44, 66, 220
meditation
    and melatonin, 80
    for inner knowing, 279
melatonin, 46, 60, 62, 73, 77–81, 84, 95, 163, 245, 249
    breast cancer link to, 46, 78
        treatment, 60
    breathing exercises and, 80, 81
    decreasing, 80
    increasing, 77–78
    interference with, 77
    meditation, 80
    production of, 78
    restoring levels of, naturally, 80
menopause, 61, 67
    What Your Doctor May Not Tell You About Menopause, 72
menstruation
    cycles, 60, 68, 71
    onset of, 67
metastases, 46, 49, 60, 244
methionine, 212
methyl chloride, 107
methylxanthine, 43, 44
MGN-3, 183
milk, 221
milk thistle, 44, 128–129
mind-body connection, 265
minerals, 194
    calcium, 127, 144, 149, 240
    cesium, 144
    daily therapeutic amounts of, 235
    how and when to take, 251
    iodine, 40, 43, 66, 72, 74, 241
    magnesium, 127, 144, 240

manganese, 243
molybdenum, 127, 242
potassium, 144, 147, 240
rubidium, 144
selenium, 72, 74, 242
zinc, 72
modified citrus pectin, 244
mung bean sprouts, 196, 207, 211
mung beans and rice, 152
mushrooms, 182, 214

N

N-acetyl cysteine (NAC), 79, 127, 246, 249
nature, connection to, 276
nipples, 39
non-toxic
    body care, 111–113
    home care, 113–115
nonylphenol ethoxylates, 105
nostril
    alternate, series, 84–85
    dominance, 80–83
nuclear industry, 92
nursing. *See* breastfeeding
nutritional
    deficiency, 234
    support for breast health, 234–251

O

obesity, 23, 27, 61, 76
olive oil, 185, 199, 202
organic food, 194
organochlorines, 28, 96, 101, 137
osteoporosis, 68
    Preventing and Reversing Osteoporosis, 68
ovaries, 58, 59, 60

P

P53 (tumor suppressor gene), 60
pain, 241
palmarosa oil, 186, 199
pancreas, 58, 59, 142
paper industry, 108
parasites, 29, 133–136
parathyroid gland, 58, 59
passion, 282
path of purification, 22

THE HEALTHY BREAST PRODUCTS ORDER FORM

Name:		Address:		
City:		**Prov./State:**		**Postal Code/Zip:**
Tel:	**Fax:**		**E-mail:**	

DESCRIPTION	QTY.	UNIT PRICE	SHIPPING (Can + U.S.)	TOTAL
A Call to Women: The Healthy Breast Program and Workbook		$35 Cdn/$25 U.S.	$5.00/book	
Recovering from Breast Cancer: A Guided Visualization Audiotape		$12 Cdn/$9 U.S.	$3.00	
The Healthy Breast Kundalini Yoga and Rebounding Video		$25 Cdn/$18 U.S.	$4.00	
The Healthy Breast Formula				
250 ml bottle		$55 Cdn/$40 U.S.	$5.00	
500 ml bottle		$90 Cdn/$65 U.S.	$6.00	
Liver Loving Formula				
250 ml bottle		$55 Cdn/$40 U.S.	$5.00	
500 ml bottle		$90 Cdn/$65 U.S.	$6.00	
Immune Power Formula				
250 ml bottle		$55 Cdn/$40 U.S.	$5.00	
500 ml bottle		$90 Cdn/$65 U.S.	$6.00	
Healthy Breast Oil				
250 ml bottle		$65 Cdn/$50 U.S.	$5.00	
500 ml bottle		$110 Cdn/$80 U.S.	$6.00	

Payment by cheque or money order to:
Healthy Breast Products
534 8th St. A East
Owen Sound, ON, Canada. N4K 1M9
Please allow 3 weeks for delivery

SUBTOTAL	
7% GST (Can. only)	
TOTAL DUE	

To order by phone or fax and for wholesale prices please call **(519) 372-2755** or **(519) 372-9212**. For other products from **The Healthy Breast Program** please visit our web site at www.healthybreastprogram.on.ca or request an order form by phone or fax. E-mail us at sdk@log.on.ca. For shipping charges to the U.S.A. add $3.00 U.S. Call for foreign shipping costs. Prices subject to change without notice.

The herbal formulas and the Healthy Breast Oil can be ordered directly by health practitioners and health food stores from St. Francis Herb Farm Inc., PO Box 29, Combermere, Ontario. tel: 1-800-219-6226 or 613-756-6279.